Integrated Hematopathology

Morphology and FCI with IHC

Integrated Hematopathology

Morphology and FCI with IHC

Cherie H Dunphy, MD, FCAP, FASCP

Professor of Pathology and Laboratory Medicine
Associate Director, Core, Flow Cytometry, and Special Procedures Laboratories
Department of Pathology and Laboratory Medicine
University of North Carolina
Chapel Hill, NC

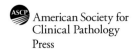
American Society for
Clinical Pathology
Press

Publishing Team

Adam Fanucci (illustration/production)
Tae Woong Moon (design/production)
Erik N Tanck (editorial content/production)
Joshua Weikersheimer (publishing direction)

Notice

Trade names for equipment and supplies described are included as suggestions only. In no way does their inclusion constitute an endorsement of preference by the Author or the ASCP. The Author and ASCP urge all readers to read and follow all manufacturers' instructions and package insert warnings concerning the proper and safe use of products. The American Society for Clinical Pathology, having exercised appropriate and reasonable effort to research material current as of publication date, does not assume any liability for any loss or damage caused by errors and omissions in this publication. Readers must assume responsibility for complete and thorough research of any hazardous conditions they encounter, as this publication is not intended to be all-inclusive, and recommendations and regulations change over time.

Printed in Hong Kong

14 13 12 11 10

Table of Contents

15 Hodgkin Lymphoma

16 Immunodeficiency-Associated Lymphoproliferative Disorders

17 Histiocytic and Dendritic Cell Neoplasms

Preface

Diagnostic hematopathology relies heavily on combining cytomorphology and histology with ancillary techniques, such as applying immunophenotyping and molecular/cytogenetic analysis. This book focuses on the applications of flow cytometric immunophenotyping (FCI) in combination with morphology for diagnostic hematopathology.

FCI is a particularly useful tool in diagnostic hematopathology. Virtually all types of specimens evaluated for hematolymphoid neoplasms (eg, peripheral blood, body fluids, bone marrow aspirates and core biopsies, fine needle aspirates, and fresh tissue biopsies) are suitable for FCI.

Of course, FCI represents only one useful tool used in diagnostic hematopathology and must never be interpreted without correlation with the cytomorphologic and histomorphologic features of each case. This comprehensive flow cytometry text appropriately covers, in depth, the technical aspects of FCI with a thorough coverage of the phenotypic markers, as well as the advantages and disadvantages of FCI. Subsequently, there is a detailed description of the phenotypic findings of normal peripheral blood, body fluids, bone marrow, and particularly lymphoid tissue elements, and then comprehensive discussions of FCI within the specific hematolymphoid neoplasms, mirroring the outline and terminology of the 2008 WHO classification. Within each discussion of a specific hematolymphoid neoplasm is a discussion of the typical immunophenotypes, which are then illustrated in variant cases, both morphologically (eg, H&E images) and immunophenotypically (eg, color dot plots). These are then correlated with molecular and cytogenetic findings as is useful. There is incorporation of the discussions of the utility of FCI in the identification of clonal B cells, at the beginning of the discussion of the B-cell neoplasms; the identification of abnormal T cells and clonality of T cells by FCI, at the beginning of the discussion of the T-cell neoplasms, the identification of myeloblasts by FCI, at the beginning of the discussion of the AMLs; the identification of B and T lymphoblasts by FCI, at the beginning of the discussions of precursor B-cell neoplasms and precursor T-cell neoplasms, respectively; and the identification of features of dyserythropoiesis by FCI, at the beginning of the discussion of the myelodysplastic syndromes. This text also has separate chapters regarding the unique applications of FCI to the evaluation of fine needle aspirate specimens and body fluids.

Also provided is a CD companion to the text that contains the listmode files of selected cases that are found within the book. The listmode files may be viewed by individuals who already have access to the software as described in the instructions for use of the CD below.

Using FACSDiva software

1. Open the Experiment that will contain the imported files
2. Files can be imported into an open Experiment only, either by opening an existing Experiment or create a new one
3. Change Area to Height for all parameters within the analysis template
4. Choose File > Import > FCS files
5. Locate the files you want to import in the dialog box that appears
6. Use the buttons in the dialog box to find the files to be imported
7. Select multiple files by holding down the Control key as you click the file names

Using CellQuest software

1. Open FACS Convert
2. Locate files on the CD
3. Select All > Convert
4. Converted files will be located in the FACS Convert folder
5. Open an analysis template
6. Edit > Select All > Plots > Change Data File
7. Select file (inside the FACS Convert folder) > Open

1 General Introduction

Chapter Contents

Organization and Purpose

Diagnostic hematopathology is a challenging field. The complexity of diagnostic hematopathology is reflected in the World Health Organization (WHO) classification of tumors of hematopoietic and lymphoid tissues, which incorporates not only morphology, as do the older classifications, but also considers the immunophenotype, cytogenetic and molecular genetic findings, as well as clinical manifestations, to define a great variety of disease-specific entities [Jaffe 2001, Swerdlow 2008]. In addition, there is an explosion of newly emerging techniques that not only aid in the accuracy of diagnosis, but also provide prognostic and therapeutic implications. In cytogenetic analyses, fluorescence in situ hybridization (FISH) has greatly expanded the versatility of traditional karyotyping. In the field of molecular pathology, polymerase chain reaction (PCR) has gradually replaced the time-consuming Southern blot technique. The branching of PCR into quantitative PCR (qPCR) and reverse transcriptase PCR (RT-PCR) brings molecular pathology to a new horizon. In situ hybridization has gradually merged into the immunohistochemical laboratories in large medical centers, and gene expression profiling (microarrays) is beginning to be incorporated into diagnostic centers.

In spite of all the exciting technological advances, morphology combined with immunophenotyping remains the mainstay in the routine diagnosis of hematolymphoid neoplasms. Most large laboratories use a combination of flow cytometric immunophenotyping (FCI) and immunohistochemical (IHC) immunophenotyping, depending on the nature of the sample and markers to be analyzed. The types of specimens suitable for FCI, as well as the advantages and disadvantages of FCI, will be discussed in a later chapter.

This book focuses on the applications of FCI in combination with morphology to diagnostic hematopathology. It represents a comprehensive flow cytometry textbook, appropriately covering, in depth, the technical aspects of FCI, phenotypic markers, as well as the advantages and disadvantages of FCI. Subsequently, there is a detailed description of the normal and abnormal phenotypic findings of peripheral blood, body fluids, bone marrow, and lymphoid tissue elements, and then detailed discussions of FCI within the specific hematolymphoid neoplasms, mirroring the outline and terminology of the WHO classification, to increase the ease of use for practicing hematopathologists/hematopathology trainees. within each of the discussions of the specific hematolymphoid neoplasms, there is discussion of the classical immunophenotypes, and then illustrative variant cases, both morphologically (ie, H&E images) and immunophenotypically (ie, color dot plots). There are discussions of morphologic correlations with illustrative images, comparisons with IHC immunophenotyping, and correlation with molecular and cytogenetic findings, when pertinent. Lastly, this textbook has separate chapters regarding the unique applications of FCI to the evaluation of fine needle aspirate specimens and body fluids.

As case review is the most efficient way of learning, this book includes large numbers of cases, covering all important clinical entities as outlined in the WHO classification, with detailed clinical history, morphologic description, and flow cytometric findings. Numerous tables summarizing diagnostic features and comparing similar diseases are furnished to facilitate the readers' understanding. This book should become a handy guidebook, used on a daily basis by practicing hematopathologists/hematopathology trainees, and ideally targets those pathologists needing a reference for their daily practice of diagnostic hematopathology, in which they routinely correlate morphology and the FCI results, which represents the standard of care.

A separate CD accompanies the text, containing the listmode data for selected cases.

Applications of Flow Cytometry to Diagnostic Hematopathology

The following list represents just some of the applications of flow cytometric immunophenotyping to diagnostic hematopathology that will be discussed in this textbook: distinguishing between follicular hyperplasia (FH) and follicular lymphoma (FL), detection of the lack of surface immunoglobulin (sIg) and light chain expression by a significant number of B-cells indicating malignancy, subtyping B-cell lymphomas/leukemias composed predominantly of small cells, identifying prognostic markers in chronic lymphocytic leukemia (CLL), differentiating lymphoplasmacytic lymphoma (LPL) or other types of B-cell lymphomas from plasma cell dyscrasias (PCD), identifying prognostic markers in PCD, differentiating various types of large B-cell lymphomas (LBCL) from anaplastic PCD and from anaplastic CD30+ large cell lymphoma (LCL), immunophenotyping B-cell lymphomas/leukemias, distinguishing between hematogones and neoplastic lymphoblasts, differentiating non-Hodgkin lymphoma (NHL) from Hodgkin lymphoma and T-cell from B-cell NHL, identifying composite lymphomas, distinguishing between T-cell lymphoblastic lymphoma (LL) and thymoma, diagnosing and subclassifying NHL in fine needle aspirate (FNA) specimens and body fluids, and immunophenotyping T-cell lymphomas/leukemias, natural killer (NK) cell lymphoproliferative disorders, post-transplant lymphoproliferative disorders (PTLD), granulocytic/monocytic sarcomas (GS/MS) (including leukemia cutis), acute myelogenous leukemias (AML), and myelodysplastic syndromes (MDS). FCI may be particularly useful in identifying markers in AML that highly correlate with specific recurring cytogenetic abnormalities and prognosis. In addition, FCI may be useful in excluding a diagnosis of NHL in cases of non-hematopoietic malignancies. These applications of FCI are useful not only in initial diagnosis, but also in staging various sites for lymphomatous involvement (ie, bone marrow) and, in certain situations, may also be extremely helpful in evaluating for relapsing or minimal residual disease. These applications and others will be discussed in detail in the following chapters of this textbook.

References

Jaffe E, Harris N, Stein H, et al [2001] *Tumors of Haematopoietic and Lymphoid Tissues.* Lyon, France: IARC Press.

Swerdlow SH, Camp E, Harris NL, et al, eds [2008] *World Health Organization Classification of Tumours. Pathology and Genetics of Tumours of the Haematopoietic and Lymphoid Tissues.* Lyon, France: IARC Press.

2 Basic Principles and Instrumentation of Flow Cytometry

John Schmitz, PhD

Chapter Contents

Flow cytometry (FC) is a technology allowing the detection and enumeration of normal and abnormal cellular components of various tissues. Understandably, this technology has proven particularly useful for the analysis of samples from patients with hematologic malignancies. FC can rapidly assess physical characteristics as well as extra- and intra-cellular immunophenotypes of individual cells in complex samples, such as peripheral blood, bone marrow, body fluid, and tissue samples, as previously discussed. As such, FC has proven to be an indispensable tool for detection and characterization of malignant cells in a background of normal cellular elements. This information is important for the diagnosis of patients with a variety of hematolymphoid malignancies, as well as for providing data relevant to prognosis and patient management.

The application of FC for hematopathology relies upon an understanding of the basic theory of FC including instrumentation as well as pre-analytic, analytic, and post-analytic factors contributing to the generation of accurate and useful FC data. This chapter provides an overview of these issues.

Basic Theory of FC

The goal of FC is to gather data on the intrinsic (size, structural complexity) and extrinsic (antigenic makeup, nucleic acid content, or functional attributes) characteristics of cells. To gather this data, FC relies on the analysis of cells in suspension that pass one by one, in rapid succession through 1 or more monochromatic light sources (lasers). As each individual cell passes through the laser light it scatters the incident light. The scattered laser light is directed to and collected in the forward (along the axis of the laser light; forward scatter) and 90 directions (perpendicular to the axis of the laser light; side scatter). Forward scatter laser light is proportional to the cross sectional area of the cell while 90° scattered light is reflective of the internal complexity of the cell (ie, nuclear lobes and cytoplasmic granules) will scatter more light in the 90° direction [f2.1a]. The incident laser light can also excite fluorochromes attached to cells or fluorescent dyes taken up by the cells. Scattered fluorescent light is collected (in the 90° direction) and directed to 1 or more photo-detectors (photomultiplier tubes). The scattered fluorescent light provides information on the antigenic makeup (if fluorochrome-labeled monoclonal antibodies are used) or other cellular characteristics (eg, nucleic acid content if DNA intercalating dyes are used) of the cell. These data are digitized and stored for later multiparameter analysis of the cell populations in the sample. The following sections provide an overview of the components of a typical clinical flow cytometer. Detailed discussions of these components can be found in [Shapiro 2001].

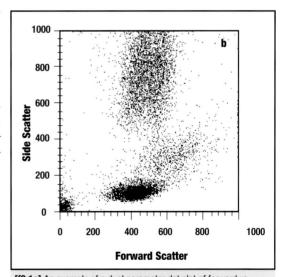

[f2.1a] An example of a dual parameter dot plot of forward vs sides scatter. A whole blood sample in which red blood cells were lysed is displayed. As indicated in the figure, the intrinsic features of peripheral white blood cells are sufficient to distinguish granulocytes, monocytes, and lymphocytes.

Fluidics

To begin the FC analysis process, a single cell suspension from the tissue of interest is injected into the fluidics system of the cytometer. The function of the fluidics system is to deliver the cells in suspension, one by one, rapidly and uniformly to the intersection point (interrogation point) of the fluidics stream and beam(s) from the laser(s). This is accomplished by hydrodynamic focusing of the sample stream within a stream of sheath fluid resulting from differential pressures of the 2 streams. The coaxial flow of cells thus generated passes through a flow cell where it intersects 1 or more laser beams. This carefully controlled process assures reproducible illumination of each cell, which is critical for reliable determination of cellular characteristics.

Optics

The optical system of the flow cytometer is responsible for illuminating the cells as they pass through the laser beam, directing the scatter light to specific photodetectors that register the amount of scattered light generated by each cell and converting that signal to a digital signal, which is then stored for later analysis. When an individual cell intersects the laser(s), incident laser light is scattered in all directions. Likewise, if the cell is labeled with a fluorochrome (antibody bound or dye) that can be excited by the incident laser light, fluorescence is emitted from the cell. In newer instruments, multiple lasers producing different wavelengths of light are common. Typical clinical flow cytometers are constructed so the sheath fluid, containing the stream of cells, intersects the laser beam within a flow cell. Upon intersecting the laser light, the cell scatters the incident light and fluorescent emissions in all directions. Scattered laser and fluorescent light is then split into distinct wavelengths that are directed to specific photodetectors which register the light received from each individual cell. Directing scatter light to photodetectors relies upon the use of several types of optical components, including collecting lenses, dichroic mirrors, and various types of filters, which will not be addressed in this chapter.

Electronics/Computer

Upon interaction with a photodetector, the incident light generates an electrical signal that is converted to a digital signal proportional to the intensity of the incident light. This signal is then stored in the computer memory for later analysis of the intrinsic and extrinsic parameters of the cell. The digital signals for each intrinsic and extrinsic parameters are stored as channel numbers, which can vary depending upon instrument resolution (eg, 0-256 channels vs 0-1024 channels). Fluorescence data are often presented on a logarithm scale in order to visualize both dimly and brightly fluorescent cells.

Multiple pieces of data on each cell are collected and stored as correlated list mode data. Typical clinical flow cytometers assess 3-6 fluorochromes on a single cell in addition to forward and side scatter parameters. As technology has evolved, flow cytometers have been developed that can assess an even larger number of parameters simultaneously, up to 17 or more, depending upon the incorporation of multiple lasers and appropriate detectors to facilitate high order analyses termed polychromatic flow cytometry [Perfetto 2004]. This correlated information is available for later computer analysis.

Data Analysis

The list mode data collected from multi-parameter analyses can be displayed and analyzed in a variety of ways depending on the specific need. The simplest means of data presentation is the single parameter histogram [f2.1b]. This display provides a frequency distribution of the light scatter or fluorescent properties of a cell population. The frequency of the positive events can be determined by computer analysis of the number of events in the positive region (higher channel numbers) divided by the total number of events analyzed. Another common method for display of dual parameter data is the dual parameter dot plot [f2.1a],[f2.1c]. This is a 2-dimensional display of 2 cellular parameters. Each dot on the display represents an individual event (cell or cell fragment) that has passed through the laser and been captured by the optical system. In some cases, it is convenient to divide the plot into 4 quadrants with the aid of user-defined cursor settings to demarcate double-negative, double-positive, and single-positive events [f2.1c]. A display, similar to the dual parameter dot plot, is the density plot. This display generates a color change related to the frequency of cells with similar intrinsic or extrinsic parameters.

An important feature of flow cytometry is its ability to assess phenotypic characteristics of specific subsets of cells in a complex mixture, such as peripheral blood or bone marrow. This is accomplished by using various combinations of intrinsic and/or extrinsic parameters to identify populations of interest in a process referred to as gating [f2.2]. Gating is followed by more detailed

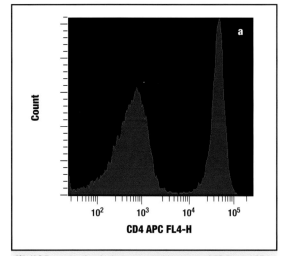

[f2.1b] Example of a single parameter histogram of CD4+ and CD4 staining cells. The peak to the right represents events (cells) that have stained positive for the presence of the CD4 antigen in the total lymphocyte population and are recorded in the higher channel numbers. The remainder of the lymphocytes (left peak, CD4) was not bound by the CD4 antibody and appears in the lower channels.

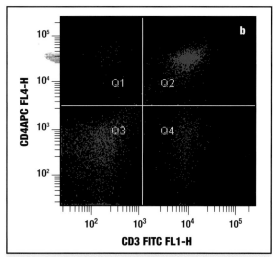

[f2.1c] An example of a dual parameter dot plot of forward vs sides scatter. A whole blood sample in which red blood cells were lysed is displayed. As indicated in the figure, the intrinsic features of peripheral white blood cells are sufficient to distinguish granulocytes, monocytes, and lymphocytes

analyses of the cells within the gate. This process allows one to assess parameters of a cell population while excluding analysis of cell populations that are not of interest. Analysis gates may be used individually or linked using Boolean logic (and/or/not) to further restrict analysis and define unique populations of cells. This approach to analysis is particularly useful for the enumeration of rare events (ie, low frequency cell populations), as it reduces the detection of non-specific cells from the population of interest thus increasing

the specificity of the analysis [Sutherland 1997]. It should be noted that current software applications typically allow the user to gate on cell populations and identify each gated population in subsequent analysis plots by assigning a unique color to the gated population. Subsequent analyses then display all populations rather than an individual gated population.

Standard flow cytometric analysis determines the percent of specific cell populations in the sample. For example, CD4 and CD8 T lymphocyte enumeration

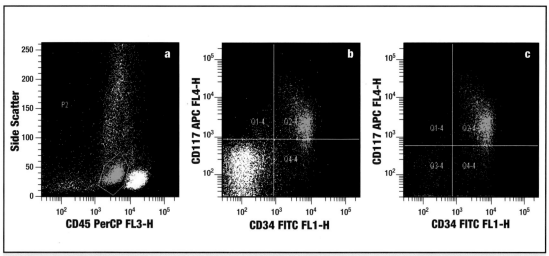

[f2.2] An example of a dual parameter dot plot of forward vs sides scatter. A whole blood sample in which red blood cells were lysed is displayed. As indicated in the figure, the intrinsic features of peripheral white blood cells are sufficient to distinguish granulocytes, monocytes, and lymphocytes

is based upon the determination of the percentages of these subsets in the total lymphocyte population. While this approach to data analysis and reporting is suitable for populations of cells stained with monoclonal antibodies that demonstrate clear and distinct bimodal distribution of fluorescence [f2.1a], some antigens display a unimodal (disperse) fluorescence pattern that may overlap what is classically considered negative and positive staining regions and are thus difficult to describe in a qualitative fashion as clearly positive or negative. There are several options used to describe the fluorescent characteristics of such populations of cells. One may describe the cell population with the aid of a discriminator based upon the use of an isotype control antibody and report as positive only those events falling outside of the cursor [f2.3]. Isotype controls are fluorochrome labeled antibodies (matched to the isotype, fluorochrome and concentration of the target specific antibodies) with binding specificity for an antigen not found on human cells. As such, isotype controls are used to assess the level of nonspecific binding of antibodies to cells. Alternatively, one may ignore the subjective application of positive and negative discriminators and describe the population in subjective terms such as negative, dim, bright, or heterogeneous [Wood 2006]. This approach is often used to describe the fluorescent characteristics of white blood cells as the level of expression of some antigens are altered characteristically in certain hematolymphoid malignancies [Craig 2008]. Alternative methods include

the use of fluorescence standards with defined levels of fluorescence (eg, MESF beads). The mean fluorescence of the cells of interest is compared to a standard cure with the resultant value used to describe the staining intensity [Kay 2006].

Antibodies and Fluorochromes

Monoclonal antibodies are the antigen specific probes used to define the immunophenotypic characteristics of cells. The power of flow cytometric analysis relies upon the use of monoclonal antibodies coupled to fluorescent compounds facilitating characterization of cell lineage, maturity, activation state, as well as viability or nucleic acid content. with the development of a wide array of fluorochromes and technologic advances in instrumentation, polychromatic analysis (>5 colors simultaneously) can be employed to define very unique and rare subsets of cells in complex mixtures. Standard clinical flow cytometers now assess up to 6 cell surface or intracellular antigens simultaneously. Antibodies used for flow cytometric immunophenotypic analysis of hematolymphoid malignancies are discussed in detail in Chapter 4.

Fluorochromes allow one to detect binding of monoclonal antibody to cells. Fluorochromes, covalently attached to antibodies, emit light when excited by incident light of the appropriate wavelength. The excitation and emission spectra vary with the specific fluorochrome. with appropriately configured instrumentation, and careful selection of fluorochrome-

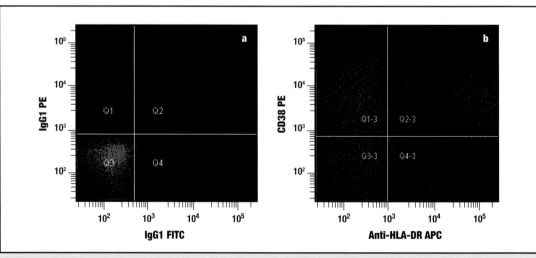

[f2.3] An example of a dual parameter dot plot of forward vs sides scatter. A whole blood sample in which red blood cells were lysed is displayed. As indicated in the figure, the intrinsic features of peripheral white blood cells are sufficient to distinguish granulocytes, monocytes, and lymphocytes

antibody combinations, a potentially large number of different cell surface and/or intra-cellular antigens can be assessed simultaneously in a single tube. A great increase in the number and types of fluorochromes (and dyes) used in flow cytometric analyses has facilitated the development of this polychromatic analysis. The ability to incorporate many uniquely labeled antibodies into 1 staining reaction has several advantages (for a detailed discussion of this topic see Wood [2007]) including the following:

1. the ability to analyze samples with limited cellularity

2. a large number of antibodies combined into 1 tube may also facilitate more refined analysis which can enhance the sensitivity and specificity of the assessment

3. combining antibodies in 1 tube reduces the need for antibody redundancy between multiple tubes, saving cost as well as technologist time.

Fluorochrome-labeled monoclonal antibodies are not the only reagents useful for flow cytometric analysis. Nucleic acid binding dyes may be employed for several purposes in flow cytometric analyses. By virtue of their ability to intercalate into DNA, they may be used to determine the DNA content of cells for assessment of DNA ploidy or cell cycle [Check 2007]. Additionally, DNA binding dyes can be used to assess cell viability [O'Brien 1995]. Intact cell membranes exclude dyes, while damaged membranes allow dyes to penetrate the cell and intercalate into DNA. Thus, fluorescence of cells stained with DNA binding dyes is an indicator of cell death. This application can prove very useful for analysis of samples that have been held or shipped prior to analysis. Cell viability may be compromised in held/shipped samples and it is well known that dead cells may non-specifically bind to antibodies [Terstappen 1988]. Viability dyes can be combined with fluorescent monoclonal antibodies, and by excluding dye positive cells with an appropriate gating strategy, one can restrict analysis to viable cells.

While instrumentation and fluorochromes have evolved extensively over the past few years, the issue of *spectral overlap* still remains and must be carefully controlled for accurate flow cytometric analysis. A challenge of multiparameter flow cytometry lies in the fact that the emission spectra of commonly used fluorochromes overlap [Tung 2004]. For example, the emission of cells stained with a FITC-labeled antibody will be detected in the appropriate FITC detector. However, a small portion of the FITC emissions may also be detected by the PMT for phycoerythrin due to overlap in the FITC emission spectra in the range of wavelengths detected by the phycoerythrin detector. In order to account for this phenomenon, the user needs to adjust the cytometer circuitry to subtract a portion of the signal generated by the PE detector to account for contaminating FITC emissions. Likewise, a portion of the signal generated by the FITC detector can be subtracted to account for contaminating PE emissions. This is referred to as compensation adjustment [Roederer 2001] and is typically performed prior to sample acquisition. More recently, software is available allowing acquisition of uncompensated data with software based compensation adjustments during data analysis.

Sample Handling and Processing

The only restriction related to type of sample submitted for flow cytometric analysis is that it must consist of a dispersed cell suspension. Peripheral blood, bone marrow, and body fluids are typical types of samples received for analysis, however lymphoid tissue may also be submitted for analysis. In this case, the tissue must be disaggregated, typically by physical means, to generate a single cell suspension.

Monoclonal antibody staining for flow cytometric analysis is relatively straight forward. Typically, the cell suspension is incubated with the monoclonal antibodies for 15-30 minutes. Red blood cells, if present, may be removed by lysis, and the sample is then washed and re-suspended in a fixative, such as paraformaldehyde. While relatively simple, there are a number of components of sample processing that must be controlled in order to generate quality data [Hultin 2006].

Samples should be submitted as expeditiously as possible to the flow laboratory for processing because some antigens may be modulated with time [Shalekoff 2001]. In addition, the viability of cells will decrease as the duration of sample storage increases. If there is to be a delay in processing or if shipment is required, appropriate temperature should be maintained and cells may be placed into an enriched medium that will help to maintain viability. Samples processed within 24 hours typically maintain acceptable viability without any additive. Samples received for processing beyond 24 hours should have their viability assessed to ensure integrity of the sample, unless the laboratory has documented no adverse effect of processing delay. Viability is an important issue because dead cells are known to non-specifically bind antibodies [Terstappen 1988]. Given that some samples may not be replaceable, poor viability does not exclude processing and analysis. However, it is important to note poor viability and account for it in the interpretation of the data or employ a method such as inclusion of a viability dye to exclude non-viable cells from analysis [CLSI 2006].

Laboratories should define the optimal number (and range of cell numbers) suitable for the concentration of antibody used. Occasionally, samples are received that may require an adjustment in the standard volume of sample used for staining due to a low or high cell number. As such, a cell count, either manual or automated, should be routine. In the situation of a low cell count, prioritization of the antibodies to be used will need to be determined. Thus communication between the laboratory and hematopathologist is critical for determination of which antibodies will provide the most useful information.

Most antibodies used for staining are directly coupled with a fluorochrome. Using directly-labeled antibodies is rapid and typically associated with low levels of non-specific binding to cells. Rarely, antibodies may be used that are not directly fluorochrome-labeled. In this case, detection of bound antibodies requires the use of an anti-immunoglobulin antibody, specific for the isotype of the target monoclonal antibody that is fluorochrome-labeled. This indirect staining approach allows the use of an unlabeled antibody, but requires additional time and quality control for staining. In addition, there may be a higher level of background staining, particularly on cells containing Fc receptors.

Some antigens of interest may be expressed intracellularly but not on the surface of the cell. There are several intracellular antigens that provide useful diagnostic and prognostic information [Rassenti 2004]. In these cases, a cell must be processed to allow internalization of the antibody to detect the presence of the cognate antigen. A number of commercially-available reagents are available for permeabilization of cells, and the choice should be based upon validation studies in the laboratory.

Samples containing a significant component of red blood cells must be treated in a fashion to eliminate the red cells as their high numbers interfere with analysis and needlessly increase the size of the list mode data file. Red cell elimination can take place during sample processing with the use of density gradients that remove the red cells. More commonly, red cells can be lysed during the staining process. Commercial lysing agents or in-house prepared reagents, such as ammonium chloride, effectively rid samples of red cells.

Quality Control

Quality control (QC) is critical for the generation of accurate and reproducible flow cytometric data. A variety of QC parameters are assessed and monitored for flow cytometric analyses. Mentioned previously were issues related to sample quality. Issues related to training and competency of staff are critical as well but will not be addressed here [Greig 2007]. Instrument maintenance and monitoring and monoclonal antibody QC are vital to reproducible flow analysis.

Several instrument parameters, including laser output, PMT performance, and compensation are monitored daily [Oldaker 2007]. Optical system alignment is not typically monitored or changeable in standard clinical flow cytometers. The performance of the laser(s), PMTs, and the compensation circuitry are monitored with fluorescent calibration beads. In 1 approach, unlabeled beads, as well as beads individually labeled with each fluorochrome used in analysis, are acquired on the instrument. PMT voltages are adjusted to set each bead at a pre-defined mean fluorescent intensity value. These values are plotted and monitored for trends over time that may indicate problems with the PMTs. In addition, the separation of the labeled beads compared to the unlabeled bead is monitored as an indicator of instrument sensitivity. Individually labeled beads are also run to monitor compensation values. The linearity of the photodetectors is monitored with bead standards of varying fluorescence intensity. This is particularly important if quantitative measurements are made.

New lots of monoclonal antibodies must be assessed for specific binding before being placed into use. Not only should they stain the correct number of cells in normal donor samples, they should also possess staining intensity similar to previous lots. It is advisable to QC new shipments of lots of antibodies previously checked for quality to confirm there were no adverse effect from the shipping process [CAP 2007].

Process controls that monitor the complete testing process are run periodically for immunophenotypic analysis of hematolymphoid malignancies. These controls assess the suitability of sample processing, as well as staining with the specific antibodies. A challenge related to analysis of hematolymphoid malignancies is that some of the antibodies used do not stain sufficient numbers of normal donor blood cells to serve as a useful monitor. As such, laboratories should monitor reactivity of antibodies with malignant and normal cells in patient samples longitudinally to assess antibody quality over time.

References

Check IJ [2007] DNA content analysis of solid tumors. Chapter 17 in: *Flow cytometry in clinical diagnosis*. 4th ed. Chicago, IL: ASCP Press;345-352.

Clinical and Laboratory Standards Institute [2006] *Clinical flow cytometric analysis of neoplastic hematolymphoid cells: Approved guideline second edition*. Wayne, PA: CLSI CLSI document H43-A2.

College of American Pathologists, Commission of Laboratory Accreditation [2007] *Flow Cytometry Inspection Checklist*. Northfield, IL College of American Pathologists.

Craig FE, Foon KA [2008] Flow cytometric immunophenotyping for hematologic neoplasms. *Blood* 111:3941-3967.

Greig B, Oldaker T, Warzynski M and Wood B [2007] 2006 Bethesda international consensus recommendations on the immunophenotypic analysis of hematolymphoid neoplasia by flow cytometry: Recommendations for training and education to perform clinical flow cytometry. *Cytometry* Part B 72B:S23-S33.

Hultin L, Hultin P [2006] Flow cytometry-based immunophenotyping method and applications. In: *Manual of Molecular and Clinical Laboratory Immunology*. 7th ed. Washington DC. ASM Press. 147-157.

Kay S, Herishanu Y, Pick M, et al [2006] Quantitative flow cytometry of ZAP-70 levels in chronic lymphocytic leukemia using molecules of equivalent soluble fluorochrome. *Cytometry* Part B. 70B:218-226.

O'Brien MC, Bolton WE [1995] Comparison of cell viability probes compatible with fixation and permeabilization for combined surface and intracellular staining in flow cytometry. *Cytometry* 19:243-55.

Oldaker T, Stone E [2007] Quality control and quality assurance in clinical flow cytometry. In: *Flow cytometry in clinical diagnosis*. 4th ed. Chicago, IL: ASCP Press; 73-98.

Perfetto SP, Chattopadhyay PK, Roederer M [2004] Seventeen-colour flow cytometry: Unravelling the immune system. *Nat Rev Immunol* 4:648-655.

Rassenti LZ, Juynh L. Toy TL, et al [2004] ZAP-70 compared with immunoglobulin heavy-chain gene rearrangement status as a predictor of disease progression in chronic lymphocytic leukemia. *N Engl J Med* 351:893-901.

Roederer M [2001] Spectral compensation for flow cytometry: visualization artifacts, limitations, and caveats. *Cytometry* 45:194-205.

Shalekoff S, Tiemessen CT [2001] Duration of sample storage dramatically alters expression of the human immunodeficiency virus coreceptors CXCR4 and CCR5. *Clin Diagn Lab Immunol* 8:432-436.

Sharpiro HM [2001] *Practical Flow Cytometry*. 4th ed. New York, NY: Wiley-Liss Inc.

Sutherland DR, Anderson L, Keeney M, Nayar R, Chin-Yee I [1997] Towards a world-wide standard for CD34+ enumeration. *J Hematother* 6:85-89.

Terstappen LWMM, Shah VO, Conrad MP, Recktenwald D, Loken MR [1988] Discriminating between damaged and intact cells in fixed flow cytometric samples. *Cytometry* 9: 477-484.

Tung JW, Parks DR, Moore WA, et al [2004] New approaches to fluorescence compensation and visualization of FACS data. *Clin Immunol* 110:277-283.

Wood B [2006] 9-color and 10-color flow cytometry in the clinical laboratory. *Arch Pathol Lab Med* 130:680-690.

Wood BL, Arroz M, Barnett D, et al [2007] 2006 Bethesda international consensus recommendations on the immunophenotypic analysis of hematolymphoid neoplasia by flow cytometry: optimal reagents and reporting for the flow cytometric diagnosis of hematopoietic neoplasia. *Cytometry* Part B72B:S14-S22.

3   Advantages and Disadvantages of FCI

Chapter Contents

Specimen Requirements

Many different types of specimens may be analyzed by flow cytometric immunophenotyping (FCI) to evaluate for hematolymphoid neoplasia. Types of specimens suitable for FCI include peripheral blood, bone marrow (BM) aspirates, and core biopsies [Dunphy 1999], fine needle aspirates (FNA), [Dunphy 1997] fresh tissue biopsies, and all types of body fluids [Dunphy 1996]. The specimen requirements for these various specimens are outlined in [t3.1].

Peripheral blood specimens and BM aspirates are particularly suitable for FCI, since the cells are present as single cells suspended in blood. FCI not only allows for the presence of circulating cells of hematolymphoid neoplasms (ie, acute leukemia or lymphoma) in the peripheral blood or involvement of the BM aspirate by hematolymphoid neoplasms, but it also allows for their quantitation in these specimens.

Likewise, FNA specimens of lymph nodes and extranodal tissues may be routinely and easily evaluated for hematolymphoid neoplasia by FCI, since the cells are again present as single cells in suspension. The applications of FCI to the evaluation of FNA specimens for hematolymphoid neoplasia will be discussed in great detail in Chapter 20. Also, all types of body fluids (ie, pleural, pericardial, ascitic, cerebrospinal, and vitreous fluids) may be evaluated for hematolymphoid neoplasia by FCI, as the cells are present singly in suspension. The applications of FCI to the evaluation of all types of body fluids for hematolymphoid neoplasia will be discussed in great detail in Chapter 21.

All other types of specimens (ie, bone marrow core biopsies and other extranodal and nodal fresh tissue specimens) must be disaggregated into single cell suspension for analysis by FCI. It is important to always prepare a touch preparation of the actual

---

t3.1   Specimen Requirements for Flow Cytometric Immunophenotyping

Specimen Type	Preservative/Anticoagulant	Storage/Delivery Time
Peripheral blood	EDTA-preferred heparin or ACD may be used	Room temperature; deliver within 24 hours
BM aspirate	Heparin	Room temperature; deliver within 24 hours
FNA	Passes into RPMI media	On wet ice within 24 hours
Body fluids	None (if immediate) or pellet in RPMI (if overnight)	On wet ice within 24 hours
Fresh tissue (nodal, extranodal, BM biopsy)	Teased into RPMI	On wet ice within 24 hours

specimen being disaggregated to confirm the presence of abnormal cells by cytomorphology. It is also important to always ensure that another portion of the tissue is submitted for routine histology. The tissue may then be disaggregated by "teasing" the BM core biopsy or other fresh tissue specimen. The tissue is generally held at the end by forceps on a small wire mesh and scraped with a scalpel blade in RPMI 1640 medium (Cellgro Mediatech Tissue Culture Media, Fisher Scientific, Pittsburgh, PA) until no more tissue will go into suspension. Teasing of BM core biopsies, as described above, to evaluate for hematolymphoid neoplasia by FCI is usually reserved for cases in which there is high suspicion of a hematolymphoid neoplasm involving the BM with a failed BM aspiration. In such cases, it may be extremely helpful in defining the cell of origin of the hematolymphoid neoplasm, as will be discussed in detail below. In addition, there is a report in the literature [Vos 2003] describing the acquisition of single cells from all of these tissue types described above by briefly vortexing until the RPMI cell culture medium becomes cloudy. This technique supposedly allows direct histologic correlation, since the tissue is not disrupted and is then recovered for routine histologic processing [Vos 2003].

Lastly, although not routinely practiced by all diagnostic hematopathology facilities, single cells may be isolated from formalin-fixed, paraffin-embedded material to determine clonality, and the reader is referred to [Leers 2000] for additional information.

Advantages of FCI

There are numerous advantages of FCI in the evaluation of hematolymphoid neoplasia, which will be considered below.

Technical Considerations

1. FCI allows for an expeditious analysis of the expression of cell surface antigens and may be evaluated sooner than histologic sections are available.

2. Distinct cell populations are defined by their size (forward light scatter) and granularity (side light scatter).

3. Dead cells may be gated out of the analysis.

4. Weakly expressed surface antigens may be detected.

5. Many antibodies, important in diagnostic hematopathology, are available for FCI and simply are not available by immunohistochemistry (eg, CD19, CD13)

6. Multi-color (2–, 3–, 4–, 6–, 9–) analysis may be performed, allowing not only for an accurate definition of the surface antigen profile of specific cells, but also for better analysis of samples limited by cellularity. In addition, distinct cell populations may be identified, important not only for the initial diagnosis but also in the evaluation of other sites for staging purposes and of subsequent specimens for involvement by minimal residual disease or recurrent disease.

Specimen Considerations

Peripheral blood, bone marrow aspirates, fine needle aspirates, and body fluids are ideally suited for evaluation of hematolymphoid neoplasia by FCI, since, as mentioned previously, they represent single cell suspensions that are not easily evaluated by immunohistochemistry.

Diagnostic Considerations

1. Two simultaneous hematolymphoid neoplasms (eg, AML and lymphoma, small lymphocytic lymphoma in a background of classical Hodgkin lymphoma) may be detected within the same tissue site.

2. Clonality in B-cell neoplasia is better evaluated by FCI than by immunohistochemistry.

3. A tissue biopsy may be obviated by the relatively noninvasive diagnostic evaluation of FNA specimens and body fluids, as will be discussed in detail in Chapters 20 and 21, respectively.

4. Due to multi-color flow cytometric analysis and adequate teasing of small biopsy samples, in some situations a definitive diagnosis may be rendered, obviating additional, more extensive biopsies or testing.

Disadvantages of FCI

Although there are numerous advantages of FCI in evaluating for hematolymphoid neoplasia, one must also be aware of the inherent disadvantages of this technique in this context, which are considered below.

Technical and Specimen Considerations

1. There are some markers that are not available by flow cytometry and/or are better analyzed by immunohistochemistry (eg, bcl-6, MUM1)

2. By teasing the tissues for disaggregation, there is disruption of tissue and architectural relationships are lost.

3. Sclerotic BM may yield too few cells for adequate analysis.

4. Likewise, if the individual performing the BM aspirate does not "re-direct" the BM aspirate needle or "re-aspirate" after obtaining the BM aspirate smears for cytomorphology, the resulting BM "aspirate" for FCI is often "hemodiluted" and not representative of the BM. Therefore, it is imperative a smear be prepared from the flow cytometry specimen of the "BM aspirate" to evaluate for adequacy and interpret the FCI results in light of these findings, in order to avoid a misdiagnosis (both under- and over-diagnoses) **[f3.1]**.

5. A markedly hypercellular or "packed" bone marrow specimen may yield too few cells for analysis.

6. Sclerotic tissue may be difficult to suspend for individual cellular analysis.

7. A small population of monoclonal B-cells may not be detected in a T-cell-rich (TCR) or lymphohistiocytic-rich (LHR) B-cell lymphoma (BCL) **[f3.2]**.

8. Limited biopsy specimens (punch skin biopsies, etc.) may yield too few cells for FCI.

Diagnostic Considerations

1. There is loss of architectural relationships, so, for example, a diagnosis of follicular vs diffuse lymphoma cannot be rendered.

2. Involvement of the bone marrow by lymphoma in a paratrabecular pattern may not be detected by FCI, since these paratrabecular infiltrates typically do not aspirate well.

3. T-cell lymphomas that do not have an aberrant immunophenotype may not be detected.

4. An aberrant T-cell immunophenotype (ie, absence or down regulation of pan-T-cell antigens, particularly CD7) does not necessarily indicate malignancy and may be observed in infectious mononucleosis,6 reactive dermatoses, and inflammatory disorders [Moll 1994, Smith 1995, Lazarovits 1992].

5. Partial tissue involvement by lymphoma with sampling differences or poor tumor preservation may result in falsely "negative" FCI results [Dunphy 2000] **[f3.3]**.

6. FNA specimens have the same issues as biopsy specimens, in regard to partial tissue involvement and poor tumor preservation, but can also potentially lose architectural relationships. FNA specimens will be discussed in much greater detail in Chapter 20.

7. A practical inability to detect/diagnose classical Hodgkin lymphoma (cHL) is due primarily to the low number of neoplastic cells normally present in this disease. A technique to evaluate for cHL by FCI will be discussed in greater detail in Chapter 16.

Due to these disadvantages, FCI data should always be correlated with light microscopy if no FCI abnormalities are detected. Immunohistochemistry may be needed in selected cases. In addition, as mentioned earlier, an aberrant T-cell immunophenotype does not necessarily indicate malignancy and requires correlation with light microscopy as well as clinical data and additional ancillary studies (ie, molecular/cytogenetic analysis) in some situations.

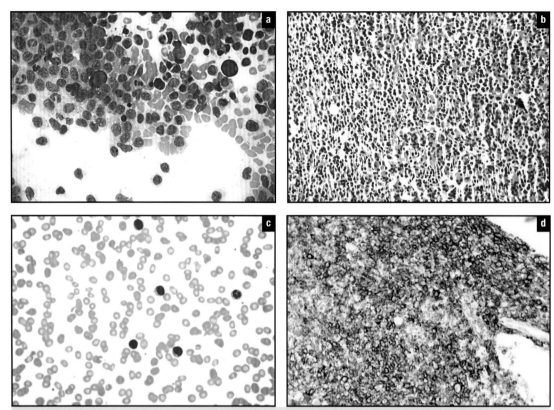

[f3.1] This case demonstrates a BM aspirate **a**, composed of sheets of lymphoid-appearing cells, some with plasmacytic features. The BM core biopsy **b** is replaced by this population of lymphoid-appearing cells. The smear prepared from the flow cytometry specimen of "bone marrow" reveals a markedly hemodiluted specimen with no spicules for evaluation **c**. Flow cytometric analysis of this sample revealed 29% of cells within the lymphocyte region. Cells within the lymphocyte region were composed of 88% T-cells with a normal immunophenotype and normal CD4:CD8 ratio. A monoclonal B-cell population was not identified. This case was initially interpreted as involvement of the BM by a T-cell lymphoma. However, subsequent immunostaining of the BM biopsy with CD138 **d** disclosed the correct diagnosis of involvement of the BM by a plasma cell myeloma. This case illustrates the importance of reviewing a prepared smear of the flow cytometry sample to determine adequacy and representation of the BM.

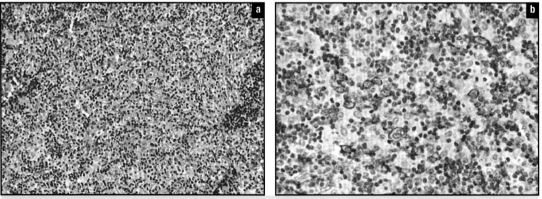

[f3.2] This case illustrates a T-cell rich large B-cell lymphoma; **a**, H&E section; **b**, CD20 immunohistochemical stain demonstrates the malignant B-cells. Flow cytometric analysis of this case did not disclose a monoclonal B-cell population, presumably due to the low number of neoplastic cells in the tissue.

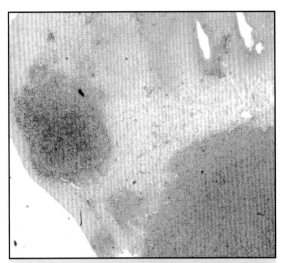

[f3.3] This case illustrates partial tissue involvement by a malignant lymphoma. The H&E section reveals large areas of tissue, composed of loose, edematous and fibrous tissue. Such partial tissue involvement could possibly result in "negative" results by flow cytometric analysis.

Also, when a monoclonal or aberrant B-cell population or an aberrant T-cell population, characterized by a loss of a T-cell antigen, is identified, cHL may be excluded only after correlation with the histology, in order to exclude the possibility of a composite lymphoma. In those cases in which FCI data is diagnostic, microscopic observations may provide additional information, not only due to sampling, but also due to patterns of involvement and the cytological features of the malignant cells.

Since all of the specific disease entities according to the WHO classification, as well as the particular nuances of fine needle aspirate specimens and body fluids, will be discussed in great detail in subsequent chapters, a more detailed discussion of the contributions of flow cytometry to evaluating tissue specimens in general, in light of the previously described advantages and disadvantages will be further discussed at this point.

FCI for Nodal and Extranodal Tissues

Large, retrospective studies have shown FCI contributes significantly to or is consistent with the final tissue diagnosis in the great majority (94% and 87%, respectively) of nodal and/or extranodal tissue specimens studied [Dunphy 2000, Ravoet 2004]. The discrepancies were due to partial tissue involvement by NHL with sampling differences, T-cell rich or lymphohistiocytic-rich variants with a small population of monoclonal B-cells, marked tumoral sclerosis, poor tumor preservation, a

T-cell NHL without an aberrant immunophenotype, and cHL. In addition, FCI may be helpful in diagnosing Ewing sarcoma/primitive neuroectodermal tumor by the detection of CD56 on the surface of the malignant cells, and may also detect carcinoma, since non-hematopoietic large cells often are detected in the CD45-negative region as large cells (high forward light scatter). In addition, epithelial membrane antigen and cytokeratin may be analyzed by FCI.

FCI for BM Specimen Evaluation

Evaluation of BM Aspirates by FCI for Lymphomatous Involvement and the Evaluation of BM Core Biopsies for Hematolymphoid Neoplasia

FCI of BM aspirates may be useful not only in the initial immunophenotyping and diagnosis of BM-based lymphomas, but it may also be useful in staging of BM specimens for lymphomatous involvement by a previously diagnosed non-BM-based lymphoma [Fineberg 1993, Dunphy 1998, Perea 2004, Mazur 2004]. Although the majority of analyses (ie, 79%-89%) show a high concordance between morphology and FCI in evaluating for lymphomatous involvement in BM specimens (ie, positive by both morphology and FCI, or negative by both morphology and FCI), there are discordant cases (either positive by FCI and negative by morphology, or positive by morphology and negative by flow cytometry). The suggested reasons for positivity by morphology and negativity by FCI mostly include paratrabecular lymphomatous involvement or sampling differences. The primary suggested reason for positivity by FCI and negativity by morphology is a low percentage (≤5%) of interstitial lymphomatous involvement. These studies have concluded that a combined approach (ie, morphological examination of the BM trephine biopsy and FCI of the BM aspirate) is better than a single method in detecting BM involvement by NHL, especially in those of B-cell origin.

As mentioned previously, BM aspirates are not always available for FCI, perhaps due to a "packed" or sclerotic bone marrow. In these situations, and when the patient has a high suspicion of a hematolymphoid malignancy, the BM core biopsy may be processed for FCI. Although architectural relationships are lost in this process and the concordance of the percentage of abnormal cells is low, this technique has been shown to be extremely useful in clearly identifying the cell of origin of the abnormal cells and in excluding other lineages of origin. In a study in which this technique was evaluated in this way, this approach was able to significantly aid in establishing a hematolymphoid neoplasm, including acute leukemias, myelodysplasias, and B-NHL [Dunphy 1998]. Again, it should be emphasized that a touch preparation of the flow cytometry sample is imperative for cytomorphologic correlation. In addition, a separate BM core biopsy sample should be simultaneously submitted for routine histology.

FCI for Evaluation of Lymphomatous Involvement of Small Biopsies

With regard to fresh tissue specimens, in addition to the issues described above (eg, partial tissue involvement, areas of necrosis, sclerotic tissue), a major limiting factor in the use of FCI in diagnostic hematopathology is the "small biopsy" specimen (eg, punch skin biopsies, gastric biopsies). As described below, vortex disaggregation has been proposed in order to obtain cells for FCI and to preserve the tissue for subsequent recovery and routine histologic processing. However, this technique is not universally employed, and there have been studies evaluating the use of FCI in diagnosing gastric lymphomas in endoscopic biopsy specimens, the use of flow cytometry in diagnosing pulmonary mucosa-associated lymphoid tissue (MALT) lymphomas in transbronchial biopsies, and the contribution of flow cytometry in diagnosing cutaneous lymphoid lesions.

Braylan et al determined FCI of freshly prepared cell suspensions obtained from endoscopic biopsy specimens may be used to reliably evaluate gastric lymphoid infiltrates [Almasri 1997]. By performing a limited panel (analyzing surface immunoglobulin-Ig light chain expression on B cells), they were able to reliably distinguish polyclonal (nonlymphoma) from clonal (lymphoma) infiltrates. This information was used as a supplement to the morphologic evaluation of the gastric biopsies. Likewise, this same group demonstrated the usefulness of a limited multiparameter FCI panel (analyzing surface Ig light chain expression on CD20+ or CD19+ cells) for confirming B-cell monoclonality [Zaer 1998].

The pathologic evaluation of mycosis fungoides (MF) and the histologic diagnosis of cutaneous lymphoid lesions in general are challenging areas in dermatopathology. As has been eluded to previously, B-cell neoplasms are easier to evaluate by FCI than are T-cell neoplasms, since not all T-cell lymphomas display an obviously aberrant immunophenotype and CD7

may be lost in some reactive conditions. In addition, skin biopsies being evaluated for lymphomatous involvement are often not very cellular.

In a relatively recent study by Wu [2003], skin specimens from 19 patients were evaluated by FCI to determine the contribution of FCI to the final diagnosis. Of interest, 88% ($^{15}/_{17}$) of cutaneous primary or secondary B-cell lymphomas showed Ig light chain restriction by FCI. The other 2 cases revealed no light chain expression (indicating clonality) and a polyclonal pattern, respectively. One patient had reactive lymphoid hyperplasia with polyclonal B cells. The last patient had a cutaneous T-cell lymphoma and revealed an aberrant T-cell population. Thus, this study demonstrated the usefulness of FCI in these skin biopsies, but one should keep in mind that B-NHLs were primarily used in this study.

Oshtory [2007] subsequently studied the usefulness of 4-color FCI in the diagnosis of MF in skin biopsy specimens from 22 patients with a "clinical suggestion" of MF. They were able to recover 20,000-30,000 cells per specimen, allowing for the evaluation of 18 antigens by 4-color FCI in all cases. A T-cell abnormality was detected by FCI in 11 patients with diagnostic International Society for Cutaneous Lymphoma (ISCL) MF diagnostic scores, whereas the 7 patients with either sub-diagnostic scores or reactive histology showed no phenotypic abnormality by FCI.

In general, to evaluate for B-cell neoplasia in small biopsy specimens, limited immunophenotyping may determine clonality and even be instrumental in subtyping small B-cell NHLs [Kaleem 2001, Xu 2002]. A limited immunophenotypic panel including a B-cell marker (ie, CD19, CD20), surface Ig light chains (κ and λ), CD5, CD10, and CD23 are useful in differentiating small lymphocytic lymphoma, mantle cell lymphoma, and follicular lymphoma. The advent of additional multi-color analysis (ie, 6- and 9-color) will allow for more markers to be analyzed on a lower number of cells, and thus increase the use of FCI in small biopsy specimens.

References

Almasri NM, Zaer FS, Iturraspe JA, Braylan RC [1997] Contribution of flow cytometry to the diagnosis of gastric lymphomas in endoscopic biopsy specimens. *Mod Pathol* 10:650-656.

Dunphy CH [1996] Combined cytomorphologic and immunophenotypic approach to evaluation of effusions for lymphomatous involvement. *Diagn Cytopathol* 15:427-430.

Dunphy CH, Ramos R [1997] Combining fine-needle aspiration and flow cytometric immunophenotyping in evaluation of nodal and extranodal sties for possible lymphoma: A retrospective review. *Diagn Cytopathol* 16:200-206.

Dunphy CH [1998] Combining morphology and flow cytometric immunophenotyping to evaluate bone marrow specimens for B-cell malignant neoplasms. *Am J Clin Pathol* 109:625-630.

Dunphy CH, Dunphy FR, Visconti JL [1999] Flow cytometric immunophenotyping of bone marrow core biopsies: Report of 8 patients with previously undiagnosed hematologic malignancy and failed bone marrow aspiration. *Arch Pathol Lab Med* 123:206-212.

Dunphy CH [2000] Contribution of flow cytometric immunophenotyping to the evaluation of tissues with suspected lymphoma? *Cytometry* 42:296-306.

Fineberg S, Marsh E, Alfonso F, et al [1993] Immuno-phenotypic evaluation of the bone marrow in non-Hodgkin's lymphoma. *Hum Pathol* 24:636-642.

Kaleem Z, White G, Vollmer RT [2001] Critical analysis and diagnostic usefulness of limited immunophenotyping of B-cell non-Hodgkin lymphomas by flow cytometry. *Am J Clin Pathol* 115:136-142.

Lazarovits AI, White MJ, Karsh J [1992] CD7– T cells in rheumatoid arthritis. *Arthritis Rheum* 35:615-624.

Leers MPG, Theunissen PHMH, Ramaekers FCS, Schutte B, Nap M [2000] Clonlity assessment of lymphoproliferative disorders by multiparameter flow cytometry of paraffin-embedded tissue: An additional diagnostic tool in surgical pathology. *Human Pathology* 31:422-427.

Mazur G, Halon A, Wrobel T, Jelen M, Kuliczkowski K [2004] Contribution of flow cytometric immunophenotyping and bone marrow trephine biopsy in the detection of lymphoid bone marrow infiltration in non-Hodgkin's lymphomas. *Neoplasma* 51:159-163.

Moll M, Reinhold U, Kukel S, et al [1994] CD7-negative helper T cells accumulate in inflammatory skin lesions. *J Invest Dermatol* 102:328-332.

Oshtory S, Apisarnthanarax N, Gilliam AC, et al [2007] Usefulness of flow cytometry in the diagnosis of mycosis fungoides. *J Am Acad Dermatol* 57:454-462.

Perea G, Altes A, Bellido M, et al [2004] Clinical utility of bone marrow flow cytometry in B-cell non-Hodgkin lymphomas (B-NHL). *Histopathology* 45:268-274.

Ravoet C, Demartin S, Gerard R, et al [2004] Contribution of flow cytometry to the diagnosis of malignant and non-malignant conditions in lymph node biopsies. *Leukemia and lymphoma* 45:1587-1593.

Smith KJ, Skelton HG, Chur WS, et al, for the Military Medical Consortium for the Advancement of Retroviral Research (MMCARR) [1995] Decreased CD7 expression in cutaneous infiltrates of HIV-1+ patients. *Am J Dermatopathol* 17:564-569.

Vos JA, Simurdak JH, Davis BJ, Myers JB, Brissette MD [2003] Vortex disaggregation for flow cytometry allows direct histologic correlation: A novel approach for small biopsies and inaspirable bone marrows. *Clinical Cytometry* 52B:20-31.

Weisberger J, Cornfield D, Gorczyca W, Liu Z [2003] Down-regulation of pan-T-cell antigens, particularly CD7, in acute infectious mononucleosis. *Am J Clin Pathol* 120:49-55.

Wu H, Smith M, Millenson MM, et al [2003] Contribution of flow cytometry in the diagnosis of cutaneous lymphoid lesions. *J Invest Dermatol* 121:1522-1530.

Xu Y, McKenna RW, Kroft SH [2002] Assessment of CD10 in the diagnosis of small B-cell lymphomas: A multiparameter flow cytometric study. *Am J Clin Pathol* 117:291-300.

Zaer FS, Braylan RC, Zander DS, Iturraspe JA, Almasri NM [1998] Multiparametric flow cytometry in the diagnosis and characterization of low-grade pulmonary mucosa-associated lymphoid tissue lymphomas. *Mod Pathol* 11:525-532.

4 Phenotypic Markers Commonly Used by FCI in Diagnostic Hematopathology

Chapter Contents

Panhematopoietic Cell Antigens

CD45 Cluster

The CD45 MAb cluster, commonly referred to as *leukocyte common antigen* (LCA), includes CD45, CD45RA, CD45RB, and CD45RO (UCHL-1). See [t4.1] for the reactivities of these antibodies in various cell types. CD45 is often used in diagnostic hematopathology to identify hematolymphoid cells by flow cytometric gating, since CD45 is expressed on the surface membrane of virtually all hematolymphoid cells and their progenitors, except megakaryocytes, erythroid cells, and plasma cells. In addition, it is well-recognized that the lymphoblasts of precursor B-cell lymphoblastic leukemia may show quite a dim expression of CD45. Nonhematolymphoid malignancies are CD45–, and thus may be identified by flow cytometric gating.

HLA-DR (Immune-Associated) Antigens

HLA-DR antigens are present on B cells, throughout B-cell ontogeny, and are lost at the plasma cell stage [f4.1], [f4.2] [Halper 1978]. They are also present on hematopoietic progenitor cells and granulocyte-macrophage, erythroid, and megakaryocytic precursors [Winchester 1977, Winchester 1945, Fitchen 1982]. HLA-DR antigens are expressed on myeloblasts, but are lost during maturation to the promyelocyte stage [Winchester 1977]. Likewise, they are expressed on proerythroblasts and megakaryocytes, but are absent from erythrocytes beyond the basophilic normoblast stage and platelets [Winchester 1977, Winchester 1978, Rabellino 1979, Belzer 1981, Robinson 1981]. They are present throughout monocyte/macrophage differentiation and on all dendritic cell populations (Langerhans cells, interdigitating dendritic cells, and follicular dendritic cells) [Foucar 1990, Steinman 1991, Rowden 1977, Klareskog 1977, Heinen 1984]. HLA-DR antigens are also expressed at the earliest

t4.1 CD45 Cluster Antibodies and Reactivities

Antibody Reactivity				Cell Expression
CD45	CD45RA	CD45RB	CD45RO	
+	+	+	–	Pre-B and B cells
+	+	+	–	Naïve T cells
+	–	+	–	T cells
+	–	+	–	Macrophages; T cells; plasma cell subset; marginal zone B cells
+	–	+	–	Macrophages; granulocytes, thymocytes; memory T cells; transformed B cells; preplasma cells

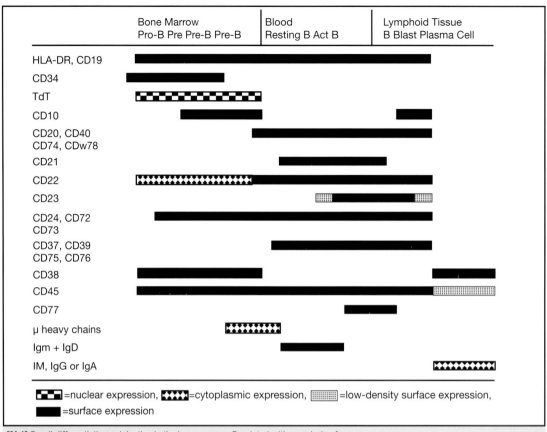

[f4.1] B-cell differentiation, originating in the bone marrow. Reprinted with permission from [Perruccello 1994].

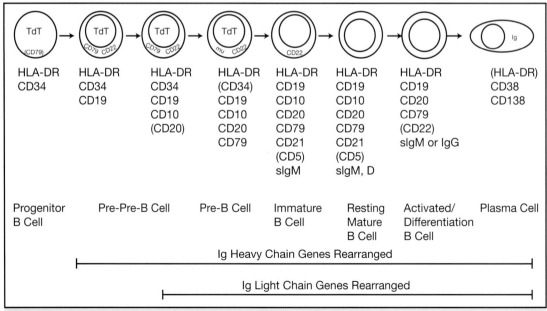

[f4.2] Schematic of B-cell differentiation. Reprinted with permission from [van Lochem 2004].

stages of T-cell ontogeny, but are quickly lost. The vast majority of thymocytes and mature peripheral T cells are HLA-DR– [Chess 1976, Winchester 1976, Hoffman 1977, Halper 1980]. Activated T cells do acquire HLA-DR expression [f4.3], [f4.4] [Evans 1978, Fu 1978, Yu 1980].

HLA-DR antigen expression on hematolymphoid malignancies mirrors the expression on benign hematolymphoid cells; although HLA-DR antigens are expressed variably by all categories of post-thymic T-cell neoplasia [Knowles 1986, Knowles 1989]. This known pattern of HLA-DR expression may be useful in differentiating acute promyelocytic leukemia (HLA-DR–) from acute monocytic leukemia (brightly HLA-DR+), differentiating AML (HLA-DR+) from precursor T-cell lymphoblastic leukemia (HLA-DR–), differentiating a small B-cell lymphoma (HLA-DR+) from a *lymphoid variant* of plasma cell myeloma, etc.

B-Cell Lineage-Associated Antigens

CD10

CD10 (common acute lymphoblastic leukemia antigen-CALLA) is a B-cell lineage-associated antigen frequently used by FCI in diagnostic hematopathology. As the name implies, it is frequently expressed by precursor B-cell lymphoblastic leukemia/lymphoma (B-LL) (up to 90%), but it may also be expressed by non-neoplastic hematolymphoid cells [ie, precursor B cells residing in the bone marrow (BM) (hematogones), thymocytes, and mature granulocytes (but not immature myeloid cells)], precursor T-cell lymphoblastic leukemia/lymphoma, various B- and T-cell non-Hodgkin lymphomas (ie, angioimmunoblastic T-cell lymphoma and other peripheral T-cell lymphomas), and chronic B-cell lymphoproliferative disorders (ie, hairy cell leukemia, as discussed below), as well as a small number (<3%) of AMLs [Arber 1997, Braun 1983, McCormack 1986, Tran-Paterson 1990, Longacre 1989]. Lack of CD10 expression in precursor B-LL is associated with decreased survival [Basso 1992, Kersey 1982, Vannier 1989]. The intensity of CD10 expression in both precursor B-LL and precursor T-LL is associated with prognosis (ie, increased intensity with better prognosis) [Glencross 1992]. CD10 is expressed in up to 80% of follicular lymphoma (more frequently lost with increasing grade), in up to 90% of Burkitt lymphoma (usually intense expression), and in rare cases of mantle cell lymphoma [Arber 1997, Dunphy 2001c]. In addition, CD10 may be expressed by otherwise typical cases of hairy cell leukemia. The CD10 co-expression does not correlate with any difference in morphology, clinical course, or therapeutic regimens [Dunphy 1999b, Jasionowski 2003, Robins 1993]. Lastly, CD10 may be expressed in up to 33% of plasma cell dyscrasias, representing a poor prognostic indicator [Durie 1985, Kurabayashi 1988, Tamura 1989].

CD19

CD19 represents the earliest B-cell lineage associated antigen and is expressed at all stages of B-cell differentiation up to the final stage of B-cell maturation (ie, normal plasma cells do not express CD19). It is not expressed by immature, mature, or activated T cells, monocytes, macrophages, or granulocytes [Nadler 1983, Meeker 1984]. It is expressed by 90% of precursor B-LL and in the great majority of various forms of B-cell non-Hodgkin lymphomas and chronic B-cell lymphoproliferative disorders [Nadler 1983, Meeker 1984, Nadler 1984]. One should keep in mind that plasma cell dyscrasias may acquire aberrant expression of CD19, as may AML, particularly AMLs associated with the 8;21 translocation or the 9;22 translocation [Reading 1993, Cueno 1992].

CD20

CD20 follows HLA-DR, TdT, CD19, and CD10 expression in B-cell ontogeny and appears on the B-cell surface between Ig light chain gene rearrangement and the expression of intact surface Ig. It is lost at the end stage of B-cell maturation (ie, at the mature plasma cell stage) [Anderson 1984, Chittal 1990, Hokland 1985 Uckun 1992, Moreau 1993]. CD20 is thus expressed by a subset of precursor B-cell LL (ie, by the early pre-B cell stage of precursor B-LL, and by LL with a mature B-cell immunophenotype). CD20 is expressed by the great majority of various forms of B-cell non-Hodgkin lymphomas and chronic B-cell lymphoproliferative disorders. It is characteristically dimly expressed, or may even be absent, in chronic lymphocytic leukemia/small lymphocytic lymphoma (CLL/SLL). It is expressed by the monoclonal small B cells and plasmacytoid lymphocytes of lymphomplasmacytic lymphoma, which may be associated with Waldenström macroglobulinemia. Although normal plasma cells do not express CD20, CD20 may be aberrantly expressed in plasma cell dyscrasias, and especially in the "small cell" or "lymphoid" variant of plasma cell myeloma [Hall 1987, Linder 1988, Chadburn 1994, San Miguel 1991, Leo 1992, Harada 1993, Ruiz-Argüelles 1994].

Although CD20 is a highly specific marker of B-cell lineage neoplasms, one should keep in mind that a subset of dim CD20+ normal T cells and rare CD20+ T-cell lymphomas have been described [Hutlin 1993, Quintanilla-Martinez 1994].

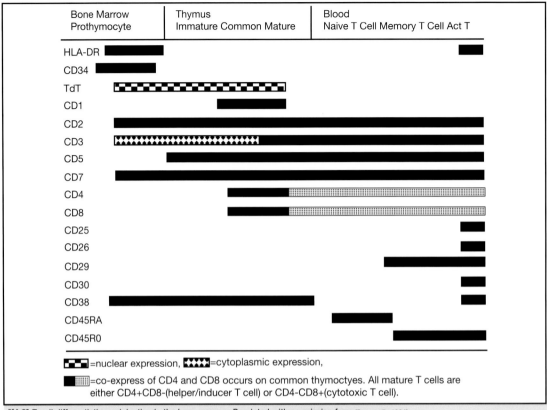

[f4.3] T-cell differentiation, originating in the bone marrow. Reprinted with permission from [Perruccello 1994]

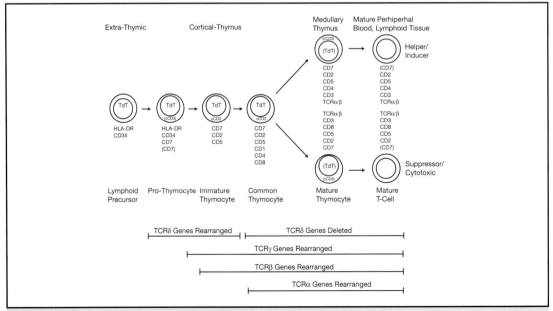

[f4.4] Schematic of T-cell differentiation. Reprinted with permission from [Lanier 1986]

CD22

CD22 is expressed in the cytoplasm at the earliest stages of pre-B cell differentiation and thus is expressed by up to 80% of precursor B cells (ie, hematogones) in the BM. Cytoplasmic CD22 and CD19 expressions occur at approximately the same time in B-cell ontogeny, prior to acquisition of CD20. Interestingly CD22 is not exported to the cell surface until the mature, resting B-cell stage, and thus, the great majority (ie, 95%) of peripheral blood B cells contain CD22, but only about 75% express surface CD22. CD22 expression then transiently increases, rapidly decreases, and is lost prior to the plasma cell stage [Campana 1985, Dörken 1987, Dörken 1986, Nadler 1986, Schwartig 1985]. In lymph nodes, tonsils, and other benign lymphoid tissues, CD22 is strongly expressed by mantle zone cells and less strongly by germinal center cells [Nadler 1986, Zola 1987]. Due to this variable expression in B-cell ontogeny, it is not surprising there is variable expression of CD22 by precursor B-cell LL (more than 50% of cases), B-cell NHL, and chronic B-cell lymphoproliferative disorders. Virtually all cases of hairy cell leukemia and prolymphocytic leukemia exhibit CD22 expression, and these 2 leukemias show the highest intensity of CD22 expression [Nadler 1984, Schwartig 1985, Mason 1987]. CD22 is not expressed in T-cell leukemias or lymphomas [Nadler 1986, Mason 1987, Boue 1988].

CD23

CD23 differs from other B-cell lineage-restricted antigens, since it is expressed weakly or not at all on resting, mature peripheral blood and lymphoid tissue B cells, but it appears on activated B cells [Nadler 1986 Thorley-Lawson 1985, Kikutani 1986]. In normal lymphoid tissue, CD23 expression is absent or intermittently present on a small fraction of mantle zone cells, is absent on marginal zone B cells, and is variably present on germinal center B cells [Nadler 1986, Zola 1987, Moldenhauer 1986, Pallesen 1987]. CD23 (type B isoform only) is also expressed by monocytes, eosinophils, Langerhan cells, follicular dendritic cells, and subpopulations of T cells, platelets, and thymic epithelium. CD23 is not expressed by precursor B cells, plasma cells, myeloid cells, or normal nonlymphoid tissue [Thorley-Lawson 1985, Pallesen 1987, Delespess 1992, Capron 1986, Hardie 1993, Yamaoka 1996]. This marker is commonly used to distinguish CLL/SLL from mantle cell lymphoma/leukemia, since CD23 is variably expressed (dim to bright) in cases of CLL/SLL and is typically negative or only dimly expressed in mantle cell lymphoma [Gong 2001]. It may be variably

expressed by follicular lymphoma and is typically not expressed by marginal zone B-cell lymphomas, lymphoplasmacytic lymphoma, plasma cell dyscrasias, hairy cell leukemia, and precursor B-cell lymphoblastic leukemia/lymphoma, as well as T-cell and myeloid neoplasms [Nadler 1984, Nadler 1986, Thorley-Lawson 1985, Pallesen 1987, Harris 1994].

CD24

CD24 is a pan-B cell antigen, expressed by CD34+ progenitor B cells in the BM, and not lost until the terminal plasma cell stage of B-cell differentiation. It is not expressed by T cells, monocytes, or red blood cells, but is expressed by mature granulocytes [Zola 1987, Abramson 1981, Melink 1983, Duperray 1990, Solvason 1992]. Thus, as may be predicted, it is expressed by the vast majority of precursor B-cell lymphoblastic leukemias/lymphomas and virtually all mature B-cell NHLs and chronic lymphoproliferative disorders (except nodal and extranodal marginal zone B cell lymphomas). It is not expressed by plasma cell dyscrasias, T-cell neoplasms, or myeloid neoplasms (except CML in blast crisis) [Nadler 1984, Zola 1987, Abramson 1981, Fischer 1990, Kersey 1982]. CD24 may be particularly useful in identifying precursor B-cell lymphoblastic leukemia/lymphoma, even when there is absence of later B-cell markers (ie, CD10 and CD20; see [f4.1]).

CD79

CD79 is present as a multimeric receptor complex on the cell surface, composed of CD79a (α) and CD79b (β). CD79 expression is restricted to B-cell lineage among normal hematopoietic cells. It begins at the progenitor B-cell stage and ceases around the onset of plasma cell differentiation [Mason 1992, Borst 1993, Venkitaraman 1997, Nakamura 1998, Mason 1991, Mason 1996, Nakamura 1992].

CD79a expression is present in nearly all cases of precursor B-cell lymphoblastic leukemia/lymphoma, more than 95% of mature B-cell NHLs and chronic lymphoproliferative disorders, and approximately 50% of plasma cell dyscrasias. In addition, CD79a may be expressed by many precursor T-cell lymphoblastic lymphomas/leukemias and a subset of AMLs (all representing acute promyelocytic leukemia) [Mason 1991, Mason 1995, Buccheri 1993, Kanavaros 1995, Pilozzi 1988, Arber 1996a].

CD79b expression has been shown useful in improving the diagnostic accuracy in subtyping chronic B-cell lymphoproliferative disorders, particularly in distinguishing CLL and mantle cell lymphoma.

CD79b appears to be absent or dimly expressed in CLL and brightly expressed in mantle cell lymphoma [McCarron 2000]; however, one should recognize that higher intensity CD79b expression may occur in 20% of CLL cases. Of interest, this expression correlates with trisomy 12 and atypical immunophenotypic features; in turn, trisomy 12 in CLL correlates with the worst prognosis [Schlette 2003].

CD138

Among hematopoietic cells, only cIg-containing plasma cells express CD138 (also referred to as syndecan-1) [Horvathova 1995, Wijdenes 1998, Wijdenes 1996]. Plasma cell dyscrasias variably express CD138, and CD138 may also be expressed by CLL, primary effusion lymphomas, and plasmablastic lymphomas [Clément 1995, Gaidano 1997, Vega 2005]. However, CD138 is not expressed by precursor B-cell lymphoblastic leukemias/lymphomas or Burkitt lymphomas, diffuse large B-cell lymphomas, T-cell neoplasms, or myeloid neoplasms. Thus, CD138 may be useful in distinguishing these entities, which may be morphologically challenging. Note that plasma cells are often underestimated in BM aspirate specimens by flow cytometric immunophenotyping, either because the cells are fragile and the cytoplasm is stripped, or because the cells are large and fall outside the gates of flow cytometric analysis.

Surface immunoglobulin (sIg) heavy chains and light chains may be analyzed on B cells to determine clonality, although light chain analysis is generally adequate for this purpose. Keep in mind that as detection of monoclonal B cells by FCI may be useful in establishing a diagnosis of a B-cell neoplasm, it should also be noted that the lack of sIg light chain expression by FCI also helps identify peripheral B-cell lymphoma. In a recent study by Li et al, cases with >25% B cells lacking sIg light chain expression all represented lymphoma [Li 2002]. By FCI, the identified sIg light chain-negative population was distinctly separate from the normal polytypic B cells; in 90% of cases, the identified population was larger by forward angle light scatter than the reactive T cells and polytypic B cells. In their review of reactive cases, no reactive case revealed >17% sIg– B cells.

Prognostic Markers in CLL

CD2, CD7, CD10, CD13, CD33, CD34, CD38, ZAP-70

In addition to subtyping B-cell lymphoma/leukemia composed predominantly of small cells, FCI can detect prognostic markers in CLL/SLL. Expression of aberrant markers by FCI, particularly CD2, CD7, CD10, CD13, CD33, and CD34, has been demonstrated to be associated with significantly shortened overall survival and increased aggressiveness [Kampalath 2003]. Expression of CD38 by >20%-30% of the neoplastic cells in CLL has been associated with an unfavorable prognosis [Ibrahim 2001, Del Poeta 2001]. Likewise, the expression of ZAP-70 as detected by FCI has been shown to correlate with immunoglobulin heavy-chain variable region (IgV$_H$) mutational status, more rapid disease progression, and poorer survival [Crespo 2003, Weistner 2003].

T-Cell Lineage-Associated Antigens

CD1

CD1 is also referred to as the common thymocyte antigen, since it is not expressed at the very early stages of T-cell ontogeny, but is expressed by the majority of CD4+/CD8+ thymocytes and not by CD4+/CD8– or CD4–/CD8+ thymocytes. Likewise, it is expressed by the majority of cortical thymocytes and not by most medullary thymocytes. CD1 is not expressed by resting mature peripheral blood and lymphoid tissue T cells [Van Dogen 1985, McMichael 1979, Cattoretti 1987]. CD1 expression by benign T cells is mirrored by T-cell neoplasms. Precursor T-cell lymphoblastic lymphoma/leukemia expressing a cortical thymocyte immunophenotype express CD1, whereas those expressing prothymocyte or medullary thymocyte immunophenotypes lack CD1 expression [t4.2]. Thymomas typically express CD1a. All mature (post-thymic) T-cell neoplasms lack expression of CD1 [Knowles 1989]. In addition, CD1a expression is characteristic of Langerhans cells and interdigitating dendritic cells [Krenacs 1993]. Of interest, benign monocytes, macrophages, and follicular dendritic cells as well as their neoplastic counterparts lack CD1 [Turner 1984, Franklin 1986, Roholl 1988].

CD2

CD2, also referred to as the sheep erythrocyte antigen, is a pan-T-cell antigen, representing 1 of the earliest T-cell lineage-restricted antigens to appear during T-cell ontogeny, appearing after CD7 and before CD1 [Van

t4.2 Immunophenotypes of T-ALL

Antigen	Pre-T ALL (I) Prothymocytes	Pre-T ALL (II) Common Thymocytes	T-ALL (III) Mature Thymocytes		T-ALL (IV) Mature T Lymphocytes	
			T-H	T-S	T-H	T-S
CD1	–	+	–	–	–	–
CD2	±	±	+	+	+	+
sCD3	–	±	+	+	+	+
CD5	+	+	+	+	+	+
CD7	+	+	+	+	+	+
CD4	–	+	+	–	+	–
CD8	–	+	–	+	–	+

Dogen 1985]. As such, it is expressed throughout T-cell ontogeny by prothymocytes throughout T-cell maturation [f4.3]. It is also expressed by true natural killer cells.

CD2 expression by benign T cells and true natural killer cells is mirrored by T-cell neoplasms. It is expressed in the vast majority of precursor and mature (post-thymic) T-cell neoplasms, as well as in neoplasms of true natural killer cell origin. Likewise, thymomas typically express CD2. As with other T-cell antigens, CD2 may be aberrantly lost by a mature T-cell neoplasm. CD2 is not expressed by precursor or most mature B-cell neoplasms. As mentioned previously, it may be expressed in B-cell CLL and represents a poor prognostic marker in that disorder. CD2 may also be aberrantly expressed by a small subset of AMLs, most commonly acute promyelocytic leukemia and acute myelomonocytic leukemia with eosinophilia associated with inversion 16 [Mirro 1985, Venditti 1997, Rovelli 1992, Adriaansen 1993]. Lastly, it may be aberrantly expressed by mast cells in mast-cell disorders, and CD2 co-expression indicates neoplastic mast cells [Pardanani 2004].

CD3

CD3 is the most lineage-specific T-cell marker. It is present within the cytoplasm (intracytoplasmic-cCD3) prior to its expression on the cell surface membrane (sCD3) [Link 1985, Campana 1987, van Dongen 1988]. Thus, cCD3 may be demonstrated in prothymocytes and in the cells in the early to mid-thymocyte stage [f4.3]. As common thymocytes develop into mature medullary thymocytes and subsequently into mature peripheral T cells, cCD3 is lost. Surface CD3 is expressed by virtually all mature peripheral blood and lymphoid tissue T cells but not by any other hematolymphoid or non-hematolymphoid cell population.

CD3 (cCD3 and sCD3) expression by benign T cells is mirrored by T-cell neoplasms. Thus, cCD3 expression is characteristic of precursor T-cell lymphoplastic lymphoma/leukemia, especially in the early stages. Surface CD3 may then be expressed by a subset of cells in the common thymocyte and medullary thymocyte stage of precursor T-cell neoplasms and is expressed by mature (post-thymic) T-cell neoplasms. As with other mature T-cell neoplasms, sCD3 may be aberrantly lost, primarily by anaplastic large cell lymphomas. The lineage specificity of CD3 is helpful in distinguishing precursor T-cell from precursor B-cell neoplasms and AMLs, and distinguishing T-cell NHLs from B-cell NHLs. It is not expressed by B-cell NHLs.

CD4 and CD8

CD4 and CD8 are discussed together, since they represent markers for mature helper and suppressor T cells, respectively. They both appear and are expressed at the common thymocyte stage and then differentiate into either helper (CD4+) or suppressor (CD8+) thymocytes at the medullary thymocyte stage. Mature helper T cells maintain CD4 expression throughout the mature T-cell stages, as mature suppressor T cells maintain CD8 expression. In addition, natural killer cell expansions do not typically demonstrate CD8 expression.

CD4 and CD8 expressions by benign T cells are somewhat mirrored by T-cell neoplasms (ie, precursor

T-cell neoplasms of the common thymocyte stage dually express CD4 and CD8, as do thymomas). Mature (post-thymic) T-cell neoplasms are most commonly CD4+, although rare cases may be CD4+/CD8+, CD4–/CD8+, or CD4–/CD8–. Natural killer cell leukemias typically express CD8, in contrast to NK-cell expansions.

CD4 and CD8 are not expressed by precursor B-cell neoplasms, although CD4 may be aberrantly expressed by B-cell CLL and by AMLs [Jani 2007, Venditti 1997]. In addition, CD8 may be aberrantly expressed by B-cell CLL [Schroers 2004, Parisi-Duchêne 2006]. There are no apparent clinical implications for aberrant expressions of CD4 and CD8 in B-cell CLL.

CD5

CD5 is another T-cell marker acquired at the immature thymocyte stage that persists throughout T-cell maturation [f4.4]. However, it is also expressed by a small but significant number of normal B cells circulating in the peripheral blood and residing in fetal and adult peripheral lymphoid tissue [Caligaris-Cappio 1982, Gadol 1986, Hardy 1986].

CD5 expression by benign T cells is mirrored by T-cell neoplasms (ie, precursor T-cell neoplasms typically strongly express CD5, as do thymomas), and most mature (post-thymic) T-cell neoplasms express CD5. As with other mature T-cell neoplasms, CD5 may be aberrantly lost.

CD5 is not lineage-specific and, as mentioned previously, may be detected on a small percentage of resting B cells. Thus, it is not surprising CD5 may be aberrantly expressed on B-cell neoplasms, and this aberrant CD5 expression is quite characteristic of B-cell CLL/SLL and mantle cell lymphoma. CD5 is not observed in precursor B-cell neoplasms; however, CD5 may be aberrantly expressed by <5% of AMLs, without any prognostic implication [Kuerbitz 1992, Smith 1992].

CD7

CD7 is the first T-cell lineage-associated antigen, acquired at the prothymocyte stage, and is maintained throughout T-cell maturation [f4.3], [f4.4]. As such, it is expressed by precursor T-cell neoplasms as well as mature (post-thymic) neoplasms. Like other T-cell antigens, it may be aberrantly lost in mature T-cell neoplasms and is the most frequently lost T-cell antigen in these disorders. In particular, CD7 is characteristically lost in mycosis fungoides (and Sézary syndrome) as well as adult T-cell leukemia/lymphoma syndrome. It may rarely be aberrantly expressed by B-cell CLL and

5%-20% of AMLs, imparting the worse prognosis in both of these disorders [Jani 2007, Kasparu 1989].

Large Granular Lymphocyte- or Natural Killer Cell-Associated Antigens

CD16

CD16 reacts with approximately 15%-20% of peripheral blood lymphocytes, <5% of lymphocytes in the tonsil, spleen, and BM, and almost no lymphocytes in the lymph node and thymus [Perussia 1983, Perussia 1984]. The CD16+ peripheral blood lymphocytes are represented by 90% large granular lymphocytes (LGLs) (bright CD16+/dim CD56+) and 10% non-LGLs (dim CD16+/bright CD56+). CD16 is also expressed by a small subset of T cells [Lanier 1985]. In addition, CD16 may also be expressed by activated monocytes, more than 95% neutrophils, and a subset of eosinophils but not by basophils [deHaas 1995, Ravetch 1989, Schmidt 1989, Robertson 1990, Stain 1987].

CD16 expression, among hematolymphoid neoplasms, largely mirrors its expression among benign hematolymphoid cells. CD16 is uniformly expressed by the cells of both NK-cell expansions and NK-cell LGL-leukemia and is variably expressed by the cells of T-cell LGL-leukemia. CD16 may also be expressed by extranodal NK/T-cell lymphomas of the nasal type, by rare precursor T-cell neoplasms, by monocytic neoplasms, and by Langerhans cell neoplasms [Jaffe 1996, Kaplan 1986, Sheibani 1987, Nadler 1984]. It is not expressed by precursor or mature B-cell neoplasms, plasma-cell neoplasms, or by AMLs [Nadler 1984].

CD16 expression in relationship to CD11b and CD13 in the granulocytes of patients with myelodysplasia (MDS) will be discussed under the CD11b section.

CD56

CD56, or neuronal cell adhesion molecule (NCAM), is a pan-NK cell marker and is expressed by peripheral blood NK cells, as described above in the CD16 section. Like CD16, CD56 is also expressed by a small subset (5%) of peripheral blood CD3+ T cells. CD56 is not normally expressed by thymocytes, B cells, plasma cells, monocytes, or granulocytes [Griffin 1983]. It is important to recognize that CD56 is also expressed by neural cells, as will be further discussed below [Edelman 1986].

Among hematolymphoid neoplasms, CD56 is expressed by a greater variety of these neoplasms than CD16. CD56 is uniformly expressed by NK-cell expansions and NK-LGL leukemia, and more variably expressed by T-cell LGL leukemia. CD56 is not expressed by B-cell NHLs (except the rare microvillous large B-cell lymphoma) [Hammer 1998], but it is characteristically expressed by extranodal NK/T-cell lymphomas of the nasal type. CD56 is also often expressed by hepatosplenic T-cell lymphoma and may be expressed by a subset of cells in enteropathy-associated T-cell lymphoma and subcutaneous panniculitis-like T-cell lymphoma (especially those of γ/δ origin), and rare cases of anaplastic large cell lymphoma [Chott 1998, Jaffe 1999, Dunphy 2006a]. In addition, CD56 may be expressed by some precursor T-cell neoplasms but has not been described in the thymocytes of thymomas. CD56 is also characteristically expressed with CD4 by the rare, highly aggressive hematodermic neoplasm, once considered "blastic NK-cell lymphoma," but now considered a neoplasm of an immature plasmacytoid dendritic cell derivation [Pillchowska 2007].

Although normal plasma cells do not express CD56, it may be expressed in plasma cell myelomas (PCMs) with varying reports of clinical significance and prognosis. It has been demonstrated that strong expression of CD56 in PCM myeloma correlates with the presence of lytic bone lesions. Indeed, others have shown that the lack of or weak expression of CD56 by PCM characterized a special subset of myeloma associated with a lower osteolytic potential and a higher tendency for circulation of the malignant plasma cells in the peripheral blood and for central nervous system involvement. This subset was also characterized by more extensive BM infiltration and significantly decreased overall survival [Ely 2002, Pellat-Deceunynck 1998, Rawstron 1999, Chang 2005, Sahara 2002].

It has also been shown that CD56 expression by plasma cells indicates clonality, being identified in PCM, lymphoplasmacytic lymphoma, rare cases of monoclonal gammopathy of undetermined significance (MGUS), but not in any reactive plasmacytosis. In this study, it was suggested that the presence of CD56+ plasma cells in an occasional case of MGUS most likely represents a clonal population, which will progress in time [Dunphy 2007a].

Likewise, although CD56 is not expressed by normal monocytes and myeloid cells, it may be aberrantly expressed in the monocytic cells of chronic myelomonocytic leukemia (CMML) and the myeloid cells of myelodysplastic syndromes and chronic myeloid neoplasms [Dunphy 2004a, Dunphy 2004b]. In addition, CD56 may be aberrantly expressed in various types of

AML. Although CD56 is often aberrantly expressed in AMLs with monocytic differentiation, it has been demonstrated that CD56 expression in AMLs is nonspecific as to the subtype and may also rarely be seen in APL [Dunphy 1999a]. The rare CD56+ APL cases should be distinguished from myeloid/NK cell acute leukemia, which may resemble APL morphologically, but lack the characteristic t(15;17) [Scott 1994].

Lastly, it is important to recognize that CD56 is characteristically expressed by neuroendocrine neoplasms (eg, small cell carcinoma, Ewing sarcoma/ primitive neuroectodermal tumor, Merkel cell carcinoma), since these small, round blue cell tumors are often included in the differential diagnosis of an NHL [Farinola 2003, Dunphy 2000a].

CD57

CD57 is expressed by 10%-24% of peripheral blood lymphocytes, including a subset of natural killer cells and a distinct T-cell population (CD2+, CD3+, and CD5+). CD57 is not expressed by peripheral blood B cells, monocytes, or granulocytes [Lanier 1983]. However, CD57 is expressed by some neural and neuroendocrine cells, similar to CD56.

In contrast to CD16, CD47 is weakly expressed by NK-cell expansions, variably expressed by NK-cell LGL leukemia, and uniformly expressed by T-cell LGL leukemia. CD57 negativity in NK-cell LGL leukemia has been associated with the worst prognosis [Pandolfi 1990]. Less than 10% of extranodal NK/T-cell lymphomas of the nasal type express CD57, and as CD16 and CD56, occasional precursor T-cell neoplasms may demonstrate CD57 expression. In addition, >95% of thymomas express CD57; however, CD57 is not expressed by B-cell NHLs or leukemias, plasma cell dyscrasia, AMLs, or Langerhans cell histiocytosis.

Like CD56, CD57 may be expressed by neuroendocrine neoplasms, but, in addition, may be expressed by a wide range of additional neoplasms of epithelial, neural, and mesenchymal origin [Arber 1995].

Monocyte- and Myeloid-Associated Antigens

CD11b

CD11b belongs to the leukocyte integrin receptor family of cellular adhesion molecules, which plays a critical role in the cellular adhesion reactions of leukocytes [Sanchez-Madrid 1983]. As such, it is expressed by more than

90% of peripheral blood monocytes, granulocytes, and NK cells, as well as follicular dendritic cells and 30% of BM cells (myeloid cells beginning with the promyelocyte stage). CD11b is not expressed by mature, resting B or T cells, erythrocytes, or platelets [Todd 1981, Griffin 1981, Lanier 1986, Schriever 1989].

Among hematolymphoid neoplasms, CD11b expression mirrors that of its normal counterparts. CD11b may be variably expressed by AMLs, with more uniform expression by AMLs with monocytic differentiation, and no expression observed in AML, M6 or AML, M7. In addition, CD11b expression in adult AML significantly predicts a shorter duration of survival [Bradstock 1994]. Abnormal patterns of expression of CD11b vs CD16 or CD13 vs CD16 among the maturing granulocytes have been considered quite useful in distinguishing benign processes from myelodysplastic processes [Olsaka 1997, Stetler-Stevenson 2001, Wells 2003]. These abnormal patterns will be discussed in more detail with illustrative images in the chapter entitled "Myelodysplastic Syndromes." Lower fluorescent intensity of CD16 has been observed on granulocytes in high-risk MDS patients and CML [Dunphy 2004b]. In addition, FCI of non-CML chronic myeloid neoplasms has identified basophils (CD11b+/CD13+/CD33+/HLA-DR-/CD15–/CD117–) with a significantly increased rate of immunophenotypic abnormalities, as well as expanded BM eosinophils with bright expression of CD11b, CD13, CD15, and CD45, without CD16, in chronic eosinophilic leukemia [Kussick 2003].

CD11b is variably expressed by NK-cell LGL and T-cell LGL leukemias and by extranodal NK/T cell lymphomas of the nasal type, as well as neoplasms of histiocytic derivation. CD11b is not expressed by other mature (post-thymic) T-cell neoplasms or B-cell neoplasms (except hairy cell leukemia and plasma cell myeloma). The presence of CD11b in myeloma cells may be related to a poor prognosis.

CD11c

CD11c is also expressed strongly by peripheral blood monocytes and less strongly by granulocytes [Giorno 1986, Cabanas 1988]. It is also expressed by NK cells, T-cell large granular lymphocytes, and interdigitating dendritic cells, but not by follicular dendritic cells or cutaneous Langerhans cells [Köller 1989].

Among hematolymphoid neoplasms, CD11c is expressed by AMLs, somewhat similarly to CD11b, with no APLs reported. It is not expressed by precursor

B-cell or T-cell neoplasms. It may also be expressed by neoplasms of histiocytic derivation [Venditti 1997].

CD11c is expressed by the majority of CD4–/CD8+ post-thymic T-cell neoplasms (including T-cell large granular lymphocytoses) and by some CD4+/CD8– post-thymic T-cell neoplasms. More importantly, CD11c is expressed in virtually all patients with hairy cell leukemia (HCL) and the prolymphocytic variant of HCL (HC-V). It may also be expressed less intensely by marginal zone B-cell lymphomas. In addition, it may rarely be expressed by distinct chronic lymphoid leukemias exhibiting features intermediate between CLL and HCL [Wormsley 1990, Hanson 1990].

CD13

CD13 is a myelomonocytic marker expressed by the majority of peripheral blood granulocytes, 25% of monocytes, and 6% of normal BM cells (all stages of myeloid differentiation from the myeloblast through the granulocyte). It is not expressed by any stage of erythroid differentiation, or any normal stage of B- or T-cell differentiation.

Among hematopoietic malignancies, CD13 is a pan-myeloid marker expressed by up to 95% of AMLs (M0-M6), with a smaller proportion of AML, M7s. The patterns of CD13 expression in MDS patients and in non-CML chronic myeloid neoplasms was discussed in the CD11b section. In addition, aberrant loss of expression of CD13 by mature monocytes may be particularly useful in establishing a diagnosis of CMML [Dunphy 2004a]. However, CD13 is not lineage-specific, since it may be aberrantly expressed in precursor B- and T-cell neoplasms, as well as in anaplastic large cell lymphoma without any apparent prognostic implications [Dunphy 2000b]. with the exception of CLL and PCM, mature B- and T-cell neoplasms are uniformly CD13– [Griffin 1984, Drexler 1986]. As mentioned previously, CD13 expression in CLL has been demonstrated to be associated with a significantly shortened overall survival and increased aggressiveness. The presence of CD13 in myeloma cells may be related to a poor prognosis.

CD14

CD14 is the most monocyte-specific (not the most sensitive) marker among myelomonocytic cells, being expressed in high density by more than 90% of peripheral blood monocytes and by 5%-10% of normal BM cells (primarily monocytes). It is weakly expressed by approximately 30% of granulocytes. CD14 appears at the promonocyte stage and is maintained throughout normal monocytic differentiation. It is not expressed by any stage of T-cell differentiation, erythrocytes, or platelets. It is, however, detectable in very low density on a variable proportion of peripheral blood B cells and mantle zone B cells [Dimitiu-Bona 1983].

Among hematopoietic neoplasms, CD14 is expressed in up to 20% of AMLs, predominantly those with monocytic differentiation. It is less sensitive than CD64 for AMLs with monocytic differentiation (see the discussion under the CD64 section). Loss of CD14 by mature monocytes may be particularly useful in establishing a diagnosis of CMML [Dunphy 2004a]. Although often not evaluated in B- or T-cell neoplasms, CD14 is detectable in approximately 90% of CLL, 80% of follicular lymphoma, and 40% of diffuse B-cell NHLs, as well as rare T-cell NHLs [Ziegler-Heitbrok 1988, Medeiros 1991, Morabito 1987]. In addition, the presence of CD14 in myeloma cells may be related to a poor prognosis.

CD33

CD33 is also a myelomonocytic marker expressed by all peripheral blood monocytes and by 30% of all normal BM cells (including myeloblasts, promyelocytes, and myelocytes). CD33-antigen density decreases from the myeloblast to the myelocyte stage and is absent or only minimally expressed by terminally differentiated granulocytes. It is present throughout monocyte differentiation. CD33 is not expressed by normal granulocytes, erythrocytes, platelets, thymocytes, or any stage of B- or T-cell differentiation. It may be expressed, however, by epidermal Langerhans cells [De Fraissinette 1990].

Among hematopoietic malignancies, CD33 is expressed by up to 100% of AMLs (M0-M7). Like CD13, it may be aberrantly expressed in precursor B- and T-cell neoplasms. with the exception of CLL and PCM, CD33 is not expressed by mature B- or T-cell neoplasms. As mentioned previously, CD33 expression in CLL has been demonstrated to be associated with significantly shortened overall survival and increased aggressiveness. The presence of CD33 in myeloma cells may be related to a poor prognosis [Ruiz-Argüelles 1994].

CD64

CD64 (FcγRI) binds IgG1 and IgG3 with high affinity and is expressed on virtually all peripheral blood monocytes. In addition, normal promyelocytes typically reveal dim expression of CD64 [Olweus 1995, Guyre 1995].

In hematopoietic malignancies, it may be expressed by AMLs. In a relatively recent study, CD64 was expressed by the blasts in all acute monocytic leukemias (AMoLs) to varying degrees; 43% showed 3+ intensity and the remaining 57% showed 1-2+ intensity. None of the other subtypes of AML demonstrated 3+ intensity expression of CD64 by the blasts, and thus, this finding may be useful in distinguishing AMoL from all other subtypes of AML. In addition, 3+ intensity CD15 expression was highly significant in the AML, M4, and M5 subtypes. Conversely, 2+ to 3+ intensity CD13 expression was highly significantly observed in the "non-M4 or M5 subtypes." The combination of any degree of CD64 expression with 3+ intensity CD15 expression and heterogeneous, or 1+ to 2+, intensity, CD13 expression was observed only in the AML, M4 or M5 subtypes [Dunphy 2007c].

Of note, 1-2+ intensity CD64 expression was also demonstrated in AML, M1s (27%), M2s(41%), and AMMLs (22%), and thus, by CD64 expression, these other AML subtypes with 1-2+ intensity CD64 expression could not be distinguished from AMoLs with <3+ intensity.

The great majority of AML, M3s (86%), demonstrated 1+ intensity expression of CD64. In addition, 14% of AML, M0s, demonstrated 1+ intensity expression of CD64. Of note, none of the AMLs with dim (1+) CD64 expression had a lack of CD34 and HLA-DR expression, other than the AML, M3s. Thus, the lack of HLA-DR and CD34 expression in AML, M3 may be very useful in distinguishing M3 from other subtypes with dim (1+) CD64 intensity. In addition, none of the AML, M6s, or M7s revealed any CD64 expression, and thus, these subtypes may possibly be excluded if CD64 expression is demonstrated.

Of particular interest was the absence of CD64 expression in 78% AMMLs. This finding suggests the blasts in AMML infrequently express CD64, and the monocytic component in the majority of these cases is represented by mature monocytes, since only the blast population was analyzed for CD64 expression.

CD64 expression has not been described in precursor or mature B- or T-cell neoplasms.

CD123

The specific α-subunit of the interleukin-3 receptor (ie, IL-3Ra, CD123) is expressed on hematopoietic cells, including monocytes, "lymphoid" or "plasmacytoid" dendritic cells, neutrophils, basophils, and megakaryocytes, but not on mature (peripheral) T cells, natural killer cells, platelets, or red blood cells [Du 2007]. In addition, there is a hypothesis that there is a common CD123+/CD11c– dendritic cell, natural killer cell, and B-cell progenitor resident in marrow, and this cell may be identical to the common lymphoid progenitor previously described in mice and/or the human CD34+/Lin–/CD10+ progenitor [Szabolcs 2003]. Also, the common β subunit (β_c) of the IL-3R (IL-3R β_c) is shared by IL-3, granulocyte-macrophage colony-stimulating factor (GM-CSF) and IL-5Rs.

Thus, it is not surprising that CD123 is strongly expressed in 45%-95% of AML, 40%-100% of precursor B-cell lymphoblastic leukemia, and 85% of hairy cell leukemia. The expression of CD123 is elevated in the primitive leukemia stem cell populations of AML, chronic myeloid leukemia, and some other myeloid malignancies, but it is not detectable in normal hematopoietic stem cells [Du 2007]. In addition, CD123 is characteristically expressed in the relatively newly described entity, "CD4+/CD56+ hematodermic neoplasm," of apparent early plasmacytoid dendritic cell origin [Jacob 2003].

CD163

CD163, a hemoglobin-scavenger receptor, is largely restricted to the monocyte/macrophage lineage. It is expressed by nonneoplastic monocytes and histiocytes and is not expressed by normal splenic littoral cells or plasmacytoid monocytes [Nguyen 2005].

CD163 expression is primarily limited to neoplasms with monocytic/histiocytic differentiation and, as such, has been observed in the majority of cases of Rosai-Dorfman disease, hemophagocytic lymphohistiocytosis, histiocytic sarcoma, Langerhans cell histiocytosis, giant cell tenosynovial tumor, juvenile xanthogranuloma, as well as a subset of AMLs with monocytic differentiation, epithelioid cell histiocytomas, fibrous histiocytomas, and atypical fibroxanthomas. In addition, it has been observed in all cases of littoral cell angioma and thus may be useful in distinguishing littoral cell angiomas from other atypical or reactive splenic proliferations. CD163 reactivity has not been observed in follicular dendritic cell tumors, carcinomas, lymphomas/hematolymphoid disorders, or mesenchymal neoplasms [Nguyen 2005, Vos 2005].

Progenitor Cell-Associated Antigens

CD34

CD34, the human progenitor cell antigen, as the name implies, is expressed selectively on hematopoietic progenitor cells but also on vascular endothelial cells and some tissue fibroblasts. CD34 is expressed by approximately 1%-2% of normal BM mononuclear cells, including lymphoblasts, myeloblasts, monoblasts, and megakaryoblasts [Civin 1984]. Erythroid precursors have been shown to be CD34– [Dunphy 2007b]. CD34 is lost progressively from hematopoietic progenitor cells in parallel with advancing maturational stage. CD34 is not expressed by normal peripheral blood B or T cells, monocytes, granulocytes, erythrocytes, or platelets [Civin 1984].

CD34 expression in hematopoietic neoplasms mirrors the expression by normal cells in the BM (ie, by blasts and vascular endothelial cells). If not, it is expressed by blasts in approximately 40% of AMLs, is preferentially expressed by morphologically and immunophenotypically less mature AMLs (ie, acute monocytic leukemia and acute promyelocytic leukemia are characteristically CD34–), and is associated with a worse prognosis in AML [Vaughan 1988]. Note that not all myeloblasts express CD34, and thus this marker by itself may not necessarily reliably quantitate the percentage of myeloblasts in peripheral blood and BM aspirate specimens [Dunphy 2007b]. In addition, CD34 is expressed by 75% of precursor B-cell lymphoblastic leukemias and by <5% of precursor T-cell lymphoblastic leukemias. CD34 expression appears to be an independent favorable prognostic indicator in precursor B-cell lymphoblastic leukemia [Borowitz 1990]. Since CD34 is expressed by vascular endothelium, it is not surprising that it is expressed by a wide spectrum of benign and malignant vascular neoplasms [Kuzu 1992].

TdT

Terminal deoxynucleotidyl transferase (TdT) is an intranuclear enzyme and marker of immaturity. It is not lineage-specific, being expressed in precursor B cells in normal BM as well as in immature thymic lymphocytes. As such, TdT may be expressed in 70%-95% of precursor B-cell and precursor T-cell lymphoblastic leukemias/lymphomas. In addition, it may be expressed by blasts in AML [Arber 1996b]. TdT may be expressed by limited subsets of AML-M0, M1, M2, and M4, as well as AML with multilineage dysplasia, but has not been shown to be present in any cases of AML-M3, M5, M6, or M7 [Dunphy 2006b].

Non-Lineage Antigens [t4.3]

CD15

CD15 is a carbohydrate antigen expressed by virtually all peripheral blood granulocytes (including eosinophils and basophils), as well as by peripheral blood monocytes and tissue histiocytes. CD15 is also expressed by the majority day 7 BMs granulocyte/monocyte-colony forming units [Andrews 1983]. Erythroid precursors, megakaryocytes, lymphocytes, and normal plasma cells lack CD15.

As such, 50%-70% of AML (M1-M3) express CD15, whereas 75%-90% of AML (M4 and M5) express CD15 [Bernstein 1982]. It is expressed by <5% of patients with precursor B-cell or T-cell lymphoblastic leukemia/lymphoma. However, precursor B-cell lymphoblastic leukemia associated with the t(4;11) is characterized by a CD19+/CD15+/CD10−/CD20− immunophenotype and is associated with a particularly poor prognosis [Dunphy 2001b]. Likewise, the presence of CD15 antigen, like other myelomonocytic antigens, in myeloma cells may be related to a poor prognosis [Ruiz-Argüelles 1994].

CD15 may also be expressed by Reed-Sternberg cells, and their identification by flow cytometry will be further discussed in the chapter discussing this topic.

CD25

CD25 (also referred to as IL-2R1) is known to be expressed by activated T and B cells, as well as monocytes and tissue macrophages [Chadburn 1992, O'Laughlin 1992]. It is not expressed by normal mast cells. CD25 expression may be useful in diagnosing both B- and T-cell neoplasms as well as mast-cell neoplasms. CD11c and CD25 (strong) are characteristically expressed in all cases of hairy cell leukemia [Oertel 1992]. However, one should keep in mind that CD25 expression is not specific for hairy cell leukemia and may also occur in other B-cell neoplasms, specifically in Waldenström macroglobulinemia and mantle cell lymphoma [San Miguel 2003, Lardelli 1990]. Hairy cell leukemia may usually be distinguished from these other B-cell neoplasms, based on the differences in morphology and other immunophenotypic markers, which will be discussed in the chapter discussing mature B-cell neoplasms. CD25 is not expressed by the prolymphocytic variant of hairy cell leukemia (ie, hairy cell variant).

In diagnosing T-cell neoplasms, CD25 may be most useful in distinguishing mycosis fungoides (MF)/ Sézary syndrome (SS) from adult T-cell leukemia/ lymphoma (ATLL). ATLL characteristically expresses CD25, whereas MF/SS is usually CD25−. However, one should keep in mind that CD25 expression in T-cell neoplasms is not specific for ATLL and may also be encountered in CD30+ anaplastic large cell lymphoma and even in cutaneous T-cell lymphoma (MF/SS) prior to and at higher risk of undergoing large cell transformation [Carbone 1990, Stefanato 1998].

Lastly, CD25 is a reliable marker for neoplastic-mast cells. Although morphologically mast-cell neoplasms may be difficult to distinguish from hairy cell leukemia in BM sections, the additional immunophenotypic markers in hairy cell leukemia, and the presence of tryptase and C-kit (CD117) in mast cell neoplasms, should distinguish these 2 entities that are typically CD25+ [Pardanani 2004].

CD26

CD26 (transmembrane serine aminopeptidase dipeptidyl peptidase IV-DDP IV) is an activation marker of thymocytes and T lymphocytes, which is associated with reactivity on naive and memory T cells [Ulmer 1992, Babusíková 1999]. CD26 is also expressed by B and NK lineages [Buhling 1995, Buhling 1994]. In addition, CD26 may be expressed by normal non-hematolymphoid cells, including cells of the small intestine, renal proximal tubules, and splenic sinus lining cells.

Although CD26 has not been studied much in human neoplasia, it has been shown to be expressed in several hematolymphoid neoplasms, all of which were of T-cell origin. CD26 expression has been described on various subsets of T-cell neoplasms, including T-cell leukemias associated with HTLV-1, CD30+ anaplastic large-cell lymphomas, hepatosplenic T-cell lymphoma, and precursor T-cell lymphoblastic leukemia/lymphoma. Interestingly, CD26 expression has been shown to be decreased in MF/SS [Carbone 1995a, Kondo 1996, Carbone 1995b, Ruiz 1998, Klobusická 1999, Sokolowska-Wojdylo 2005]. In fact, the absence of CD26 expression on skin-homing peripheral blood CD4+ T-helper cells is a very sensitive and highly specific marker for early diagnosis and therapeutic monitoring of patients with SS.

CD30

CD30 (Ki-1; Ber-H2) expression is associated with activation and is not expressed by resting peripheral blood B or T cells or monocytes, or by germinal center T cells, mantle zone B cells, cortical thymocytes, thymic epithelium, cutaneous Langerhans cells, interdigitating

t4.3 Non-Lineage Specific Antigens with Indications/Applications of Flow Cytometric Detection in Diagnostic Hematopathology

	Antigen Reactive Hematolymphoid Cells	Hematolymphoid Malignancy with Reactivity Pattern
CD15	Peripheral blood granulocytes, eosinophils, basophils, monocytes, and tissue histiocytes	AML (M1-M3): 50%-70% express CD15 AML (M4 and M5): 75%-90% express CD15 Precursor B-LL with t(4;11): CD19+/CD15+/CD1– IP PCM: CD15+ correlates with poor prognosis
CD25	Activated T and B cells, monocytes, and tissue histiocytes	HCL: CD25 is strongly expressed ATLL: CD25 is characteristically expressed MCD: CD25 reliably detects neoplastic mast cells
CD26	Activated thymocytes and T lymphocytes, B and NK lineages	T-cell neoplasms (except MF/SS): CD26 is variably + MF/SS: CD26 is decreased or absent
CD30	Immunoblasts, activated tissue histiocytes, occasional medullary thymocytes, and plasma cells	B-NHLs: 15%-20% express CD30 T-NHLs: 30% express CD30 PEL and plasmablastic lymphoma: CD30+ ALCL: Strongly and uniformly CD30+
CD36	Monocytes, platelets, and erythroblasts	AML (M4, M5, and M6): CD36 expression higher than in AML (M1-M3) AML (M7): Increased CD36 expression correlates with increased mega-karyoblastic maturation CD4+/CD56+; hematodermic neoplasm: CD36+ MDS: Granulocytes may aberrantly express CD36
CD38	Pre-B lymphocytes, plasma cells, thymocytes, activated T lymphocytes, NK cells, myeloblasts, and erythroblasts	Precursor T- and B-LL: Both may express CD38 with T-LL cases more likely to express than B-LL cases; CLL: CD38+ by >30% of CLL cells associated with unfavorable prognosis; WM, BL, PCM, plasmablastic lymphoma, PEL, PTLD, CD4+/CD56+ hematodermic neoplasm, indolent NK cell large granular lymphocytosis, blasts and granulocytes of MDS, and AML: CD38 may be expressed in all of these entities
CD43	Thymocytes, mature T cells, activated B cells, plasma cells, NK cells, monocytes/histiocytes, CD34+ cord blood cells, erythroblasts, megakaryocytes, and BM CD34+ cells	Mature T-cell lymphomas: 85% express CD43 Precursor T-LL: most express CD43 Precursor B-LL: 75% express CD43 Mature B-NHLs: 30% express CD43 AML: >95% express CD43 PCM: express CD43 Co-expression of CD43 and CD20 indicates a B-cell neoplasm
CD71	Actively proliferating cells, erythroblasts	Precursor T-LL: express CD71; precursor B-LL: variably express CD71 Immunoblastic B-NHLs: variably express CD71 Higher grade lymphomas associated with increased CD71 expression
CD103	Intestinal intraepithelial lymphocytes, dendritic epidermal T cells, and thymocytes	EATL: express CD103 ATLL: express CD103 HCL: express CD103
CD117	Myeloblasts, promyelocytes, mast cells	De-novo AMLs: 65%-85% express CD117 Precursor T-LL: 11% express CD117; precursor B-LL: 2% express CD117; Mast cell disorders: express CD117; PCM: may express CD117
Bcl-2	Normal T and B cells (>80%)	B-NHLs: majority (except BL) express bcl-2 T-cell neoplasms: mature and T-LL may express bcl-2

ALCL, anaplastic large cell lymphoma; AML, acute myeloid leukemia; ATLL, adult T-cell leukemia/lymphoma; BL, Burkitt lymphoma; CLL, chronic lymphocytic leukemia; EATL, enteropathy-associated T-cell lymphoma; HCL, hairy cell leukemia; IP, immunophenotype; LL, lymphoblastic leukemia/lymphoma; MCD, mast cell disorders; MDS, myelodysplastic syndrome; MF/SS, mycosis fungoides/Sézary syndrome; NHLs, non-Hodgkin lymphomas; NK, natural killer; PCM, plasma cell myeloma; PEL, primary effusion lymphoma; PTLD, post-transplant lymphoproliferative disorder; WM, Waldenström macroglobulinemia.

dendritic cells, and developing hematolymphoid cells in fetal liver and BM. CD30 may be expressed by immunoblasts, activated tissue macrophages, and occasional medullary thymocytes, and may show cytoplasmic staining of plasma cells (although possibly artifactual) [Schwarting 1989].

In hematolymphoid neoplasms, CD30 may be expressed by 15%-20% of B-cell NHL and 30% of T-cell NHL, including primary effusion lymphomas and plasmablastic lymphomas. However, the expression is usually variable and on a subset of the cells. The neoplasm in which CD30 expression is characteristically strong and uniform is anaplastic large cell lymphoma, and this expression may be detected by flow cytometry [Juco 2003]. One should keep in mind that embryonal carcinoma may also express CD30, but these cells are not usually able to be disaggregated to pass through the flow cytometer as single cells. As stated previously, CD30 expression by flow cytometry should always be correlated with the light microscopic features, as well as additional immunophenotypic, cytogenetic, and molecular features of each case.

CD30 may also be expressed by Reed-Sternberg cells, and their identification by flow cytometry will be further discussed in the chapter discussing this topic.

CD30 is not expressed by acute or chronic leukemias of myeloid or lymphoid origin.

CD36

CD36 (thrombosplondin receptor) is a membrane glycoprotein that may be expressed by monocytes, platelets, and endothelial cells, as well as mammary epithelial cells and some tumor cell lines. It is also a very early marker of erythroid differentiation but is not expressed by granulocytes and lymphocytes [Greenwalt 992].

As such, it may be expressed by AMLs, particularly those with monocytic differentiation (M4 and M5), erythroid differentiation (M6), or megakaryocytic differentiation (M7). CD36 expression has been shown to be significantly higher in M4, M5, and M6 than in M1, M2, and M3 [Tang 2007]. In M7, CD36 expression has been shown to increase gradually according to the differentiation and maturation of the cells (ie, increased CD36 expression with megakaryoblast maturation) [Imamura 1994]. In addition, CD36-high cases had a superior outcome compared with CD36– cases in childhood M7 cases (not associated with Down syndrome) [Savaşan 2006]. However, of interest, AMLs associated with the FLT3 internal tandem duplication (and poor prognosis) very often expressed CD36 (and

CD11b) [Muñoz 2003]. CD36 is also expressed by the CD4+/CD56+ hematodermic neoplasm and may be aberrantly expressed by granulocytes in myelodysplastic syndromes [Feuillard 2002, Maynadié 2002].

CD38

CD38 is recognized as an integral membrane glycoprotein and is expressed on essentially all pre-B lymphocytes, plasma cells, and thymocytes [Babusíková 1999]. The antigen is expressed during the early stages of T- and B-lymphocyte differentiation, is lost during the intermediate stages of maturation, and then reappears during the final stages of maturation. It is also present on activated T lymphocytes, NK cells, myeloblasts (in regenerating BM), and erythroblasts [Weisberger 2003, Zelenznikova 2007]. As such, it is non-lineage restricted and may be expressed in the following:

- ▶ T- and B-cell precursor lymphoblastic leukemia/lymphoma (T-cell cases were more likely than B-cell cases to express CD38) [Koehler 1993]
- ▶ chronic lymphocytic leukemia (expression of CD38 by > 20%-30% of the neoplastic cells by FCI in CLL has been associated with an unfavorable prognosis) [Ibrahim 2001, Del Poeta 2001]
- ▶ Waldenström macroglobulinemia [Konoplev 2005]
- ▶ Burkitt lymphoma
- ▶ multiple myeloma [Ruiz-Argüelles 1994]
- ▶ plasmablastic lymphoma [Vega 2005]
- ▶ primary effusion lymphoma
- ▶ post-transplant lymphoproliferative disorders
- ▶ CD4+/CD56+ hematodermic neoplasm [Feuillard 2002]
- ▶ indolent NK cell large granular lymphocytosis [Lima 2004]
- ▶ myelodysplastic syndromes in the blasts and granulocytes [Maynadié 2002]
- ▶ AML

CD138 is much more specific for plasma cell differentiation than CD38. There has not been any prognostic significance associated with CD38 expression in any of these disorders except CLL, as described above.

CD43

CD43 (ie, MT-1, Leu22), often considered a T-cell lineage-associated antigen, is expressed by >95% thymocytes (all cortical thymocytes and approximately half of medullary thymocytes), and 95% and 85% mature T cells in the peripheral blood and tonsil, respectively.

However, CD43 is expressed by essentially all WBCs (except resting mature B cells—follicle center and mantle zone B cells), including activated B cells, plasma cells, NK cells, granulocytes, monocytes/macrophages, CD34+ cord blood cells (ie, partially committed myeloid, erythroid, and lymphoid progenitors and stem cells), erythroblasts, megakaryocytes, and BM CD34+ cells [West 1986].

In hematolymphoid neoplasms, CD43 is expressed by approximately 85% mature (post-thymic) T-cell lymphomas, most precursor T-cell neoplasms, 75% of precursor B-cell neoplasms, 30% of non-lymphoblastic B-cell NHLs (67% of SLL/CLL and mantle cell lymphoma, most Burkitt lymphomas, 10%-20% large B-cell lymphomas, 10% follicle center cell lymphomas), >95% of AMLs (M1-M5; CD43 is not expressed by M6), and plasma cell dyscrasias [West 1986]. Hairy cell leukemia does not express CD43 [Stoll 1989]. CD43 co-expression on normal B cells is distinctly unusual, and thus, CD20 and CD43 co-expression may be extremely useful in distinguishing a non-neoplastic lymphoid proliferation from a B-cell neoplasm [Contos 1992]. In addition, CD5 and CD43 co-expression may be useful in distinguishing SLL (CD5+/CD43+) from a CD5+ marginal zone B-cell lymphoma (CD5+/CD43–).

CD71

CD71 (the transferrin receptor) is a prototypic-activation antigen associated with increased proliferative activity in most tissues. CD71 is expressed by actively proliferating cells belonging to all hematopoietic lineages, as well as some nonhematopoietic lineages. The transferrin receptor is also present on early erythroid cells (erythroblasts) but is lost as reticulocytes differentiate into mature erythrocytes. It is not expressed by resting peripheral blood and lymphoid tissue B and T cells, monocytes, granulocytes, and erythrocytes [Schwarting 1989, Trowbridge 1995].

Among lymphoid neoplasms, CD71 is expressed by precursor T-cell lymphoblastic leukemia/lymphoma and more variably by mature (post-thymic) T-cell neoplasms and large B-cell immunoblastic lymphomas [Knowles 1986, Aisenberg 1980]. Low-grade NHLs and chronic lymphoproliferative disorders do not typically express CD71 [Habeshaw 1983]. In this regard, CD71 fluorescence intensity by flow cytometric analysis is extremely useful in distinguishing CD10+ low- from high-grade lymphomas, and also in distinguishing follicular lymphoma (FL) from non-FL high-grade

lymphomas (since grade 3 FL has a lower proliferative activity than non-FL high-grade lymphomas), and thus CD71 may be used as a surrogate marker for proliferative activity [Wu 2006]. Although decreased CD71 expression may be observed on nucleated red blood cells in myelodysplastic syndromes, there are no significant reports of the diagnostic or prognostic usefulness of CD71 in acute leukemias [Malcovati 2005].

CD103

CD103 (mucosa lymphocyte antigen-MLA) has a unique and fairly restricted tissue distribution. It is expressed on almost all (>90%) intestinal intraepithelial lymphocytes, in about 40% of lamina propria T lymphocytes in the intestine, in the majority of intraepithelial lymphocytes in extra-intestinal sites, and by 0.5%-5% T lymphocytes in peripheral blood and peripheral lymphoid tissues. CD103 is also expressed on dendritic epidermal T cells and on distinct subsets of fetal, neonatal, and adult thymocytes [Kilshaw 1988, Kilshaw 1991, LeFrançois 1994, Kilshaw 1990, Andrew 1996]. It is not expressed by resting B cells.

Not surprisingly, CD103 is expressed by enteropathy-associated T-cell lymphomas but also by adult T-cell leukemia/lymphoma and hairy cell leukemia. In addition, CD103 is not typically expressed by splenic, nodal, or extranodal marginal zone lymphomas and may also be negative in the hairy cell variant. Thus, this marker may be particularly useful in the differential diagnoses of these lymphoid neoplasms [Micklem 1991].

CD117

CD117 (or c-kit, the stem cell receptor ligand) is a tyrosine kinase receptor that may be expressed by myeloblasts and promyelocytes but not by myeloid cells beyond the promyelocytic stage of differentiation [van Lochem 2004]. It is expressed by 40%-60% of the CD34+ BM mononuclear cells, including primitive and granulo-monocytic progenitor cells. In contrast, B-lymphoid committed progenitor cells (CD34+CD19+) express low levels of CD117. Among CD34– BM cells, only a small number of cells (mostly erythroid) express the receptor [Olweus 1996]. CD117 is also normally expressed by mast cells, skin basal cells and melanocytes, breast epithelium, ovary and interstitial cells of Cajal [Tsuura 1994].

As such, approximately 65%-85% of de-novo AMLs may show expression of CD117 in the blast population [Dunphy 2001a, Hans 2002]. CD117 expression in AML does not correlate with the French American

British (FAB) or World Health Organization (WHO) subtype, although CD117 expression in AML has been shown to be associated with a poor prognosis and is expressed in up to 95% of relapsed AMLs [Dunphy 2001a, Hans 2002, Ashman 1988]. Although CD117 expression is a relatively specific marker for myeloid lineage of acute leukemia, a large study has revealed 11% CD117+ cases within precursor T-cell lymphoblastic leukemia/ lymphoma and 2% CD117+ cases within precursor B-cell leukemia/lymphoma [Bene 1998]. It has been suggested that CD117 in these precursor T– and B-cell neoplasms may identify a subgroup of cases, which may correspond to leukemias either arising from early prothymocytes and/or early hematopoietic cells, both of which are able to differentiate to the lymphoid and myeloid pathways. As expected, CD117 is also expressed by all cases of mast-cell disorders [Natkunam 2000]. The only other hematolymphoid disorder that may show CD117 expression is plasma cell dyscrasia [Bayer-Garner 2003]. CD117 expression has not been demonstrated in Hodgkin lymphoma, anaplastic large cell lymphoma, or other peripheral T- or B-cell NHLs [Natkunam 2000, Rassidakis 2004]. CD117 may also be expressed in non-hematolymphoid neoplasms, including strong, diffuse staining in synovial sarcomas, osteosarcomas, Ewing sarcomas, and gastric stromal tumors, and more variable staining in neuroblastomas, Wilms' tumors, rhabdomyosarcomas, and lung tumors with neuroendocrine differentiation [Smithey 2002, Sarlomo-Rikala 1998, Butnor 2004].

Bcl-2

Bcl-2 is considered to be a novel proto-oncogene because it blocks apoptosis in many cell types [Yang 1997]. Bcl-2 is thought to provide a selective survival advantage for cells by blocking apoptosis and thus may contribute to tumorigenesis [Reed 1991]. Bcl-2 is a 26 kD intracellular, integral membrane protein found primarily in the nuclear envelope, endoplasmic reticulum, and outer mitochondrial membrane [Krajewski 1993]. It is expressed by >80% of normal T and B cells in peripheral blood, interfollicular areas, and mantle zones of lymph nodes and the thymic medulla [Aiello 1992, Pezzella 1995]. Bcl-2 protein expression has also been observed in normal colonic crypts and normal epidermal melanocytes [Flohil 1996, Saenz-Santamaría 1994, van den Oord 1994].

Bcl-2 protein expression is often used to distinguish follicular hyperplasia from FL. Bcl-2 is non-reactive in reactive germinal centers and is typically strongly reactive in the malignant nodules of FL. In addition,

flow cytometric analysis using simultaneous staining of cytoplasmic bcl-2 and cell surface CD20 and multicolor flow cytometric analysis may be extremely useful in diagnosing FL in lymph and BM specimens [Cornfield 2000, Cook 2003]. However, it should be noted that there are rare cases of FL that are comprised of bcl-2– malignant nodules. Bcl-2+ reactive germinal centers have not been described [Pezzella 1995]. Bcl-2 may also represent a useful marker for distinguishing reactive monocytoid B-cell hyperplasia from marginal zone lymphoma in other sites. However, one should keep in mind bcl-2 has also been shown to be consistently expressed by reactive marginal zone B cells of the spleen, abdominal lymph nodes, and ileal lymphoid tissue; thus, bcl-2 expression should not be used as a criterion for discriminating between benign and malignant marginal zone B-cell proliferations involving these sites [Meda 2003].

Although expression of the bcl-2 protein is associated with the t(14;18) chromosome translocation and is expressed on a significantly higher percentage of follicular lymphomas associated with this translocation, expression of the bcl-2 oncogene protein is not specific for the t(14;18) chromosomal translocation [Ngan 1998, Skinnider 1999, Pezzella 1990]. Bcl-2 protein expression may be detected in a substantial number of B-cell as well as T-cell lymphoproliferative disorders not associated with the t(14;18) [Wheaton 1998 Lai 1998]. Bcl-2 protein expression has been described in 100% of SLLs, 80% of FLs, 38% of diffuse LCLs, 33% of high-grade B-cell Burkitt-like lymphomas, 0% of Burkitt lymphomas, and 0% of B-cell lymphoblastic lymphomas [Wheaton 1998]. Thus, the significant difference in bcl-2 expression between Burkitt-like high-grade BCL and BL was suggested as an additional use of bcl-2. Bcl-2 positivity may rarely occur in BL and has been described when there is a coexistent t(14;18) and Burkitt translocation. In addition, although T-cell lymphoproliferative disorders have a significantly lower bcl-2 expression than B-cell disorders, peripheral T-cell lymphoma, including anaplastic CD30+ LCL and angioimmunoblastic-type, and lymphoblastic lymphomas, may reveal expression of the bcl-2 protein.

In addition, bcl-2 protein expression may be observed in a variety of non-hematolymphoid neoplasms, including breast carcinoma, gastric carcinoma, prostatic carcinoma, thyroid carcinoma, basal cell carcinoma, trichoepithelioma, soft tissue sarcomas, ameloblastomas, and melanoma [Bhargava 1994, Lauwers 1995, Tulunay 2004, Puglisi 2000, Poniecka 1999, Sabah 2007, Kumamoto 1999, Ramsay 1995].

Erythrocyte-Associated Antigens

CD235a (Glycophorin A)

CD235a (glycophorin A) is a sialoglycoprotein present on human red blood cells (RBCs) and erythroid precursor cells. This antibody recognizes human RBCs and erythroid precursors and is useful in erythroid cell development studies. Mature, non-nucleated RBCs are also characteristically glycophorin A (Gp A) positive [Langlois 1985]. Gp A is not expressed by B- or T lymphocytes, thymocytes, myeloid cells, or megakaryocytes.

As such, Gp A is a highly sensitive and specific probe for erythroleukemias. In a large study of Gp A expression in malignant hematopoiesis, Gp A expression was observed in only 2 cases of acute erythroid leukemia and was not demonstrated in the 121 non-erythroid leukemias [Liszka 1983]. In an even larger study, AML and precursor B-cell lymphoblastic leukemia were shown to very rarely express Gp A, and it was concluded that these cases probably represented genuine "cryptic" erythroleukemias [Greaves 1983].

Platelet-Associated Antigens

CD41

CD41a reacts with a calcium-dependent complex of CD41/CD61 (GPIIb/IIIa), the receptor for fibrinogen, fibronectin, and von Willebrand factor, mediating platelet adhesion and aggregation. CD41a is expressed on normal platelets and megakaryocytes, and its detection is useful in the morphological and physiological studies of platelets and megakaryocytes. However, CD41a is also expressed by erythroid burst-forming units (BFU-E) [Nakahata 1994].

CD41b reacts with GPIIb, also known as aIIb integrin, of the complex GPIIb/IIIa expressed on normal platelets and megakaryocytes. This antibody appears to be a weak aggregation inducer. CD41b is also expressed by erythroid burst-forming units (BFU-E) [Nakahata 1994].

CD42b

CD42b reacts with a 170 kdalton (kDa) 2 chain membrane glycoprotein, GPIb, that forms a non-covalent complex with GPIX (CD42a), found on platelets and megakaryocytes. The GPIb/IX complex serves as the vWF surface receptor involved in the adhesion of platelets to the subendothelium of damaged vascular walls. Of note, monoclonal antibodies to GPIb do not react with the earliest megakaryocytes and are not as sensitive as monoclonal antibodies to GPIIB/IIIa (ie, CD41a) or GPIIIa (ie, CD61) in detecting the earliest megakaryocytes, and thus acute megakaryoblastic leukemia and AML/transient myeloproliferative disorder in Down syndrome.

CD61

CD61 recognizes an Mr 110-kDa protein, also known as GPIIIa [Halper 1978, Winchester 1977, Winchester 1978].

With the CD41 antigen (GPIIb), the CD61 antigen forms the GPIIb/IIIa complex, which acts as a receptor for fibrinogen, von Willebrand factor (vWf), fibronectin, and vitronectin on activated platelets [von dem Borne 1989a, Modderman 1989, Modderman 1989, Fitzgerald 1987, Fijnheer 1990, von dem Borne 1989b]. The CD61 antigen is found on all normal resting and activated platelets. Platelets from individuals with Glanzmann thrombasthenia show a >90% reduction of binding of CD61, and heterozygote carriers of the disorder show approximately 50% reduction [Jennings 1986, Shattil 1985]. The CD61 antigen is also found on endothelial cells, megakaryocytes, and on some myeloid, erythroid, and T-lymphoblastic leukemic cell lines. It should also be noted that intracellular expression of CD61 in the megakaryoblasts of acute megakaryoblastic leukemia precedes surface expression, and thus cytoplasmic expression of CD61 by permeabilization of the cell membrane and flow cytometry should be performed in all cases of AML with undifferentiated morphology and negative cytochemistries to differentiate M0 form M7 [Käfer 1999].

Comparison of these 3 markers (ie, CD41, CD42, and CD61) has shown CD42 is the least sensitive for early megakaryoblasts (due to the lack of CD42 expression by early megakaryoblasts), CD41a is the most sensitive but least specific, and CD61 is the most specific marker of megakaryoblastic differentiation [Käfer 1999, Karandikar 2001].

Paroxysmal Nocturnal Hemoglobinuria (PNH)-Associated Deficient Antigens

CD55 and CD59

Paroxysmal nocturnal hemoglobinuria is an acquired clonal expansion of BM stem cells that are deficient in the decay-accelerating factor, which is a complement regulatory glycoprotein (CD55), as well as in the membrane inhibitor of reactive lysis (CD59) and the C8-binding protein. These proteins are deficient on the membranes of red blood cells, granulocytes, monocytes, and platelets. The disorder is associated with intermittent hemolytic anemia, hemoglobinuria, infection, a tendency toward BM aplasia, and venous thromboses and, thus, must be differentiated from other hematologic disorders. This distinction is most easily accomplished by flow cytometric analysis of peripheral WBCs and RBCs for CD55 and CD59, which will both be deficient in PNH. PNH patients will demonstrate either completely (PNH III) or partially (PNH II) deficient RBCs and granulocytes. Anti-CD59 best demonstrates PNH II red cells, which are present in 50% of PNH patients. The proportion of abnormal granulocytes is usually greater than the proportion of abnormal red cells. Anti-CD55 does not delineate the erythrocyte populations as well as anti-CD59. Either anti-CD55 or anti-CD59 could be used equally to analyze granulocytes. Platelets are not generally used for detailed analysis, as the normal and abnormal populations are not well distinguished. Flow cytometry of erythrocytes using anti-CD59 or of granulocytes using either anti-CD55 or anti-CD59 provides the most accurate technique for the diagnosis of PNH; it is clearly more specific, more quantitative, and more sensitive than the tests for PNH depending on hemolysis by complement (the acidified serum lysis [Ham] test, the sucrose lysis test, and the complement lysis sensitivity [CLS] test) [Hall 1996].

Monoclonal Antibodies as Targeted Therapy for Hematolymphoid Malignancies

CD20

Rituximab is a mouse/human chimeric IgG(1)-κ monoclonal antibody that targets the CD20 antigen found on the surface of malignant and normal B lymphocytes. CD20 is expressed on >90% of B-cell NHLs and to a lesser degree on B-cell chronic lymphocytic leukemia (CLL) cells. Clinical trials with rituximab indicate the drug has broad application for B-cell malignancies, although further clarification is needed to determine its optimal use in many of these clinical settings. More importantly, rituximab in combination with CHOP chemotherapy, has emerged as a new treatment standard for previously untreated diffuse large B-cell lymphoma, at least in elderly patients. Compared with conventional chemotherapy, rituximab is associated with markedly reduced hematological events, such as severe neutropenia, as well as

associated infections. Rituximab may be particularly suitable for elderly patients or those with poor performance status, and its tolerability profile facilitates its use in combination with cytotoxic drugs. In addition, rituximab also demonstrates significant activity in relapsed or refractory, low-grade or follicular, B-cell NHL, including refractory CLL, and should be used in patients with a disease that is refractory to purine nucleoside analogs (PNAs). Combination therapies with PNAs and cyclophosphamide, and especially with rituximab, are more active than monotherapy with PNAs in regard to response rate and possible survival [Rao 2007].

CD22

BL22 is an immunotoxin targeting CD22 and has been shown to induce complete remissions in a high proportion of cases of hairy cell leukemia [Kreitman 2006].

CD25 (IL-2R)

The anti-CD25 recombinant immunotoxin LMB-2 and/or anti-Tac is active in several CD25+ hematolymphoid malignancies, including adult T-cell leukemia/lymphoma (ATLL) and hairy cell leukemia [Kreitman 2006, Zhang 2005, Kiyokawa 1989]. Of interest, high-affinity IL-2R presents on acute and lymphoma type ATLL cells resulting in higher sensitivity to anti-CD25 monoclonal antibody in these cells than in those from chronic or smoldering disease.

CD33

Calicheamicin, a highly potent antitumor antibiotic that cleaves double-stranded DNA at specific sequences, has been conjugated to a humanized anti-CD33 MAb to produce gemtuzumab ozogamicin. Gemtuzumab ozogamicin is directed against the CD33 antigen expressed by the hematopoietic cells. It has been approved for use in patients with CD33+ AML in first relapse who are aged >60 years and who are not considered candidates for other cytotoxic chemotherapy [Rao 2007].

CD52

Alemtuzumab is a recombinant DNA-derived, humanized MAb directed against the 21- to 28-kD cell surface glycoprotein, CD52. CD52 is expressed on the surface of normal and malignant B and T lymphocytes, NK cells, monocytes, macrophages, and tissues of the male reproductive system. The proposed mechanism of action is antibody-dependent lysis of leukemic cells after cell surface binding. Alemtuzumab is indicated for the treatment of B-CLL in patients treated with alkylating agents who have failed to respond to fludarabine therapy [Rao 2007].

Recommended "concensus" reagents for initial and secondary evaluations of hematopoietic neoplasms, as determined at the 2006 Bethesda International Concensus Conference on Flow Cytometric Immunophenotyping of Hematolymphoid Neoplasia, are provided in [t4.4] and [t4.5], respectively [Wood 2007].

In addition, recommended, less extensive FCI panels are outlined in [t4.6]. Of course, additional markers may be analyzed, as indicated and based on the results of these recommended panels outlined.

t4.4 Consensus Reagents for Initial Evaluation for Hematopoietic Neoplasia [Wood 2007]

Lineage	Primary Reagents
B cells	CD5, CD10, CD19, CD20, CD45, κ, λ
T cells and NK cells	CD2, CD3, CD4, CD5, CD7, CD8, CD45, CD56
Myelomonocytic cells	CD7, CD11b, CD13, CD14, CD15, CD16, CD33, CD34, CD45, CD56, CD117, HLA-DR
Myelomonocytic cells (limited)	CD13, CD33, CD34, CD45
Plasma cells	CD19, CD38, CD45, CD56

t4.5 Reagents for Secondary Evaluation of Specific Hematopoetic Cell Lineages

Lineage	Secondary Reagents
B cells	CD9,* CD11c, CD15, CD22, cCD22, CD23, CD25, CD13, CD33, CD34, CD38, CD43, CD58,** cCD79a, CD79b, CD103, FMC7, Bcl-2, cKappa, cLambda, cMPO, TdT, Zap-70, cIgM
T cells and NK cells	CD1a, cCD3, CD10, CD16, CD25, CD26, CD30, CD34, CD45RA, CD45RO, CD57, ab-TCR, gd-TCR, cMPO, cTIA-1, T-beta chain isoforms, TdT
Myelomonocytic cells	CD2, cCD3, CD4, cCD22, CD25, CD36, CD38, CD41, CD61, cCD61, CD64, CD71, cCD79a, cMPO, CD123, CD163, CD235a
Plasma cells	CD10, CD117, CD138, cKappa, cLambda

*CD9, an accessory molecule having a molecular weight of about 27 kD present on activated T cells

**CD58, also known as lymphocyte function-associated antigen 3 (LFA-3) is a 45-70 kD cell surface protein that is a member of the immunoglobulin superfamily CD58 is expressed on both hematopoietic and non-hematopoietic cells including B cells, T cells, monocytes, erythrocytes, endothelial cells, epithelial cells, and fibroblasts. High levels are observed on memory T cells and dendritic cells. CD58 expressed on antigen presenting cells and target cells enhances T cell recognition via the binding of its cognate ligand, CD2, on the T cell surface.

t4.6 Recommended Panels for Flow Cytometric Immunophenotyping

Acute Screen

BMA/PB/LN
G1/G1/45/G1
G2/G2/45/G2
71/33/45/14
10/19/45/20
34/56/45/117
7/64/45/HLA-DR
15/13/45/11b
5/2/45/3
L/K/45/19*

*not performed on follow-up AML specimens

Follow-Up to Acute Screen

B cell	T cell	Myeloid
22/24/45	3/8/45/4	36/GlyA/45
	3/1a/45	61/14/45

Intracellular
3/MPO/45

Chronic/Lymphoma Screen

BMA/PB/LN	**PLASMA CELL**
G1/G1/45/G1	G1/G1/45/G1
G2/G2/45/G2	G2/G2/45/G2
71/33/45/14	71/33/45/14
10/5/45/23	3/138/45/56
3/2/45/20	20/38/45/HLA-DR
52/7/45/19	L/K/45/19
3/8/45/4	
L/K/45/19	

Hematopoietic
3/19/45

Follow-Up to Chronic/Lymphoma Screen

Hairy Cell	Adult T cell	LGL
22/11c/45	7/25/45/3	3/16+56/45/-
103/25/45		57/3/45/56

ALCL
30/19/45/3

+CLL*
20/38/45
5/79b/45
3/ZAP-70/19

Plasma Cell
3/138/45/56
20/38/45/HLA-DR

*automatically performed on all newly diagnosed CLL.

ALCL, anaplastic large cell lymphoma; AML, acute myeloid leukemia; BMA, bone marrow aspirate; CLL, chronic lymphocytic leukemia; LGL, large granular lymphocyte; LN, lymph node; MPO, myeloperoxidase; PB, peripheral blood.

References

Abramson CS, Kersey JH, LeBien TW [1981] A monoclonal antibody (BA-1) reactive with cells of human B lymphocyte lineage. *J Immunol* 126:83-88.

Adriaansen HJ, te Boekhorst PAW, Hagemeijer AM, et al [1993] Acute myeloid leukemia M4 with BM eosinophilia (M4Eo) and inv(16)(p13q22) exhibits a specific immunophenotype with CD2 expression. *Blood* 81:3043-3051.

Aiello A, Delia D, Borrello MG, et al [1992] Flow cytometric detection of the mitochondrial bcl-2 protein in normal and neoplastic human lymphoid cells. *Cytometry* 13:502-509.

Aisenberg AC, Wilkes B [1980] Unusual human lymphoma phenotype defined by monoclonal antibody. *J Exp Med* 152:1126-1131.

Anderson KC, Bates MP, Slaughenhoupt BL, et al [1984] Expression of human B cell-associated antigens on leukemias and lymphomas: A model of human B cell differentiation. *Blood* 63:1424-1433.

Andrew DP, Rott LS, Kilshaw PJ, Butcher EC [1996] Distribution of α4β7 and αEβ7 integrins on thymocytes, intestinal epithelial lymphocytes and peripheral lymphocytes. *Eur J Immunol* 26:897-905.

Andrews RG, Torok-Storb B, Bernstein ID [1983] Myeloid-associated differentiation antigens on stem cells and their progeny identified by monoclonal antibodies. *Blood* 62:124-132.

Arber DA, Weiss LM [1995] CD57: A review. *Appl Immunohistochem* 3:137-152.

Arber DA, Jenkins KA, Slovak ML [1996a] CD79α expression in acute myeloid leukemia. High frequency of expression in acute promyelocytic leukemia. *Am J Pathol* 149:1105-1110.

Arber DA, Jenkins KA [1996b] Paraffin section immunophenotyping of acute leukemias in BM specimens. *Am J Clin Pathol* 106:462-468.

Arber DA, Weiss LM [1997] CD10: A review. *Appl Immunohistochem* 5:125-140.

Ashman LK, Roberts MM, Gadd SJ, et al [1988] Expression of 150-kD cell surface antigen identified by monoclonal antibody YB5.B8 is associated with poor prognosis in acute non-lymphoblastic leukaemia. *Leuk Res* 12:923-928.

Babusíková O, Ondráčková V, Prachar J, et al [1999] Flow cytometric analysis of some activation/proliferation markers on human thymocytes and their correlation with cell proliferation. *Neoplasma* 46:349-355.

Basso G, Putti MC, Cantù-Rajnoldi A, et al [1992] The immunophenotype in infant acute lymphoblastic leukaemia: Correlation with clinical outcome. An Italian multicentre study (AIEOP). *Br J Haematol* 81:184-191.

Bayer-Garner IB, Schwartz MR, Lin P, et al [2003] CD117, but not lysozyme, is positive in cutaneous plasmacytoma. *Arch Pathol Lab Med* 127:1596-1598.

Belzer MB, Fitchen JH, Ferrone S, et al [1981] Expression of Ia-like antigens on human erythroid progenitor cells as determined by monoclonal antibodies and heteroantiserum to Ia-like antigens. *Clin Immunol Immunopath* 20:111-115.

Bene MC, Bernier M, Casasnovas RO, et al [1998] The reliability and specificity of c-kit for the diagnosis of acute myeloid leukemias and undifferentiated leukemias. *Blood* 92:596-599.

Bernstein ID, Andrews RG, Cohen SF, et al [1982] Normal and malignant human myelocytic and monocytic cells identified by monoclonal antibodies. *J Immunol* 128:876-881.

Bhargava V, Kell DL, van de Rijn M, et al [1994] Bcl-2 immunoreactivity in breast carcinoma correlates with hormone receptor positivity. *Am J Pathol* 145:535-540.

Borowitz MJ, Shuster JJ, Civin CI, et al [1990] Prognostic significance of CD34 expression in childhood B-precursor acute lymphocytic leukemia: A pediatric oncology group study. *J Clin Oncol* 8:1389-1398.

Borst J, Brouns GS, deVries E, et al [1993] Antigen receptors on T and B lymphocytes: Parallels in organization and function. *Immunol Rev* 132:49-84.

Boue DR, LeBein TW [1988] Expression and structure of CD22 in acute leukemia. *Blood* 71:1480-1486.

Bradstock K, Matthews J, Benson E, et al [1994] Australian Leukaemia Study Group. Prognostic value of immunophenotyping in acute myeloid leukemia. *Blood* 84:1220-1225.

Braun MP, Martin PJ, Ledbetter JA, et al [1983] Granulocytes and cultured human fibroblasts express common acute lymphoblastic leukemia-associated antigens. *Blood* 61:718-725.

Buccheri V, Mihaljevic B, Matutes E, et al [1993] mb-1: A new marker for B-lineage lymphoblastic leukemia. *Blood* 82:853-857.

Buhling F, Dunz D, Reinhold D, Ulmer AJ, Ernst M, Flad HD, Ansorge S [1994] Expression and functional role of dipeptidyl peptidase IV on human natural killer cells. *Nat Immun* 13:270-279.

Buhling F, Junker U, Reinhold D, Neubert K, Jager L, Ansorge S [1995] Functional role of CD26 on human B lymphocytes. *Immunol Lett* 45:47-51.

Butnor KJ, Burchette JL, Sporn TA, et al [2004] The spectrum of kit (CD117) immunoreactivity in lung and pleural tumors: A study of 96 cases using a single-source antibody with a review of the literature. *Arch Pathol Lab Med* 128:538-543.

Cabanas D, Sanches-Madrid F, Acevedo A, et al [1988] Characterization of a CD11c-reactive monoclonal antibody (HC1/1) obtained by immunizing with phorbol ester differentiated U937 cells. *Hybridoma* 7:167-176.

Caligaris-Cappio F, Gobbi M, Bonfill M, et al [1982] Infrequent normal B lymphocyte express features of B chronic lymphocytic leukemia. *J Exp Med* 155:623-628.

Campana D, Janossy G, Bofill M, et al [1985] Human B cell development: I. Phenotypic differences of B lymphocytes in the BM and peripheral lymphoid tissue. *J Immunol* 134:1524-1530.

Campana D, Thompson JS, Amlot P, et al [1987] The cytoplasmic expression of CD3 antigens in normal and malignant cells of the T lymphoid lineage. *J Immunol* 138:648-655.

Capron M, Jouault T, Prin L, et al [1986] Functional study of monoclonal antibody to IgE Fc receptor (FceR2) of eosinophils, platelets and macrophages. *J Exp Med* 164:72-89.

Carbone A, Gloghini A, De Re V, et al [1990] Histopathologic, immunophenotypic, and genotypic analysis of Ki-1 anaplastic large cell lymphomas that express histiocyte-associated antigens. *Cancer* 66:2547-2456.

Carbone A, Gloghini A, Zagonel V, Aldinucci D, Gattei V, Degan M, Improta S, Sorio R, Monfardini S, Pinto A [1995a] The expression of CD26 and CD40 ligand is mutually exclusive in human T-cell non-Hodgkin's lymphomas/leukemias. *Blood* 86:4617-4626.

Carbone A, Gloghini A, Zagonel V, Pinto A [1995b] An update on the diagnostic relevance of CD26 antigen expression in CD30 positive anaplastic large cell lymphomas. *Hum Pathol* 26:1169-1170.

Cattoretti G, Berti E, Mancuso A, et al [1987] A MHC class 1 related family of antigens with widespread distribution on resting and activated cells. In: McMichael AJ, Beverley PCL, Cobbold S, et al, eds. *Leukocyte Typing III: White Cell Differentiation Antigens.* Oxford: Oxford University Press;89-92.

Chadburn A, Inghirami G, Knowles DM [1992] The kinetics and temporal expression of T-cell activation-associated antigens CD15 (LeuM1), CD30 (Ki-1), EMA, and CD11c (LeuM5) by benign activated T cells. *Hematol Pathol* 6:193-202.

Chadburn A, Knowles DM [1994] Paraffin-resistant antigens detectable by antibodies L26 and polyclonal CD3 predict the B- or T-cell lineage of 95% of diffuse aggressive non-Hodgkin's lymphoma. *Am J Clin Pathol* 102:284-291.

Chang H, Bartlett E, Patterson B, Chen CI, Yi QL [2005] The absence of CD56 on malignant plasma cells in the cerebrospinal fluid is the hallmark of multiple myeloma involving central nervous system. *Br J Haematol* 129:539-541.

Chess L, Evans R, Humphreys RD, et al [1976] Inhibition of antibody dependent cellular cytoxitiy and immunoglobulin synthesis by an antiserum prepared against a human B-cell Ia-like molecule. *J Exp Med* 144:113-122.

Chittal SM, Alard C, Rossi R-F, et al [1990] Further phenotypic evidence that nodular, lymphocyte-predominant Hodgkin's disease is a large B-cell lymphoma in evolution. *Am J Surg Pathol* 14:1024-1035.

Chott A, Haedicke W, Mosberger I, et al [1998] Most CD56+ intestinal lymphomas are CD8+CD5–T-cell lymphomas of monomorphic small to medium size histology. *Am J Pathol* 153:1483-1490.

Civin CI, Strauss LC, Brovall C, et al [1984] Antigenic analysis of hematopoiesis: III. A hematopoietic progenitor cell surface antigen defined by a monoclonal antibody raised against KG-Ia cells. *J Immunol* 133:157-165.

Clément C, Vouijs WC, Klein B, et al [1995] B-B2 and B-B4, two new mAb against secreting plasma cells. In Schlossman SF, Boumsell L, Gilks WR, et al, eds. *Leukocyte Typing V: White Cell Differentiation Antigens.* New York: Oxford University Press:714-715.

Contos MJ, Kornstein MJ, Innes DJ, et al [1992] The utility of CD20 and CD43 in subclassification of low-grade B-cell lymphoma on paraffin sections. *Mod Pathol* 5:631-633.

Cook JR, Craig FE, Swerdlow SH [2003] Bcl-2 expression by multicolor flow cytometric analysis assists in the diagnosis of follicular lymphoma in lymph node and BM. *Am J Clin Pathol* 119:145-151.

Cornfield DB, Mitchell DM, Almasri NM, et al [2000] Follicular lymphoma can be distinguished from benign follicular hyperplasia by flow cytometry using simultaneous staining of cytoplasmic bcl-2 and cell surface CD20. *Am J Clin Pathol* 114:258-263.

Crespo M, Bosch F, Villamor N, Bellosilla B, et al [2003] ZAP-70 expression as a surrogate for immunoglobulin-variable-region mutations in chronic lymphocytic leukemia. *N Engl J Med* 348:1767-1775.

Cueno A, Michaux JL, Ferrant A, et al [1992] Correlation of cytogenetic patterns and clinicobiological features in adult myeloid leukemia expressing lymphoid markers. *Blood* 79:720-727.

De Fraissinette A, Dezutter-Dambuyant C, Schmitt D, et al [1990] Ontogeny of Langerhans cells: Phenotypic differentiation from the BM to the skin. *Dev Comp Immunol* 14:335-346.

deHaas M, Kleijer M, Roos D, et al [1995] Characterization of mAb of the CD16 cluster and six newly generated CD16 mAb. In: Schlossman SF, Boumsell L, Gilks WR, et al, eds. *Leukocyte Typing V: White Cell Differentiation Antigens*. New York: Oxford University Press:811-814.

Del Poeta G, Maurillo L, Venditti A, et al [2001] Clinical significance of CD38 expression in chronic lymphocytic leukemia. *Blood* 98:2633-2639.

Delespess G, Sarfati M, Wu CY, et al [1992] The low-affinity receptor for IgE. *Immunol Rev* 125:77-97.

Dimitiu-Bona A, Burmester GR, Waters SJ, et al [1983] Human mononuclear phagocyte differentiation antigens: I. Patterns of antigenic expression on the surface of human monocytes and macrophages defined by monoclonal antibodies. *J Immunol* 130:145-152.

Dörken B, Moldenhauer G, Pezzutto A, et al [1986] HD39 (B3), a B lineage-restricted antigen whose cell surface expression is limited to resting and activated human B lymphocytes. *J Immunol* 136:4470-4479.

Dörken B, Pezzutto M, Kohler M, et al [1987] Expression of cytoplasmic CD22 in B-cell ontogeny. In: McMichael AJ, Beverley PCL, Cobbold S, et al, eds. *Leukocyte Typing III: White Cell Differentiation Antigens*. Oxford: Oxford University Press: 474-476.

Drexler HG, Sagawa K, Menon M, et al [1986] Phenotyping of malignant hematopoietic cells: II. Reactivity pattern of myeloid monoclonal antibodies with emphasis on MCS-2. *Leuk Res* 10:17-23.

Du X, Ho M, Pastan I [2007] New immunotoxins targeting CD123, a stem cell antigen on acute myeloid leukemia cells. *J Immunother* 30:607-613.

Dunphy CH [1999a] Comprehensive review of adult acute myelogenous leukemia: Cytomorphological, enzyme cytochemical, flow cytometric immunophenotypic, and cytogenetic findings. *J Clin Lab Anal* 13:19-26.

Dunphy CH, Oza YU, Skelly ME [1999b] An otherwise typical case of non-Japanese hairy cell leukemia with CD10 and CDw75 expression: Response to cladaribine phosphate therapy. *J of Clin Lab Anal* 13:141-144.

Dunphy CH [2000a] Contribution of flow cytometric immunophenotyping to the evaluation of tissues with suspected lymphoma. *Cytometry* 42:296-306.

Dunphy CH, Garder LJ, Manes JL, et al [2000b] CD30+ anaplastic large-cell lymphoma with aberrant expression of CD13: Case report and review of the literature. *J Clin Lab Anal* 14:299-304.

Dunphy CH, Polski JM, Evans HL, et al [2001a] Evaluation of BM specimens with acute myelogenous leukemia for CD34, CD15, CD117, and myeloperoxidase. *Arch Pathol Lab Med* 125:1063-1069.

Dunphy CH, Gardner LJ, Evans HL, Javadi N [2001b] CD15(+) acute lymphoblastic leukemia and subsequent monoblastic leukemia: Persistence of t(4;11) abnormality and B-cell gene rearrangement. *Arch Pathol Lab Med* 125:1227-1230.

Dunphy CH, Polski JM, Evans HL, Gardner LJ [2001c] Paraffin immunoreactivity of CD10, CDw75, and Bcl-6 in follicle center cell lymphoma. *Leuk Lymphoma* 41:585-592.

Dunphy CH, Orton SO, Mantell J [2004a] Relative contributions of enzyme cytochemistry and flow cytometric immunophenotying to the evaluation of acute myeloid leukemias with a monocytic component and of flow cytometric immunophenotyping to the evaluation of absolute monocytoses. *Am J Clin Pathol* 122:865-874.

Dunphy CH [2004b] Applications of flow cytometry to chronic myeloproliferative disorders and myelodysplastic syndromes. *J Clin Ligand Assay* 27:170-179.

Dunphy CH, DeMello, DE, Gale GB [2006a] Pediatric CD56+ anaplastic large cell lymphoma. *Arch Pathol Lab Med* 130:1859-1864.

Dunphy CH, Kang LC [2006b] Immunoreactivity of MIC2 (CD99) and terminal deoxynucleotidyl transferase (TdT) in BM clot and core specimens of acute myeloid leukemias and myelodysplastic syndromes. *Arch Path Lab Med*. 130:153-157.

Dunphy CH, Nies MK, Gabriel DA [2007] Correlation of plasma cell percentages by CD138 immunohistochemistry, cyclin D1 status, and CD56 expression with clinical parameters and overall survival in plasma cell myeloma. *Appl Immunohistochem Mol Morphol* 15:248-254.

Dunphy CH, O'Malley DP, Perkins SL, Chang CC [2007a] Analysis of immunohistochemical markers in BM sections to evaluate for myelodysplastic syndromes and acute myeloid leukemias. *Appl Immunohistochem Mol Morphol* 15:154-159.

Dunphy CH, Tang W [2007b] The value of CD64 expression in distinguishing acute myeloid leukemia with monocytic differentiation from other subtypes of acute myeloid leukemia: A flow cytometric analysis of 64 cases. *Arch Pathol Lab Med* 131:748-754.

Duperray C, Boiron JM, Boucheix C, et al [1990] The CD24 antigen discriminates between pre-B and B cells in the human BM. *J Immunol* 145:3678-3683.

Durie BGM, Grogan TM [1985] CALLA-positive myeloma: An aggressive subtype with poor survival. *Blood* 66:229-232.

Edelman GM [1986] Cell adhesion molecules in the regulation of animal form and tissue pattern. *Ann Rev Cell Biol* 2:81-116.

Ely SA and Knowles DM [2002] Expression of CD56/neural cell adhesion molecule correlates with the presence of lytic bone lesions in multiple myeloma and distinguishes myeloma from monoclonal gammopathy of undetermined significance and lymphomas with plasmacytoid differentiation. *Am J Pathol* 160:1293-1299.

Evans RL, Faldetta TJ, Humphreys RE, et al [1978] Peripheral human T cells sensitized in mixed leukocyte culture synthesize and express Ia-like antigens. *J Exp Med* 148:1440-1445.

Farinola MA, Weir EG, Ali SZ [2003] CD56 expression of neuroendocrine neoplasms on immunophenotyping by flow cytometry: A novel diagnostic approach to fine-needle aspiration biopsy. *Cancer* 99:240-246.

Feuillard J, Jacob MC, Valensi F, et al [2002] Clinical and biologic features of CD4(+)CD56(+) malignancies. *Blood* 99:1556-1563.

Fijnheer R, Modderman PW, Veldman H, et al [1990] Detection of platelet activation with monoclonal antibodies and flow cytometry. *Transfusion*. 30:20-25.

Fischer GF, Majdic O, Gadd S, et al [1990] Signal transduction in lymphocytic and myeloid cells via CD24, a new member of phosphoinositolanchored membrane molecules. *J Immunol* 144:638-641.

Fitchen JH, LeFevre C, Ferrone S, et al [1982] Expression of Ia-like and HLA-A, B antigens on human multipotential hematopoietic progenitor cells. *Blood* 59:188-190.

Fitzgerald LA, Steiner B, Rall Jr SC, Lo S-S, Phillips DR [1987] Protein sequence of endothelial glycoprotein IIIa derived from a cDNA clone. *J Biol Chem* 262:3936-3939.

Flohil CC, Janssen PA, Bosman FT [1996] Expression of bcl-2 protein in hyperplastic polyps, adenomas, and carcinomas of the colon. *J Pathol* 178:393-397.

Foucar K, Foucar E [1990] The mononuclear phagocyte and immunoregulatory effector (M-PIRE) system: Evolving concepts. *Semin Diagn Pathol* 7:4-18.

Franklin WA, Mason DY, Pulford K, et al [1986] Immunohistological analysis of human mononuclear phagocytes and dendritic cells by using monoclonal antibodies. *Lab Invest* 54:322-335.

Fu SM, Chiorazzi N, Wang CY, et al [1978] Ia-bearing T lymphocytes in man: Their identification and role in the generation of allogeneic helper activity. *J Exp Med* 148:1423-1428.

Gadol N, Ault KA [1986] Phenotypic and functional characterization of human Leu1 (CD5) B cells. *Immunol Rev* 93:23-34.

Gaidano G, Gloghini A, Gattai V, et al [1997] Association of Kaposi's sarcoma-associated herpes virus-positive primary effusion lymphoma with expression of the CD138/syndecan-1 antigen. *Blood* 90:4894-4900.

Giorno R [1986] Immunohistochemical analysis of human peripheral blood and lymphoid tissues using monoclonal antibodies immunoreactive with non-lymphoid cells. *Histochemistry* 84:241-245.

Glencross KD, Adam F, Poole J, et al [1992] CD10 antigen density in childhood common acute lymphoblastic leukaemia: Comparisons of race and sex. *Leuk Res* 16:1197-1201.

Gong JZ, Lagoo AS, Peters D, et al [2001] Value of CD23 determination by flow cytometry in differentiating mantle cell lymphoma from chronic lymphocytic leukemia/small lymphocytic lymphoma. *Am J Clin Pathol* 116:893-897.

Greaves MF, Sieff C, Edwards PAW [1983] Monoclonal antiglycophorin as a probe for erythroleukemias. *Blood* 61:645-651.

Greenwalt DE, Lipsky RH, Ockenhouse CF, et al [1992] Membrane glycoprotein CD36: A review of its roles in adherence, signal transduction, and transfusion medicine. *Blood* 80:1105-1115.

Griffin JD, Ritz J, Nadler LM, et al [1981] Expression of myeloid differentiation antigens on normal and malignant myeloid cells. *J Clin Invest* 68:932-941.

Griffin JD, Hercend T, Beveridge RP, et al [1983] Characterization of an antigen expressed by human natural killer cells. *J Immunol* 130:2947-2951.

Griffin JD, Linch D, Sabbath K, et al [1984] A monoclonal antibody reactive with normal and leukemic human myeloid progenitor cells. *Leuk Res* 8:521-534.

Guyre PM, Von Dem Borne AEG [1995] CD64 cluster workshop report. In: Schlossmann SF, Boumsell L, Gilks W, et al, eds. *Leucocyte Typing V: White Cell Differentiation Antigens*. New York, NY: Oxford University Press; 778-782.

Habeshaw JA, Lister TA, Greaves MF [1983] Correlation of transferrin receptor expression with histologic class and outcome in non-Hodgkin's lymphoma. *Lancet* i:498-500.

Hall PA, D'Ardenne AJ, Richards MA, et al [1987] Lymphoplasmacytoid lymphoma: an immunohistological study. *J Pathol* 153:213-223.

Hall SE, Rosse WF [1996] The use of monoclonal antibodies and flow cytometry in the diagnosis of paroxysmal nocturnal hemoglobinuria. *Blood* 87:5332-5340.

Halper J, Fu SM, Wang CY, et al [1978] Patterns of expression of human "Ia-like" antigens during the terminal stages of B cell development. *J Immunol* 120:1480-1484.

Halper JP, Knowles DM, Wang CY [1980] Ia antigen expression by human malignant lymphomas: Correlation with conventional lymphoid markers. *Blood* 55:373-382.

Hammer RD, Vnencak-Jones CL, Manning SS, et al [1998] Microvillous lymphomas are B-cell neoplasms that frequently express CD56. *Mod Pathol* 11:239-246.

Hans CP, Finn WG, Singleton TP, et al [2002] Usefulness of anti-CD117 in the flow cytometric analysis of acute leukemia. *Am J Clin Pathol* 117:301-305.

Hanson CA, Gribbin TE, Schnitzer B, et al [1990] CD11c (LeuM5) expression characterizes a B cell chronic lymphoproliferative disorder with features of both chronic lymphocyte leukemia and hair cell leukemia. *Blood* 76:2360-2367.

Harada H, Kawana MM, Huang N, et al [1993] Phenotypic difference of normal plasma cells from mature myeloma cells. *Blood* 81:2658-2663.

Hardie DL, Johnson GD, Khan M, et al [1993] Quantitative analysis of molecules which distinguish functional compartments within germinal centers. *Eur J Immunol* 23:997-1004.

Hardy RR, Hayakawa K [1986] Development and physiology of Ly-1 B and its human homolog, Leu-1 B. *Immunol Rev* 83:53-79.

Harris NL, Jaffe ES, Stein H, et al [1994] A revised European-American classification of lymphoid neoplasms: A proposal from the International Lymphoma Study Group. *Blood* 84:1361-1392.

Heinen E, Lilet-Leclercq C, Mason DY, et al [1984] Isolation of follicular dendritic cells from human tonsils and adenoids: II. Immunocytochemical characterization. *Eur J Immunol* 14:267-273.

Hoffman T, Wang CY, Winchester RJ, et al [1977] Human lymphocytes bearing "Ia-like" antigens: Absence in patients with infantile agammaglobulinemia. *J Immunol* 119:1520-1524.

Hokland P, Ritz J, Schlossman SF, et al [1985] Orderly expression of B cell antigens during the in vitro differentiation of non-malignant human pre-B cells. *J Immunol* 135:1746-1751.

Horvathova M, Gailard JP, Liautard J, et al [1995] Identification of novel and specific antigens of human plasma cells by mAb. In: Schlossman SF, Boumsell L, Gilks WR, et al, eds. *Leukocyte Typing V: White Cell Differentiation Antigens*. New York: Oxford University Press; 713-714.

Hutlin LE, Hausner MA, Hutlin PM, et al [1993] CD20(pan-B cell) antigen is expressed at a low level on a subpopulation of human T lymphocytes. *Cytometry* 14:196-204.

Ibrahim S, Keating M, Kim-Anh D, et al [2001] CD38 expression as an important prognostic factor in B-cell chronic lymphocytic leukemia. *Blood* 98:181-186.

Imamura N, Ota H, Abe K, et al [1994] Expression of the thrombospondin receptor (CD36) on the cell surface in megakaryoblastic and promegakaryocytic leukemias: Increment of the receptor by megakaryocyte differentiation in vitro. *Am J Hematol* 45:181-184.

Jacob MC, Chaperot L, Mossuz P, et al [2003] CD4+ CD56+ lineage negative malignancies: A new entity developed from malignant early plasmacytoid dendritic cells. *Haematologica* 88:941-955.

Jaffe ES, Chan JKC, Su I-J, et al [1996] Report of the workshop on nasal and related extranodal angiocentric T/natural killer cell lymphomas: Definitions, differential diagnosis and epidemiology. *Am J Surg Pathol* 20:103-111.

Jaffe ES, Krenacs L, Kumar S, et al [1999] Extranodal peripheral T-cell and NK-cell neoplasms. *Am J Clin Pathol* 111:S46-S55.

Jani P, Qi XY, Chang H [2007] Aberrant expression of T-cell-associated markers CD4 and CD7 on B-cell chronic lymphocytic leukemia. *Am J Hematol* 82:73-76.

Jasionawski TM, Hartung L, Greenwood JH, Perkins SL, Bahler DW [2003] Analysis of CD10+ hairy cell leukemia. *Am J Clin Pathol* 120:228-235.

Jennings LK, Ashmun RA, Wang WF, Dockter ME [1986] Analysis of human platelet glycoproteins IIb-IIIa and Glanzmann thrombasthenia in whole blood by flow cytometry. *Blood* 68:173-179.

Juco J, Holden JT, Mann KP, et al [2003] Immunopheno- typic analysis of anaplastic large cell lymphoma by flow cytometry. *Am J Clin Pathol* 119:205-212.

Käfer G, Willer A, Ludwig W, et al [1999] Intracellular expression of CD61 precedes surface expression. *Ann Hematol* 78:472-474.

Kampalath B, Barcos MP, Stewart C [2003] Phenotypic heterogeneity of B cells in patients with chronic lymphocytic leukemia/small lymphocytic lymphoma. *Am J Clin Pathol* 119:824-832.

Kanavaros P, Gaulard P, Charlotte F, et al [1995] Discordant expression of immunoglobulin and its associated molecule mb-1/CD79a is frequently found in mediastinal large B cell lymphomas. *Am J Pathol* 146:735-741.

Kaplan J, Ravindranath Y, Inoue S [1986] T cell acute lymphoblastic leukemia with natural killer cell phenotype *Am J Hematol* 22:355-364.

Karandikar NJ, Aquino DB, McKenna RW, et al [2001] Transient myeloproliferative disorder and acute myeloid leukemia in Down syndrome: An immunophenotypic analysis. *Am J Clin Pathol* 116:204-210.

Kasparu H, Koller U, Krieger O, et al [1989] Significance of gp40/CD7 or TdT positivity in AML patients. In: Knapp W, Dorken B, Gilks WR, et al, eds. *Leucocyte Typing IV: White Cell Differentiation Antigens.* New York: Oxford University Press, 936-937.

Kersey J, Abramson C, Perry G, et al [1982] Clinical usefulness of monoclonal antibody phenotyping in childhood acute lymphoblastic leukemia. *Lancet* ii:1419-1423.

Kikutani H, Suemura M, Owaki H, et al [1986] Fce receptor, a specific differentiation marker transiently expressed on mature B cells before isotype switching. *J Exp Med* 164:1455-1469.

Kilshaw PJ, and Baker KC [1988] A unique surface antigen on intraepithelial lymphocytes in the mouse. *Immunol Lett* 18:149-154.

Kilshaw PJ, Murant SJ [1990] A new surface antigen on intraepithelial lymphocytes in the intestine. *Eur J Immunol* 20:2201-2207.

Kilshaw PJ, Murant SJ [1991] Expression and regulation of β7(βp) integrins on mouse lymphocytes: Relevance to the mucosal immune system. *Eur J Immunol* 21:2591-2597.

Kiyokawa T, Shirono K, Hattori T, et al [1989] Cytotoxicity of interleukin 2-toxin toward lymphocytes from patients with adult T-cell leukemia. *Cancer Res* 49:4042-4046.

Klareskog L, Tjeinlund UM, Forsum U, et al [1977] Epidermal Langerhans cells express Ia antigens. *Nature* 268:248-250.

Klobusická M, Babusíková O [1999] CD26 and DPP IV expression in T acute lymphoblastic leukemia cells: Immunocytochemistry and enzyme cytochemistry. *Gen Physiol Biophys* 18 (Suppl 1):34-37.

Knowles, DM [1986] The human T-cell leukemias: Clinical, cytomorphologic, immunophenotypic, and genotypic characteristics. *Hum Pathol* 17:14-33.

Knowles, DM [1989] Immunophenotypic and antigen receptor gene rearrangement analysis in T cell neoplasia. *Am J Pathol* 134:761-785.

Koehler M, Behm F, Hancock M, et al [1993] Expression of activation antigens CD38 and CD71 is not clinically important in childhood acute lymphoblastic leukemia. *Leukemia* 7:41-45.

Köller U [1989] Summary of immunohistology studies. In: Knapp W, Dörken B, Gilks WR, et al, eds. *Leukocyte Typing IV: White Cell Differentiation Antigens.* Oxford: Oxford University Press, 862-867.

Kondo S, Kotani T, Tamura K, Aratke Y, Uno H, Tsubouchi H, Inoue S, Niho Y, Ohtaki S [1996] Expression of CD26/dipeptidyl peptidase IV in adult T cell leukemia/lymphoma (ATLL). *Leuk Res* 20:357-363.

Konoplev S, Medeiros LJ, Bueso-Ramos CE, et al [2005] Immunophenotypic profile of lymphoplasmacytic lymphoma/Waldenström macroglobulinemia. *Am J Clin Pathol* 124:414-420.

Krajewski S, Tanaka S, Takayama S, Schibler MJ, Fenton W, Reed JC [1993] Investigation of the subcellular distribution of the Bcl-2 oncoprotein: Residence in the nuclear envelope, endoplasmic reticulum, and outer mitochondrial membranes. *Cancer Res* 53:4701-4714.

Kreitman RJ, Pastan I [2006] Immunotoxins in the treatment of refractory hairy cell leukemia. *Hematol Oncol Clin North Am* 20:1137-1151.

Krenacs L, Tiszalvicz L, Krenacs T, et al [1993] Immunohistochemical detection of CD1a antigen in formalin-fixed and paraffin-embedded tissue sections with monoclonal antibody O10. *J Pathol* 171:99-104.

Kuerbitz SJ, Civin CI, Krischer JP, et al [1992] Expression of myeloid-associated and lymphoid-associated cell-surface antigens in acute myeloid leukemia of childhood: A pediatric oncology group study. *J Clin Oncol* 10:1419-1429.

Kumamoto H, Ooya K [1999] Immunohistochemical analysis of bcl-2 family proteins in benign and malignant ameloblastomas. *J Oral Pathol Med* 28:343-349.

Kurabayashi H, Kuboto K, Murakami H, et al [1988] Ultrastructure of myeloma cells in patients with common acute lymphoblastic leukemia antigen (CALLA)-positive myeloma. *Cancer Res* 48:6234-6237.

Kussick SJ, Wood BL [2003] Four-color flow cytometry identifies virtually all cytogenetically abnormal BM samples in the workup of non-CML myeloproliferative disorders. *Am J Clin Pathol* 120:854-865.

Kuzu I, Bicknell R, Harris AL, et al [1992] Heterogeneity of vascular endothelial cells with relevance to diagnosis of vascular tumours. *J Clin Pathol* 45:143-148.

Lai R, Arber DA, Chang KL, Wilson CS, Weiss LM [1998] Frequency of bcl-2 expression in non-Hodgkin's lymphoma: A study of 778 cases with comparison of marginal zone lymphoma and monocytoid B-cell hyperplasia. *Mod Pathol* 11:864-869.

Langlois RG, Bigbee WL, Jensen RH [1985] Flow cytometric characterization of normal and variant cells with monoclonal antibodies specific for glycophorin A. *J Immunol* 134:4009-4017.

Lanier LL, Le AM, Phillips JH, et al [1983] Subpopulations of human natural killer cells defined by expression of the Leu-7 (HNK-1) and Leu-11 (NK-15) antigens. *J Immunol* 131:1789-1796.

Lanier LL, Kipps TJ, Phillips JH [1985] Functional properties of a unique subset of cytotoxic CD3+ T lymphocytes that express Fc receptors for IgG (CD16/Leu-11 antigen). *J Exp Med* 162:2089-2106.

Lanier LL, Phillips JH [1986] A map of the cell surface antigens expressed on resting and activated human natural killer cells. In: Reinherz El, Haynes BF, Nadler LM, et al, eds. *Leucocyte Typing II: Human, Myeloid and Hematopoietic Cells*. New York: Springer-Verlag, 157-170.

Lardelli P, Bookman MA, Sundeen J, et al [1990] Lymphocytic lymphoma of intermediate differentiation. Morphologic and immunophenotypic spectrum and clinical correlations. *Am J Surg Pathol* 14:752-763.

Lauwers GY, Scott GV, Karpeh MS [1995] Immunohistochemical evaluation of bcl-2 protein expression in gastric adenocarcinomas. *Cancer* 75:2209-2213.

LeFrançois, L, Barrett TA, Havran WL, Puddington L [1994] Developmental expression of the αIELβ7 integrin on T cell receptor γδ and T cell receptor αβ T cells. *Eur J Immunol* 24:635-640.

Leo R, Boecker M, Peest D, et al [1992] Multiparameter analyses of normal and malignant human plasma cells: CD38+, CD56+, CD54+, cIg+ is the common phenotype of myeloma cells. *Ann Hematol* 64:132-139.

Li S, Eshleman JR, Borowitz MJ [2002] Lack of surface immunoglobulin light chain expression by flow cytometric immunophenotyping can help diagnose peripheral B-cell lymphoma. *Am J Clin Pathol* 118:229-234.

Lima M, Almeida J, Montero AG, et al [2004] Clinicobiological, immunophenotypic, and molecular characteristics of monoclonal CD56–/+dim chronic natural killer cell large granular lymphocytosis. *Am J Pathol* 165:1117-1127.

Linder J, Ye Y, Armitage JO, et al [1988] Monoclonal antibodies marking B-cell non-Hodgkin's lymphoma in paraffin-embedded tissue. *Mod Pathol* 1:29-34.

Link MP, Stewart SJ, Warnke RA, et al [1985] Discordance between surface and cytoplasmic expression of the Leu-4 (T3) antigen in thymocytes and in blast cells from childhood T lymphoblastic malignancies. *J Clin Invest* 76:248-253.

Liszka K, Majdic O, Bettelheim P, et al [1983] Glycophorin A expression in malignant hematopoiesis. *Am J Hematol* 15:219-226.

Longacre TA, Foucar K, Crago S, et al [1989] Hematogones: A multiparameter analysis of BM precursor cells. *Blood* 73:543-552.

Malcovati L, Della Porta MG, Lunghi M, et al [2005] Flow cytometry evaluation of erythroid and myeloid dysplasia in patients with myelodysplastic syndrome. *Leukemia* 19:776-783.

Mason DY, Stein H, Gerdes J, et al [1987] Value of monoclonal anti-CD22 (p135) antibodies for the detection of normal and neoplastic B lymphoid cells. *Blood* 69:836-840.

Mason DY, Cordell JL, Tse AG, et al [1991] The igM-associated protein mb-1 as a marker of normal and neoplastic B cells. *J Immunol* 147:2474-2482.

Mason DY, van Noesel CJM, Cordell JL, et al [1992] The B29 and mb-1 polypeptides are differentially expressed during human B cell differentiation. *Eur J Immunol* 22:2753-2756.

Mason DY, Cordell JL, Brown MH, et al [1995] CD79a: A novel marker for B-cell neoplasms in routinely processed tissue samples. *Blood* 86:1453-1459.

Maynadié M, Picard F, Husson B, et al [2002] Immunophenotypic clustering of myelodysplastic syndromes. *Blood* 100:2349-2356.

McCarron KF, Hammel JP, Hsi ED [2000] Usefulness of CD79b expression in the diagnosis of B-cell chronic lymphoproliferative disorders. *Am J Clin Pathol* 113:805-813.

McCormack RT, Nelson RD, LeBien TW [1986] Structure/function studies of the common acute lymphoblastic leukemia antigen (CALLA/CD10) expressed on human neutrophils. *J Immunol* 137:1075-1082.

McMichael AJ, Pilch JR, Galfre G, et al [1979] A human thymocyte antigen defined by a hybrid myeloma monoclonal antibody. *Eur J Immunol* 9:205-210.

Meda BA, Frost M, Newell J, et al [2003] Bcl-2 is consistently expressed in hyperplastic marginal zones of the spleen, abdominal lymph nodes, ileal lymphoid tissue. *Am J Surg Pathol* 27:888-894.

Medeiros LJ, Herrington RD, Gonzalez CL, et al [1991] My4 antibody staining of non-Hodgkin's lymphomas. *Am J Clin Pathol* 95:363-368.

Meeker TC, Miller RA, Link MP, et al [1984] A unique human B lymphocyte antigen defined by a monoclonal antibody. *Hybridoma* 3:305-320.

Melink GB, LeBien TW [1983] Construction of an antigenic map for human B cell precursors. *J Clin Immunol* 3:260-267.

Micklem KJ, Dong Y, Willis A, et al [1991] HML-1 antigen on mucosa-associated T cells, activated cells, and hairy leukemic cells is a new integrin containing the β 7 subunit. *Am J Pathol* 139:1297-1301.

Mirro J, Antouin GR, Zipf TF, et al [1985] The E-rosette associated antigen of T cells can be identified on blasts from patients with acute myeloblastic leukemia. *Blood* 65:363-367.

Modderman PW [1989] Cluster report: CD61. In: Knapp W, Dörken B, Gilks WR, et al, eds. *Leucocyte Typing IV: White Cell Differentiation Antigens*. New York: Oxford University Press, 1025.

Modderman PW [1989] New clusters: CD29/CDw49, CD47, CD51, CD55, and CD61. In: Knapp W, Dörken B, Gilks WR, et al, eds. *Leucocyte Typing IV: White Cell Differentiation Antigens*. New York: Oxford University Press, 1017-1019.

Moldenhauer G, Dorken B, Schwartz R, et al [1986] Analysis of ten B lymphocyte specific workshop monoclonal antibodies. In: Reinherz EL, Haynes BF, Nader LM, eds. *Leukocyte Typing*, vol 2. New York: Springer-Verlag, 61-67.

Morabito F, Prasthofer EF, Dunlap NE, et al [1987] Expression of myelomonocytic antigens on chronic lymphocytic leukemia B cells correlates with their ability to produce interleukin 1. *Blood* 70:1750-1757.

Moreau I, Duivert V, Bachereau J, et al [1993] Culture of human fetal B-cell precursors on BM stroma maintains highly proliferative CD20dim cells. *Blood* 81:1170-1178.

Muñoz L, Aventín A, Villamor N, et al [2003] Immunophenotypic findings in acute myeloid leukemia with FLT3 internal tandem duplication. *Haematologica* 88:637-645.

Nadler LM, Anderson KC, Marti G, et al [1983] B4, a human B lymphocyte-associated antigen expressed on normal, mitogen-activated, and malignant B lymphocytes. *J Immunol* 131:244-250.

Nadler LM, Korsmeyer SJ, Anderson KC, et al [1984] B cell origin of non-T cell acute lymphoblastic leukemia: A model for discrete stages of neoplastic and normal pre-B cell differentiation. *J Clin Invest* 74:332-340.

Nadler LM [1986] B cell/leukemia panel workshop: Summary and comments. In: Reinherz EL, Haynes BF, Nadler LM, et al, eds. *Leukocyte Typing II*, vol 2. New York: Springer Verlag, 3-43.

Nakamura T, Kubagawa H, Cooper MD [1992] Heterogeneity of immunoglobulin-associated molecules on human B cells identified by monoclonal antibodies. *Proc Natl Acad Sci USA* 89:8522-8526.

Nakahata T, Okumura N [1994] Cell surface antigen expression in human erythroid progenitors: Erythroid and megakaryocytic markers. *Leuk Lymphoma* 13:401-409.

Nakamura T [1998] CD79 workshop panel report. In Kishimoto T, Kikutani H, von dem Borne AEGK, et al, eds. *Leukocyte Typing VI: White Cell Differentiation Antigens*. New York: Garland Publishing, 180-182.

Natkunam Y, Rouse RV [2000] Utility of paraffin section immunohistochemistry for c-kit (CD117) in the differential diagnosis of systemic mast cell disease involving the BM. *Am J Surg Pathol* 24:81-91.

Ngan BY, Chen-Levy Z, Weiss LM, Warnke RA, Cleary ML [1998] Expression in non-Hodgkin's lymphoma of the bcl-2 protein associated with the t(14;18) chromosomeal translocation. *N Engl J Med* 318:638-644.

Nguyen TDT, Schwartz EJ, West RB, et al [2005] Expression of CD163 (Hemoglobin scavenger receptor) in normal tissues, lymphomas, carcinomas, and sarcomas is largely restricted to the monocyte/macrophage lineage. *Am J Surg Pathol* 29:617-624.

O'Laughlin S, Braverman M, Smith-Jefferies M, et al [1992] Macrophages (histiocytes) in various reactive and inflammatory conditions express different antigenic phenotypes. *Hum Pathol* 23:1410-1418.

Oertel J, Kastner M, Bai AR, et al [1992] Analysis of chronic lymphoid leukaemias according to FAB. *Leuk Res* 16:919-927.

Olsaka A, Saionji K, Igari J, Watanabe N, Iwabuchi K, Nagaoka I [1997] Altered surface expression of effector cell molecules on neutrophils in myelodysplastic syndromes. *Br J Haematol* 98:108-113.

Olweus J, Lund-Johansen F, Terstappen LWMM [1995] CD64/F$_c$RI is a granulo-monocytic lineage marker on CD34+ hematopoietic progenitor cells. *Blood* 85:2402-2413.

Olweus J, Terstappen LWMM, Thompson PA, Lund-Johansen F [1996] Expression and function of receptors for stem cell factor and erythropoietin during lineage commitment of human hematopoietic progenitor cells. *Blood* 88:1594-1607.

Pallesen G [1987] The distribution of CD23 in normal human tissues and in malignant lymphomas. In McMichael AJ, Beverley PCL, Cobbold S, et al, eds. *Leukocyte Typing III: White Cell Differentiation Antigens*. Oxford: Oxford University Press, 383-386.

Pandolfi F, Loughran TP, Starkebaum G, et al [1990] Clinical course of prognosis of the lymphoproliferative disease of granular lymphocytes: A multicenter study. *Cancer* 65:341-348.

Pardanani A, Kimlinger T, Reeder T, et al [2004] Bone marrow mast cell immunophenotyping in adults with mast cell disease: A prospective study of 33 patients. *Leuk Res* 28:777-783.

Parisi-Duchêne E, Mazurier I, Moskovtchenko P [2006] Aberrant CD8 expression in B-chronic lymphocytic leukemia: Report of five cases. *Acta Haematol* 115:74-77.

Pellat-Deceunynck C, Barille S, Jego G, et al [1998] The absence of CD56(NCAM) on malignant plasma cells is a hallmark of plasma cell leukemia and of a special subset of multiple myeloma. *Leukemia* 12:1977-1982.

Perruccello SJ, Johnson DR [1994] In Keren DK, Hanson CA, Hurtubise PE, eds. *Flow Cytometry and Clinical Diagnosis*. Chicago: ASCP Press.

Perussia B, Starr S, Abraham S, et al [1983] Human natural killer cells analyzed by B73.1, a monoclonal antibody blocking Fc receptor functions: I. Characterization of the lymphocyte subset reactive with B73.1. *J Immunol* 130:2133-2141.

Perussia B, Trinchieri G, Jackson A, et al [1984] The Fc receptor for IgG on human natural killer cells: Phenotypic, functional, and comparative studies with monoclonal antibodies. *J Immunol* 133:180-189.

Pezzella F, Tse GD, Cordell JL, Pulford KAF, Gatter KC, Mason DY [1990] Expression of the bcl-2 oncogene protein is not specific for the 14;18 chromosomal translocation. *Am J Pathol* 137:225-232.

Pezzella F, Gatter K [1995] What is the value of bcl-2 protein detection for histopathologists? *Histopathology* 26:89-93.

Pillchowska ME, Fleming MD, Pinkus JL, et al [2007] CD4+/CD56+ hematodermic neoplasm ("blastic natural killer cell lymphoma"): Neoplastic cells express the immature dendritic cell marker BDCA-2 and produce interferon. *Am J Clin Pathol* 128:445-453.

Pilozzi E, Pulford K, Jones M, et al [1988] Co-expression of CD79a (JCB117) and CD3 by lymphoblastic lymphoma. *J Pathol* 186:140-143.

Poniecka AW, Alexis JB [1999] An immunohistochemical study of basal cell carcinoma and trichoepithelioma. *Am J Dermatopathol* 21:332-336.

Puglisi F, Cesselli D, Damante G, et al [2000] Expression of Pax-8, p53 and bcl-2 in human benign and malignant thyroid diseases. *Anticancer Res* 20:311-316.

Quintanilla-Martinez L, Preffer F, Rubin D, et al [1994] CD20+ T-cell lymphoma: Neoplastic transformation of a normal T-cell subset. *Am J Clin Pathol* 102:483-489.

Rabellino EM, Nachman RL, Williams W, et al [1979] Human megakaryocytes: I. Characterization of the membrane and cytoplasmic components of isolated BM megakaryocytes. *J Exp Med* 149:1273-1287.

Ramsay JA, From L, Kahn HJ [1995] Bcl-2 protein expression in melanocytic neoplasms of the skin. *Mod Pathol* 8:150-154.

Rao AV, Schmader K [2007] Monoclonal antibodies as targeted therapy in hematologic malignancies in older adults. *Am J Geriatr Pharmacother* 5:247-262.

Rassidakis GZ, Georgakis GV, Oyarzo M, et al [2004] Lack of c-kit (CD117) expression in CD30+ lymphomas and lymphomatoid papulosis. *Mod Pathol* 17:946-953.

Ravetch JV, Perussia G [1989] Alternative membrane forms of Fc gamma RIII (CD16) on human natural killer cells and neutrophils: Cell type-specific expression of two genes that differ in single nucleotide substitutions. *J Exp Med* 170:481-497.

Rawstron A, Barrans S, Blythe D, et al [1999] Distribution of myeloma plasma cells in peripheral blood and BM correlates with CD56 expression. *Br J Haematol* 104:138-143.

Reading CL, Estey EH, Huh YO, et al [1993] Expression of unusual immunophenotype combinations in acute myelogenous leukemia. *Blood* 81:3083-3090.

Reed JC, Meister L, Tanaka S, Cuddy M, Yum S, Geyer C, Pleasure D [1991] Differential expression of bcl-2 protooncogene in neuroblastoma and other human tumor cell lines of neural origin. *Cancer Res* 51:6529-6538.

Robertson MJ, Ritz J [1990] Biology and clinical relevance of human natural killer cells. *Blood* 76:2421-2438.

Robins BA, Ellison DJ, Spinosa JC, et al [1993] Diagnostic application of two-color flow cytometry in 161 cases of hairy cell leukemia. *Blood* 82:1277-1287.

Robinson J, Sieff C, Deila D, et al [1981] Expression of cell-surface HLA-DR, HLA-ABC and glycophorin during erythroid differentiation. *Nature* 289:68-71.

Roholl PJM, Kleyne J, Prins MEF, et al [1988] Immunologic marker analysis of normal and malignant histiocytes: A comparative study of monoclonal antibodies for diagnostic purposes. *Am J Clin Pathol* 89:187-194.

Rovelli A, Biondi A, Rajnoldi AC, et al [1992] Microgranular variant of acute promyelocytic leukemia in children. *J Clin Oncol* 10:1413-1418.

Rowden G, Lewis MG, Sullivan AK [1977] Ia antigen expression on human epidermal Langerhans cells. *Nature* 268:247-248.

Ruiz P, Mailhot S, Delgado P [1998] CD26 expression and dipeptidyl peptidase IV activity in an aggressive hepatosplenic T-cell lymphoma. *Cytometry* 34:30-35.

Ruiz-Argüelles GJ, San Miguel JF [1994] Cell surface markers in multiple myeloma. *Mayo Clin Proc* 69:684-690.

Sabah M, Cummins R, Leader M, et al [2007] Immunoreactivity of p53, Mdm2, p21(WAF1/CIP1) Bcl-2, and Bax in soft tissue sarcomas: Correlation with histologic grade. *Appl Immunohistchem Mol Morphol* 15:64-69.

Saenz-Santamaría MC, Reed JA, McNutt NS, et al [1994] Immunohistochemical expression of bcl-2 in melanomas and intradermal nevi. *J Cutan Pathol* 21:393-397.

Sahara N, Takeshita A, Shigeno K, et al. Clinicopathological and prognostic characteristics of CD56-negative multiple myeloma. *Br J Haematol* 2002;117:882-885.

San Miguel JF, González M, Gascón A, et al [1991] Immunophenotypic heterogeneity of multiple myeloma: Influence on the biology and clinical course of the disease. *Br J Haematol* 77:185-190.

San Miguel JF, Vidriales MB, Ocio E, et al [2003] Immunophenotypic analysis of Waldenström macroglobulinemia. *Semin Oncol* 30:187-195.

Sanchez-Madrid F, Nagy JA, Robbins E, et al [1983] A human leukocyte differentiation antigen family with distinct α-subunits and a common β-subunit; The lymphocyte function-associated antigen (LFA-1), the C3bi complement receptor (OKM1/Mac-1), and the p150,95 molecule. *J Exp Med* 158:1785-1803.

Sarlomo-Rikala M, Kovatich AJ, Barusevicius A, et al [1998] CD117: A sensitive marker for gastrointestinal stromal tumors that is more specific that CD34. *Mod Pathol* 11:728-734.

Savaşan S, Buck S, Raimondi SC, et al [2006] CD36 (thrombospondin receptor) expression in childhood acute megakaryoblastic leukemias: In vitro drug sensitivity and outcome. *Leuk Lymphoma* 47:2076-2083.

Schlette E, Medeiros LJ, Keating M, Lai R [2003] CD79b expression in chronic lymphocytic leukemia. Association with trisomy 12 and atypical immunophenotype. *Arch Pathol Lab Med* 127:561-566.

Schmidt RE, Perussia B [1989] Cluster report: CD16. In Knapp W, Dörken B, Gilks WR, et al, eds. *Leukocyte Typing IV: White Cell Differentiation Antigens*. New York: Oxford University Press, 574-578.

Schriever F, Freedman AS, Freeman G, et al [1989] Isolated human follicular dendritic cells display a unique antigenic phenotype. *J Exp Med* 169:2043-2058.

Schroers R, Pukrop T, Durig J, et al [2004] B-cell chronic lymphocytic leukemia with aberrant CD8 expression: Genetic and immunophenotypic analysis of prognostic factors. *Leukemia and Lymphoma* 45:1677-1681.

Schwartig R, Stein H, Wang CY [1985] The monoclonal antibodies α-S-HCL1 (α-Leu-14) and α-S-HCL3 (α-LeuM5) allow the diagnosis of hairy cell leukemia. *Blood* 65;974-983.

Schwarting R, Gerdes J, Dürkop H, et al [1989] Ber-H2: A new anti-Ki-1 (CD30) monoclonal antibody directed at a formol-resistant epitope. *Blood* 74:1678-1689.

Schwarting R, Stein H [1989] Cluster report: CD71. In Knapp W, Dorken B, Gilks WR, et al, eds. *Leucocyte Typing IV: White Cell Differentiation Antigens*. New York: Oxford University Press, 455-460.

Scott AA, Head DR, Kopecky KJ, et al [1994] HLA-DR−CD33+CD56+CD16− myeloid/natural killer cell acute leukemia: A recently unrecognized form of acute leukemia potentially misdiagnosed as French-American-British acute myeloid leukemia-M3. *Blood* 84:244-255.

Shattil SJ, Hoxie JA, Cunningham M, Brass L [1985] Changes in the platelet membrane glycoprotein IIb-IIIa complex during platelet activation. *J Biol Chem* 260:11107-11114.

Sheibani K, Winberg CD, Burke JS, et al [1987] Lymphoblastic lymphoma expressing natural killer cell-associated antigens: A clinicopathologic study of six cases. *Leuk Res* 11:371-377.

Skinnider BF, Horsman DE, Dupuis B, Gascoyne RD [1999] Bcl-6 and Bcl-2 protein expression in diffuse large B-cell lymphoma and follicular lymphoma: Correlation with 3q27 and 18q21 chromosomal abnormalities. *Human Pathol* 30:803-808.

Smith FO, Lampkin BC, Versteeg C, et al [1992] Expression of lymphoid-associated cell surface antigens by childhood acute myeloid leukemia cells lacks prognostic significance. *Blood* 79:2415-2422.

Smithey BE, Pappo AS, Hill DA [2002] C-kit expression in pediatric solid tumors: A comparative immunohistochemical study. *Am J Surg Pathol* 26:486-492.

Sokolowska-Wojdylo M, Wenzel J, Gaffal E, et al [2005] Absence of CD26 expression on skin-homing CLA+CD4+ T lymphocytes in peripheral blood is a highly sensitive marker for early diagnosis and therapeutic monitoring of patients with Sézary syndrome. *Clin Exp Dermatol* 30:702-706.

Solvason N, Kearny JF [1992] The human fetal omentum: A site of B cell generation. *J Exp Med* 175:397-404.

Stain C, Jager U, Majdic O, et al [1987] The phenotyping of human basophils with the myeloid workshop panel. In: McMichael AJ, Beverley PCL, Cobbold S, et al, eds. *Leukocyte Typing III: White Cell Differentiation Antigens*.Oxford: Oxford University Press, 720-722.

Stefanato CM, Tallini G, Crotty PL [1998] Histologic and immunophenotypic features prior to transformation in patients with transformed cutaneous T-cell lymphoma: Is CD25 expression in skin biopsy samples predictive of large cell transformation in cutaneous T-cell lymphoma? *Am J Dermatopathol* 20:1-6.

Steinman RM [1991] The dendritic cell system and its role in immunogenicity. *Annu Rev Immunol* 9:271-296.

Stetler-Stevenson M, Arthur DC, Jabbour N, Xie XY, Molidrem J, Barrett AJ, et al [2001] Diagnostic utility of flow cytometric immunophenotyping in myelodysplastic syndrome. *Blood* 98:979-987.

Stoll M, Dalchau R, Schmidt R [1989] Cluster report: CD43. In: Knapp W, Dorken G, Gilks WR, et al, eds. *Leukocyte Typing V: White Cell Differentiation Antigens.* Oxford: Oxford University Press, 604-608.

Szabolcs P, Park KD, Reese M, et al [2003] Absolute values of dendritic cell subsets in BM, core blood, and peripheral blood enumerated by a novel method. *Stem Cells* 21:296-303.

Tamura J, Kurabayashi H, Sawamura M, et al [1989] Clinical features of common acute lymphoblastic leukemia antigen (CALLA)-positive myeloma: A report of four cases. *Blut* 58:229-233.

Tang HR, Wang FC, Jian YW, et al [2007] CD36 expression in leukemia cells checked with multiparameter flow cytometry and its significance. *Zhongguo Shi Yan Xue Ye Xue Za Zhi* 15:29-34.

Thorley-Lawson DA, Nadler LM, Bhan AK, et al [1985] BLAST-2 [EBVCS], an early surface marker of human B cell activation is superinduced by Epstein-Barr virus. *J Immunol* 134:3007-3012.

Todd RF, Nadler LM, Schlossman SF [1981] Antigens on human monocytes identified by monoclonal antibodies. *J Immunol* 126:1435-1442.

Tran-Paterson R, Boileau G, Giguère V, et al [1990] Comparative levels of CALLA/neutral endopeptidase on normal granulocytes, leukemic cells, and transfected COS-1 cells. *Blood* 76:775-782.

Trowbridge IS [1995] Overview of CD71. In: Schlossman SF, Boumsell I, Gilks WR, et al, eds. *Leukocyte Typing V: White Cell Differentiation Antigens.* New York: Oxford University Press, 1139-1141.

Tsuura Y, Hiraki H, Watanabe K, et al [1994] Preferential localization of c-kit product in tissue mast cells, basal cells of skin, epithelial cells of breast, small cell lung carcinoma and seminoma/dysgerminoma in human: Immunohistochemical study on formalin-fixed, paraffin-embedded tissues. *Virchows Arch* 424:135-141.

Tulunay O, Orhan D, Baltaci S, et al [2004] Prostatic ductal adenocarcinoma showing bcl-2 expression. *Int J Urol* 11:805-808.

Turner RR, Wood GS, Beckstead JH, et al [1984] Histiocytic malignancies: Morphologic immunologic and enzymatic heterogeneity. *Am J Surg Pathol* 8:485-500.

Uckun FM, Haissig S, Ledbetter JA, et al [1992] Developmental hierarchy during early human B-cell ontogeny after autologous BM transplantation using autografts depleted of CD19+ B-cell precursors by anti-CD19 pan-B-cell immunotoxin containing pokeweed antiviral protein. *Blood* 79:3369-3379.

Ulmer AJ, Mattern T, Flad HD [1992] Expression of CD26 (dipeptidyl peptidase IV) on memory and naïve T lymphocytes. *Scand J Immunol* 35:551-559.

van den Oord JJ, Vandeghinste N, De Ley M, et al [1994] Bcl-2 expression in human melanocytes and melanocytic tumors. *Am J Pathol* 145:294-300.

van Dogen JJM, Hooijkaas H, Comans-Bitter M, et al [1985] Human BM cells positive for terminal deoxynucleotidyl transferase (TdT), HLA-DR, and a T cell marker may represent prothymocytes. *J Immunol* 135:3144-3150.

van Dongen JJM, Krissansen GW, Wolvers-Tettero ILM, et al [1988] Cytoplasmic expression of the CD3 antigen as a diagnostic marker for immature T-cell malignancies. *Blood* 71:603-612.

van Lochem EG, van der Velden VHJ, Wind HK, et al [2004] Immunophenotypic differentiation patterns of normal hematopoiesis in human BM: Reference patterns for age-related changes and disease-induced shifts. Cytometry Part B. *Clin Cytometry* 60B:1-13.

Vannier JP, Bene MC, Faure GC, et al [1989] Investigation of the CD10 (cALLA) negative acute lymphoblastic leukaemia: Further description of a group with a poor prognosis. *Br J Haematol* 72:156-160.

Vaughan WP, Civin CI, Weisenburger DD, et al [1988] Acute leukemia expressing the normal human hematopoietic stem cell membrane glycoprotein CD34 (MY10). *Leukemia* 2:661-666.

Vega F, Chang C-C, Medeiros L, et al [2005] Plasmablastic lymphomas and plasmablastic plasma cell myelomas have nearly identical immunophenotypic profiles. *Mod Pathol* 18:806-815.

Venditti A, Del Poeta G, Buccisano F, et al [1997] Minimally differentiated acute myeloid leukemia (AML-M0): Comparison of 25 cases with other French-American-British subtypes. *Blood* 89:621-629.

Venkitaraman AR, Williams GT, Dariavich P, et al [1997] The B-cell antigen receptor of the five immunoglobulin classes. *Nature* 352:777-781.

von dem Borne AEGKR, Modderman PW [1989a] Cluster report: CD41. In: Knapp W, Dörken B, Gilks WR, et al, eds. *Leucocyte Typing IV: White Cell Differentiation Antigens.* New York: Oxford University Press; 997-999.

von dem Borne AEGKR, Modderman PW, Admiraal LG, Nieuwenhuis KH [1989b] Platelet antibodies, the overall results. In: Knapp W, Dörken B, Gilks WR, et al, eds. *Leucocyte Typing IV: White Cell Differentiation Antigens*. New York: Oxford University Press; 950-966.

Vos JA, Abbondanzo SL, Barekman CL, et al [2005] Histiocytic sarcoma: A study of five cases including the histiocyte marker CD163. *Mod Pathol* 18:693-704.

Weisberger J, Cornfield D, Gorczyca W, et al [2003] Down-regulation of pan-T-cell antigens, particularly CD7, in acute infectious mononucleosis. *Am J Clin Pathol* 120:49-55.

Weistner A, Rosenwald A, Barry TS, et al [2003] ZAP-70 expression identifies a chronic lymphocytic leukemia subtype with unmutated immunoglobulin genes, inferior clinical outcome, and distinct gene expression profile. *Blood* 101:4944-4951.

Wells DA, Benesch M, Loken MR, et al [2003] Myeloid and monocytic dyspoiesis as determined by flow cytometric scoring in myelodysplastic syndrome correlates with the IPSS and with outcome after hematopoietic stem cell transplantation. *Blood* 102:394-403.

West KP, Warford A, Fray L, et al [1986] The demonstration of B-cell, T-cell and myeloid antigens in paraffin sections. *J Pathol* 150:89-101.

Wheaton S, Netser J, Guinee D, Rahn M, Perkins S [1998] Bcl-2 and bax protein expression in indolent vs aggressive B-cell non-Hodgkin's lymphomas. *Hum Pathol* 29:820-825.

Wijdenes J, Vouijs WC, Clement C, et al [1996] A plasmocyte selective monoclonal antibody (B-B4) recognizes syndecan-1. *Br J Hematol* 94:318-323.

Wijdenes J, Clément C, Klein B, et al [1998] CD138 (syndecan-1) workshop panel report. In: Kishimoto T, Kikutani H, von dem Borne AEGKr, et al, eds. *Leukocyte Typing VI: White Cell Differentiation Antigens*. New York: Garland Publishing, 249-252.

Winchester RJ, Wang CY, Halper JP, et al [1976] Studies with B-cell allo- and heteroantisera: Parallel reactivity and special properties. *Scand J Immunol* 5:745-757.

Winchester RJ, Ross GD, Jarowski CI, et al [1977] Expression of Ia-like antigen molecules on human granulocytes during early phases of differentiation. *Proc Natl Acad Sci USA* 74:4012-4016.

Winchester RJ, Meyers PA, Broxmeyer HE, et al [1978] Inhibition of human erythropoietic colony formation in culture by treatment with Ia antisera. *J Exp Med* 148:613-618.

Wood BL, Arroz M, Barnett D, et al [2007] 2006 Bethesda International Concensus recommendations on the immunophenotypic analysis of hematolymphoid neoplasia by flow cytometry: Optimal reagents and reporting for the flow cytometric diagnosis of hematopoietic neoplasia. *Clinical Cytometry* 72B:S14-S22.

Wormsley SB, Baird SM, Gadol N, et al [1990] Characteristics of CD11c+ CD5+ chronic B cell leukemias and the identification of novel peripheral blood B cell subsets with chronic lymphoid leukemia immunophenotypes. *Blood* 76:123-130.

Wu JM, Borowitz MJ, Weir EG [2006] The usefulness of CD71 expression by flow cytometry for differentiating indolent from aggressive CD10+ B-cell lymphomas. *Am J Clin Pathol* 126:39-46.

Yamaoka KA, Arock M, Issaly F, et al [1996] Granulocyte macrophage colony stimulating factor induces Fc epsilon RII/CD23 expression on normal human polymorphonuclear neutrophils. *Int Immunol* 8:479-490.

Yang J, Liu X, Bhalla K, Kim CN, Ibrado AM, Cai J, Peng T, Jones DP, Wang X [1997] Prevention of apoptosis by Bcl-2: Release of cytochrome c from mitochondria blocked. *Science* 275:1129-1132.

Yu DTY, Winchester RJ, Fu SM, et al [1980] Peripheral blood Ia-positive T cells. Increase in certain diseases and after immunization. *J Exp Med* 151:91-100.

Zelenznikova T, Stevulova L, Kovarikova A, et al [2007] Increased myeloid precursors in regenerating BM; implications for detection of minimal residual disease in acute myeloid leukemia. *Neoplasma* 54:471-477.

Zhang M, Zhang Z, Goldman CK, et al [2005] Combination therapy for adult T-cell leukemia-xenografted mice: Flavopiridol and anti-CD25 monoclonal antibody. *Blood* 105:1231-1236.

Ziegler-Heitbrok HWL, Passlick B, Flieger D [1988] The monoclonal antimonocyte antibody My4 stains B lymphocytes and two distinct monocyte subsets in human peripheral blood. *Hybridoma* 7:521-527.

Zola H [1987] The surface antigens of human B lymphocytes. *Immunol Today* 8:308-315.

5 Normal vs Abnormal FCI Findings: Peripheral Blood, Body Fluids, Bone Marrow, and Lymph Node

Chapter Contents

Introduction

Flow cytometric immunophenotyping (FCI) is a useful tool in diagnostic hematopathology. It is primarily based on the analysis of surface marker expression on cells that defines their immunophenotype and origin. Distinct cell populations are first defined by their size (forward light scatter properties) and granularity (side light scatter properties). Forward light scatter evaluates cell size. Small to medium-sized cells include lymphocytes and the most mature erythroid precursors; medium-sized to large cells include monocytes and neutrophils [f5.1]. Hematogones, or B-lymphocyte precursors, are relatively small cells; plasma cells may vary from small/medium to large; blasts (lymphoid and myeloid) are generally medium-sized to large; and nonhematopoietic cells are generally large to very large [f5.1]. Side light scatter is based on the "reflectivity" of internal cell components and, thus, measures cytoplasmic complexity or granularity. Lymphocytes are the least complex cells, followed by hematogones and erythroid precursors. The most granular cells are neutrophils (granulocytes) and eosinophils. Monocytes reside in the middle. Blasts may vary from low cytoplasmic granularity (generally lymphoblasts) to medium complexity (generally myeloblasts, depending on their morphology) [f5.2]. Of interest, some highly granular cells (ie, mast cells and basophils) will actually absorb light (instead of reflecting light) and appear with low side light scatter.

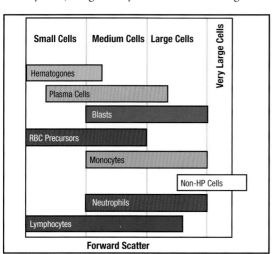

[f5.1] Cell size vs forward light scatter. From left to right on this axis, cell size increases. Small cells, such as lymphocytes and the most mature erythroid precursors, are on the left. Moderate to large cells include monocytes, neutrophils, as well as lymphocytes. Hematogones, or B-lymphocyte precursors, will be small cells with a size that overlaps the lymphocyte population. Plasma cells may vary in size from small/medium to large, which could correlate with the degree of differentiation. Blasts (both lymphoblasts and myeloblasts) are medium to a larger size. Finally, non-hematopoietic cells are generally much larger than hematopoietic cells, although there may be some overlap with other large hematopoietic cells.

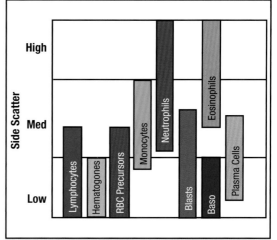

[f5.2] Cell cytoplasmic granularity/complexity vs side light scatter: From left to right on this axis, cell cytoplasmic complexity/ granularity increases. Cells with low side scatter, and low cytoplasmic complexity, would include most lymphocytes, hematogones, erythroid precursors. Lymphoblasts would generally have low side scatter, while myeloid leukemias would have either low or moderate, depending on the morphology of the blasts. Monocytes sit in the middle and more granularity seems to indicate more "activation." Finally, as mentioned previously, basophils have numerous granules, but these absorb rather than reflect light, so have low side scatter.

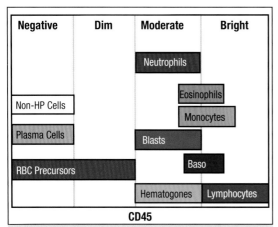

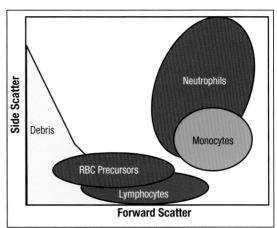

[f5.3] Degree of CD45 expression. From left to right on this axis, CD45 expression increases in intensity. CD45 is a surface marker that is present to varying degrees on almost all hematopoietic cells. Lymphocytes have the highest degree of CD45 positivity. There is an overlap in the intensity of CD45 expression of hematogones, lymphoblasts, myeloblasts, and neutrophils. Erythroid precursors start with brighter CD45 expression and lose it as they mature. Non-malignant plasma cells are CD45 negative and non-hematopoietic cells, such as stromal cells or carcinoma cells, are also negative. Blasts may dimly express CD45 or be CD45–, particularly lymphoblasts.

[f5.4] An integrated diagram of an idealized bone marrow scatter pattern evaluating forward vs side scatter demonstrates that lymphocytes are generally small to medium-sized with low side scatter; neutrophils are moderate to large in size with moderate to high levels of side scatter.

Expression of CD45 may also be useful in characterizing cells by flow cytometry. Lymphocytes have the highest degree of CD45 expression. There may be an overlap in the degree of CD45 expression by hematogones, blasts (lymphoid and myeloid), and neutrophils (all with moderate intensity). However, blasts may occasionally dimly express CD45 or be CD45– (particularly lymphoblasts). Erythroid precursors may initially dimly express CD45, but become CD45– as they mature. Nonmalignant plasma cells and nonhematopoietic cells are CD45– [f5.3].

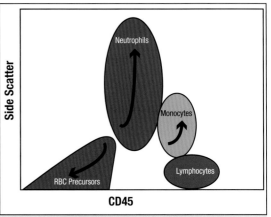

[f5.5] An integrated diagram of an idealized bone marrow demonstrating CD45 expression vs side scatter. Lymphocytes have the highest degree of CD45 with low levels of side scatter. Neutrophils have moderate CD45 expression and moderate to high levels of side scatter. As they mature, the granularity tends to increase. Monocytes tend to lie between lymphocytes and neutrophils. As they mature or become activated, they generally increase in side scatter. Erythroid precursors start out somewhat larger with moderate to low levels of CD45 expression. As they mature, they decrease in size and lose CD45 positivity.

Patterns of Light Scatter and CD45 Expression

Normal Bone Marrow

An integrated diagram of an idealized bone marrow (BM) scatter pattern, plotting forward vs side light scatter [f5.4], reveals lymphocytes and erythroid precursors in the region with low forward light scatter and low side light scatter; monocytes with moderate to marked forward light scatter and low to moderate side light scatter; and neutrophils with moderate to marked forward and side light scatter. A diagram of CD45 expression vs side light scatter [f5.5] reveals erythroid precursors with low side light scatter and decreasing CD45 expression with maturity; lymphocytes, low side light scatter and strong expression of CD45; monocytes with low to moderate side light scatter and increasing CD45 expression with maturity/activation; and neutrophils with moderate CD45 expression and moderate to high levels of side light scatter.

Some cell populations in normal BM may appear increased in reactive conditions (ie, plasma cells, hematogones, eosinophils, and basophils). They would appear in the regions depicted in the diagram of side

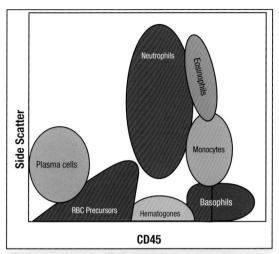

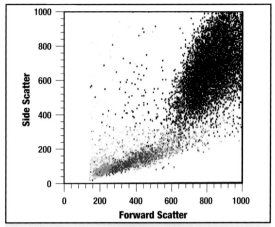

[f5.6] Same diagram as [f5.5] with overlaid rare "normal" populations. These are cells that are present in significant amounts in only some, but not all marrows. When they are increased in reactive conditions, they can often present confusing populations for evaluation. The first group is the plasma cell. These are generally CD45 negative and have low to moderate side scatter. They may be increased in a variety of reactive conditions or increased in plasma cell dyscrasias. Hematogones are benign B cell precursors that are generally small with moderate CD45 positivity and low side scatter. Finally, eosinophils and basophils are relatively rare granulocytes compared to neutrophils. They have a tendency to be slightly higher in CD45 expression than neutrophils, but basophils absorb laser light from side scatter, so they tend to fall next to lymphocytes. The have dimmer CD45 expression than lymphocytes. Mast cells have similar side scatter and CD45 properties (CD45 is moderately expressed by mast cells) to basophils.

[f5.7] Forward vs side light scatter properties of an actual normal bone marrow demonstrate lymphocytes (red), monocytes (green), and maturing myeloid cells (black).

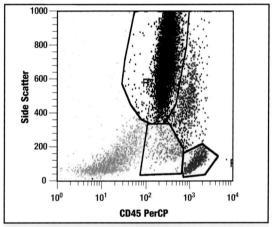

[f5.8] Side light scatter vs CD45 expression of an actual normal bone marrow demonstrates lymphocytes (red), monocytes (orange), and maturing myeloid cells (black).

light scatter vs CD45 expression [f5.6] (ie, plasma cells with no CD45 expression and low side light scatter; hematogones with moderate CD45 expression and low side light scatter; eosinophils with strong CD45 expression and high levels of side light scatter; and basophils with moderate CD45 expression but low side light scatter, as previously discussed). Actual normal patterns of BM are depicted in [f5.7] and [f5.8].

Abnormal Bone Marrow

Involvement of the BM by various lymphoid disorders may result in abnormal patterns of BM scatter plots. Involvement by chronic lymphocytic leukemia (CLL) results in marked expansion of the "lymphocyte" region with decreases in populations of cells in the "monocyte" and "granulocyte" regions [f5.9]. A similar pattern may be seen in involvement of the BM by other types of lymphoid disorders, composed predominantly of small cells. Involvement by lymphomas composed of a mixture of small and large cells or composed predominantly of large cells may result in expansions of both the "typical

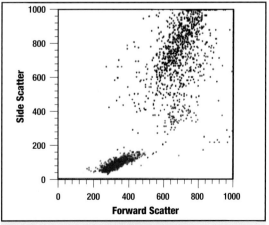

[f5.9] Pattern of chronic lymphocytic leukemia in bone marrow: side vs forward light scatter

lymphocyte" region and a "larger lymphocyte" region, characterized by higher forward light scatter (due to a larger size) and low side light scatter (due to a relatively low complexity); again, there may be decreases in the populations of cells in the "monocyte" and "granulocyte" regions **[f5.10]**. The cells of hairy cell leukemia (HCL) generally fall within a region characterized by higher forward light scatter (due to their larger size, primarily due to their more abundant cytoplasm and "hairy" projections) and slightly increased side light scatter **[f5.11]** and **[f5.12]**. In acute leukemia, there will be an increase in cells within various regions, depending on the size of the blasts, their cytoplasmic complexity, and their degree of CD45 expression. Acute lymphoblastic leukemia (ALL) usually shows a continuum of cells expanding from the small lymphocyte region to the intermediate and large cell regions, and may show decreased CD45 expression 0when compared to the CD45 expression of small lymphocytes **[f5.13]** and **[f5.14]**. Acute myeloid leukemia (AML) will often show an increase of cells within the large cell and/or monocyte region(s) **[f5.15]**. The blasts may also show decreased CD45 expression when compared to the CD45 expression of the small lymphocytes **[f5.16]**. Acute promyelocytic leukemia (APL) is often composed of hypergranular promyelocytes and blasts resulting in an expansion of the blast/promyelocyte

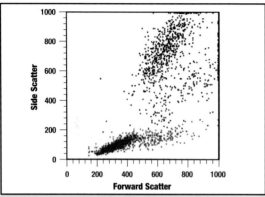

[f5.10] Pattern of follicle center cell lymphoma, mixed small and large cell type: side scatter vs CD45 expression

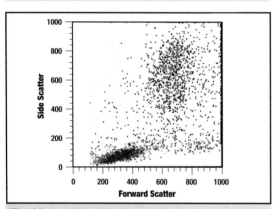

[f5.11] Pattern of chronic lymphocytic leukemia in bone marrow: side vs forward light scatter

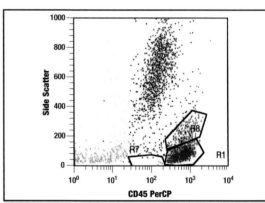

[f5.12] Pattern of hairy cell leukemia: side scatter vs CD45 expression

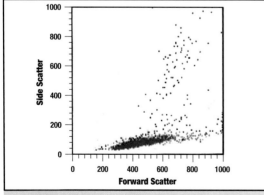

[f5.13] Pattern of acute lymphoblastic leukemia: side vs forward light scatter

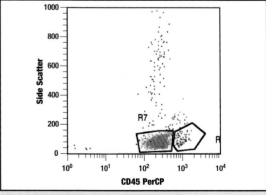

[f5.14] Pattern of acute lymphoblastic leukemia: side scatter vs CD45 expression

region [f5.17], again with possible decreased CD45 expression [f5.18]. The blasts of AML, M0 often have a very small amount of cytoplasm that is hypogranular and thus will show an expansion of cells falling within what appears to be a "larger lymphoid" region [f5.19], again showing decreased CD45 expression [f5.20].

Chronic myelomonocytic leukemia (CMML) is characterized by a prominent monocytic component and thus often shows an expansion of the monocytic region [f5.21]. Chronic myeloid leukemia (CML) is characterized by a marked increase in myeloid cells at all stages of differentiation, with the chronic phase

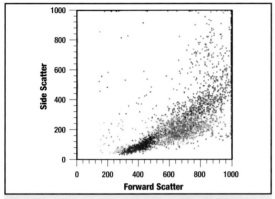

[f5.15] Pattern of acute myeloid leukemia: side vs forward light scatter

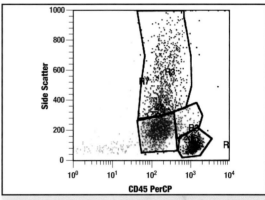

[f5.16] Pattern of acute myeloid leukemia: side scatter vs CD45 expression

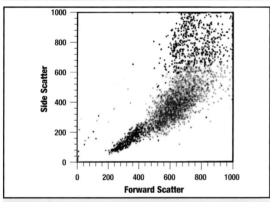

[f5.17] Pattern of acute promyelocytic leukemia: side vs forward light scatter

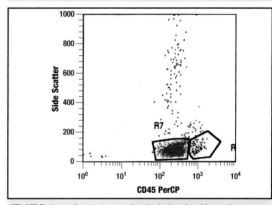

[f5.18] Pattern of acute promyelocytic leukemia: side scatter vs CD45 expression

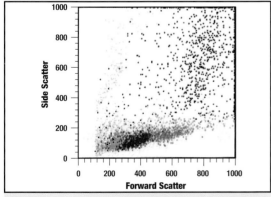

[f5.19] Pattern of acute myeloid leukemia, M0: side vs forward light scatter

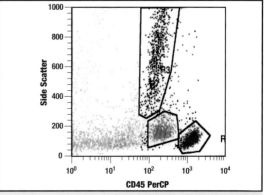

[f5.20] Pattern of acute myeloid leukemia, M0: side scatter vs CD45 expression showing <5% blasts. The remaining elements in the BM (eg, the lymphocyte region) are typically markedly depleted. Flow cytograms of myelodysplastic syndromes may show an increase of cells in the "blast" region and/or may show an increase in hypogranular myeloid cells, resulting in a shift of myeloid cells towards the region with lower side light scatter properties [f5.22]. Neoplastic plasma cells (ie, those of plasma cell myeloma [PCM]) are often stripped of their cytoplasm and do not fall within the gates of flow cytometric analysis. However, if they do survive processing, neoplastic plasma cells in BM will typically reveal an increase of cells within the region where normal plasma cells fall (ie, with low side scatter and no CD45 expression); however, one should keep in mind that neoplastic plasma cells may show dim CD45 expression. Involvement of the BM by a metastatic nonhematolymphoid malignancy may reveal an increase of cells in the CD45–, large cell (high forward light scatter) region; one should keep in mind that metastatic nonhematolymphoid malignancies may be cohesive and

may not disaggregate into single cells to pass through the flow cytometer.

Normal Lymph Node

In contrast to an idealized BM, a normal lymph node (LN) scatter pattern, plotting forward vs side light scatter [f5.23], reveals a spectrum of cells, demonstrating low to high forward light scatter and low side light scatter; the great majority of cells have low forward light scatter, representing small lymphocytes.

Abnormal Lymph Node

Abnormal scatter plots of LN may be seen in various types of lymphomatous involvement. CLL/small lymphocytic lymphoma (SLL) demonstrates a dense, distinct population of cells in the "small lymphocyte" region [f5.24]; this pattern may also be seen in B- or T-cell lymphomas composed predominantly of small lymphocytes [f5.25]. Lymphomas composed of intermediate-sized and/or large cells may demonstrate

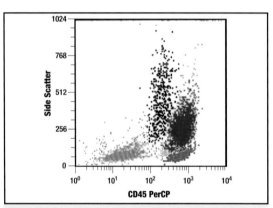

[f5.21] Pattern of chronic myelomonocytic leukemia: side scatter vs CD45 expression; green, lymphocytes; red, monocytes

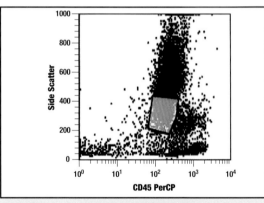

[f5.22] Pattern of myelodysplastic syndrome with increase in low-side scatter myeloid cells: side scatter vs CD45 expression

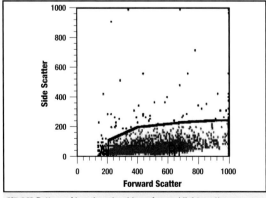

[f5.23] Pattern of lymph node: side vs forward light scatter

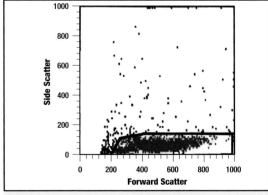

[f5.24] Pattern of small lymphocytic lymphoma: side vs forward light scatter expansions of these regions on the scatter plots of the involved LNs; they will have varying degrees of forward light scatter (dependent on their size) and low side light scatter [f5.26] and [f5.27]. Nodal involvement by granulocytic sarcoma will reveal an increase of cells characterized by high forward light scatter (large size) and variable side light scatter, depending on the granularity within their cytoplasm and variable degrees of CD45 expression, similar to myeloblasts of AML [f5.28] and [f5.29].

Normal Peripheral Blood

Normal peripheral blood reveals a white blood cell (WBC) count in the range of $4.5\text{-}6.2 \times 10^3/\text{mm}^3$ ($4.5\text{-}6.2 \times 10^9/\text{L}$) with 43%-58% neutrophils and 30%-35% lymphocytes [Bain 1996].

Abnormal Peripheral Blood

Involvement of the peripheral blood by CLL, HCL, ALL, AML, CML, CMML, and MDS would show similar patterns to those depicted of BM. Both B- and

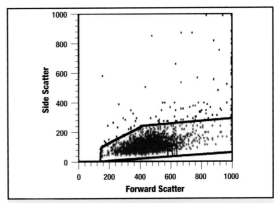

[f5.25] Pattern of peripheral T-cell lymphoma composed of predominantly small lymphocytes: side vs forward light scatter

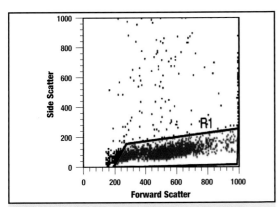

[f5.26] Pattern of peripheral T-cell lymphoma composed of predominantly intermediate-sized lymphocytes: side vs forward light scatter

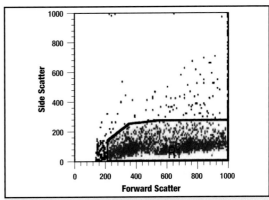

[f5.27] Pattern of diffuse large B-cell lymphoma: side vs forward light scatter

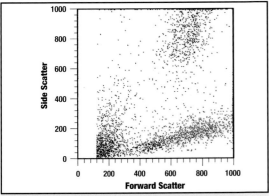

[f5.28] Pattern of granulocytic sarcoma: side vs forward light scatter

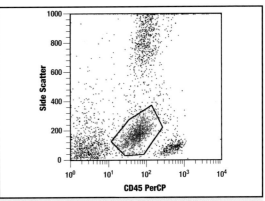

[f5.29] Pattern of granulocytic sarcoma: side scatter vs CD45 expression

T-cell NHLs may peripheralize. Examples are shown of involvement of the peripheral blood by classical mantle cell lymphoma (MCL) and the blastoid variant of MCL [f5.30] [f5.31] and [f5.32] [f5.33] respectively.

"Negative" Body Fluids

Since accumulation of fluid in pleural, ascitic, or pericardial sites is always abnormal, they will be referred to as "negative," rather than "normal," if nonneoplastic. Negative body fluids (ie, pleural, ascitic, and pericardial fluids) contain approximately 75% macrophages, 23% lymphocytes, and marginally present mesothelial cells, neutrophils, and eosinophils [Noppen 2004]. Negative cerebrospinal fluid (CSF) contains only a few lymphocytes. These are the only cells observed in a "negative" CSF, unless there is peripheral blood contamination.

Abnormal Body Fluids

Obviously, all of these above-described body cavities may be involved by various lymphomas and acute leukemias. The applications of flow cytometric immunophenotyping to body fluids will be covered in detail in Chapter 20. Dot plot patterns of forward light scatter vs side light scatter and forward light scatter vs CD45 expression reflect the type of hematolymphoid neoplasm involving the particular body fluid. Examples are shown of involvement of various body fluids by MCL (pleural fluid [f5.34] [f5.35]), large B-cell lymphoma (ascitic fluid [f5.36] [f5.37]), Burkitt lymphoma (pleural fluid [f5.38] [f5.39]), ALL (CSF [f5.40] [f5.41]), and AML (CSF [f5.42] [f5.43]).

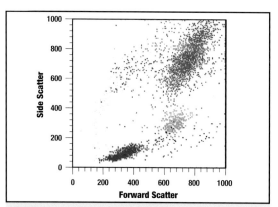

[f5.30] Pattern of mantle cell lymphoma: side vs forward light scatter. The classical mantle cell lymphoma shows an expanded lymphocyte region.

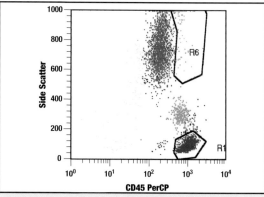

[f5.31] Pattern of mantle cell lymphoma: side scatter vs CD45 expression. The classical mantle cell lymphoma shows an expanded lymphocyte region.

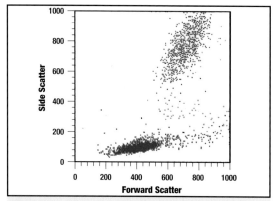

[f5.32] Pattern of blastoid variant of mantle cell lymphoma: side vs forward light scatter. The blastoid variant of mantle cell lymphoma shows an expanded region including small and larger lymphoid forms.

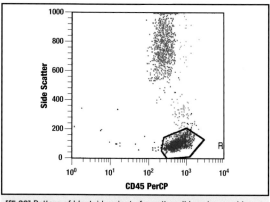

[f5.33] Pattern of blastoid variant of mantle cell lymphoma: side scatter vs CD45 expression. The blastoid variant of mantle cell lymphoma shows an expanded region including small and larger lymphoid forms.

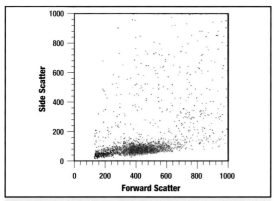

[f5.34] Pattern of mantle cell lymphoma involvement of pleural fluid: side vs forward light scatter.

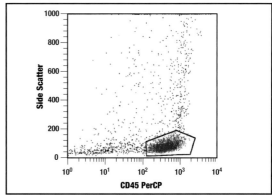

[f5.35] Pattern of mantle cell lymphoma involvement of pleural fluid: side scatter vs CD45 expression.

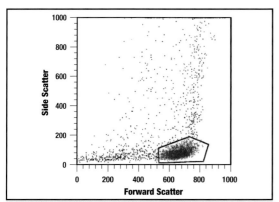

[f5.36] Pattern of large B-cell lymphoma involvement of ascitic fluid: side vs forward light scatter.

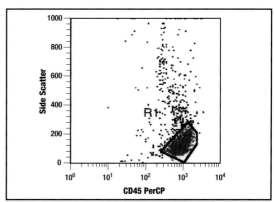

[f5.37] Pattern of large B-cell lymphoma involvement of ascitic fluid: side scatter vs CD45 expression.

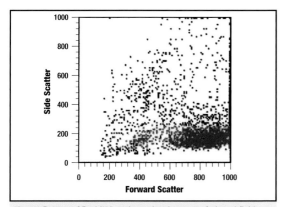

[f5.38] Pattern of Burkitt lymphoma involvement of pleural fluid: side vs forward light scatter.

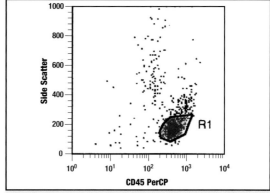

[f5.39] Pattern of Burkitt lymphoma involvement of pleural fluid: side scatter vs CD45 expression.

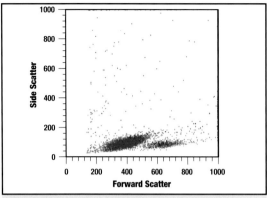

[f5.40] Pattern of acute lymphoblastic leukemia lymphoma involvement of cerebrospinal fluid: side vs forward light scatter

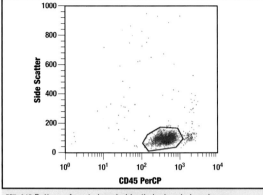

[f5.41] Pattern of acute lymphoblastic leukemia lymphoma involvement of cerebrospinal fluid: side scatter vs CD45 expression

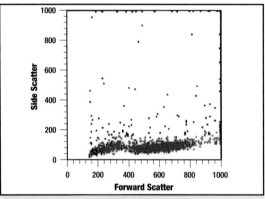

[f5.42] Pattern of acute myeloid leukemia lymphoma involvement of cerebrospinal fluid: side vs forward light scatter

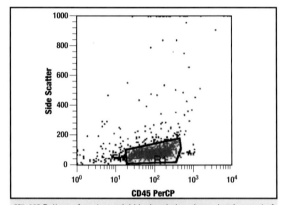

[f5.43] Pattern of acute myeloid leukemia lymphoma involvement of cerebrospinal fluid: side scatter vs CD45 expression

Patterns of Antigen Expression

"Normal Cells" and "Normal Reactive Cells" vs "Abnormal Counterparts"

Definitions of antigen expression

The recommended descriptions of antibody distribution are *negative*, *positive*, or *partially expressed*, and are relative to an appropriate negative control population. The recommended descriptions of antibody fluorescence intensity are *dim*, *bright*, and *heterogeneous*, with the intensity relative to the closest normal hematolymphoid population [Wood 2007].

Hematogones and Blasts of Precursor B-Cell Lymphoblastic Leukemia

Hematogones (B-lymphocyte precursors), originally recognized by their morphologic features in BM smears, may occur in large numbers in some healthy infants and young children and in a variety of diseases in both children and adults. Hematogones may be particularly prominent in the regeneration phase following chemotherapy or BM transplantation and in patients with autoimmune and congenital cytopenias, neoplasms, and acquired immunodeficiency syndrome (AIDS). In some instances, they may constitute 5% to more than 50% of cells in the BM. In particular, increased numbers of hematogones may cause problems in diagnosis, due to the morphologic features they commonly share with the neoplastic lymphoblasts of ALL and lymphoblastic lymphoma. Their immunophenotype also has features in common with neoplastic B-cell precursor lymphoblasts [t5.1] [t5.2]. Although single- and 2-color flow cytometry do not reliably differentiate hematogones from leukemic lymphoblasts, appropriately applied 3- and 4-color multiparametric flow cytometry are reported to distinguish between these cell populations in nearly all instances [f5.44] [f5.45] [f5.46] [McKenna 2001]. Hematogones always exhibit a typical complex spectrum of antigen expression that defines

t5.1 Normal Maturational Sequence of Bone Marrow Hematogones

Hematogones				Mature B-Cells
Increasing maturation →				
TdT				
CD34				
CD10 (brt)	CD10	CD10	CD10	
CD19	CD19	CD19	CD19	CD19
CD22 (dm)	CD22 (dm)	CD22 (dm)	CD22 (dm)	CD22
CD38 (brt)	CD38 (brt)	CD38 (brt)	CD38 (brt)	CD38 (brt/–)
		CD20 (dm)	CD20	CD20
		sIg	sIg	sIg

t5.2 Immunophenotypes of B-Lineage Lymphoblastic Leukemias

Early Pre-B	Pre-B	Mature B (Burkitt)
CD19+, CD20–	CD19+, CD20+	CD19+, CD20–
CD24+	CD24+	CD24+
CD10±	CD10±	Intense CD10
sIg/light chain –	sIg/light chain –	sIg/light chain +
TdT+	TdT+	TdT–

brt, bright; dm, dim; sIg, surface immunoglobulin

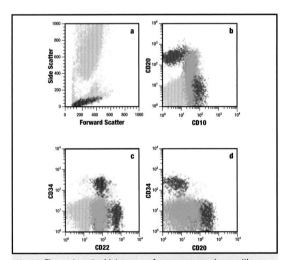

[f5.44] Flow cytometry histograms of a marrow specimen with increased hematogones. The histograms illustrate the normal pattern of maturation of B-lymphocyte precursors (hematogones) with the 4-color antibody combination of CD10, CD20, CD22, and CD34. Violet indicates early-stage hematogones; green, intermediate and late-stage hematogones; and blue, mature B cells (reprinted with permission from [McKenna 2001]).

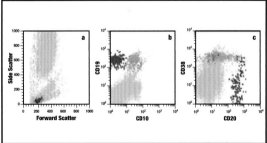

[f5.45] Flow cytometry histograms of a marrow specimen with increased hematogones. The histograms illustrate the normal pattern of maturation of B-lymphocyte precursors (hematogones) with the 4-color antibody combination of CD10, CD20, CD19, and CD38. The CD10-CD20 histogram was similar to the one illustrated in [f5.44]. Violet indicates early-stage hematogones; green, intermediate and late-stage hematogones; blue, mature B cells (reprinted with permission from [McKenna 2001]).

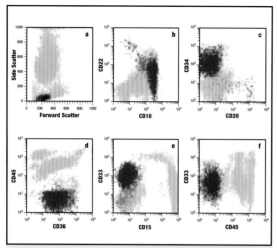

[f5.46] Flow cytometry histograms of bone marrow from a patient with relapse of precursor B-acute lymphoblastic leukemia illustrating multiple antigenic aberrancies. The lymphoblasts (red) exhibit an abnormal spectrum of expression of CD22 and overexpression of CD10 relative to the normal hematogone population (violet). They are uniformly CD34+ and negative for CD20 and CD45. The lymphoblasts express the myeloid-associated antigens CD36 and CD33 and underexpress CD38. Red indicates neoplastic lymphoblasts; violet, hematogones; and blue, mature B lymphocytes.

the normal antigenic evolution of B-cell precursors and lacks aberrant expression [f5.44] [f5.45]. In contrast, lymphoblasts in precursor B-ALL show maturation arrest, according to their stage [t5.2], and exhibit varying numbers of immunophenotypic aberrancies (eg, expression of CD13, CD33) [f5.46] [McKenna 2001].

Mature B Cells

Aberrant T-cell antigen expression

Aberrant CD5 expression is characteristic of SLL/CLL and MCL. However, one should keep in mind there is a significant population of CD5+ B cell subsets that exist in human B cell ontogeny during fetal development (ie, fetal spleen, fetal BM, and fetal liver B lineage lymphoid cells). In addition, CD5+ B cells may exist as minor populations in adult spleens in post-BM transplantation settings [Valente 1990, Waddick 1993].

Aberrant expression of CD8 has also been described in CLL [Koelliker 1994]. In addition, expression of aberrant T-cell markers by FCI, particularly CD2 and CD7, has been demonstrated to be associated with significantly shortened overall survival and increased aggressiveness [Kampalath 2003].

Other authors have also reported aberrant expression of CD5 on diffuse large cell lymphoma as well as diffuse mixed lymphoma, and CD2 and CD7 expressions in 5% and 2% of B-NHLs, respectively [Inaba 2000].

Clonality

Clonality is defined as a κ:λ ratio of >3:1 or <1:2. However, one should keep in mind that significant lack of surface light chain expression is also indicative of a clonal process. In a recent study by Li et al [2002], cases with >25% B cells lacking sIg light chain expression all represented malignant lymphoma. By FCI, the identified sIg light chain-negative population was distinctly separate from the normal polytypic B cells; in 90% of cases, the identified population was larger (by forward light scatter) than the reactive T cells and polytypic B cells. In their review of reactive cases, no reactive case revealed >17% sIg-negative B cells.

Benign monoclonal B-cell lymphocytoses

Very low levels of circulating monoclonal B-cell subpopulations may be detected in apparently healthy individuals using flow cytometry [Marti 2005]. The term "monoclonal B-cell lymphocytosis" has been proposed to describe this finding, although there is no evidence of lymphocytosis, and the finding is detected only by flow cytometry. Such monoclonal CD5+ and CD5– B-lymphocyte expansions are particularly frequent in the peripheral blood of the elderly [Ghia 2004]. More recently, a monoclonal B-cell lymphocytosis has been described as a clinically benign (persistent, but not progressive) clonal B-cell lymphocytosis (mild to moderate lymphocytosis) with a CD5– (non-CLL) immunophenotype. The clonal population accounts for 95%-99% of the B cells and appears to have a germinal center or post-germinal center B-lymphocyte origin. In addition, clonal cytogenetic aberrations have been described in the majority of cases. Such cases likely represent an intermediate condition between covert clonal expansions and overt malignancy [Amato 2007].

Plasma Cells

As discussed previously, normal plasma cells are CD45–. In addition, they do not express any B-cell associated antigens, surface light chains, or CD56, but do express CD138. On the other hand, neoplastic plasma cells may show dim CD45+ and dim selective surface light chain expression. In the vast majority of cases, neoplastic plasma cells are negative for the mature B-cell antigen, CD20 (ie, <⅓ show weak expression and <10% of cases show strong expression in the majority of plasma cells) [Robillard 2003, Lin 2004]. Many recent studies have correlated the "lymphoid" morphology of neoplastic plasma cells with CD20-positivity [Fonseca 2002, Hoyer 2000, Matsuda 2005]. The "lymphoid" morphology, combined with a strong expression of CD20, especially when it occurs in the majority of the neoplastic cells, may present a diagnostic pitfall, mimicking more typical CD20+ mature B-cell lymphoproliferative disorders, such as CLL/SLL, MCL, marginal zone lymphoma, follicular lymphoma, as well as lymphoplasmacytic lymphoma, which may all demonstrate variable numbers of plasmacytic and lymphoplasmacytic cells. An extended immunophenotypic panel, including CD138 for plasma cell differentiation, may be particularly informative. Strong membrane positivity with CD138 is typically present in >90% of the neoplastic cells in all morphologic variants of PCM.

CD56 expression has been evaluated in PCM with varying reports of significance and prognosis. Ely et al reported that strong CD56 expression by plasma cells correlated with a diagnosis of PCM, in comparison to reactive plasmacytoses, MGUS, or NHLs with plasmacytoid differentiation [Ely 2002]. However, Mathew et al [1995] reported that strong CD56 expression could also be seen in MGUS and did not help to distinguish MGUS from plasma cell myeloma. Likewise, Martin et al reported CD56 expression in 1 of 5 samples of polyclonal plasmacytosis [Martin 2004]. A recent study by Dunphy et al [2007] showed CD56 expression by plasma cells indicated clonality, since they were identified in PCM and lymphoplasmacytic lymphoma but not in any cases of reactive plasmacytosis. Perhaps the 1 case of polyclonal

plasmacytosis previously reported by Martin et al [2004] contained a low level clonal population of plasma cells. The presence of CD56+ plasma cells in an occasional case of MGUS most likely represents a clonal population, which will progress in time. Based on the results of Dunphy et al [2007], the presence of CD56+ plasma cells does not help distinguish PCM from MGUS or lymphoplasmacytic lymphomas, as previously reported.

Ely also demonstrated the strong expression of CD56 by plasma cells of PCM correlated with the presence of lytic bone lesions. Indeed, others have shown the lack of or weak expression of CD56 by plasma cells in PCM characterized a special subset of myeloma associated with a lower osteolytic potential and a higher tendency for circulation of the malignant plasma cells in the peripheral blood. This subset was also characterized by more extensive BM infiltration and significantly decreased OS [Waddick 1993, Koelliker 1994, Lin 2004]. Chang et al also demonstrated recently the absence of CD56 on malignant plasma cells in the cerebrospinal fluid is the hallmark of central nervous system involvement in plasma cell myeloma [Kampalath 2003].

Precursor T-Cell Lymphoblastic Lymphoma/Leukemia

The immunophenotypes of T-cell ALL are outlined in [t5.3] and are best evaluated by FCI [Keren 1994]. T-cell lymphoblastic lymphoma (T-LL) most often has an

t5.3 Immunophenotypes of T-ALL

Antigen	Pre-Thymocytes	Pre-T ALL (I) Prothymocytes	Pre-T ALL (II) Common Thymocytes	T-ALL (III) Mature Thymocytes	
				T-H	T-S
CD1	−	−	+	−	−
CD2	±	±	±	+	+
cCD3	±	+	±	−	−
sCD3	−	−	±	+	+
CD5	±	+	+	+	+
CD7	+	+	+	+	+
CD4	−	−	+	+	−
CD8	−	−	+	−	+
HLA-DR	±	−	−	−	−
CD34	±	−	−	−	−
TdT	+	+	+	+	+

ALL, acute lymphocytic leukemia; cCD3, cytoplasmic CD3; sCD3, surface CD3; T-H, helpter T cell; T-S, suppressor T cell

immunophenotype corresponding to the common thymocyte stage of ALL; the immunophenotype of thymoma is identical to this stage. In addition, it should be noted that T-cell lymphoblastic lymphoma/leukemia and thymoma may also aberrantly express CD10 [Nakajima 2000]. However, FCI allows for the distinction between thymoma and T-LL. FCI features characteristic of thymoma include a smear pattern of CD4/CD8 co-expression **[f5.47a]**, a smear pattern of CD3 and TdT expression **[f5.47b]**, and lack of T-cell antigen deletion (with the exception of partial CD3). In contrast, T-LL shows much more variability in expression patterns and is characterized by a tight pattern of CD4/CD8 expression **[f5.47c]**, significant T-cell antigen deletion, and absence of the CD3 or TdT smear pattern **[f5.47d]** [Cessna 2002]. In addition, distinguishing between thymoma and T-LL must always also rely on correlation of the FCI data with the morphology.

Mature T Cells

Normal mature T cells show expression of the pan T-cell antigens, CD2, CD3, CD5, and CD7. The normal CD4:CD8 ratio is between 1 and 4. Mature T-cell lymphomas may have variable immunophenotypes by FCI. There may be variable loss of a pan T-cell antigen (ie, CD2, CD3, CD5, or CD7). Most cases are CD4+, and some are CD8+, CD4–/CD8–, or CD4+/CD8+.

Mature (and immature) T-cell lymphomas/leukemias may rarely aberrantly express the mature B-cell marker, CD20 as well as CD10. CD20+ T-cell lymphoma/leukemia is rare and the clinical significance is uncertain [Yokose 2001, Buckner 2007]. However, it is important to recognize this entity, in order to avoid potential diagnostic pitfalls, and to consider possible treatment with rituximab in this entity. A representative case is demonstrated in **[f5.48]**, with listmode data available on the accompanying disk. There is, in addition, a rare primary CD20+CD10+CD8+ T-cell lymphoma of the skin that has been described with IgH and TCR β gene rearrangements [Magro 2006]. This-ty may represent the malignant counterpart of a benign population of weakly CD20+ T cells of the CD8 subset. CD10-positivity has also been described in other peripheral T-cell lymphomas, particularly in angioimmunoblastic T-cell lymphoma, but also in occasional cases of peripheral T-cell lymphoma, unspecified. In fact, a small number of CD10+ T cells in reactive LNs may represent the normal counterpart of the neoplastic T cells in these peripheral T-cell lymphomas [Stacchini 2007].

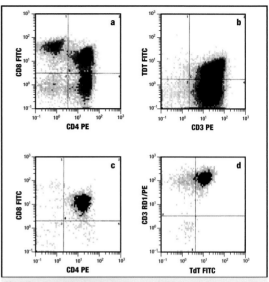

[f5.47] a, Smear pattern of CD4 (x-axis)/CD8 (y-axis) characteristic of thymoma; **b**, smear pattern of TdT (y-axis)/CD3 (x-axis) characteristic of thymoma; **c**, tight pattern of CD4 (x-axis)/CD8 (y-axis) characteristic of T-cell lymphoblastic lymphoma; **d**, tight pattern of TdT (x-axis)/CD3 (y-axis) characteristic of T-cell lymphoblastic lymphoma.

Large Granular Lymphocytes

Large granular lymphocytes (LGLs) may be of natural killer (NK) cell or T-cell lineage [Loughran 1993]. Most LGLs are NK cells (ie, CD2+, CD7+, CD3-, CD5-, CD4-, heterogeneous expression of low density CD8, CD16+, CD56+, and CD57+). CD3+ LGLs (associated with CD8 expression) represent a minor component of normal blood cells. The definition of LGL leukemia is a chronic clonal proliferation of LGL >2 × 10^9/L and persistent for 6 months. Neoplastic entities associated with this proliferation include: NK-cell expansion, NK-LGL leukemia (NK-LGLL), and T-LGL leukemia (T-LGLL) [Zambello 1993, Semenzato 1997]. Chronic NK-cell expansions and T-LGLL have a more chronic, indolent course than NK-LGLL. Patients with NK-LGL leukemia present at a younger age and have an acute clinical course with systemic disease. These entities must be differentiated from secondary or "reactive" LGL expansions. In secondary LGL expansions, the absolute NK-cell count rarely exceeds 2 × 10^9/L. Clonality in NK-cell processes may be defined by the detection of a single band for the joined termini of the EBV genome or by the analyses of NK antigens (ie, EB6 and GL183) or killer cell immunoglobulin receptors (KIRs). Normal NK cells express EB6 and GL183 as 4 subsets (EB6+/GL183+, EB6+/GL183–, EB6–/GL183–, and EB6–/GL183+); however, clonality is defined by the expression of a restricted phenotype [Zambello 1993]. Likewise, the uniform expression of a single (or multiple) KIR isoform correlates with clonality. The immunophenotypes of the NK cell processes and T-cell LGL process are outlined in [t5.4].

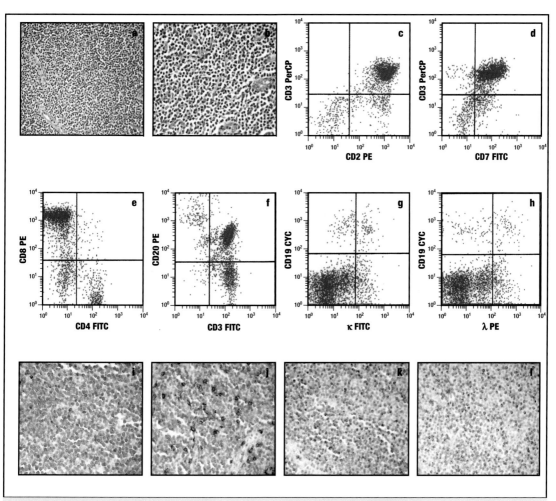

[f5.48] This case represents a peripheral (mature) T-cell lymphoma with aberrant CD20 expression. The clinical history reveals a 61-year-old male who presents with airway obstruction secondary to a base of tongue and hypopharyngeal soft tissue mass. The patient undergoes bilateral tonsillectomies, and the biopsies undergo a complete lymphoma work-up. Low power **a** and high power **b** H&E sections demonstrate the histologic features. By flow cytometric analysis, the malignant lymphocytes express CD3 **c, d, f**, CD2 **c**, CD7 **d**, CD8 **e**, and CD20 **f** and are negative for CD4 **e** and CD19 **g, h**, as well as κ **g** and λ **h**. The immunophenotype is confirmed by positive immunohistochemical (IHC) staining with CD3 **i** and CD20 **j** (T cells brightly staining and B cells with fainter staining). Furthermore, the malignant lymphocytes express TIA-1 **k** and granzyme B **l** by IHC staining. The cytogenetic results are essentially normal. The diagnosis of peripheral (mature) T-cell lymphoma with aberrant CD20 expression is made.

t5.4 Immunophenotypes of NK and T-Cell LGL Processes

Disorder	Immunophenotype
Chronic NK cell expansion	CD2+, CD3–, CD4–, CD8–, CD16+, CD56+, CD57 wk
NK-LGL leukemia	CD2+, CD3–, CD4–, CD8+, CD16+, CD56+, CD57v
T-LGL leukemia	CD2+, CD3+, CD4–, CD8+, CD16+/–, CD56–/+, CD57+

LGL, large granular lymphocytic; NK, natural killer; v, variable; wk, weak

Mature and Immature Myeloid Cells

The expression patterns of normal granulocytes in BM are depicted in **[f5.49]**. In comparison, patients with myelodysplasia (MDS) may show hypogranular granulocytes and display various aberrancies in the granulocytic lineage, as demonstrated in **[f5.50]** [van Lochem 2004]. Also of interest, the use of 4 color flow cytometry has allowed for the identification of abnormal myeloid populations

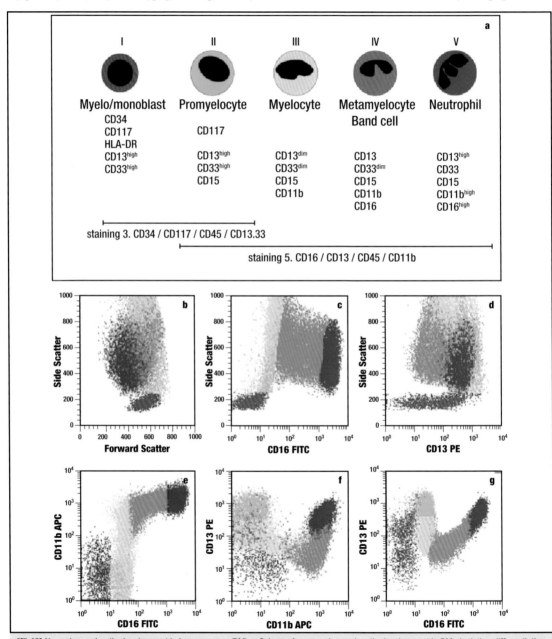

[f5.49] Normal granulocytic development in bone marrow (BM): **a** Scheme for normal granulocytic development in BM, depicting differentiation stages that can be identified by the two selected four-color immunostainings 3 and 5. The colors in the differentiation scheme globally correspond to the colors in the underlying dot plots and represent different subpopulations. The expression profiles of immunostaining 3 (CD34/CD117/CD45/CD13.33) are not presented in this image. Light scatter characteristics in combination with the intermediate CD45 expression are used to identify the granulocytic lineage **b**, in immunostaining 5 (CD16/CD13/CD45/CD11b). Five differentiation stages are distinguishable, based on the gradual increase of CD11b **e, f** and CD16 expression **c, e, g** and the dynamic CD13 expression **f, g** in combination with side scatter characteristics **d**. CD16 expression is preceded by the CD11b expression **e** (used with permission [van Lochem 2004]).

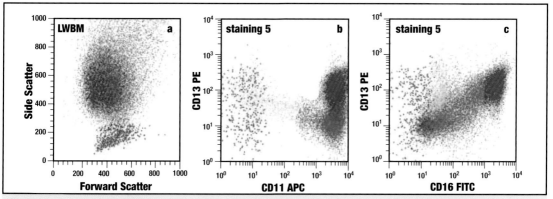

[f5.50] Hypogranular granulocytes in bone marrow (BM) of a myelodysplasia (MDS) patient. BM of an MDS patient displays various aberrancies in the granulocytic lineage. Hypogranularity of the granulocytes results in a reduced SSC **a**. Furthermore, the staining patterns in the CD11b/CD13 and CD13/CD16 dot plots are clearly changed with strongly reduced promyelocytic and myelocytic subsets **b**, **c** (used with permission [van Lochem 2004]).

in more than 90% of nonchronic myeloid leukemia (CML) myeloproliferative neoplasms (MPN) and myelodysplastic syndromes (MDS) with a clonal cytogenetic abnormality, supporting the use of FCI in the diagnosis of these disorders [Kussick 2003]. The most useful combinations of these myeloid markers in the study by Kussick et al [2003] include the following: HLA-DR and CD33; CD11b and CD16, or CD13 and CD16. The reader is referred to this reference for more detailed descriptions. In addition, the applications of flow cytometry to diagnosing chronic myeloproliferative disorders, myelodysplastic syndromes, and the overlap myelodysplastic/myeloproliferative disorders are discussed in much more detail in Chapters 7, 8, and 9, respectively.

Normal and "recovery" myeloblasts typically express the myelomonocytic markers, CD13 and CD33, as well as HLA-DR. They may show variable expressions of CD34. Neoplastic myeloblasts on the other hand may show aberrant loss of a myelomonocytic marker and show variable expressions of both HLA-DR and CD34. In fact, APL is characterized by the lack of both HLA-DR and CD34. CD117 has been considered an extremely useful marker by FCI in the evaluation of acute leukemias, since this marker has been previously reported as expressed only in AML [Newell 2003], although we and others have recently encountered CD117 expression in precursor T-cell lymphoblastic leukemia [Paietta 2004].

Normal and "recovery" myeloblasts do not co-express B-, T-, or NK-cell antigens, and such expressions by myeloblasts are considered aberrant and indicative of a clonal process. Neoplastic myeloblasts may aberrantly express T-cell markers (ie, CD2, CD5, and CD7, but not CD3, which is considered

lineage specific), a B-cell marker (ie, CD19), and an NK-cell antigen (ie, CD56). Of course, these markers should be considered in concert with a complete immunophenotypic panel. Distinction must be made between AML with aberrant T-cell or aberrant B-cell antigen expression and acute biphenotypic and/or acute mixed lineage leukemia (acute leukemias of ambiguous lineage), which will be discussed in much greater detail in Chapter 10.

FCI allows for the detection of CD19+ AML, characteristically associated with t(8;21); the myeloblasts in this type of leukemia also typically express CD34 as well as CD56 [Kita 1992]. Aberrant expression of CD19 may also be observed in AML of monocytic lineage [Brandt 1997]. However, the pattern of CD19 expression is distinctly unique in AML with a substantial monocytic/monoblastic component. In 50% of these AML cases, CD19 expression was evident only with the B4 (lytic) antibody and was not observed with B4 89B or SJ25-C1, whereas in the t(8;21)-associated AML M2 cases, CD19 was detected with all 3 antibodies. As mentioned above, CD56 is often also aberrantly expressed in CD19+ AMLs associated with t(8;21). However, CD56 may also be aberrantly expressed in other subtypes of AML and is not specific for a particular AML subtype [Dunphy 1999].

An aberrant AML immunophenotype (ie, CD7+, CD19+, CD56+) is particularly useful in detecting residual or relapsing disease and in distinguishing leukemic from recovery blasts.

Monocytes

Mature monocytes typically strongly express CD11b, CD13, CD14, CD15, CD33, CD64, and HLA-DR.

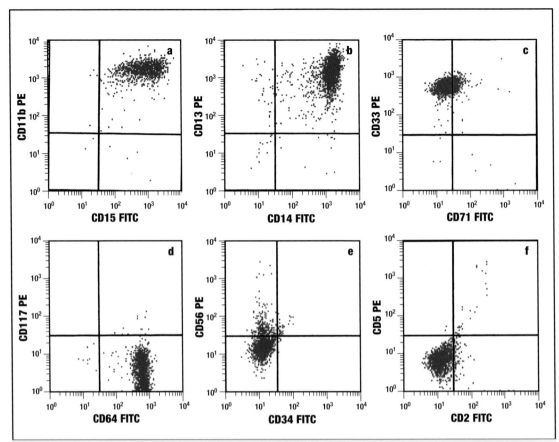

[f5.51] The samples of normal monocytes all revealed the same immunophenotype: Uniform bright expression of CD11b **a**, CD13 **b**, CD14 **b**, CD15 **a**, CD33 **c**, and CD64 **d**, with no associated expression of CD34 **e**, CD56(+<20%) **e**, CD117 **d**, or aberrant expression of CD2 **f** [Dunphy 2004].

They do not express CD56 or aberrantly express CD2 **[f5.51]**. On the other hand, CD14 is often absent or frequently diminished in expression by the blasts of AML with monocytic differentiation (ie, AMoL and AMML). In addition, other markers characteristically expressed by monocytic cells (ie, CD11b, CD13, CD15, CD33, and CD64) are absent or at least partially diminished in AMML and AMoL) **[f5.52]** [Dunphy 2004]. Thus, correlation with nonspecific esterase staining, particularly α-naphthyl acetate esterase (ANAE), is crucial in diagnosing AMLs with monocytic differentiation. In addition to revealing loss or absence of characteristic markers of monocytic cells in AMML and AMoL, CD56 might be expressed aberrantly in 50% of AMML and AMoL cases. This marker, as well as CD34 and CD117, are indicative of monocytic malignancy. In addition, aberrant expression of CD2 has been demonstrated in neoplastic immature monocytic cells.

Also CMML might be a difficult diagnosis to establish, particularly if there are no significant immature monocytic cells and no cytogenetic abnormalities. FCI studies have shown that the blast populations of CMML reveal FCI findings similar to those of the monoblasts of AMoL. Of particular interest, the FCI abnormalities detected in the monoblasts of the AMoL cases were also detected in the mature monocytes of CMML. In fact, although the CMML-1 cases were composed of mature monocytes, the FCI data revealed variable abnormalities (partial loss of CD13, CD14, and CD15 and aberrant expression of CD56 and CD2), as in the monoblasts of AMoL and not seen in normal peripheral blood and BM monocytes **[f5.53]** [Dunphy 2004]. Of particular interest, it has been demonstrated that morphologically mature monocytes might have abnormalities detected by FCI techniques. Thus FCI may be very helpful in identifying FCI abnormalities in the mature monocytes of an absolute monocytosis, indicating clues to the correct diagnosis of CMML.

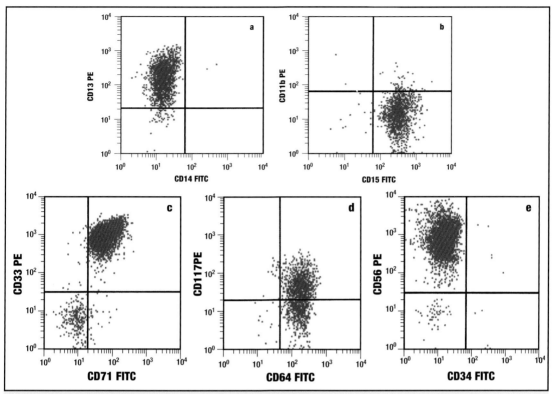

[f5.52] This M5b acute monocytic leukemia demonstrated 98% immature monocytic cells (blasts and promonocytes) by morphology. The flow cytometric immunophenotyping data revealed the "immature cells" invariably expressed CD13 **a**, CD15 **b**, and CD33 **c**, with complete loss of expression of CD11b **b** and CD14 **a** and partial loss of CD64 **d** with associated dim expression of CD117 **d** and strong expression of CD56 **e** [Dunphy 2004].

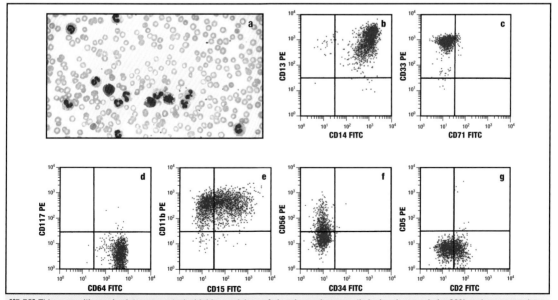

[f5.53] This case with an absolute monocytosis, highly suspicious of chronic myelomonocytic leukemia, revealed **a** 23% mature monocytes by morphology. The flow cytometric immunophenotyping data revealed uniform bright expression of CD13 **b**, CD14 **b**, CD33 **c**, CD64 **d**, moderate to bright expression of CD11b **e**, and partial loss of expression of CD15 **e** with associated partial expression of CD56(+33%) **f** and dim aberrant expression of CD2 **g**. [Dunphy 2004].

Eosinophils

Normal eosinophils, when present in sufficient numbers, may be identified within a region characterized by extremely high side light scatter (due to their markedly granular cytoplasm) and low forward light scatter (lower than granulocytes). Normal eosinophils express slightly brighter CD45 than granulocytes.

Normal eosinophils express CD11b (dimmer than most mature granulocytes), CD13 (dimmer than most mature granulocytes), CD15 (dimmer than most mature granulocytes), and CD33 (dimmer than most mature granulocytes) and HLA-DR (HLA-DR is not typically expressed on granulocytes). They do not express CD16, which is expressed on granulocytes. Since there is a certain degree of overlap of marker expression by eosinophils and granulocytes, analysis of these markers by forward light scatter seems most appropriate in evaluating these markers in these 2 distinct cell populations, since eosinophils have a lower forward light scatter than granulocytes [Kussick 2003]. In addition, eosinophils express functional IL-2R receptors (detected by CD25) and low levels of high affinity IgE receptor [Rand 1991, Kayaba 2001].

An extremely prominent eosinophil population is a rare occurrence, and massive eosinophilia in the peripheral blood or BM suggests a hypereosinophilic syndrome (HES), which may be clonal or nonclonal. Hypogranular eosinophils may occur in clonal and nonclonal (reactive) eosinophilic processes. Hypogranular eosinophils would obviously fall in a region characterized by both low forward and side light scatter. The distinction between HES and secondary eosinophilia may be determined by evaluation of surface IgE by flow cytometry, since all cases of secondary eosinophilia show surface IgE expression on the surface of the eosinophils, whereas the eosinophils of HES patients are negative for surface IgE [Berki 2001]. Other than this finding, there are no reported specific antigenic profiles distinguishing clonal from nonclonal, or neoplastic from reactive eosinophils. One should also keep in mind that secondary eosinophilia or idiopathic eosinophilia (nonclonal) may be associated with clonal T cells that express aberrant immunophenotypes by flow cytometry, and thus the lymphocyte population should also be evaluated in these cases. It has been suggested that these expanded clonal T cells have the potential to transform into malignant cells and that they should represent the major target for therapeutic interventions in these patients [Simon 2001].

Mast cells and basophils

Mast cells and basophils are the offspring of the multipotential hematopoietic stem cell; however, they are distinguishable by morphology and surface antigenicity. Basophils express CD13, CD33, dim CD45 (as compared to lymphocytes), and CD25, as well as a specific marker combination (ie, CD22+/CD19–) [Han 1999]. This specific marker combination may be used by flow cytometric analysis to easily and reliably detect basophils. Basophils are negative for CD2, CD3, CD14, CD16, CD64, HLA-DR, and C-kit (CD117) [Takahashi 1993].

Normal mast cells, on the other hand, moderately express CD45, are strongly positive for CD117, and are negative for CD25. Mast cells from patients with mastocytosis display unique aberrant characterisitics (ie, aberrant expression of CD25 and CD2 and abnormally low levels of CD117), defining the neoplastic nature of the mastocytosis [Escribano 2004].

References

Amato D, Oscier DG, Davis Z [2007] Cytogenetic aberrations and immunoglobulin V_H gene mutations in clinically benign CD5- monoclonal B-cell lymphocytosis. *Am J Clin Pathol* 128:333-338.

Bain BJ [1996] Ethnic and sex differences in the total and differential white cell count and platelet count. *J Clin Pathol* 49:664-666.

Berki T, David M, Bone B, Losonczy H, Vass J, Nemeth P [2007] New diagnostic tool for differentiation of idiopathic hypereosinophilic syndrome (HES) and secondary eosinophilic states. *Pathology Oncology Research* 7:292-297.

Brandt JT, Tisone JA, Bohman JE, Thiel KS [1997] Aberrant expression of CD19 as a marker of monocytic lineage in acute myelogenous leukemia. *Am J Clin Pathol* 107:283-291.

Buckner CL, Christiansen LR, Bourgeois D, Lazarchick JJ, Lazarchick J [2007] CD20 positive T-cell lymphoma/leukemia: A rare entity with potential diagnostic pitfalls. *Ann Clin Lab Sci* 37:263-267.

Cessna MH, Dunphy C, Brown M, et al [2002] Differentiation of thymoma from T-lymphoblastic lymphoma by flow cytometry. *Mod Pathol* 15:234A(981).

Chang H, Bartlett E, Patterson B, Chen CI, Yi QL [2005] The absence of CD56 on malignant plasma cells in the cerebrospinal fluid is the hallmark of multiple myeloma involving central nervous system. *Br J Haematol* 129:539-541.

Dunphy CH [1999] Comprehensive review of adult acute myelogenous leukemia: Cytomorphological, immunophenotypic, and cytogenetic findings. *J Clin Lab Anal* 13:19-26.

Dunphy CH, Orton SO, Mantell J [2004] Relative contributions of enzyme cytochemistry and flow cytometric immunophenotyping to the evaluation of acute myeloid leukemias with a monocytic component and of flow cytometric immunophenotyping to the evaluation of absolute monocytoses. *Am J Clin Pathol* 122:865-874.

Dunphy CH, Nies MK, Gabriel DA [2007] Correlation of plasma cell percentages by CD138 immunohistochemistry, cyclin D1 status, and CD56 expression with clinical parameters and overall survival in plasma cell myeloma. *Appl Immunohistochem Mol Morphol* 15:248-254.

Ely SA and Knowles DM [2002] Expression of CD56/ neural cell adhesion molecule correlates with the presence of lytic bone lesions in multiple myeloma and distinguishes myeloma from monoclonal gammopathy of undetermined significance and lymphomas with plasmacytoid differentiation. *Am J Pathol* 160:1293-1299.

Escribano L, Diaz-Agustin B, Lopez A, et al [2004] Immunophenotypic analysis of mast cells in mastocytosis: When and how to do it. Proposals of the Spanish Network on Mastocytosis (REMA). *Clinical Cytometry* 58B:1-8.

Fonseca R, Blood EA, Oken MM, et al [2002] Myeloma and the t(11;14)(q13;q32); Evidence for a biologically defined unique subset of patients. *Blood* 99:3735-3741.

Ghia P, Prato G, Scielzo C, et al [2004] Monoclonal CD5+ and CD5– B-lymphocyte expansions are frequent in the peripheral blood of the elderly. *Blood* 103:2337-2342.

Han K, Kim Y, Lee J, et al [1999] Human basophils express CD22 without expression of CD19. *Cytometry* 37:178-183.

Hoyer JD, Hanson CA, Fonseca R, Greipp PR, Dewald GW, Kurtin PJ [2000] The (11;14)(q13;q32) translocation in Multiple Myeloma. A morphological and immunohistochemical study. *Am J Clin Pathol* 113:831-837.

Inaba T, Shimazaki C, Sumikuma T, et al [2000] Expression of T-cell-associated antigens in B-cell non-Hodgkin's lymphoma. *Br J Haematol* 109:592-599.

Kampalath B, Barcos MP, Stewart C [2003] Phenotypic heterogeneity of B cells in patients with chronic lymphocytic leukemia/small lymphocytic lymphoma. *Am J Clin Pathol*. 119:824-832.

Kayaba H, Dombrowicz D, Woerly G, Papin JP, Loiseau S, Capron M [2001] Human eosinophils and human high affinity IgE receptor transgenic mouse eosinophils express low levels of high affinity IgE receptor, but release IL-10 upon receptor activation. *J Immunol* 167:995-1003.

Keren DF, Hanson CA, Hurtubise PE eds [1994] *Flow Cytometry and Clinical Diagnosis*. Chicago, IL: ASCP Press 214.

Kita K, Nakase K, Miwa H, et al [1992] Phenotypical characteristics of acute myelocytic leukemia associated with the t(8;21)(q22;q22) chromosome abnormality: Frequent expression of immature B-cell antigen CD19 together with stem cell antigen CD34. *Blood* 80:470-477.

Koelliker DD, Steele PE, Hurtubise PE, Flessa HC, Sheng YP, Swerdlow SH [1994] CD8-positive B-cell chronic lymphocytic leukemia. A report of two cases. *Am J Clin Pathol* 102:212-216.

Kussick SJ, Wood BL [2003] Using 4-color flow cytometry to identify abnormal myeloid populations. *Arch Pathol Lab Med* 127:1140-1147.

Li S, Eshleman JR, Borowitz MJ [2002] Lack of surface immunoglobulin light chain expression by flow cytometric immunphenotyping can help diagnose peripheral B-cell lymphoma. *Am J Clin Pathol* 118:229-234

Lin P, Mahdavy M, Zhan F, Zhang HZ, Katz RL, Shaughnessy JD [2004] Expression of PAX5 in CD20-positive multiple myeloma assessed by immunohistochemistry and oligonucleotide microarray. *Mod Pathol* 17:1217-1222.

Loughran TP [1993] Clonal diseases of large granular lymphocytes. *Blood* 82:1-14.

Magro CM, Seilstad KH, Porcu P, Morrison CD [2006] Primary CD20+CD10+CD8+ T-cell lymphoma of the skin with IgH and TCR β gene rearrangement. *Am J Clin Path* 126:14-22.

Marti GE, Rawstrom AC, Ghia P, et al [2005] Diagnostic criteria for monoclonal B-cell lymphocytosis. *Br J Haematol* 130:325-332.

Martin P, Santon A, Bellas C [2004] Neural cell adhesion molecule expression in plasma cells in BM biopsies and aspirates allows discrimination between multiple myeloma, monoclonal gammopathy of uncertain significance and polyclonal plasmacytosis. *Histopathology* 44:375-380.

Mathew P, Ahmann GJ, Witzig TE, et al [1995] Clinicopathological correlates of CD56 expression in multiple myeloma: A unique entity? *Br J Haemato* 90:459-461.

Matsuda I, Mori Y, Nakagawa Y, Sawanobori M, Uemura N, Suzuki K [2005] Close correlations between CD20 expression, a small mature plasma cell morphology and t(11; 14) in multiple myeloma. *Rinsho Ketsueki* 46:1293-1297.

McKenna RW, Washington LT, Aquino DB, et al [2001] Immunophenotypic analysis of hematogones (B-lymphocyte precursors) in 662 consecutive BM specimens by 4-color flow cytometry. *Blood* 98:2498-2507.

Nakajima J, Takamoto S, Oka T, Tanaka M, Takeuchi E, Murakawa T [2000] Flow cytometric analysis of lymphoid cells in thymic epithelial neoplasms. *Eur J Cardiothorac Surg* 18:287-292.

Newell JO, Cessna MH, Greenwood J, Hartung L, Bahler DW [2003] Importance of CD117 in the evaluation of acute leukemias by flow cytometry. *Clin Cytometry* 52B:40-43.

Noppen M [2004] Normal volume and cellular contents of pleural fluid. *Paediatric Respiratory Reviews* 5:S201-S203.

Paietta E. Ferrando AA, Neuberg D, et al [2004] Activating FLT3 mutations in CD117/KIT+ T-cell ALLs. *Blood* 104:558-560.

Pellat-Deceunynck C, Barille S, Jego G, et al [1998] The absence of CD56 (NCAM) on malignant plasma cells is a hallmark of plasma cell leukemia and of a special subset of multiple myeloma. *Leukemia* 12:1977-1982.

Rand TH, Silberstein DS, Kornfeld H, Weller PF [1991] Human eosinophils express functional interleukin 2 receptors. *J Clin Invest* 88:825-832.

Rawstron A, Barrans S, Blythe D, et al [1999] Distribution of myeloma plasma cells in peripheral blood and BM correlates with CD56 expression. *Br J Haematol* 104:138-143.

Robillard N, Avet-Loiseau H, Garand R, et al [2003] CD20 is associated with a small mature plasma cell morphology and t(11;14) in multiple myeloma. *Blood* 102:1070-1071.

Sahara N, Takeshita A, Shigeno K, et al [2002] Clinicopathological and prognostic characteristics of CD56– multiple myeloma. *Br J Haematol* 117:882-885.

Semenzato G, Zambello R, Starkebaum G, et al [1997] The lymphoproliferative disease of granular lymphocytes: Updated criteria for diagnosis. *Blood* 89:256-260.

Simon HU, Plotz SG, Simon D, Dummer R, Blaser K [2001] Clinical and immunological features of patients with interleukin-5-producing T cell clones and eosinophilia. *Allergy and Immunology* 124:242-245.

Stacchini A, Demurtas A, Aliberti S, et al [2007] The usefulness of flow cytometric CD10 detection in the differential diagnosis of peripheral T-cell lymphomas. *Am J Clin Path* 128:854-864.

Takahashi K, Takata M, Suwaki T, et al [1993] New flow cytometric method for surface phenotyping basophils from peripheral blood. *Journal of Immunological Methods* 162:17-21.

Valente G, Geuna M, Novero D, Arisio R, Palestro G, Stramignoni A [1990] CD5-positive B-cells of the fetal and adult spleen lymphoid tissue: An immunophenotypical study. *Verh Dtsch Ges Pathol* 74:155-158.

van Lochem EG, van der Velden VHJ, Wind HK, te Marvelde JG, Westerdaal NAC, van Dongen JJM [2004] Immunophenotypic differentiation patterns of normal hematopoiesis in human BM: Reference patterns for age-related changes and disease-induced shifts. *Clin Cytometry* 60B:1-13.

Waddick KG, Uckun FM [1993] CD5 antigen-positive B lymphocytes in human B cell ontogeny during fetal development and after autologous BM transplantation. *Exp Hematol* 21:791-798.

Wood BJ, Arroz M, Barnett D, et al [2007] 2006 Bethesda International consensus recommendations on the immunophenotypic analysis of hematolymphoid neoplasia by flow cytometry: Optimal reagents and reporting for the flow cytometric diagnosis of hematopoietic neoplasia. *Clinical Cytometry* 72B:S14-S22.

Yokose N, Ogata K, Sugisaki Y, Mori S, Yamada T, An E, Dan K [2001] CD20-positive T cell leukemia/lymphoma: Case report and review of the literature. *Ann Hematol* 80:372-375.

Zambello R, Trentin L, Ciccone E, et al [1993] Phenotypic diversity of natural killer (NK) populations in patients with NK-type lymphoproliferative disease of granular lymphocytes. *Blood* 81:2381-2385.

6 Classification of Hematolymphoid Neoplasms

Chapter Contents

The applications of flow cytometry to diagnostic hematopathology will be discussed in the framework of the World Health Organization (WHO) classification of tumors of hematopoietic and lymphoid tissues [Jaffe 2001]. Therefore, we provide this classification in this chapter for future reference. The WHO classification was recently revised [Swerdlow 2008], and the comparisons are seen in parentheses. The revisions of the WHO classification are primarily based on molecular genetic features, and the flow cytometric findings in these entities are similar to their original descriptions.

Chronic Myeloproliferative Diseases (Myeloproliferative Neoplasms, 2008)

Chronic myelogenous leukemia

Chronic neutrophilic leukemia

Chronic eosinophilic leukemia/hypereosinophilic syndrome (Chronic eosinophilic leukemia, NOS, 2008; also see below: myeloid and lymphoid neoplasms with eosinophilia and abnormalities of PDGFRA, PDGFRB, or FGFR1, 2008)

Polycythemia vera

Chronic idiopathic myelofibrosis (Primary myelofibrosis, 2008)

Essential thrombocythemia

Chronic myeloproliferative disease, unclassifiable (Myeloproliferative neoplasm, unclassifiable, 2008)

(Myeloid and lymphoid neoplasms with eosinophilia and abnormalities of PDGFRA, PDGFRB, or FGFR1, 2008)

(Myeloid and lymphoid neoplasms with PDGFRA rearrangement, 2008)

(Myeloid neoplasms with PDGFRB rearrangement, 2008)

(Myeloid and lymphoid neoplasms with FGFR1 abnormalities, 2008)

Myelodysplastic/Myeloproliferative Diseases

Chronic myelomonocytic leukemia

Atypical chronic myeloid leukemia (Atypical chronic myeloid leukemia, BCR-ABL1 negative, 2008)

Juvenile myelomonocytic leukemia

Myelodysplastic/myeloproliferative diseases, unclassifiable

Refractory anemia with ringed sideroblasts associated with marked thrombocytosis

Myelodysplastic Syndromes

(Refractory cytopenia with unilineage dysplasia, 2008)

Refractory anemia

(Refractory neutropenia, 2008)

(Refractory thrombocytopenia, 2008)

Refractory anemia with ringed sideroblasts

Refractory cytopenia with multilineage dysplasia

Refractory anemia with excess blasts

Myelodysplastic syndrome associated with isolated del(5q) chromosome abnormality

Myelodysplastic syndrome, unclassifiable

(Childhood myelodysplatic syndrome, 2008)

(Refractory cytopenia of childhood, 2008)

Acute Myeloid Leukemia (and Related Precursor Neoplasms, 2008)

Acute myeloid leukemia with recurrent cytogenetic abnormalities

    AML with t(8;21)(q22;q22), (AML1/ETO)

    AML with inv(16)(p13q22) or t(16;16)(p13;q22), (CBFβ/MYH11)

    Acute promyelocytic leukemia (AML with t(15;17) (q22;q12), PML/RARα) and variants, 2008)

    AML with 11q23 (MLL) abnormalities (only AML with t(9;11)(p22;q23); MLLT3-MLL included, 2008)

    (AML with t(6;9)(p23;q34); DEK-NUP214, 2008)

    (AML with inv(3)(q21q26.2) or t(3;3) (q21;q26.2);RPN1-EVI1, 2008)

    (AML (megarkaryoblastic) with t(1;22) (p13;q13);RBM15-MKL1, 2008)

    (AML with mutated NPM1, 2008)

    (AML with mutated CEBPA, 2008)

    Acute myeloid leukemia with multilineage dysplasia (AML with myelodysplasia-related changes, 2008)

Acute myeloid leukemia and myelodysplastic syndrome, therapy related (Therapy-related myeloid neoplasms, 2008)

    Alkylating agent related

    Topoisomerase II inhibitor-related

Acute myeloid leukemia not otherwise categorized (Acute myeloid leukemia, NOS, 2008)

AML, minimally differentiated (AML with minimal differentiation, 2008)

AML without maturation

AML with maturation

Acute myelomonocytic leukemia

Acute monoblastic and monocytic leukemia

Acute erythroid leukemia

Acute megakaryoblastic leukemia

Acute basophilic leukemia

Acute panmyelosis with myelofibrosis

Myeloid sarcoma (separate category, 2008)

Acute leukemias of ambiguous lineage (separate category—see below, 2008)

(Myeloid proliferations related to Down syndrome, 2008)

    (Transient abnormal myelopoiesis, 2008)

    (Myeloid leukemia associated with Down syndrome, 2008)

(Blastic plasmacytoid dendritic cell neoplasm, 2008—previously Blastic NK cell lymphoma or CD4+ CD56+ hematodermic tumor, 2008)

(Acute leukemias of ambiguous lineage, 2008)

    (Acute undifferentiated leukemia, 2008)

    (Mixed phenotype acute leukemia with t(9;22) (q34;q11.2); BCR-ABL1, 2008)

    (Mixed phenotype acute leukemia with t(v;11q23); MLL rearranged, 2008)

    Mixed phenotype acute leukemia, B/myeloid, NOS

    Mixed phenotype acute leukemia, T/myeloid, NOS

Precursor B-Cell Neoplasms

Precursor B-lymphoblastic leukemia/lymphoma (NOS and with recurrent genetic abnormalities, t(9;22), MLL rearrangements, t(12;21), hyperploidy, hypodiploidy, t(5;14), and t(1;19), 2008)

Precursor T-Cell Neoplasms

Precursor T-lymphoblastic leukemia/lymphoma

Mature B-Cell Neoplasms

Chronic lymphocytic leukemia/small lymphocytic
  lymphoma
B-cell prolymphocytic leukemia
Lymphoplasmacytic lymphoma/Waldenström
  macroglobulinemia
Splenic B-cell marginal zone lymphoma
Hairy cell leukemia
Plasma cell neoplasms
Plasma cell myeloma
Plasmacytoma
Monoclonal immunoglobin deposition diseases
Heavy chain diseases
Extranodal marginal zone B-cell lymphoma (MALT
  lymphoma)
Nodal marginal zone B-cell lymphoma
Follicular lymphoma
Mantle cell lymphoma
Diffuse large B-cell lymphoma (DLBCL associated with
  chronic inflammation, 2008; Large B-cell lymphoma
  arising in HHV8-associated multicentric Castleman
  disease, 2008)
Mediastinal (thymic) large B-cell lymphoma
Intravascular large B-cell lymphoma
(ALK+ large B-cell lymphoma, 2008)
(Plasmablastic lymphoma, 2008—also under
  Lymphomas associated with HIV-infection; see
  below)
Primary effusion lymphoma
Burkitt lymphoma/leukemia
Lymphomatoid granulomatosis
(B-cell lymphoma, unclassifiable, with features
  intermediate between DLBCL and Burkitt lymphoma,
  2008)
(B-cell lymphoma, unclassifiable, with features
  intermediate between DLBCL and classical Hodgkin
  lymphoma, 2008)

Mature T-Cell and NK-Cell Neoplasms

Leukemic/disseminated
    T-cell prolymphocytic leukemia
    T-cell large granular lymphocytic leukemia
    (Chronic lymphoproliferative disorders of NK cells,
      2008)
    Aggressive NK-cell leukemia
    (Systemic EBV+ T-cell lymphoproliferative disease of
      childhood, 2008)
    Adult T-cell leukemia/lymphoma
Primary cutaneous (WHO-EORTC classification)
    Mycosis fungoides (indolent)
    Sézary syndrome (aggressive)
    Primary cutaneous CD30+ T-cell lymphoproliferative
      disorders (indolent)
        Primary cutaneous anaplastic large cell
          lymphoma
        Lymphomatoid papulosis
    Subcutaneous panniculitis-like T-cell lymphoma
      (indolent)
    (Hydroa vacciniforme-like lymphoma, 2008)
    Provisional entities (no longer provisional, 2008)
        Primary cutaneous CD4+ small/medium-sized
          pleomorphic T-cell lymphoma (indolent))
        Primary cutaneous aggressive epidermotropic
          CD8+ cytotoxic T-cell lymphoma
          (aggressive)
    Primary cutaneous γδ T-cell lymphoma (aggressive)
    Primary cutaneous NK/T-cell lymphoma, nasal type
      (aggressive)
    Primary cutaneous peripheral T-cell lymphoma,
      unspecified (aggressive)
Other extranodal
    Extranodal NK/T-cell lymphoma, nasal type
    Enteropathy-type T-cell lymphoma (Enteropathy-
      associated T-cell lymphoma, 2008)
    Hepatosplenic γδ T-cell lymphoma (Hepatosplenic
      T-cell lymphoma, 2008)
    Primary extranodal peripheral T-cell lymphoma,
      unspecified
Nodal
    Angioimmunoblastic T-cell lymphoma
    Peripheral T-cell lymphoma, unspecified
    Anaplastic large cell lymphoma (ALK+ and ALK-,
      2008)
Neoplasm of uncertain lineage and stage of differentiation
    Blastic NK cell lymphoma (ie, CD4+CD56+
      hematodermic tumor) (Blastic plasmacytoid
      dentritic cell neoplasm, 2008)

Hodgkin Lymphoma

Nodular lymphocyte predominant Hodgkin lymphoma
Classical Hodgkin lymphoma
Nodular sclerosis Hodgkin lymphoma
Mixed cellularity Hodgkin lymphoma
Lymphocyte-rich classical Hodgkin lymphoma
Lymphocyte depleted Hodgkin lymphoma

Immunodeficiency-Associated Lymphoproliferative Disorders

Lymphoproliferative diseases associated with primary immune disorders
Human immunodeficiency virus-related lymphomas
(Lymphomas associated with HIV infection, 2008)
Post-transplant lymphoproliferative disorders

Histiocytic and Dendritic Cell Neoplasms

Histiocytic sarcoma
Langerhans cell histiocytosis
Langerhans cell sarcoma
Interdigitating dendritic cell sarcoma/tumor (no tumor, 2008)
Follicular dendritic cell sarcoma/tumor (no tumor, 2008)
Dendritic-cell sarcoma, not otherwise specified (not categorized as such, 2008)
(Fibroblastic reticular cell tumor, 2008)
(Indeterminate dendritic cell tumor, 2008)
(Disseminated juvenile xanthogranuloma, 2008)

Mastocytosis

Cutaneous mastocytosis
Systemic mastocytosis
Mast cell sarcoma
(Mast cell leukemia, 2008)
Extracutaneous mastocytoma

References

Jaffe E, Harris N, Stein H, et al [2001] *World Health Organization Classification of Tumours. Tumours of Haematopoietic and Lymphoid Tissues.* Lyon, France: IARC Press.

Swerdlow SH, Camp E, Harris NL, et al [2008] *World Health Organization Classification of Tumours. Pathology and Genetics of Tumours of the Haematopoietic and Lymphoid Tissues.* Lyon, France: IARC Press.

7 Myeloproliferative Neoplasms

Chapter Contents

Classification

- Chronic myelogenous leukemia (Ph chromosome, t(9;22)(q34;q11), BCR/ABL positive) (CML)
- Chronic neutrophilic leukemia
- Chronic eosinophilic leukemia (and the hypereosinophilic syndrome) (Chronic eosinophilic leukemia, NOS, 2008; also see below: Myeloid and lymphoid neoplasms with eosinophilia and abnormalities of *PDGFRA, PDGFRB,* or *FGFRI,* 2008)
- Polycythemia vera (PV)
- Chronic idiopathic myelofibrosis (with extramedullary hematopoiesis) (Primary myelofibrosis [PMF], 2008)
- Essential thrombocythemia (ET)
- Chronic myeloproliferative disease, unclassifiable (Myeloproliferative neoplasm, unclassifiable, 2008)
- (Myeloid and lymphoid neoplasms with eosinophilia and abnormalities of *PDGFRA, PDGFRB,* or *FGFRI,* 2008)
  - (Myeloid and lymphoid neoplasms with *PDGFRA* rearrangement, 2008)
  - (Myeloid neoplasms with *PDGFRA* rearrangement, 2008)
  - (Myeloid and lymphoid neoplasms with *FGFRI* abnormalities, 2008)

Introduction

The diagnosis of myeloproliferative neoplasms (MPNs) [including chronic myelogenous leukemia (CML), polycythemia vera (PV), essential thrombocythemia (ET), and primary myelofibrosis (PMF) has traditionally and primarily relied on morphologic findings in the peripheral blood and bone marrow combined with available cytogenetic data and clinical correlation. This approach is partially due to the fact that blasts in most cases of MPNs represent a minor population in clinical

samples, making their analysis problematic, and also due to the fact there has not been a specific marker for the various subtypes of non-CML MPNs.

However, recently the Janus kinase 2 (JAK-2) mutation has been described as a marker for non-CML MPNs. Janus kinase 2 is a cytoplasmic protein-kinase catalyzing the transfer of the gamma-phosphate group of adenosine triphosphate to the hydroxyl groups of specific tyrosine residues in signal transduction molecules. A mutation involving a valine ➔ phenylalanine substitution at codon 617 (JAK2V617F) has been described in varying frequencies in the non-CML MPNs (ie, PV: 77%-97% of patients studied; ET: 34%-57%; and primary myelofibrosis: 43%-50%). It is not present in CML [Michiels 2007]. Nevertheless, even with the discovery of this new marker, correlation of morphology with clinical features and additional ancillary studies are necessary to reach a definitive final subtype of MPN, since it is not subtype specific nor present in all non-CML MPNs. Thus, flow cytometric findings in these cases may provide important diagnostic data.

Previous studies have analyzed peripheral blood (PB) as well as bone marrow (BM) non-blast cells by flow cytometry (FC) in MPNs and identified abnormalities that have provided clues to the pathogenesis of these disorders, as well as diagnostic and prognostic implications. A review of these findings is provided.

Chronic Myelogenous Leukemia [t7.1]

Diagnosis/Differentiation from Reactive Conditions and Other MPNs

The density of CD16 antigen (FCRIII) has been shown to be significantly decreased on granulocytes in CML, as compared to healthy donors, patients with bacterial infections, and patients with other MPNs (PV and ET) [Kabutomori 1992, Carulli 1992, Kant 1997, Kabutomori 1997]. In addition, CD56 may be aberrantly expressed in CML. Aberrant CD56 expression in CML has been

t7.1 Summary of FC Abnormalities in CML: Clinical Utility

Type of Cell	FC Abnormality	Clinical Utility	References
Granulocyte	Decreased CD16 expression	Differentiation from reactive conditions and other MPNs (PV and ET)	[Kabutomori 1992, 1997, Carulli 1992, Kant 1997]
Myelocyte through metamyelocyte stages	Aberrant CD56 expression	Differentiation from benign conditions and indicator of early relapse	[Lanza 1997]
CD34+ blasts	Aberrant CD7 expression	Differentiation from benign conditions and associated with increased likelihood of disease progression	[Martin-Henago 1999, Kosugi 2000, Normann 2003]
PB myeloid cells	HLA-DR –/ OKMI+		
IP	Associated with myeloid BC	9,10	
BM mononuclear cells	CD15/HLA-DR ratio <1.0	Associated with evolution to AP of CML	[Chen 1993]

AP, accelerated phase. BC, blast crisis; BM, bone marrow; CML, chronic myelogenous leukemia; MPNs, myeloproliferative neoplasms; ET, essential thrombocythemia; FC, Flow cytometric; IP, immunophenotype; PB, peripheral blood; PV, polycythemia vera.

demonstrated from the myelocyte stage with the strongest staining in the metamyelocyte stage; granulocytes were CD56– in CML. CD56 expression has not been demonstrated in myeloid cells from BMs of healthy donors [Lanza 1993]. Also of interest, a study of purified BM CD34+ cells from chronic phase CML patients revealed a significantly increased percentage of CD34+/ CD7+ cells, compared to healthy donors (p<.05). CD7+ myeloid blast crisis of CML may represent the maturation arrest of immature myeloid progenitor cells when CD7 is transiently expressed [Martin-Henao 1999, Kosugi 2000].

Prognosis/Disease Progression

In 1985, Ligler et al determined that significant numbers of abnormal (HLA-DR–, OKM1+) myeloid cells in the peripheral blood of chronic phase CML patients in combination with cytogenetic findings predicted a myeloblastic acute phase [Ligler 1985a]. Subsequently, it was determined a CD15/HLA-DR ratio, performed on BM mononuclear cells, of <1.0 appeared earlier than morphology in the evolution of the accelerated phase of CML [Chen 1993]. Aberrant CD56 expression in CML

may also be used to monitor CML patients undergoing bone marrow transplantation, since its reappearance is associated with early relapse [Lanza 1993]. The Sokal and Hasford risk scores did not differ between CD34+/CD7– CML and CD34+/CD7+ CML, but all patients with signs of disease progression clustered in the CD34+/CD7+ population (ie, none of 10 patients with CD7– CML showed any signs of disease progression). Seven of the 10 patients with CD7+ CML showed some signs of disease progression [Normann 2003].

Clues to Pathogenesis

Of interest, neutrophils with decreased expression of CD16 show more defective chemiluminescence and phagocytosis than neutrophils with normal CD16 expression [Carulli 1992]. In addition, the decreased expression of transcripts for FcRII and FcRIII (CD16) by CML granulocytes, detected by FC, has been shown to be due to their faster degradation. This decreased steady state level of the mRNA for these Fc receptors has been shown to result in a defect in receptor-mediated endocytosis of FITC-conjugated heat-aggregated

t7.2 Summary of FC Abnormalities in Non-CML MPNs: Clinical Utility

Type of MPN	Type of Cell	FC Abnormality	Clinical Utility	References
PV	Erythroid	Increased Glycophorin A expression	Differentiation from benign conditions and other MPNs (CML and ET)	[Silva 1998]
	Erythroid	Increased Bcl-XL expression	Differentiation from benign conditions and other MPNs (CML and ET)	[Silva 1998]
ET	Platelets	Increased CD62p expression	Differentiation from benign conditions	[Griesshammer 1999]
	Platelets	Increased TSP expression	Differentiation from benign conditions	[Griesshammer 1999]
	Platelets	Decreased TPO receptors	Thrombocytosis	[Li 2000]
	Platelets	Decreased GPIa/IIa, GPIb, and GPIIb/IIIa	Bleeding complications due to defect in platelet aggregation and adhesion	[Handa 1995, Jensen 2000]
Non-CML MPNs, NOS	BM myeloid cells	1) Deviations in myeloid antigen intensity* 2) Dyssynchronous expression of 2 myeloid antigens 3) Aberrant nonmyeloid antigen expression	Differentiation of benign from neoplastic BM	[Kussick 2003]

*Flow-normal, no FC abnormalities; flow-abnormal, aberrant nonmyeloid antigen expression and/or a number of or severe myeloid antigen abnormalities; flow-indeterminate, single or mild myeloid antigenic abnormality.

CML, chronic myelogenous leukemia; ET, essential thrombocythemia; FC, flow cytometric; MPNs, myeloproliferative neoplasms; PV, polycythemia vera; TPO, thrombopoietin; TSP, thrombospondin.

IgG by CML granulocytes [Ligler 1985b]. It has also been demonstrated that expression of adhesion molecules, including L-selectin (CD62L), are decreased by CD34+ myeloid cells in CML. This finding likely explains the abnormal interaction between BM stroma and progenitors in CML, which results in unregulated proliferation [Kawaishi 1996].

Evaluation of Accelerated Phase and Blast Crises

Flow cytometric analysis is also particularly useful in determining the lineage of blasts (myeloid vs lymphoid) in the accelerated phase and blast crisis of CML. The blast crisis in CML is of lymphoid origin in one third of cases, is most often of precursor B-cell origin, and has a better prognosis than myeloid blast crisis.

Non-CML MPNs [t7.2]

Polycythemia Vera

PV is characterized by an abnormal clone of erythroid progenitors, independent of erythropoietin (EPO). In a study by Silva et al [1998], it was demonstrated that the erythroid cells in PV had a significantly increased expression of Glycophorin A and Bcl-X_L, an inhibitor of apoptosis, when compared to normal donors, patients with secondary erythrocytosis, as well as patients with other MPNs, including CML and ET. Deregulating the expression of Bcl-X_L averts apoptosis in an erythropoietin-dependent erythroblast cell line when EPO is withdrawn. Therefore, deregulated expression of Bcl-X_L may contribute to the EPO-independent survival of erythroid cells in PV and pathogenesis of this disease [Silva 1998].

PV may rarely undergo blastic transformation, usually after a very long chronic course (longer than in CML). Flow cytometric analysis may be useful in determining the type of blastic transformation (myeloid vs lymphoid), although most cases are of myeloid origin.

Essential Thrombocythemia

ET is a clonal MPN characterized by marked thrombocytosis associated with an increased risk of thromboembolism and bleeding complications. It has been shown that platelet activation plays a crucial role in the pathogenesis of prothrombotic conditions. Platelet surface expression of p-selectin (CD62p) and thrombospondin (TSP) has been shown to directly correlate with activation of platelets. In a study by Griesshammer et al [1999], it was demonstrated that the proportion of platelets expressing CD62p and TSP was significantly higher in patients with ET than in healthy controls; however, the increased expression did not correlate with symptomatology [Griesshammer 1999]. A later study by Li et al [2000] demonstrated a markedly decreased number and function of surface platelet (TPO) receptors in patients with ET. It was suggested that the thrombocytosis in ET was due to an alteration of the normal feedback interaction between TPO and its receptor [Li 2000]. The bleeding complications in ET may be due to platelet dysfunction, since a platelet defect of collagen-induced platelet aggregation and adhesion has been demonstrated in this disorder. In addition, decreased levels of platelet glycoprotein (GP) Ia/IIa, GPIb, and GPIIb/IIIa have also been demonstrated in ET [Handa 1995, Jensen 2001].

Similar to PV, ET may rarely undergo blastic transformation, and flow cytometric analysis may be useful in determining the type of blastic transformation (myeloid vs lymphoid), although most cases are of myeloid origin.

Primary Myelofibrosis

PMF is a clonal stem cell defect characterized by panmyelosis with intact maturation, progressive bone marrow fibrosis, and splenomegaly with multiorgan extramedullary hematopoiesis. It has been clearly demonstrated that the absolute number of circulating CD34+ cells in the peripheral blood, as detected by flow cytometric analysis, is useful in distinguishing PMF from non-CML MPNs, in determining prognosis in PMF, and in predicting blastic transformation in PMF [Barosi 1998]. Overall survival and interval-to-blast transformation from the time of CD34+ cell analysis were significantly shorter in patients with >0.3 × 10^3/mm³ (>0.3 × 10^9/L) CD34+ cells (p=.005 and .0005, respectively). The absolute number of CD34+ circulating cells PMF to be distinguished from other non-CML MPNs is strongly associated with the extent of myeloproliferation and predicts evolution toward blastic transformation.

As in PV and ET, flow cytometric analysis may be useful in determining the type of blastic transformation (myeloid vs lymphoid) in PMF, although most cases are of myeloid origin. In addition, one should keep in mind the risk of blastic transformation in PMF is significantly increased in patients who have undergone splenectomy [Barosi 1998].

Non-CML MPNs, Not Otherwise Specified (NOS)

Flow cytometric abnormalities have also been described in PV, ET, and in non-CML MPNs-NOS, as a group, and as detailed below.

A relatively recent study by Kussick et al [2003] analyzed BM specimens, which were performed to evaluate for a MPN, by 4-color FC. They compared the antigenic profiles of these cases with normal BM controls. They identified the following 3 major types of antigenic abnormalities:

1. deviations in myeloid antigen intensity defined as an increase or decrease of at least 1/3 of a log scale decade, compared with normal, in ≥10% of cells in the population of interest (PI);

2. dyssynchronous expression of 2 myeloid antigens, which was typically seen in most of the cells in the PI

3. aberrant expression of non-myeloid antigens defined as ≥10% of cells in the PI

The abnormalities were then assessed to classify a particular case into the following categories: flow-normal, flow-indeterminate, or flow-abnormal. Flow-normal cases had absolutely no FC abnormalities as described above. Flow-indeterminate cases were characterized by single or mild myeloid antigenic alterations, most commonly CD13 and CD33 expression. Flow-abnormal cases included all cases with an aberrant expression of non-myeloid antigens as well as cases with >1 or severe myeloid antigenic abnormalities. Of interest, both the blasts and the maturing granulocytes were immunophenotypically abnormal in most of the flow-abnormal cases, and more than half of the flow-abnormal cases revealed immunophenotypically-abnormal monocytes. In addition, the flow-abnormal cases were characterized by basophils (CD11b+/CD13+/CD33+/HLA-DR−/CD15−/CD117−) with a significantly increased rate of immunophenotypic abnormalities. There was no obvious correlation between specific antigenic abnormalities and the specific type of non-CML MPNs; however, the identification of marrow eosinophils, identified by bright expression of CD11b, CD13, CD15, and CD45, without CD16, were markedly expanded in patients with putative chronic eosinophilic leukemia. Cytogenetic correlation revealed all of the flow-normal and flow-indeterminate cases were cytogenetically normal, whereas 37% of the flow-abnormal cases revealed striking clonal cytogenetic abnormalities [Kussick 2003]. Thus, this study concluded that 4-color FC represents a useful method to distinguish benign from neoplastic marrow in the workup of non-CML MPNs.

Summary

Abnormalities have been described which may be detected by FC in morphologically mature myeloid cells, as well as in blasts, in MPNs. These abnormalities should be considered in concert and correlated with available clinical data, as well as data from additional ancillary techniques (ie, cytogenetic and molecular studies). These abnormalities may aid in earlier diagnosis and in differentiating cases with indeterminate morphology and normal cytogenetic results from benign conditions and from other hematopoietic disorders. In addition, the abnormalities may explain the clinical findings in patients with these disorders and indicate future therapeutic options and approaches.

References

Barosi G, Ambrosetti A, Centra A, et al [1998] Splenectomy and risk of blast transformation in yelofibrosis with myeloid metaplasia. Italian Cooperative Study Group on Myeloid with Myeloid Metaplasia. *Blood* 91:3930-3936.

Barosi G, Viarengo G, Pecci A, et al [2001] Diagnostic and clinical relevance of the number of circulating CD34(+) cells in myelofibrosis with myeloid metaplasia. *Blood* 98:3249-3255.

Carulli G, Gianfaldoni ML, Azzora A, Papineschi F, Vanacore R, Minnucci S, et al [1992] FcR III (CD16) expression on neutrophils from chronic myeloid leukemia. A flow cytometric study. *Leuk Res* 16:1203-1209.

Chen SS, Zhang HF, Xue WT, Li K, Wang P, Lui Y [1993] Predictors for prognosis of chronic myelocytic leukemia *Chin Med J* 106:760-762.

Griesshammer M, Beneke H, Nussbaumer B, Grunewald M, Bangerter M, Bergmann L [1999] Increased platelet surface expression of P-selectin and thrombospondin as markers of platelet activation in essential thrombocythaemia. *Thrombosis Research* 96:191-196.

Handa M, Watanabe K, Kawai Y, Kamata T, Koyama T, Nagai H, et al [1995] Platelet unresponsiveness to collagen: Involvement of glycoprotein Ia-IIa (alpha 2, beta 1 integrin) deficiency associated with myeloproliferative disorder. *Thromb Haemost* 73:521-528.

Jensen MK, Brown PDN, Lund BV, Nielsen OJ, Hasselbalch HC [2001] Increased platelet activation and abnormal membrane glycoprotein content and redistribution in myeloproliferative disorders. *Br J Haematol* 110:116-124.

Kabutomori O, Koh T, Iwatani Y, Fushimi R, Amino N, Miyai K [1992] Decrease of CD16 antigen density on granulocytes in chronic myeloid leukemia. *Rinsho Byori* 40:997-998.

Kabutomori O, Iwatani O, Koh T, Yanagihara T [1997] CD16 antigen density on neutrophils in chronic myeloproliferative disorders *Am J Clin Pathol* 107:661-664.

Kant AM, Advani SH, Zingle SM [1997] Heterogeneity in the expression of FcRIII in morphologically mature granulocytes from patients with chronic myeloid leukemia. *Leuk Res* 23:225-234.

Kawaishi K, Kimura A, Katoh O, Sasaki A, Ojuma N, Ihara A, et al [1996] Decreased L-selectin expression in CD34-positive cells from patients with chronic myelocytic leukaemia. *Br J Haematol* 93:367-374.

Kosugi N, Tojo A, Shinzaki H, Nagamura-Inoue T, Asano S [2000] The preferential expression of CD7 and CD34 in myeloid blast crisis in chronic myeloid leukemia. *Blood* 95:2188-2189.

Kussick SJ, Wood BL [2003] Four-color flow cytometry identifies virtually all cytogenetically abnormal bone marrow samples in the workup of non-CML myeloproliferative disorders. *Am J Clin Pathol* 120:854-865.

Lanza F, Bi S, Castoldi G, Goldman JM [1993] Abnormal expression of N-CAM (CD56) adhesion molecule on myeloid and progenitor cells from chronic myeloid leukemia. *Leukemia* 7:1570-1575.

Li J, Xia Y, Kuter DJ [2000] The platelet thrombopoietin receptor number and function are markedly decreased in patients with essential thrombocythaemia. *Br J Haematol* 111:943-953.

Ligler FS, Brodsky I, Schlam ML, Fuscaldo KE [1985a] Cytogenetics and cell surface marker analysis in CML-1. Prediction of phenotype of acute phase transformation. *Leuk Res* 9:1093-1098.

Ligler FS, Brodsky I, Schlam ML, Fuscaldo KE [1985b] Cytogenetics and flow cytometry may predict phenotype of CML blast crisis. *Cancer Detect Prev* 8:317-323.

Martin-Henao GA, Quiroga R, Sureda A, Garcia J [1999] CD7 expression on CD34+ cells from chronic myeloid leukemia in chronic phase. *Am J Hematol* 61:178-186.

Michiels JJ, Bernema Z, Van Bockstaele D, DeRaeve H, Schroyens W [2007] Current diagnostic criteria for the chronic myeloproliferative disorders (MPD) essential thrombocythemia (ET), polycythemia vera (PV) and chronic idiopathic myelofibrosis (CIMF). *Pathol Biol* (Paris) 55:92-104.

Normann AP, Egeland T, Madshus IH, Heim S, Tjonnfjord GE [2003] CD7 expression by CD34+ cells in CML patients of prognostic significance? *Eur J Haematol* 71:266-275.

Silva M, Richard C, Benito A, Sanz C, Olalla I, Fernandez-Luna JL [1998] Expression of Bcl-x in erythroid precursors from patients with polycythemia vera. *NEJM* 338:564-571.

8   Myelodysplastic Syndromes

Chapter Contents

Classification

- (Refractory cytopenia with unilineage dysplasia, 2008)
  - Refractory anemia (RA)
  - (Refractory neutropenia, 2008)
  - (Refractory thrombocytopenia, 2008)
- Refractory anemia with ringed sideroblasts (RARS)
- Refractory cytopenia with multilineage dysplasia (RCMD)
- Refractory anemia with excess blasts (RAEB)
  - RAEB-1
  - RAEB-2
- Myelodysplastic syndrome, unclassifiable
- Myelodysplastic syndrome associated with isolated del(5q) chromosome abnormality
- (Childhood myelodysplatic syndrome, 2008)
  - (Refractory cytopenia of childhood, 2008)

Introduction

Similar to the chronic myeloproliferative disorders (MPNs) discussed in the previous chapter, the diagnosis of low-grade myelodysplastic syndromes (MDSs) (ie, refractory anemia, refractory anemia with ringed sideroblasts, and refractory cytopenia with multilineage dysplasia) has relied primarily on the morphologic findings in the peripheral blood and bone marrow combined with available cytogenetic data and clinical correlation. This approach is due to the fact there is not a significant increase in blasts in the low-grade myelodysplastic syndromes. However, previous studies have analyzed peripheral blood (PB) as well as bone marrow (BM) non-blast cells and blasts by flow cytometry in MDSs and identified abnormalities which have provided clues to the pathogenesis of these disorders, as well as diagnostic and prognostic implications.

In addition, there are a significantly larger number of studies applying FC analysis to PB and BM samples of patients with MDS than to the chronic MPNs. As in the chronic MPNs, the findings have implied various applications of FC to diagnosing MDS, including differentiating low-grade MDS from various benign conditions, correlation of the French-American-British (FAB) subtype and grade of MDS with FC abnormalities, determining prognosis, predicting leukemic transformation and relapse, and providing clues to the pathogenesis of MDS. A review of these findings is provided [t8.1].

Diagnosis/Differentiation from Various Benign Conditions

Detection of Hypogranularity

Since, even in the low-grade MDSs, the myeloid series is often hypogranular, there may be detectable shifts in the scattergrams of forward light scatter (FSC) vs side light scatter (SSC, which detects complexity and granularity of the cytoplasm) and SSC vs CD45 expression. The comparisons of the scattergrams (SSC vs CD45 expression) of normal BM cells and hypogranular myeloid cells, as may be seen in MDS, are illustrated in [f8.1].

Detection of Aberrant Antigen Expression

Myeloid/monocytic/myeloblast abnormalities

A study, by Baumann et al, of the PB myeloid population in MDS patients has demonstrated the persistence of CD33 expression on dysplastic granulocytes in higher-grade MDSs (ie, RAEB-1 and RAEB-2), to

t8.1 Summary of FC Abnormalities in MDSs with Clinical Utility

Type of MDS	Type of Cell	FC Abnormality	Clinical Utility	References
RAEB, RAEBt	PB myeloid cells	Persistence of CD33 to later myeloid stages	Differentiation from benign conditions	1
MDS, NOS	PB and BM granulocytes	Increased intensity of CD33 expression	Differentiation from benign conditions	2
MDS, NOS	Myeloblasts	Anomalous CD56 expression	Differentiation from benign conditions	3
MDS, NOS	PB granulocytes	Increased surface LAP expression	Differentiation from benign conditions and higher in RA than in RAEB and RAEBt	4
MDS, NOS	BM granulocytes	Decreased CD10 expression	Differentiation from benign conditions	5
High-risk MDS, NOS	Granulocytes	Persistent CD64 expression Low-intensity CD32 expression Lower-intensity CD16 expression	Differentiation from benign conditions	6
RA	BM non-erythroid mononuclear cells	CD34/CD45 dull+/side scatter low cells with wide antigenic distribution	Differentiation from aplastic anemia (AA)	12
Hypoplastic MDS	BM blasts	Normal or increased number of CD34+ cells	Differentiation from AA	13
MDS, NOS	BM granulocytes	Abnormal patterns of CD11b vs CD16 expression or CD13 vs CD16 expression Loss of CD64 expression	Differentiation from benign conditions, including AA	7
MDS	BM myeloid cells	Phenotypically abnormal myeloblasts (blasts with markers of mature granulocytes) Phenotypically abnormal myeloid cells and monocytes (abnormal pattern of CD13 vs CD16 expression, asynchronous left-shifts, anomalous CD56 expression)	Differentiation from benign conditions, including AA	8
MDS	BM myeloid cells	1) Deviations in myeloid antigen intensity* 2) Dyssynchronous expression of 2 myeloid antigens 3) Aberrant non-myeloid antigen expression	Differentiation of benign from neoplastic BM	9
MDS, NOS	BM mature, non-blast cells	Higher HLA-DR expression Decreased CD10 expression Lower side scatter properties Higher CD34 expression	Differentiation from benign conditions	10

		IP Clusters	Correlation with FAB Subtype	
MDS, all types	BM myeloid cells	CD45lo cells with CD34hi/CD38+, CD34lo/CD38+, and CD56hi/CD71+	RAEB-1, RAEB-2	16
		CD45hi/SSChi granulocyte with CD71+	RA, RARS	
		CD45hi/SSChi granulocyte with CD36+	RAEB-1, RAEB-2	
MDS,NOS	BM myeloblasts	Abnormal patterns of CD34 and CD117 expression. Decreased CD45 density, increased CD13 and CD34 density, and increased expression of CD11c and CD4 (dim) correlated with increasing MDS grade	Grading of MDS	17
MDS, NOS	BM myeloid cells	HLA-DR + patients. Low CD11b expression. HLA-DR+/low CD11b expression	Shorter median time to leukemic transformation. Worst prognosis	22
MDS, NOS	BM CD45lo blasts	Increased CD34 expression	High-risk MDS	16
MDS, NOS	BM myeloid cells	Increased CD13 and CD33 expression	High-risk MDS	23
MDS, all types	Blasts	CD10 and CD15 expression. CD7 and CD117 expression	Low-risk MDS (RA, RARS). High-risk MDS (RAEB-1, RAEB-2)	24
MDS, NOS	Myeloid cells	Aberrant nonmyeloid antigen expression	Predictive of relapse	25
MDS, NOS	BM myeloid cells	Increasing number of phenotypically abnormal myeloblasts, myeloid cells, and monocytes	Increased likelihood of relapse and worse overall survival	8
MDS, NOS	BM myeloid cells	CD95 expression	Longer overall survival	26
MDS, NOS	BM blasts	Increased P-glycoprotein expression	Worse survival	27-29
MDS, NOS	PB lymphocytes	Low CD3 and CD8 percentages	Worse survival	30, 31

aFlow-normal, no FC abnormalities; flow-abnormal, aberrant nonmyeloid antigen expression and/or a number of or severe myeloid antigen abnormalities; flow-indeterminate, single or mild myeloid antigenic abnormality. BM, bone marrow; CMML, chronic myelomonocytic leukemia; FC, flow cytometry; ; MDS, myelodysplastic syndrome; NOS, not otherwise specified; PB, peripheral blood; RA, refractory anemia; RAEB, RA with excess blasts; RAEBt, RAEB in transformation; RARS, RA with ringed sideroblasts.

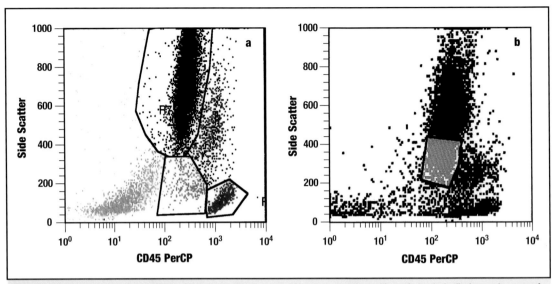

[f8.1] Flow cytograms of side light scatter vs CD45 expression: **a** normal BM pattern; **b** patient with myelodysplasia displays an increase of myeloid cells with low side light scatter (highlighted in purple).

later myeloid stages than in normal myeloid maturation [Baumann 1986]. A later study of the concentration of CD33 levels on the surface of PB and BM cells revealed that the overall CD33 intensity in BM samples was higher than in PB samples. CD33 intensity in PB and BM granulocytes was higher in MDS and lower in normal controls. In addition, the concentration of CD33 on CD33+ cells was significantly increased on CD34+ cells in MDS patients <60 years, compared with patients ≥60 years. However, there was no correlation of CD33 intensity with cytogenetic findings or response to therapy [Jilani 2002]. There may also be anomalous expression of CD56 by the myeloblasts of MDS that may aid in establishing the diagnosis [Mann 1997]. In addition, the percentage of surface leukocyte alkaline phosphatase (LAP)+ PB granulocytes has been shown to be significantly increased in MDS patients, in comparison to normal controls. Of interest, this study also concluded that the percentage of LAP+ cells was higher in RA than in RAEB-1 and RAEB-2. The higher percentage of LAP+ cells directly correlated with increased serum G-CSF levels detected in these patients [Takemoto 1999]. Also, in comparison to normal controls, the percentage of CD10+ BM mature granulocytes is significantly decreased in MDS patients, in comparison to normal controls [Chang 2000]. Also, dyssynchronous expression of CD11b and CD16 has been described in the maturing granulocytes in MDS patients. Olsaka et al [2007] described changes in a variety of leukocyte activation

antigens, including FcRI (CD64), FcRII (CD32), and FcRIII (CD16) in MDS. They described persistent expression of CD64, low-intensity CD32 expression, and lower fluorescent intensity of CD16 on granulocytes in high-risk MDS patients [Olsaka 1997].

A study by Stetler-Stevenson et al [2001] made the important observation that FC may be used for distinguishing reactive from dysplastic BM samples in morphologically equivocal cases of MDS. FC was informative in 75% of cases with normal cytogenetics and indeterminate morphology by demonstrating dual-lineage or trilineage FC abnormalities. This study found that abnormal patterns of expression of CD11b vs CD16 or CD13 vs CD16 among the maturing granulocytes were particularly useful for distinguishing benign from dysplastic processes, while aberrant expression of non-myeloid antigens and loss of CD10 among the granulocytes were less common findings [f8.2]. In addition, the study demonstrated loss of CD64 on the granulocytes in about two thirds of MDS patients. FC for myeloid dysplasia was more sensitive than morphology [Stetler-Stevenson 2001].

In a more recent study by Wells et al [2003], BM cells of myeloid lineage were studied by FC in a large series of MDS patients and compared to healthy donors. Among 115 MDS patients, 78% revealed abnormalities., with the most common abnormality being the presence of phenotypically abnormal myeloblasts, defined as myeloblasts with expression of markers of mature

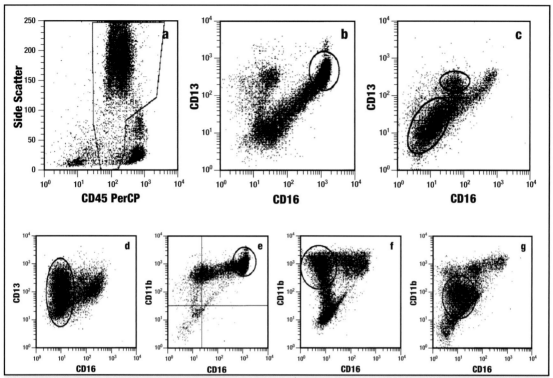

[f8.2] Immunophenotypic myeloid abnormalities in MDS. **a** The analysis gate used is based on CD45 (x-axis) vs side light scatter and includes granulocytes and precursors (CD45 dim and spectrum of SSC) **b** CD13 (y-axis) vs CD16 (x-axis). Oval indicates the majority of cells in this gate in normal BM. **c, d** MDS BM: CD13 vs CD16 Ovals highlight abnormal populations. **e** CD11b vs CD16. Oval indicates the majority of cells in this gate in normal BM **f-g** MDS BM: CD11b vs CD16. Ovals highlight abnormal populations.

granulocytes (ie, CD11b, CD15, and CD16). The most common phenotypic aberrancies in maturing myeloid cells were the abnormal relationship between CD13 and CD16 in myeloid cells, asynchronous shifts to the left (ie, the expression of antigens that appear on immature cells in concert with antigens identified only on mature cells), and the presence of CD56 on maturing myeloid cells. None of the healthy donors had abnormal myeloid or myeloblast findings. Of note, 23% of patients with Hodgkin lymphoma revealed CD56+ maturing myeloid cells and monocytes, while 1 of 15 (7%) patients with nonhematopoietic malignancies revealed CD56+ maturing myeloid cells and monocytes. Overall, CD56 expression on maturing myeloid cells was much less frequent in non-MDS patients than in MDS patients (p <.05) [Wells 2003].

The most recent study by Kussick et al [2003] used 4-color FC to analyze a large series of BM samples submitted for evaluation of MDS. They compared the antigenic profiles of these cases with normal BM

controls. They identified 3 major types of antigenic abnormalities:

1. deviations in myeloid antigen intensity, defined as an increase or decrease of at least ⅓ of a log scale decade, compared with normal, in ≥10% of cells in the population of interest (PI)

2. dyssynchronous expression of 2 myeloid antigens, which was typically seen in most of the cells in the PI

3. aberrant expression of non-myeloid antigens, defined as ≥10% of cells in the PI

The abnormalities were then assessed to classify a particular case into the following categories: flow-normal, flow-indeterminate, or flow-abnormal. Flow-normal cases had absolutely no FC abnormalities as described above. Flow-indeterminate cases were characterized by single or mild myeloid antigenic alterations, most commonly CD13 and CD33 expression. Flow-abnormal cases included all cases with aberrant expression of non-myeloid antigens as well as cases with >1 or severe myeloid antigenic abnormalities. Their study of MDS cases revealed cytogenetic abnormalities in 54% of the flow-abnormal cases, 6.5% in the flow-indeterminate cases, and 3% of the flow-normal cases. Thus, they concluded that 4-color FC was valuable in the workup of MDSs [Kussick 2003].

Xu et al later confirmed the presence of antigenic abnormalities in mature, non-blast cells in the BM of MDS cases (higher HLA-DR expression, decreased CD10 expression, lower side scatter properties, and higher expression of CD34), that were not present in the normal controls [Xu 2003].

Unrelated to antigenic abnormalities on mature or mature myeloid cells, a recent study has also demonstrated the enumeration of hematogones by flow cytometric analysis of bone marrow aspirates as a biomarker to aid in the diagnosis of MDS. The percentages of total hematogones and stage I hematogones have been shown to be significantly lower in MDS, compared with non-MDS samples (including 1 control group with cytopenias and another control group of noncytopenic lymphoma staging BMs). In addition, the decreased percentage of hematogones was not significantly between MDS subgroups or between those with and without associated cytogenetic abnormalities [Maftoun-Banankhah 2008].

Erythroid abnormalities

Loss of erythrocyte A, B, and H antigens have been described in MDS [Braneo 2001]. However, there was no statistical difference in the detection of erythroid dysplasia by FC vs morphology in the study by Stetler-Stevenson et al [Stetler-Stevenson 2001].

Platelet/megakaryocytic abnormalities

Decreased expression of c-Mpl, GPIIb/IIIa, and GPIb on platelets has been described in patients with RA [Braneo 2001]. However, in the study by Stetler-Stevenson et al, morphology was more sensitive than FC in detecting megakaryocytic abnormalities [Stetler-Stevenson 2001].

Differentiation between Hypoplastic MDS and Aplastic Anemia

Flow cytometric patterns of BM hematopoietic progenitors with a CD34+/CD45^{dull+}/SSC^{low} immunophenotype has been shown to be useful in distinguishing RA

and aplastic anemia (AA). The percentages of CD34+/CD45^{dull+}/SSC^{low} cells in BM non-erythroid mononuclear cells with or without the expression of CD38, CD71, CD33, and CD13 in these progenitors were all significantly decreased in AA, when compared to normal BM controls. In contrast, in RA BMs, the percentage of CD34+/CD45^{dull+}/SSC^{low} cells showed wide distribution; cell surface antigen expression patterns varied among each cell. Some showed high expression frequency of specific antigens, possibly reflecting the clonal expansion of an abnormal clone in the BM [Otawa 2001]. A more recent study has confirmed the usefulness of quantitative analysis of BM CD34+ cells in distinguishing AA from hypoplastic MDS. All patients with a normal or increased percentage of CD34+ cells were ultimately diagnosed with hypoplastic MDS, whereas all patients with low BM CD34+ cell numbers met standard clinical criteria for AA [Matsui 2006]. These flow cytometric studies support the finding that hypoplastic MDS may be distinguished from AA by detecting the presence of increased CD34+ cells by immunohistochemical staining of BM sections in hypoplastic MDS (not seen in BM sections of AA) [Horny 2007].

The 2001 Stetler-Stevenson study also demonstrated the usefulness of FC in differentiating MDS from AA. Multiple myeloid abnormalities were detected in 95% of MDS cases with adequate myeloid FC data and in only 1/15 (7%) of AA cases and in no normal marrows [Stetler-Stevenson 2001]. Also, in the 2003 study by Wells et al, only 12% of AA cases showed an abnormal relationship between CD13 and CD16; 1 had CD56+ maturing myeloid cells, and 1 lacked CD33 expression. In addition, there was an increased lymphoid:myeloid ratio of BM cells in 73% of AA patients, compared to 33% in MDS patients [Wells 2003].

Grading of MDS

Traditionally, most studies have not found a correlation of specific abnormalities by FC with the grade of MDS. However, a 2002 French study by Maynadie et al of BM samples of MDS patients demonstrated that patients with MDS could be clustered according to their immunophenotype of both CD45^{lo} blasts and CD45^{hi}/SSC^{hi} granulocytes. The immunophenotypic (IP) clustering of patients with MDS correlated with FAB subtype, the percentage of blasts in BM smears, and cytogenetic data. Expression of CD34 and CD36 on CD45^{lo} blasts or expression of CD36 and CD71 on CD45^{hi}/SSC^{hi} granulocytes identified specific IP subgroups of patients with MDS. Clustering of CD45^{lo} BM cells revealed a correlation of CD16+ with chronic myelomonocytic leukemia and CD34^{hi}/CD38+, CD34^{lo}/CD38+, and CD36^{hi}/CD71+ with RAEB-1 and RAEB-2. Clustering of CD45^{hi}/SSC^{hi} granulocytes revealed a correlation of CD71+ with RA and RARS and a correlation of CD36+ with RAEB-1 and RAEB-2 [Maynadie 2002].

In addition, more recently Pirrucello et al demonstrated a statistically significant correlation between the presence of decreased myeloblast CD45 intensity, increased CD13 and CD34 density, and increased expression of CD11c and dim CD4 with MDS grade. There was a direct relationship between the number of myeloblast phenotypic abnormalities and MDS grade. Abnormal patterns of CD34 and CD117 expression were present in 50% RARS, 68% RCMLD, and 100% RAEB cases [Pirrucello 2006]. These abnormal patterns are demonstrated in [f8.3].

Quantitation of Myeloblasts and Recognition of "Microblasts"

Accurate BM blast counts (BCs) are obviously essential for a diagnosis of myelodysplasia and to distinguish a high-grade MDS from an acute myeloid leukemia (AML). It may be difficult to determine an accurate percentage of myeloblasts to establish a diagnosis of MDS or AML, based on a BM aspirate alone. This is particularly true if the BM is hemodiluted or not able to be aspirated, due to a myriad of causes including marked

reticulin fibrosis, a "packed" marrow, the technique of obtaining the BM specimen, and other causes. In addition, erythroid precursors may be difficult to morphologically distinguish from myeloblasts in BM sections (aspirate clot and needle core biopsies) and high-grade MDS or AML arising in a background of MDS may have small blasts (or "microblasts") that appear lymphoid by cytomorphologic examination. It should also be kept in mind that all subtypes of AML (including acute promyelocytic leukemia) and rare cases of precursor B-cell lymphoblastic leukemia may arise in myelodysplasia [Ogawa 1989, Najfeld 1994, Pajor 1998]. For all of these reasons, ancillary techniques (ie, flow cytometry and immunohistochemical staining-IHCS) may be necessary to accurately identify, subtype, and quantify the percentage of BM blasts. Obviously, if the bone marrow is not able to be aspirated or is markedly hemodiluted, flow cytometric analysis will underestimate the percentage of BM blasts. However, even in this situation, flow cytometric analysis may provide useful information, since not all myeloblasts express CD34 and/or CD117. If the blasts are CD34+ and/or CD117+ by flow cytometric analysis (even of a hemodiluted sample), IHCS with CD34 and/or CD117 should be performed on the BM sections in order to accurately determine the percentage of BM blasts. CD34 and CD117 IHCS of BM sections may be particularly useful when BMA smears are insufficient or equivocal [Dunphy 2007].

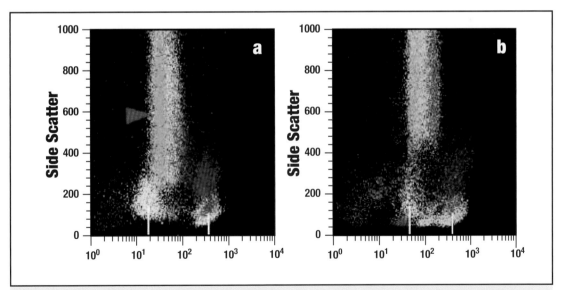

[f8.3] Antigen map of patient with refractory anemia with multilineage dysplasia **a** and normal bone marrow **b** illustrating phenotypic changes in MDS. The antigen expression color map is shown at the right. In the RCMLD, the myeloblasts (representing 5% of cells) exhibit decreased CD45 density in comparison with the normal myeloblasts (white metric). There is an increase in CD117+CD34– precursors (ie, promyelocytes) (green, red arrowhead). The immature granulocytes exhibit a decrease in side light scatter.

Predicting Prognosis, Leukemic Transformation, and Relapse

Several studies have reported the usefulness of abnormalities detected by FC in MDS in predicting prognosis and the likelihood of leukemic transformation and relapse. Mittelman et al analyzed BM cells (not further distinguished) from MDS patients and demonstrated HLA-DR+ patients had a shorter median time to leukemic transformation (p= .004) and low CD11b expression correlated with development of AML (p< .05); HLA-DR+ patients with low CD11b expression had the poorest prognosis with short median time to leukemic transformation (p= .017) [Mittelman 1993]. Increased expression of CD34 on CD45^{lo} blasts has been shown to correlate with poor International Prognostic Scoring System (IPSS), a poor cytogenetic risk factor, and high blast count on BM smears [Maynadie 2002]. An increased percentage of BM cells expressing CD13 and CD33 has also been shown to indicate a worse outcome and an increased likelihood of progression to a higher risk MDS or leukemic transformation [Kristensen 1990]. Ogata et al demonstrated that CD10 expression and CD15 expression were more prevalent on blasts of low-risk MDS (RA and RARS), whereas CD7 expression and CD117 expression were more prevalent on those of high-risk MDS (RAEB-1 and RAEB-2) and leukemic transformation of MDS [Ogata 2002]. In addition, aberrant antigen expression has been shown to be useful in predicting early relapse [Ito 2001]. In the study previously described above by Wells et al, an increasing number of abnormalities by FC (FC scores classified as mild, moderate, and severe) correlated with the likelihood of predicting relapse and overall survival (OS); relapse rate and OS were 3% and 74% in the mild group, 15% and 40% in the moderate group, and 33% and 36% in the severe group, respectively [Wells 2003].

CD95 (FAS/APO-1), a regulator of apoptosis, is not present on normal BM cells. However, analysis of CD95 on BM cells from MDS patients has demonstrated that CD95+ MDS patients have longer OS; CD95– MDS patients have a worse OS and increased likelihood of leukemic transformation [Polosukhina 1998]. Increased p-glycoprotein (PGP) expression by BM blasts has been associated with an immature blast immunophenotype, a low blast peroxidase activity, a higher risk of acute leukemic transformation, and a worse response to anthracycline-containing intensive chemotherapy [Lepelley 1994, Sonneveld 1993, List 1991]. Lastly, low PB CD3 and CD8 percentages have been shown to correlate with leukemic transformation and poor survival [Symeonidis 1991, Carpani 1989].

Clues to Pathogenesis

Although increased percentages of BM CD13+ and CD33+ cells (not further distinguished) have been associated with higher-risk MDS, as previously mentioned, a concomitant decrease in the proliferative activity in the immature myeloid cells has been demonstrated, indicating the block in differentiation may be coupled to a simultaneous block in proliferation, particularly in advanced stages [Jensen 1994]. This hypothesis has been supported by a number of studies, which have generally found abnormally increased apoptosis in RA/RARS, with associated increases in caspase 3 activation and expression of pro-apoptotic Bcl-2 family members [Delia 1992, Parker 2000, Matthes 2000, Boudard 2000, Boudard 2002, Lindberg 2001, Merchant 2001]. As mentioned earlier, caspase 3 has been implicated in the increased apoptosis seen in MDS; of interest, inhibition of its activity has been shown to at least partially restore the growth of committed progenitors. In addition, surface expression of phosphatidylserine (PS) has been used as an early marker of apoptosis; PS expression has been shown to be markedly increased in MDS patients, compared to controls. High PS expression in MDS has been correlated with unfavorable cytogenetic findings (ie, monosomies 5 and 7, trisomy 8, or complex cytogenetic abnormalities) [Raza 1996, Kliche 1997]. However, other studies have demonstrated a tendency in higher-grade MDS (RAEB-1 and RAEB-2) to decreased apoptosis and increased proliferation. Based on these studies, the grade of MDS appears to depend, to some degree, on the prevailing mechanism of increased apoptosis vs increased proliferation [Delia 1992, Parker 2000, Matthes 2000, Boudard 2000, Boudard 2002, Lindberg 2001, Merchant 2001]. Flow cytometry has also revealed decreased numbers of transferrin receptors on erythroblasts in MDS, possibly contributing to the decreased response of MDS patients to iron therapy [Kaiper-Kramer 1997].

Summary

Abnormalities have been described that may be detected by FC in morphologically mature myeloid cells and blasts in MDSs. These abnormalities should be considered in concert and correlated with available clinical data, as well as data from additional ancillary techniques (ie, cytogenetic and molecular studies). These abnormalities may aid in an earlier diagnosis and in differentiating cases with indeterminate morphology and normal cytogenetic results from benign conditions and from other hematopoietic disorders. In addition, the abnormalities may explain the clinical findings in patients with these disorders and indicate prognosis and the likelihood to leukemic transformation, thus affecting therapeutic options and approaches.

References

Baumann MA, Keller RH, McFadden PW, Libnoch JA, Patrick CW [1986] Myeloid cell surface phenotype in myelodysplasia: Evidence for abnormal persistence of an early myeloid differentiation antigen. *Am J Hematol* 22:251-257.

Boudard D, Sordet O, Vasselou C, Revol V, Bertheas MF, Freyssenet D, et al [2000] Expression and activity of caspases 1 and 3 in myelodysplastic syndromes. *Leukemia* 14:2045-2051.

Boudard D, Vasselon C, Bertheas MF, Jaubert J, Mounier C, Reynaud J, et al [2002] Expression and prognostic significance of bcl-2 family proteins in myelodysplastic syndromes. *Am J Hematol* 70:115-125.

Braneo T, Farmer BJ, Sage RE, Dobrovic A [2001] Loss of red cell A, B, and H antigens is frequent in myeloid malignancies. *Blood* 97:3633-3639.

Carpani G, Rosti A, Vozzo N [1989] T lymphocyte subpopulations in myelodysplastic syndromes. *Acta Haematol* 81:173-175.

Chang CC, Cleveland RP [2000] Decreased CD10-positive mature granulocytes in bone marrow from patients with myelodysplastic syndrome. *Arch Pathol Lab Med* 124:1152-1156.

Delia D, Aiello A, Soligo D, Fontanella E, Melani C, Pezzella F, et al [1992] Bcl-2 proto-oncogene expression in normal and neoplastic human myeloid cells. *Blood* 79:1291-1298.

Dunphy CH, O'Malley DP, Perkins SL, Chang CC [2007] Analysis of immunohistochemical markers in bone marrow sections to evaluate for myelodysplastic syndromes and acute myeloid leukemias. *Applied Immunohistochemistry and Molecular Morphology* 15:154-159.

Horny HP, Sotlar K, Valent P [2007] Diagnostic value of histology and immunohistochemistry in myelodysplastic syndrome. *Leuk Res* 31:1609-1616.

Ito S, Ishida Y, Murai K, Kuriya S [2001] Flow cytometric analysis of aberrant antigen expression of blasts using CD45 blast gating for minimal residual disease in acute leukemia and high-risk myelodysplastic syndrome. *Leuk Res* 25:205-211.

Jensen IM, Hokland P [1994] The proliferative activity of myelopoiesis in myelodysplasia evaluated by multiparameter flow cytometry. *Br J Haematol* 87:477-482.

Jilani I, Estey E, Huh Y, Joe Y, Manshouri T, Yared M, et al [2002] Differences in CD33 intensity between various myeloid neoplasms. *Am J Clin Pathol* 118:560-566.

Kaiper-Kramer PA, Huisman CM, Van der Molen-Sinke J, Abbes A, Van Eijk HG [1997] The expression of transferrin receptors on erythroblasts in anaemia of chronic disease, myelodysplastic syndromes, and iron deficiency. *Acta Haematol* 97:127-131.

Kliche KO, Andreef M [1997] High expression of phosphatidylserine in MDS, secondary AML and normal progenitors: comparison with primary AML. *Blood* 90(S1):202a.

Kristensen JS, Hokland P [1990] Monoclonal antibody ratios in malignant myeloid diseases: Diagnostic and prognostic use in myelodysplastic syndromes. *Br J Haematol* 74:270-276.

Kussick SJ, Wood BL [2003] Using four-color flow cytometry to identify abnormal myeloid populations. *Arch Pathol Lab Med* 127:1140-1147.

Lepelley P, Soenen V, Preudhomme C, Lai JL, Cosson A, Fenaux P [1994] Expression of the multidrug resistance P-glycoprotein and its relationship to hematological characteristics and response to treatment in myelodysplastic syndromes. *Leukemia* 8:998-1004.

Lindberg EH, Schmidt-Mende J, Forsblom AM, Christensson B, Fadeel B, Zhivotovsky B [2001] Apoptosis in refractory anaemia with ringed sideroblasts is initiated at the stem cell level and associated with increased activation of caspases. *Br J Haematol* 112:714-726.

List AF, Spier CM, Cline A, et al [1991] Expression of the multidrug resistance gene product (P-glycoprotein) in myelodysplasia is associated with a stem cell phenotype. *Br J Haematol* 78:28-34.

Maftoun-Banankhah S, Maleki A, Karandikar NJ, et al [2008] Multiparameter flow cytometric analysis reveals low percentage of bone marrow hematogones in myelodysplastic syndromes. *Am J Clin Pathol* 129:300-308.

Mann KP, DeCastro CM, Liu J, Moore JO, Bigner SH, Traweek ST [1997] Neural cell adhesion molecule (CD56)-positive acute myelogenous leukemia and myelodysplastic and myeloproliferative syndromes. *Am J Clin Pathol* 107:653-660.

Matsui WH, Brodsky RA, Smith BD, Borowitz MJ, Jones RJ [2006] Quantitative analysis of bone marrow CD34 cells in aplastic anemia and hypoplastic myelodysplastic syndromes. *Leukemia* 20:458-462.

Matthes TW, Meyer G, Samii K, Beris P [2000] Increased apoptosis in acquired sideroblastic anaemia. *Br J Haematol* 111:843-852.

Maynadie M, Picard F, Husson B, Chatelain B, Comet V, Le Roux G, et al, and the Groupe d'Etude Immunologique des Leucemies (GEIL) [2002] Immunophenotypic clustering of myelodysplastic syndromes. *Blood* 100:2349-2356.

Merchant SH, Gonchoroff NJ, Hutchison RE [2001] Apoptotic index by Annexin V flow cytometry: Adjunct to morphologic and cytogenetic diagnosis of myelodysplastic syndromes. *Cytometry* 46:28-32.

Mittelman M, Karcher DS, Kammerman LA, Lessin LS [1993] High Ia (HLA-DR) and low CD11b (Mo1) expression may predict early conversion to leukemia in myelodysplastic syndromes. *Am J Hematol* 43:167-171.

Najfeld V, Chen A, Scalise A, et al [1994] Myelodysplastic syndrome transforming to acute promyelocytic-like leukemia with trisomy and rearrangement of chromosome 11. *Genes Chromosomes Cancer* 10:15-25.

Ogata K, Nakamura K, Yokose N, Tamura H, Tachibana M, Taniguichi O, et al [2002] Clinical significance of phenotypic features of blasts in patients with myelodysplastic syndrome. *Blood* 100:3887-3896.

Ogawa K, Shineha H, Abe R, et al [1989] Acute promyelocytic leukemia with a history of RAEB in transformation and the 15/17 translocation. *Rinsho Ketsueki* 10:67-71.

Olsaka A, Saionji K, Igari J, Watanabe N, Iwabuchi K, Nagaoka I [1997] Altered surface expression of effector cell molecules on neutrophils in myelodysplastic syndromes. *Br J Haematol* 98:108-113.

Otawa M, Kawanishi Y, Iwase O, Shoji N, Miyazawa K, Ohyashiki K [2001] Comparative multi-color flow cytometric analysis of cell surface antigens in bone marrow hematopoietic progenitors between refractory anemia and aplastic anemia. *Leuk Res* 24:359-366.

Pajor L, Matolcsy A, Vass JA, et al [1998] Phenotypic and genotypic analyses of blastic cell population suggest that pure B-lymphoblastic leukemia may arise from myelodysplastic syndrome. *Leuk Res* 22:13-17.

Parker JE, Mufti GJ, Rasool F, Mijovic A, Devereux S, Pagluica A [2000] The role of apoptosis, proliferation, and the bcl-2 related proteins in the myelodysplastic syndromes and acute myeloid leukemia secondary to MDS. *Blood* 96:3932-3938.

Pirruccello SJ, Young KH, Aoun P [2006] Myeloblast phenotypic changes in myelodysplasia. CD34 and CD117 expression abnormalities are common. *Am J Clin Pathol* 125:884-894.

Polosukhina ER, Kuznetsov SV, Logcheva NP, Zabotina TN, Tenuta MR, Shirin AD, et al [1998] An evaluation of the prognostic significance of antigen CD95 (FAS/APO-1) expression on the cells of patients with a myelodysplastic syndrome, acute myeloid leukemia, and chronic myeloleukemia. *Ter Arkh* 70:21-25.

Raza A, Gregory SA, Preisler HD [1996] The myelodysplastic syndromes in 1996: Complex stem cell disorders confounded by dual actions of cytokines. *Leuk Res* 20:881-890.

Sonneveld P, van Dongen JJM, Hagemeijer A, et al [1993] High expression of the multidrug resistance P-glycoprotein in high-risk myelodysplasia is associated with immature phenotype. *Leukemia* 7:963-969.

Stetler-Stevenson M, Arthur DC, Jabbour N, Xie XY, Molidrem J, Barrett AJ, et al [2001] Diagnostic utility of flow cytometric immunophenotyping in myelodysplastic syndrome. *Blood* 98:979-987.

Symeonidis A, Kourakli A, Katevas P, et al [1991] Immune function parameters at diagnosis in patients with myelodysplastic syndromes: Correlation with the FAB classification and prognosis. *Eur J Haematol* 47:277-281.

Takemoto Y, Masuhara K, Yamada S, Fujmori Y, Takemoto Y, Masuhara K, et al [1999] Flow-cytometric analysis of leukocyte alkaline phosphatase in myelodysplastic syndromes. *Acta Haematol* 102:89-93.

Wells DA, Benesch M, Loken MR, Vallejo C, Myerson D, Leisenring WM, et al [2003] Myeloid and monocytic dyspoiesis as determined by flow cytometric scoring in myelodysplastic syndrome correlates with the IPSS and with outcome after hematopoietic stem cell transplantation. *Blood* 102:394-403.

Xu D, Schultz C, Akker Y, Cannizzaro L, Ramesh KH, Du J, et al [2003] Evidence for expression of early myeloid antigens in mature, non-blast myeloid cells in myelodysplasia. *Am J Hematol* 74:9-16.

Chapter Contents

Classification

- Chronic myelomonocytic leukemia
- Atypical chronic myeloid leukemia (Atypical chronic myeloid leukemia, BCR-ABL1–, 2008)
- Juvenile myelomonocytic leukemia
- Myelodysplastic/myeloproliferative disease, unclassifiable
  - Refractory anemia with ringed sideroblasts associated with marked thrombocytosis

Introduction

This group of disorders characteristically demonstrates myelodysplastic as well as myeloproliferative features at the initial diagnosis. Thus, flow cytometric analysis may reveal hypogranular myeloid cells, as described in the myelodysplastic syndromes, and/or may reveal a monocytosis, as characteristically seen in chronic myelomonocytic leukemia (CMML) and juvenile myelomonocytic leukemia (JMML), as will be described below. There does not appear to be any significant data regarding the specific flow cytometric features of atypical chronic myeloid leukemia. As with the myelodysplastic syndromes, flow cytometric analysis may be useful in identifying and quantitating the percentage of myeloblasts, in order to recognize transformation to an acute leukemia.

Chronic Myelomonocytic Leukemia

CMML is defined as a persistent peripheral absolute monocytosis ($>1.0 \times 10^3/mm^3$ [$1.0 \times 10^9/L$]) for at least 3 months with the exclusion of other causes. In the WHO classification, CMML is divided morphologically into CMML-1 and CMML-2, based on the percentage of blasts in the PB and bone marrow (BM). CMML-1 has fewer than 5% blasts in the PB and fewer than 10% blasts in the BM; CMML-2 has 5%-19% blasts in the PB and 10%-19% blasts in the BM. Of note, promonocytes are counted as blast equivalents for diagnostic (CMML vs acute monocytic/monoblastic leukemia-AMoL) and subtyping (CMML-1 vs CMML-2) purposes.

In regard to distinguishing CMML from AMoL, it may be difficult to morphologically distinguish promonocytes (ie, blast equivalents) from mature monocytes. Flow cytometric analysis cannot distinguish between these 2 cell types, since they have the same immunophenotype. However, flow cytometric analysis may be useful in detecting monoblasts, if they express CD34, as in AML-M5a.

When establishing a diagnosis CMML and differentiating CMML from an absolute monocytosis, flow cytometric analysis may be quite useful. CMML might be a difficult diagnosis to establish, particularly when there are no significant immature forms of monocytic cells (MCs) and no cytogenetic abnormalities. Morphologically, the MCs in the PB and BM may appear mature without any atypical features. Flow cytometric analysis has been shown to aid in establishing a diagnosis of CMML in such situations.

Defining Aberrant Monocytic Cells

It has been demonstrated that normal PB/BM monocytes reveal invariable, bright expression of CD11b, 13, 14, 15, 33, and 64, and HLA-DR with lack of expression of CD34, 56, 117, and 2 **[f9.1]** [Dunphy 2004]. In this same study, which also analyzed AMoLs, CMMLs, and "absolute monocytoses" of undetermined significance by morphology alone, the blast populations in CMML-1 and CMML-2 revealed flow cytometric findings similar to those of the monoblasts of AMoL. Of particular

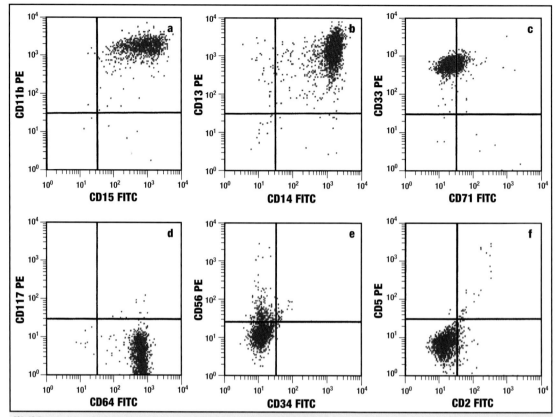

[f9.1] The samples of normal monocytes all revealed the same immunophenotype: uniform bright expression of CD11b **a**, CD13 **b**, CD14 **b**, CD15 **a**, CD33 **c**, and CD64 **d** with no associated expression of CD34 **e**, CD56 (+<20%) **e**, CD117 **d**, or aberrant expression of CD2 **f**.

interest, this study also demonstrated the flow cytometric abnormalities detected in the monoblasts of the AMoLs also were detected in the mature MCs of the CMML cases. Although the CMML-1 cases were composed of mature MCs, the FCI data revealed variable abnormalities (partial loss of CD13, 14, and 15, and expression of CD56), as in the monoblasts of AMoL and not seen in normal PB and BM monocytic cells. The MCs of CMML revealed invariable expression of CD33, 11b, and 64, with some cases showing partial loss of CD13, 14, and 15 **[f9.2]**. In addition, the MCs of some CMML cases revealed variable expression of CD56 and lack of expression of CD34 and CD117.

Of particular interest, 1 CMML-2 case (with 14% immature and 26% mature MCs by morphologic examination) revealed no "blast population" by FCI techniques. However, by flow cytometric analysis, all of the cells within the increased population of "MCs" revealed an identical abnormal immunophenotype, again confirming that morphologically mature MCs

might have abnormalities detected by FCI techniques **[f9.3]**.

In addition, cases with an absolute monocytosis of undetermined significance by morphology alone, but highly suspicious of CMML, revealed invariable expression of CD11b, 14, 33, and 64. Some of these showed variable expression of CD56, dim aberrant expression of CD2, and partial loss of expression of CD13 and CD15. They lacked expression of CD34 and CD117 **[f9.4]**. These absolute monocytoses were able to be correctly classified as CMML since they revealed flow cytometric abnormalities, indicating clues to their correct classification as CMML.

One should also always keep in mind that a diagnosis of CMML should never be rendered based on examination of a peripheral blood specimen alone. A bone marrow examination is always indicated to exclude a more acute process.

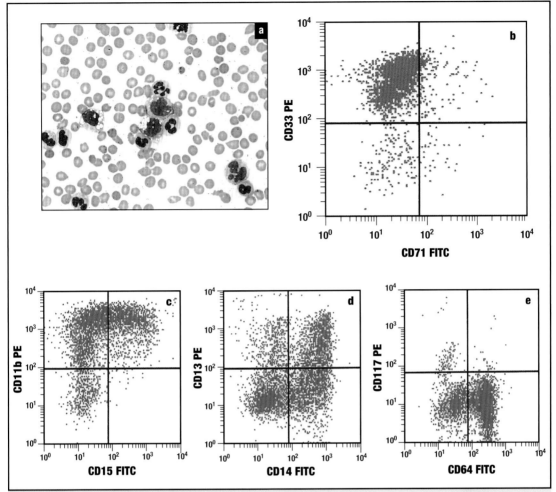

[f9.2] This CMML-1 was composed predominantly of **a** mature monocytes. The FCI data revealed bright expression of CD33 **b** and CD11b **c** with partial loss of expression of CD13 **d**, CD14 (+56%) **d**, CD15 **c**, and CD64 (+72%) **e**.

Juvenile Myelomonocytic Leukemia

Juvenile myelomonocytic leukemia (JMML) is defined as a clonal hematopoietic disorder of childhood characterized by a principal proliferation of granulocytic and monocytic lineages. Occasional dysplastic myeloid cells (pseudo-Pelger Huet cells, promyelocytes and myelocytes with macronucleoli) may be observed and dyseythropoiesis is minimal. The diagnostic criteria include the following:

1. peripheral blood monocytosis $>1 \times 10^3/mm^3$ $(1 \times 10^9/L)$

2. blasts (including promonocytes) <20% of the peripheral WBCs and nucleated marrow cells

3. no Ph chromosome or BCR/ABL fusion gene, plus 2 or more of the following: hemoglobin F increased for age; immature granulocytes in peripheral blood; a white blood cell count $>10 \times 10^3/mm^3$ $(>10 \times 10^9/L)$; a clonal chromosomal abnormality (ie, may be monosomy 7, seen in 30%-40% of cases); or in-vitro hypersensitivity of myeloid progenitors to GM-CSF.

Antibodies directed against GM-CSF have been shown to selectively inhibit growth of JMML colonies, whereas antibodies against a variety of other growth factors do not. Cultured nonadherent peripheral blood cells are approximately 10× more sensitive to exogenous GM-CSF than controls but show normal sensitivity to

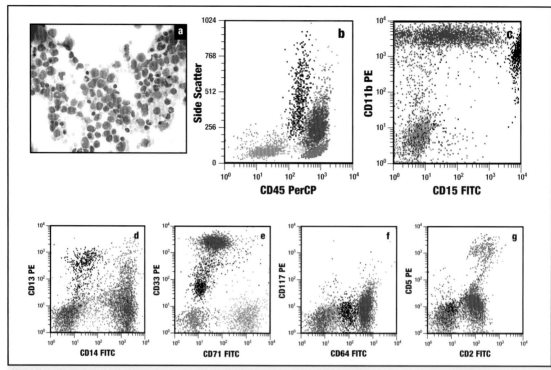

[f9.3] This CMML-2 was morphologically composed of **a** 14% immature monocytic cells (blasts + promonocytes) and 26% mature monocytes. The FCI data revealed **b** 54% of cells within the "monocytic" region (bright red), which revealed uniform bright expression of CD11b **c**, CD14 **d**, andCD33 **e** with moderate expression of CD64 **f**, partial loss of expression of CD15 **c**, complete loss of expression of CD13 **d**, and aberrant dim expression of CD2 **g**.

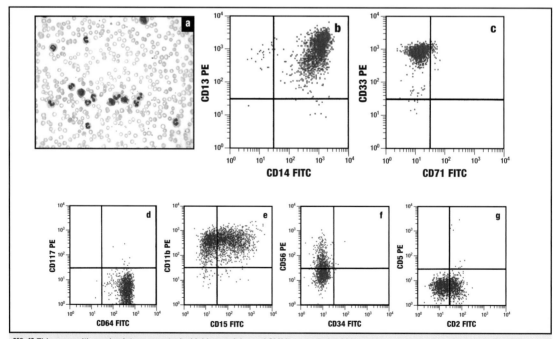

[f9.4] This case with an absolute monocytosis, highly suspicious of CMML, revealed **a** 23% mature monocytes by morphology. The FCI data revealed uniform bright expression of CD13 **b**, CD14 **b**, CD33 **c**, CD64 **d**, moderate to bright expression of CD11b **e**, and partial loss of expression of CD15 **e** with associated partial expression of CD56 (+33%) **f** and dim aberrant expression of CD2 **g**.

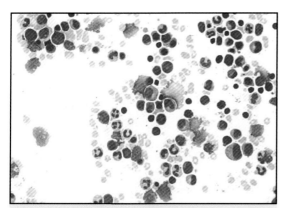

[f9.5] This Wright-stained BM aspirate smear is of a case of JMML which morphologically did not reveal an apparent increase in monocytic cells, nor significant dyerythropoiesis.

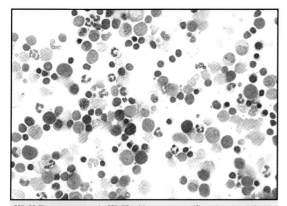

[f9.6] The same case in **[f9.5]** with a non-specific esterase stain reveals <20% of cells staining.

interleukin-3 and G-CSF [Gualtieri 1989, Emmanuel 1991]. It is important to recognize and correctly diagnose JMML, since this disorder has an overall poor prognosis. If untreated, 30% rapidly progress, dying within 1 year of diagnosis. with therapy, the median survival ranges from 5 months to more than 4 years.

Although there are no descriptions of flow cytometric features of JMML in the literature, the author has encountered a case of JMML that was difficult morphologically and by traditional enzyme cytochemistry to initially characterize. The patient was a 28-month-old female who had a WBC of $8.8 \times 10^3/mm^3$ ($8.8 \times 10^9/L$) (monocytes $0.8 \times 10^3/mm^3$ [$0.8 \times 10^9/L$]; basophils $0.1 \times 10^3/mm^3$ [$0.1 \times 10^9/L$]; neutrophils $3.6 \times 10^3/mm^3$ [$3.6 \times 10^9/L$]), a hemoglobin of 8.6 g/dL (MCV 83), and a platelet count of $124 \times 10^3/mm^3$ ($124 \times 10^9/L$). Morphologically, there was not an apparent increase in monocytic cells, although there were myeloid cells with possibly decreased granularity. There was not a significant degree of dyserythropoiesis **[f9.5]**. The non-specific esterase stain (α-napthhyl butyrate esterase [ANBE]) did not reveal a significantly increased percentage of monocytic cells (<20%) **[f9.6]**. Although flow cytometric analysis of the bone marrow revealed only 7% monocytes, there was an aberrant, identical immunophenotype of both the monocytes and the low side scatter myeloid cells, as demonstrated in **[f9.7]** and **[f9.8]**, respectively. The flow cytometric findings established a diagnosis of JMML, prior to ancillary studies, which later revealed a normal female karyotype, an increased Hemoglobin F for age, and in vitro hypersensitivity of myeloid progenitors to GM-CSF.

As with myelodysplastic syndromes and CMML, flow cytometric analysis may aid in identifying and quantitating the percentage of myeloblasts in JMML, in order to recognize transformation to an acute leukemia.

Comparison with Enzyme Cytochemistry and Immunohistochemistry

One should keep in mind that, as demonstrated, flow cytometric analysis may aid in identifying monocytic cells in morphologically challenging cases of CMML and JMML, but if the bone marrow aspirate submitted for flow cytometric analysis is hemodiluted, then enzyme cytochemical staining with non-specific esterases (ie, ANBE and alpha naphthyl acetate esterase-ANAE) may aid in detecting a monocytic component in CMML and JMML. Recently, CD14 has become available for paraffin immunohistochemistry, and comparisons with detection by flow cytometric analysis are not to this author's knowledge yet available.

References

Dunphy CH, Orton SO, Mantell J [2004] Relative contributions of enzyme cytochemistry and flow cytometric immunophenotyping to the evaluation of acute myeloid leukemias with a monocytic component and the contribution of flow cytometric immunophenotyping to the evaluation of absolute monocytoses. *Am J Clin Pathol* 122:865-874.

Emmanuel PD, Bates LJ, Castleberry RP, Gualtieri RJ, Zuckerman KS [1991] Selective hypersensitivity to granulocyte-macrophage colony-stimulating factor by juvenile chronic myelogenous leukemia hematopoietic progenitors. *Blood* 77:925-929.

Gualtieri RJ, Castleberry RP, Gibbons J, et al [1989] Granulocyte-macrophage colony stimulating factor is an endogenous regulator of cell proliferation in juvenile chronic myelogenous leukemia. *Blood* 74:2360-2367.

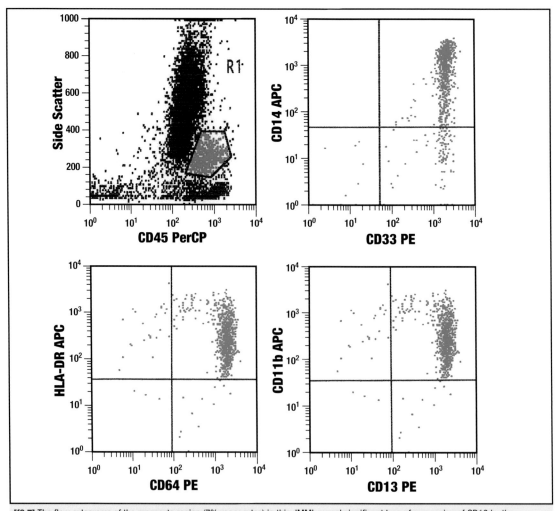

[f9.7] The flow cytograms of the monocyte region (7% monocytes) in this JMML reveal significant loss of expression of CD13 by the monocytes.

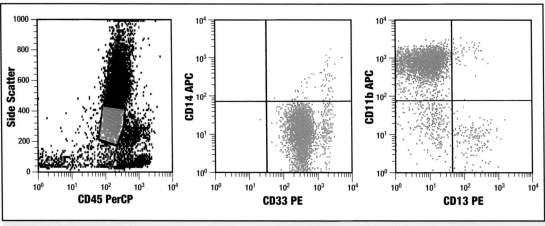

[f9.8] The flow cytograms of the low side scatter myeloid cell region in the JMML again reveal significant loss of expression of CD13 by these myeloid cells.

Chapter Contents

Classification

AML with Recurrent Cytogenetic Abnormalities and AML, Not Otherwise Specified (NOS)

- AML, minimally differentiated
- AML, minimally differentiated
- AML without maturation
- AML with maturation [AML with t(8;21) (q22;q22);(AML/ETO), 2008]
- Acute promyelocytic leukemia [AML with t(15;17)(q22;q12); (PML/RARα) and variants, 2008]
- Acute myelomonocytic leukemia (AMML) AMML, Eo
- [AML with inv(16)(p13q22) or t(16;16) (p13;q22);(CBFβ/MYH11)]
- Acute monoblastic leukemia
- Acute monocytic leukemia
- [AML with t(9;11)(p22;q23), 2008]
- (AML with inv(3)(q21q26.2) or t(3;3)(q21;q26.2);RPN1-EVI1, 2008]
- Acute erythroid leukemias
- Erythroleukemia (erythroid/myeloid)
- Pure erythroid leukemia
- Acute megakaryoblastic leukemia
- [AML (megakaryoblastic) with t(1;22)(p13;q13);RBM15-MKL1, 2008]
- Variant: Acute myeloid leukemia/transient myeloproliferative disorder in Down syndrome
- (Myeloid proliferations related to Down syndrome, 2008)
  - (Transient abnormal myelopoiesis, 2008)
  - (Myeloid leukemia associated with Down syndrome, 2008)
- Acute basophilic leukemia
- Acute panmyelosis with myelofibrosis
- (AML with mutated NPM1, 2008)
- (AML with mutated CEBPA, 2008)

Introduction

Flow cytometric analysis is particularly useful in the initial diagnosis of acute myeloid leukemia (AML), as well as in providing immunophenotypic data that may be used in subtyping the AML and detecting relapse or residual disease. These applications will be discussed and compared to immunohistochemical methods, which may need to be used when a bone marrow aspirate is not available for flow cytometric analysis and other ancillary studies (ie, cytogenetic and/or molecular analyses).

Diagnosis

Differentiation between AML and Reactive Condition or Myelodysplastic Syndrome

Flow cytometric analysis (FCA) may be particularly useful in distinguishing leukemic myeloblasts from those increased in an acute bacterial infection, since leukemic myeloblasts may show aberrant antigen expression (ie, expression of a non-lineage antigen, eg, CD2, CD5, CD7, CD19, CD56). In addition, FCA may help distinguish AML from a myelodysplastic syndrome (MDS) by quantitating myeloblasts (in an adequate, representative bone marrow sample) and by distinguishing microblasts (often seen in MDS) from lymphocytes [f10.1].

Differentiation between AML and Precursor (B- or T-Cell) Lymphoblastic Leukemia (LL)

FCA is obviously useful in differentiating AML from precursor B- or T-cell LL, which is important in determining the appropriate therapy. The distinction between AML with aberrant B-cell antigen expression (ie, CD19) and a precursor B-cell LL with aberrant myeloid antigen expression (ie, CD13, CD33, and/or CD15) may usually be made by the combination of markers expressed and review of the cytomorphology of the blasts in the peripheral blood and/or bone marrow (BM) aspirate smear. AML with aberrant CD19

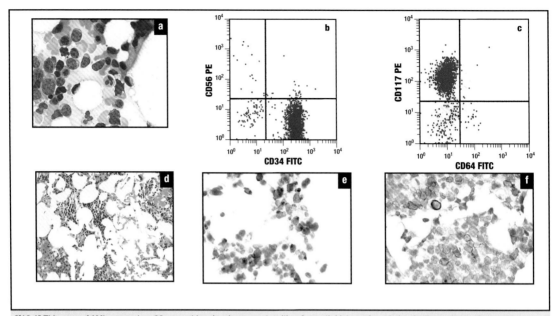

[f10.1] This case of AML occurs in a 63-year-old male who presents with a 9-month history of myelodysplastic syndrome. At current presentation, his CBC data reveals a WBC count of $3.8 \times 10^3/mm^3$ ($3.8 \times 10^9/L$), a hemoglobin of 11.6 g/dL, and a platelet count of $40 \times 10^3/mm^3$ ($40 \times 10^9/L$). A bone marrow aspirate is performed to evaluate status of current disease and is characterized by small blasts, or "microblasts" **a**. Flow cytometric analysis of the bone marrow revealed a hemodiluted bone marrow with 14% of cells within the immature cell region. The immature cells expressed CD13, CD33, CD34 **b**, CD117 **c**, and HLA-DR without expression of any other markers analyzed. The bone marrow section **d** reveals lymphoid-appearing cells. CD34 **e** and CD117 IHC **f** were extremely helpful in confirming the greatly increased percentage of blasts in this case. The cytogenetic results demonstrated that 4 of 17 cells analyzed had chromosomal abnormalities; 3 of 17 had deleted chromosome 20q; 1 of 17: extra copy of chromosome 22; and the remaining 13 cells were normal (46, XY). Diagnosis of AML with multilineage dysplasia arising from a previous myelodysplastic syndrome in a hypocellular bone marrow is made.

expression is often associated with CD56 and CD34 expressions, with AML, M2 morphology, and with a t(8;21), discussed in the corresponding section below.

Likewise, the distinction between AML with aberrant T-cell antigen expression and precursor T-cell LL with aberrant myeloid antigen expression may again usually be made by the combination of markers expressed and review of the cytomorphology of the blasts in the peripheral blood and/or BM aspirate smear. AML with aberrant T-cell antigen expression (ie, CD2, CD7, or CD5 but not CD3) is HLA-DR+, whereas precursor T-cell LL is generally HLA-DR– **[f10.2]**. However, occasional cases of AML may also be HLA-DR– **[f10.4]** and **[f10.5]** and thus must be distinguished from precursor T-cell LL with aberrant myeloid antigen expression, which occasionally may also express HLA-DR **[f10.5]**. Among AMLs, CD2 co-expression is almost exclusively restricted to 2 AML subtypes: M3 variant (AML, M3v) and M4-eos and their related molecular aberrations. The most valuable markers to differentiate between myeloperoxidase (MPO)-negative AML (subtype M0) and precursor LLs

include CD13, CD33, and CD117, typical of M0, and intracytoplasmic CD79a (cCD79a), intracytoplasmic CD3 (cCD3), CD10, and CD2, typical of B-cell– or T-cell-lineage ALL [Thalhammer-Scherrer 2002]. Although cCD79a and CD10 are characteristically expressed in precursor B-cell LL, up to 60% of precursor T-cell LL may also express cCD79a and up to 47% of precursor T-cell LL, CD10 **[f10.6]** [Lewis 2006].

Note that, although CD117 has previously been considered an extremely useful marker of AML by FCA, subsequent reports have demonstrated CD117 expression in a small proportion of precursor T-cell LL (9%), mainly consisting of those of immature pro-T/pre-T-cell origin **[f10.7]**. CD117 expression is rare in precursor B-cell LL and occurs in <3%-5% of cases [Newell 2003, Suggs 2007, Sperling 1997].

In the study by Suggs [2007], of the 27% of precursor B-cell LLs expressing myeloid markers, 53% expressed CD13; 89%, CD33; and only 5%, CD117. Up to 42% of those expressing myeloid markers expressed both CD13 and CD33; and only 5%, all 3-CD13, CD33, and CD117 **[f10.8]**. Of the 29% of precursor T-cell LLs

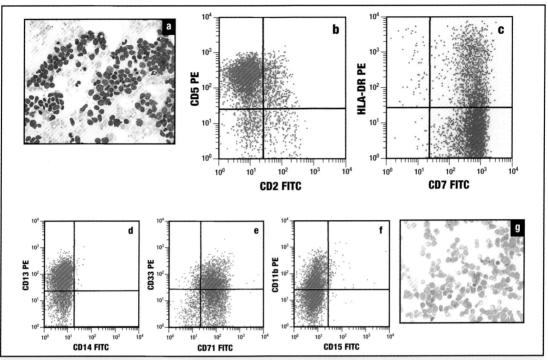

[f10.2] This case of AML demonstrates aberrant expression of CD5 and CD7. The clinical history reveals a 47-year-old male with a history of cervical lymphadenopathy, night sweats, and weight loss for the past few months. The blasts are characterized by high nuclear: cytoplasmic ratios a. By flow cytometric analysis, they express CD5 b, CD7 c, CD13 d, CD33 e, CD11b f, CD34, and show heterogeneous expression of HLA-DR c. They are negative for CD2 b, CD14 d, CD15 f, as well as CD3, CD64, CD117, and B-cell antigens. MPO is staining >3% of blasts g. Conventional cytogenetic studies are normal. The diagnosis of AML with aberrant CD5 and CD7 expressions is made.

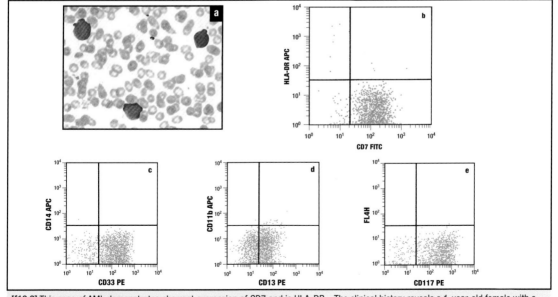

[f10.3] This case of AML demonstrates aberrant expression of CD7 and is HLA-DR–. The clinical history reveals a 1-year-old female with a history of trisomy 21 and pancytopenia. The blasts have markedly increased nuclear:cytoplasmic ratios a. The blasts variably express CD7 b, CD33 c, CD13 d, CD117 e, CD34, and CD56, and are negative for HLA-DR b, CD14 c, CD11b d, CD15, CD64, CD2, CD3, and CD5, as well as B-cell antigens. Conventional cytogenetic studies demonstrate a trisomy 21 and pericentric inversion of chromosome 3. The diagnosis of the peripheral blood specimen is AML with aberrant CD7 and HLA-DR-negativity. A subsequent bone marrow revealed >50% of cells staining with CD61, and was diagnosed as AML, M7.

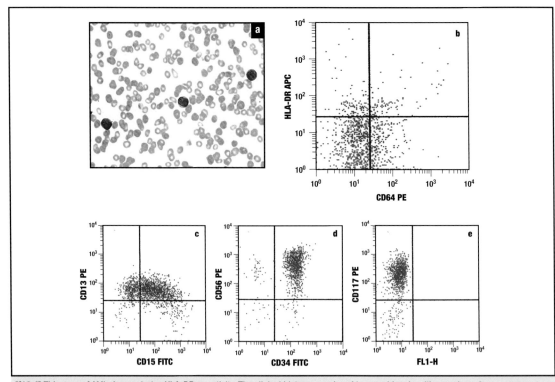

[f10.4] This case of AML demonstrates HLA-DR-negativity. The clinical history reveals a 41-year-old male with anemia and thrombocytopenia. The blasts have markedly increased nuclear:cytoplasmic ratios **a**. The blasts express CD64 (dim, **b**), CD13 **c**, CD15 **c**, CD33, CD34 **d**, and CD56 **d**, and CD117 **e**. They are negative for HLA-DR **b**, CD11b, CD14, and all T-cell and B-cell antigens. FISH (trisomy 8) results are abnormal, and the diagnosis of AML lacking HLA-DR is made.

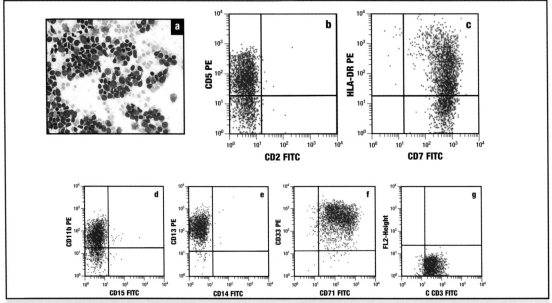

[f10.5] This case of precursor T-cell lymphoblastic leukemia/lymphoma demonstrates aberrant myeloid antigen expression. The clinical history reveals a 28-year-old with an elevated WBC count and anemia. The blasts have increased nuclear:cytoplasmic ratios with some "hand-mirror" forms **a**. The blasts express CD5 **b**, CD7 **c**, CD11b **d**, CD13 **e**, CD33 **f**, CD34, heterogeneous HLA-DR **c**, and cytoplasmic CD3 **g**. They are negative for CD1a, CD2 **b**, sCD3, CD4, CD8, CD15 **d**, CD14 **e**, CD64, CD117, and all B-cell antigens. IHC stains reveal negativity with MPO and positivity with TdT. The conventional cytogenetic results show del (16)(q11q21). The diagnosis of precursor T-cell lymphoblastic leukemia with aberrant myeloid antigen expression is made.

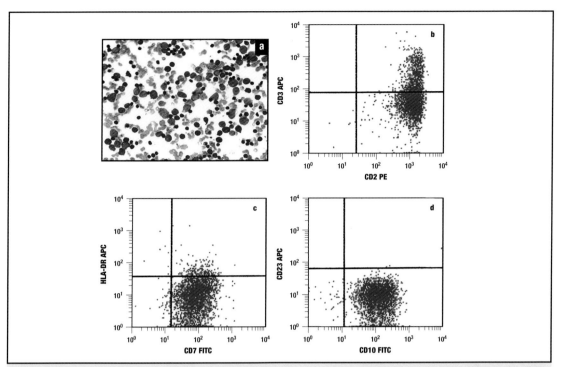

[f10.6] This case of precursor T-cell lymphoblastic leukemia/lymphoma demonstrates aberrant CD10 expression. The clinical history reveals a 38-year-old male with diffuse lymphadenopathy, night sweats, and lower extremity edema, rule out lymphoma. The blasts have increased nuclear:cytoplasmic ratios with some "hand-mirror" forms **a**. The blasts express CD1a, CD2 **b**, CD3 (subset-C), CD4, CD7 **c**, CD8, and aberrant CD10 **d**. They are negative for HLA-DR **c**, CD34, B-cell, and myeloid antigens. The conventional cytogenetic results demonstrated an abnormal polyploid clone. The diagnosis of precursor T-cell lymphoblastic leukemia/lymphoma with aberrant CD10 expression is made.

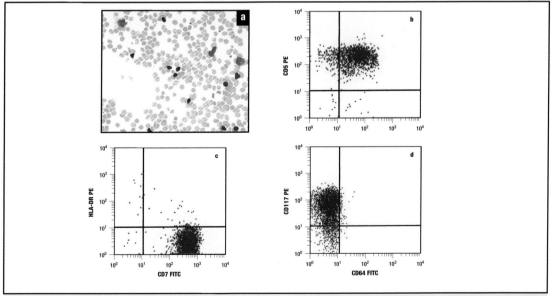

[f10.7] This case of precursor T-cell lymphoblastic leukemia/lymphoma demonstrates aberrant CD117 expression. The clinical history reveals a 66-year-old female with anemia and numerous blasts on the peripheral blood smear. The blasts have increased nuclear:cytoplasmic ratios with some "hand-mirror" forms **a**. The blasts express CD2 **b**, CD5 **b**, CD7 **c**, and CD117 **d**. They are negative for CD3, CD4, CD8, HLA-DR **c**, CD34, and all B-cell and additional myeloid antigens. MPO is negative in the blasts by enzyme cytochemical staining. TdT is positive by IHC. Conventional cytogenetic results are normal. The diagnosis of precursor T-cell lymphoblastic leukemia/lymphoma with aberrant CD117 expression is made.

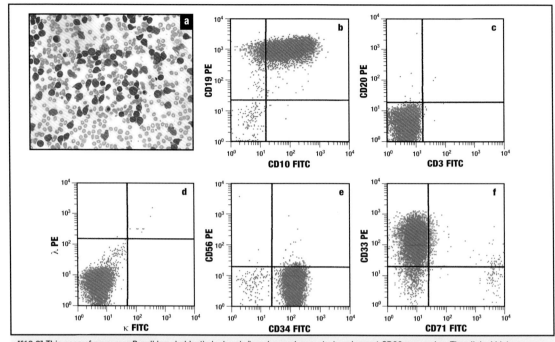

[f10.8] This case of precursor B-cell lymphoblastic leukemia/lymphoma demonstrates aberrant CD33 expression. The clinical history reveals an 8-year-old female with anemia, thrombocytopenia, and blasts on the peripheral blood smear. The blasts have increased nuclear: cytoplasmic ratios with some "hand-mirror" forms **a**.The blasts express CD10 **b**, CD19 **b**, CD34, HLA-DR, and aberrant CD33 **c**. They are negative for CD20, surface light chains, and all T-cell and additional myeloid antigens. Conventional cytogenetic studies show a hyperdiploid clone. The diagnosis of precursor B-cell lymphoblastic leukemia/lymphoma with aberrant CD33 expression is made.

expressing myeloid markers, 67% expressed CD13; 67%, CD33; and 50%, CD117 (ie, only 14% of the total T-cell LLs studied). Up to 17% of those expressing myeloid markers expressed both CD13 and CD117; 17%, both CD13 and CD33; and 17%, all 3-CD13, CD33 and CD117. The distinction between acute leukemia of ambiguous lineage vs precursor T-cell LL with aberrant myeloid antigen expression may be made by applying the criteria from the section below entitled "Differentiation of AML with Aberrant Antigen Expression from Acute Leukemias of Ambiguous Lineage (ie, Mixed Lineage and Mixed Phenotype Acute Leukemia)."

Of interest, there is a unique subset of de-novo adult T-cell LLs that co-express CD117 and cCD3, and are associated with activating mutations in the FLT3 RTK gene. Activating FLT3 mutations are the most common genetic aberrations in AML, resulting in the constitutive activation of the receptor tyrosine kinase (RTK), but such mutations have been rarely found in LL. This unique subset of T-cell LL indicates the need for clinical trials to test the efficacy of drugs inhibiting the FLT3 RTK in this subset of patients [Paietta 2004].

Quantitation of Myeloblasts

As mentioned above, FCA is useful in immunophenotyping MDS and differentiating MDS from an AML, since it allows for the detection of an accurate percentage of myeloblasts. Microblasts are characteristic of MDS and often difficult to morphologically differentiate from lymphocytes. However, note that the quantitation of myeloblasts in BM samples may only be reliably determined if the BM sample submitted for FCA is representative of the BM and not hemodiluted. For this reason, one must always prepare and review a smear of the "bone marrow" sample submitted for flow cytometry to ensure the adequacy of the sample and the presence of abnormal cells. Because not all myeloblasts express CD34 and/or CD117, there is not a single marker that may be used to quantitate the percentage of myeloblasts in the flow cytometry sample.

Nevertheless, even in "hemodiluted" samples of BM, FCA may be useful to determine if blasts are CD34+ and/or CD117+, since if they are expressed, these markers may then be analyzed by immunohistochemistry (IHC) of the BM clot and/or core biopsy sections, in order to quantitate the percentage of myeloblasts for diagnostic purposes [Wells 1996, Dunphy 2001, Dunphy 2007].

Correlation of FCI with AML Subtype

AML, M0 [t10.2]

In regards to immunophenotyping and subtyping AMLs, FCA defines AML, M0 (MPO-negative AML by enzyme cytochemical staining), which requires expression of myelomonocytic markers (ie, CD13, CD33) by FCA. Obviously, there is no expression of intracytoplasmic MPO, CD3, or lineage-specific B-cell markers [f10.9].

AML, M2 Associated with t(8;21)

FCI allows for the detection of CD19+ AML, characteristically associated with t(8;21); the myeloblasts in this type of leukemia also typically express CD34 as well as CD56 [f10.10] [Kita 1992]. Aberrant expression of CD19 may also be observed in AML of monocytic lineage [Brandt 1997]. However, the pattern of CD19 expression is distinctly unique in AML with a substantial monocytic/monoblastic component. In 50% of these AML cases, CD19 expression was evident only with the B4 (lytic) antibody and was not observed with B4 89B or SJ25-C1, whereas in the t(8;21)-associated AML M2 cases, CD19 was detected with all 3 antibodies.

In addition, it has been demonstrated that FCA may further distinguish between KIT-mutated and KIT-unmutated cases of AML with t(8;21). KIT-mutated cases show diminished CD19 and positive CD56 expression on the leukemic blasts, compared to cases without KIT mutations, which show stronger

CD19 expression and more variable CD56 expression [De 2007].

APL (Classical and Hypogranular or Microgranular Variant-M3v)

Flow cytometric analysis most often differentiates the hypogranular variant of acute promyelocytic leukemia from acute monocytic leukemia (AMoL, or AML, M5) [t10.1] [Krasinska 1998]. These AMLs may be difficult to morphologically distinguish from each other. By FCA, both the classical (hypergranular) and microgranular or hypogranular variants of APL uniformly lack expression of CD14, typically lack expression of HLA-DR, CD34, and CD56, and may have dim expression of CD64

t10.1 Immunophenotype of AML, M3 vs M5

AML, M3	AML, M5
CD13++	CD13++
CD33+++	CD33++
HLA-DR–/+ (27%)	HLA-DR+++
CD34–/+(rare)	CD34–/+(M5a)
CD14–	CD14–/+
CD64 dim+	CD64 +-+++
CD117+	CD117–/+
CD4–; CD56–/+(rare)	CD4+; CD56+

t10.2 Correlation of Flow Cytometric Markers and AML Subtype

AML Subtype	Marker Expression
AML, M0	Requires expression of CD13 or CD33; no expression of cMPO, cCD3, or B-cell markers
AML, M2	Aberrant CD19 expression correlates with CD34+, CD56+ and t(8;21)
AML, M3	CD13+, CD33+, HLA-DR–/+ (27%), CD34–/+(rare), CD14–, CD64 dim+, CD117+, CD4–, CD56–/+(rare)
AMML, M4 and AMoL, M5	CD14 is frequently negative in monoblasts; CD11b, CD13, CD15, CD33, and CD64 may be partially loss or absent in monoblasts; aberrant expression of CD34, CD56, and CD117 may be observed in monoblasts, indicating clonality; intense expression (3+) of CD64 distingusihes AMoL from other AML subtypes; dimmer (1+-2+) expression of CD13 is characteristic of blasts of AMML and AMoL; combined expression of CD64 (any degree of intensity) with intense expression of CD15 and less intense expression of CD13 is seen only in AMML or AMoL.
AML, M6b	Glycophorin A is expressed by erythroblasts in pure erythroid leukemia
AML, M7	Requires expression of CD41, CD42b, and/or CD61

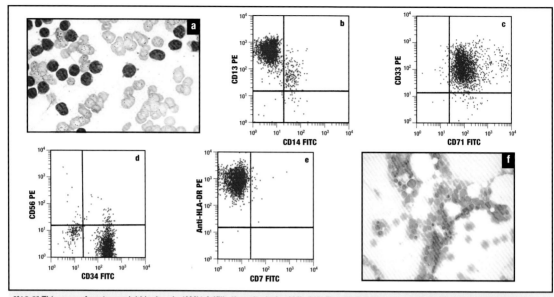

[f10.9] This case of acute myeloid leukemia (AML) fulfills the criteria for AML, M0. The clinical history reveals a 55-year-old female with a previous history of treated breast cancer with "blasts" in the peripheral blood. The clinician has concerns about their morphologic resemblance to lymphoblasts, and the submitting diagnosis is rule out secondary ALL. The blasts have increased nuclear:cytoplasmic ratios with some "hand-mirror" forms **a**. The flow cytometric analysis of the bone marrow aspirate reveals a hypercellular specimen (173 × 10³ cells/mm³ [173 × 10⁹ cells/L]) with 99% of cells within a combined lymphocyte and large cell region, which represents a continuum of cell sizes. The blasts express CD13 **b**, CD33 **c**, CD71 **c**, CD34 **d**, HLA-DR **e**, and CD117 (not shown). They were negative for CD7 **e**, CD14 **b**, CD56 **d**, and all T-cell and B-cell antigens. MPO stains <3% of blasts **f**. The diagnosis of AML, M0 is made.

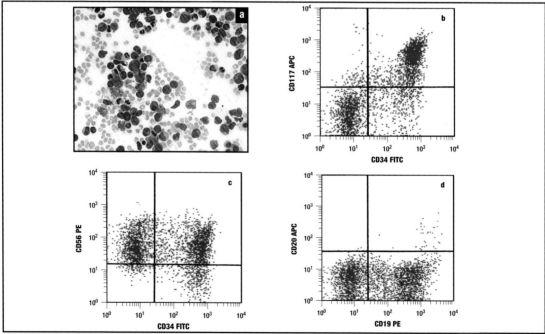

[f10.10] This case of AML reveals aberrant expression of CD19 and CD56 associated with CD34-positivity, characteristic of AML associated with t(8;21). The clinical history reveals a 38-year-old female with a 3-month history of fatigue and easy bruising associated with anemia, thrombocytopenia, and leukocytosis with numerous blasts on the peripheral blood smear. The blasts have abundant granular cytoplasm **a**. The blasts express CD34 **b**, CD117 **b**, HLA-DR, CD11b, CD13, CD15, CD33, CD64, and aberrant expressions of both CD56 **c**, and CD19 **d**. They are negative for CD20, surface light chains, and all T-cell antigens. They stain with MPO and SBB in >3% of blasts. The cytogenetic results show t(8;21), and the diagnosis of AML with t(8,21) is made.

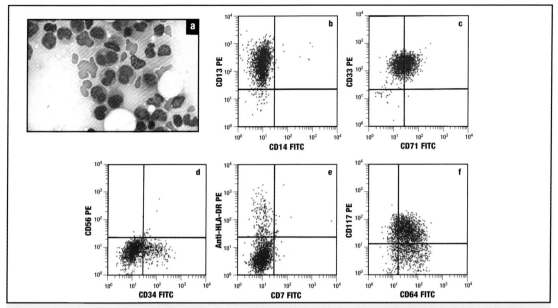

[f10.11] This case of AML demonstrates the characteristic immunophenotype of APL. The clinical history reveals a 46-year-old female presents with pancytopenia and rare blasts on the peripheral blood smear. The blasts reveal abundant cytoplasm and convoluted nuclei **a**. The blasts express CD13 **b**, CD33 **c**, and dim CD64 f and CD117 **f**. They are negative for CD34 **d**, HLA-DR **e**, and CD56, as well as all T-cell and B-cell antigens. The blasts stain intensely for MPO, SBB, and CAE and are negative for ANAE and ANBE. The cytogenetic show t(15;17), and the diagnosis of acute promyelocytic leukemia, hypogranular variant, is made.

as well as CD117 **[f10.11]**, whereas AMoL uniformly expresses HLA-DR, often expresses CD56 and CD64, may express CD34, and variably expresses CD117.

It should be kept in mind, however, that occasional cases of APL may express HLA-DR (27% of cases), and rare cases, CD34 [Carey 1994]. In AMLs, other than APL, expression of CD34 has been demonstrated in 62% of cases, and expression of HLA-DR, in 86% of cases. In a large study by Kaleem et al, 10% of 259 non-APL AMLs were negative for both CD34 and HLA-DR, as opposed to 80% of 41 APL cases. None of the APL cases were positive for both CD34 and HLA-DR, in contrast to 58% of the non-APL AMLs [Kaleem 2003].

In addition, although CD14 is a monocyte-specific marker, depending on the FCI technique and the epitopes analyzed, CD14 is often absent or frequently diminished in expression of AMLs with monocytic differentiation (ie, acute myelomonocytic leukemia—AMML or AML, M4 and AMoL or AML, M5) [Krasinska 1998, Dunphy 2004]. Thus, CD14 expression alone is not helpful in differentiating APL from AMoL and must be interpreted in light of a complete immunophenotypic panel, combined with cytomorphological examination of the immature cells.

AMLs with Monocytic Component (AMoL and AMML)

CD14 expression in AMoL and AMML

As alluded to above, although CD14 is a monocyte-specific marker, CD14 is often absent or frequently diminished in expression in AMLs with monocytic differentiation (ie, AMML and AMOL). Although CD14 has been touted as commonly expressed in AMML and AMoL, it has also been demonstrated that CD14 is negative in most cases of AMML and AMoL. The study by Eschoa et al concluded that although mature monocytes strongly express CD14, most immature leukemic monocytes (ie, monoblasts) lack CD14 expression [Eschoa 1999].

Diminished expressions of CD11b, CD13, CD15, CD33, and/or CD64 in AMoL and AMML

In addition, other markers characteristically expressed by normal monocytic cells (ie, CD11b, CD13, CD15, CD33, and CD64) may be absent or at least partially diminished in AMML and AMoL [Dunphy 2004].

Aberrant expressions of CD34, CD56, and CD117 in AMoL and AMML

CD56 may be aberrantly expressed in up to 50% of AMML and AMoL. Detection of CD34 and CD117 expression by FCA has also been shown to be indicative of malignancy in monocytic disorders and thus, may be observed in AMML and AMoL [Dunphy 2004].

CD64 and CD15 expressions in AMoL and AMML

A relatively recent study has concluded that CD64 is a sensitive and specific marker for distinguishing AMML and AMoL from other AML subtypes [Krasinska 1998]. A subsequent study further evaluated the usefulness of CD64 by FCA in distinguishing AMML and AMoL from other AML subtypes [Dunphy 2007]. In this subsequent study, CD64 was expressed in all AMoLs to varying degrees; 43% showed 3+ intensity and the remaining 57% of cases showed 1-2+ intensity. None of the other subtypes of AML demonstrated 3+ intensity expression of CD64, and thus, this feature was considered significant and useful, when present, in distinguishing AMoL from all other subtypes of AML.

Of note, 1-2+ intensity CD64 expression was also demonstrated in AML, M1s (27%), M2s (41%), and AMMLs (22%). The great majority of APLs (86%) and a subset of AML, M0s (14%) demonstrated 1+ intensity expression of CD64. Thus, by FCA of CD64 expression alone, these other AML subtypes with 1-2+ or 1+ intensity CD64 expression could not be distinguished from AMoLs with <3+ intensity. Of note, none of the AMLs with dim (1+) CD64 expression had lack of CD34 and HLA-DR expression, other than the APLs. Thus, the lack of HLA-DR and CD34 expression in APL may be very useful in distinguishing APL from other subtypes with dim (1+) CD64 intensity. In addition, none of the AML, M6s, or M7s revealed any CD64 expression, and thus, these subtypes may possibly be excluded if CD64 expression is demonstrated.

In addition, 3+ intensity CD15 expression was also highly significant in the AMML and AMoL subtypes. Conversely, 2+ to 3+ intensity CD13 expression was significantly observed in the "non-AMML or AMoL subtypes." The combination of any degree of CD64 expression with 3+ intensity CD15 expression and heterogeneous, or 1+ to 2+ intensity, CD13 expression was observed only in the AMML and AMoL subtypes. A case of AML, M5a is demonstrated in [f10.12], showing the immunophenotypic features described above.

In this study, analysis of expression of other markers (ie, CD11b, CD14, CD117, and CD56) showed no significant difference among the AML subtypes. This finding again supports the study by Krasinkas et al, illustrating that CD14 is only moderately specific for monocytic differentiation [Krasinska 1998].

AML, M5a vs M5b

Mature monocytes cannot be distinguished from promonocytes or monoblasts by FCA, unless the monoblasts express CD34. In a recent study, it was determined there were no statistically significant differences in the immunophenotypes of the M5a and M5b populations. CD34 and CD117 were the least prevalent antigens, detected in only 30% and 11% of the M5 samples analyzed, respectively [Villeneuve 2008].

AML, M6a vs M6b

The leukemic blasts in AML, M6a are myeloblasts, whereas those in M6b are erythroblasts. Thus, FCA may be quite useful in distinguishing these 2 subtypes, since erythroblasts will demonstrate surface expression of glycophorin A.

AML, M7

Flow cytometric analysis defines acute megakaryocytic leukemia, which requires demonstration of megakaryocytic antigen expression (ie, CD41, CD42b, and/or CD61) by the blasts. Since acute megakaryocytic leukemia may resemble ALL in pediatric patients, FCA may be particularly useful [f10.13] [Gassmann 1995].

Comparison of these 3 markers (ie, CD41, CD42, and CD61) has shown that CD42 is the least sensitive for early megakaryoblasts (due to the lack of CD42 expression by early megakaryoblasts), and CD41a is the most sensitive but least specific, and that CD61 is the most specific marker of megakaryoblastic differentiation [Käfer 1999, Karandikar 2001].

Tissue Forms of AML Subtypes

The tissue presentation of AML may be termed granulocytic sarcoma (ie, chloroma) if infiltrated and forming a tumor mass by myeloblasts; monocytic sarcoma, if composed of monocytic blasts; or erythroid sarcoma, if composed of the malignant erythroblasts of AML, M6b (ie, pure erythroid leukemia). They have the same immunophenotypes, as described above. A representative case of erythroid (erythroblastic) sarcoma is illustrated in [f10.14], with listmode output available on the accompanying disk.

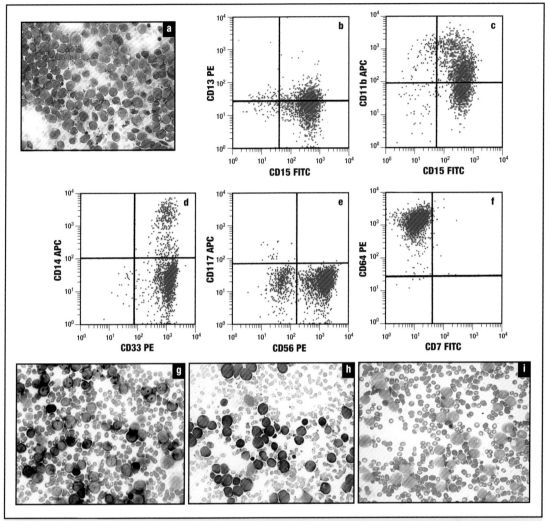

[f10.12] This case of AML reveals immunophenotypic features characteristic of monoblastic leukemia. The clinical history demonstrates a 48-year-old male with a history of hepatitis C, abdominal pain, gross hematuria, and leukocytosis, with disseminated intravascular coagulation. The blasts reveal abundant cytoplasm with numerous cytoplasmic vacuoles **a**. The blasts show strong expression of CD15 **b, c** with some loss of expression of CD13 **b**, some loss of expression of CD11b **c**, expression of CD33 **d**, lack of expression of CD14 **d**, aberrant expression of CD56 **e**, and strong expression of CD64 **f** and HLA-DR. They are negative for CD34, and CD117 **e**, as well as B-cell and T-cell antigens. The enzyme cytochemical stains are demonstrated in **g** (ANAE), **h** (ANBE), and **i** (CAE). The blasts intensely stain with ANAE and ANBE and show fine granular staining with CAE. The cytogenetic results reveal trisomy 8 and other abnormalities, but no t(15;17). The diagnosis of AML, M5a is made.

Differentiation of AML with Aberrant Antigen Expression from Acute Leukemias of Ambiguous Lineage (ie, Mixed Lineage and Mixed Phenotype Acute Leukemia) [t10.3]

Flow cytometric analysis is useful in distinguishing AML with aberrant antigen expression from acute leukemias of ambiguous lineage (ie, mixed lineage [f10.15] and mixed phenotype acute leukemias), which generally have a poor prognosis. This distinction is based on a scoring system as demonstrated in [t10.3]. Acute leukemia of ambiguous lineage is established when the score from 2 separate lineages is each >2 [Anon 1998].

Differentiation between AML with Aberrant CD56 Expression and Myeloid/Natural Killer Cell Precursor Acute Leukemia

AMLs may aberrantly express CD56, and CD56 expression has been described as a fairly common finding in M0, M2, M4, and M5 [Reuss-Borst 1992]. Although CD56 expression is more commonly expressed in AMLs

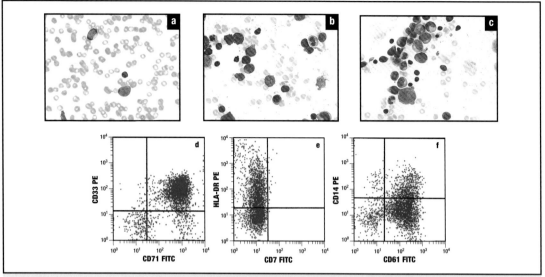

[f10.13] This case of AML, M7 is defined by flow cytometric analysis. The clinical history reveals an 18-month-old female who presents with 12% blasts in the peripheral blood. The blasts have increased nuclear:cytoplasmic ratios with rare cytoplasmic blebs a-c. The blasts strongly express CD33 d and show heterogeneous expression of HLA-DR e. The blasts are negative for CD14 f, CD34, CD64, CD117, and CD13, as well as T-cell and B-cell antigens. They strongly express CD61 f. The diagnosis acute megakaryoblastic leukemia, M7 is made.

t10.3 Scoring System for the Definition of Acute Leukemias of Ambiguous Lineage

Acute leukemia of ambiguous lineage is established when the score from two separate lineages is each >2.

Score	B-lymphoid	T-lymphoid	Myeloid
2	cCD79a*	cCD3 or sCD3	MPO
	cIgM	Anti-TCR	
	cCD22		
1	CD19	CD2	CD117
	CD20	CD5	CD13
	CD10	CD8	CD33
		CD10	CD65
0.5	TdT	TdT	CD14
	CD24	CD7	CD15

c, cytoplasmic; s, surface.

*CD79a may also be expressed in some cases of precursor T lymphoblastic leukemia/lymphoma.

with monocytic differentiation [AMML (67%), and AMoL (100%)], it may be nonspecifically expressed in other AML subtypes, including M0 (15%), M2 (22%), and even APL (17%) [Mann 1997, Dunphy 1999]. CD56 expression has also been described in a unique subtype of AML (CD56+, CD33+, CD13+/−, CD34−, HLA-DR−, CD16−), characterized by a high white blood cell count and marked nuclear foldings with variable cytoplasmic granularity resembling APL-M3v [Scott 1994]. Obviously, this entity would need to be distinguished from a CD56+ APL-M3v by exclusion of a t(15;17). Of interest, the CD56+ AMLs had the

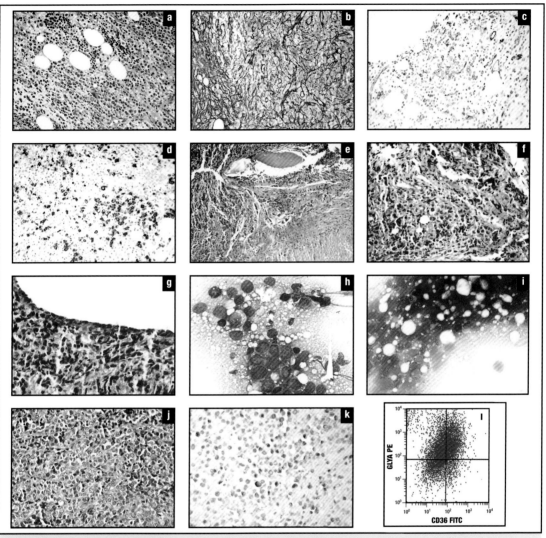

[f10.14] This case of erythroid (erythroblastic) sarcoma is characterized by flow cytometric analysis of a lymph node. The clinical history reveals a 42-year-old HIV-negative male with a history of alcohol abuse, a 7-month history of myelodysplastic syndrome, and pancytopenia, presenting with a new-onset lytic bone lesions and left supraclavicular lymphadenopathy. He has been treated with anti-thymocyte globulin, prednisone, and cyclosporine, as well as subsequent thalidomide for the myelodysplastic syndrome. The original diagnosis of a myelodysplastic syndrome is reviewed in the BM section **a** and demonstrates the abnormal localization of immature precursors interstitially associated with marked BM reticulin fibrosis **b**. The immature precursors are CD34+ and MPO+ by IHC stains (**c** and **d**, respectively). The cytogenetic data of this original BM specimen 44,X,–Y,der(5)t(5;?15)(q?22;q12),–7,–15,+?r[3]/46,XY[1], and diagnosis of myelodysplastic syndrome with marked reticulin fibrosis is made. The disease progresses, and the cytogenetic data from a subsequent BM performed 4 months later shows that each of the 23 cells analyzed are abnormal, representing 4 clones. These cells contain an unbalanced t(5;15), trisomy 8, a deleted chromosome 10q, and a derivative chromosome 19p. All cells contain additional abnormalities, including a 20p with additional material and an isochromosome of 20 long arm. The patient then developed lytic bone lesions and lymphadenopathy. A BM biopsy is again performed and reveals necrosis **e** and crush artifact **f**. PAS stain of the BM biopsy reveals positivity within large malignant-appearing cells **g**, consistent with erythroleukemia. The concurrent CBC data reveals a marked pancytopenia (WBC $0.4 \times 10^3/mm^3$ [$0.4 \times 10^9/L$], ANC 0, ALC $0.3 \times 10^3/mm^3$ [$0.3 \times 10^9/L$], Hgb 8 g/dL, Plt $16 \times 10^3/mm^3$ [$16 \times 10^9/L$]). The concurrent left supraclavicular lymphadenopathy is biopsied ($2.6 \times 1.7 \times 0.8$ cm red-tan lymph node tissue) and reveals sheets of large cells with basophilic cytoplasm on the touch preparation **h**, which show cytoplasmic positivity with the PAS stain **i**. The lymph node section reveals effacement by the sheets of large cells **j**. By IHC staining, the large cells are HbA1+ **k** and negative for CD45, CD20, CD3, HMB.45, S-100, AE1/AE3, CD138, CD30, κ, and λ. By FCI, 70% of cells fall within "region of interest," 74% of these cells express Glycophorin A **l** and "dim" CD45, as well as dim partial expression of CD36 **l** and heterogeneous expression of CD71. No additional markers, including T-cell, B-cell, or mylemonocytic markers are expressed. The cytogenetic data of this lymph node demonstrates that each of the 7 cells analyzed is abnormal, including extra copies of chromosomes 5 and 8 and monosmies Y and 15. Also seen are an unbalanced t(5;15), a deleted chromosome 8q, a deleted chromosome 10q, derivative chromosomes 19 and 20, and an isochromosome 20q. 1/7 cells: broken tetraploid with the above abnormalities. Additional ring and marker chromosomes are present. The diagnosis of erythroblastic sarcoma is rendered. The patient is treated for AML with 7+3+7 chemotherapy. At 6 weeks post-therapy, the bone marrow showed 80% malignant-appearing erythroblasts as seen previously. No additional follow-up is available.

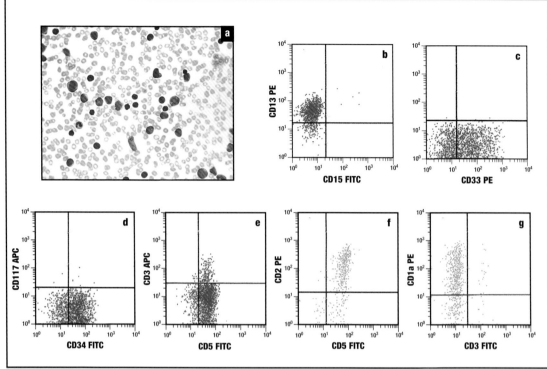

[f10.15] This case of bilineage acute leukemia (AML and precursor T-cell LL) is detected by flow cytometric analysis. The clinical history reveals a 56-year-old female with anemia, thrombocytopenia, and a marked leukocytosis, with numerous blasts on the peripheral blood smear. There are 2 populations morphologically on the peripheral blood smear. One population of blasts is relatively smaller with increased nuclear:cytoplasmic ratios; the other population of blasts is larger with more abundant cytoplasm and with some nuclear convolutions **a**. The population of "larger" blasts represents 58% of the peripheral white blood cells and show expression of CD13 **b**, CD33 **c**, CD34 **d**, and HLA-DR with aberrant expression of CD5 **e** and CD7. These blasts are negative for CD15 **b**, CD14 **c**, CD117 **d**, CD2, CD3 **e**, CD3, CD4, and CD8 as well as all B-cell antigens. The population of "smaller" blasts represents 20% of the peripheral white blood cells and show expression of CD2 **f**, CD5 **f**, CD1a **g**, CD4, and CD7. These blasts are negative for HLA-DR, CD3 **g**, and CD8, as well as all B-cell and myeloid antigens. The diagnosis of AML and precursor T-cell lymphoblastic leukemia/lymphoma: bilineage acute leukemia is made.

highest incidence of trisomy 22 (67% of cases studied) and trisomy 21 (75% of cases studied) [Dunphy 1999].

AMLs with CD56 expression must also be differentiated from CD7+/CD56+ myeloid/natural killer cell precursor acute leukemia. This distinct entity was described in 1997 by Suzuki et al and is characterized by the following immunophenotype: CD7+, CD33+, CD34+, CD56+, and frequently HLA-DR+ [Suzuki 1997]. A subset of these cases are cCD3+ by flow cytometry with additional cases cCD3+ by northern blotting. The majority show germline configurations of the T-cell receptor β and γ chain genes and Ig heavy chain gene. They are characteristically negative for MPO by cytochemical staining and negative for other NK, T-cell, and B-cell markers by flow cytometry. Morphologically, they are distinct from APL-M3v, being characterized by lymphoblastic morphology (L2 type with variation in size), round to moderately irregular nuclei and prominent nucleoli, pale cytoplasm, and a lack of azurophilic granules. It is important to recognize this entity, since it is more responsive to chemotherapeutic regimens for AML than to those for LL, although it often subsequently pursues a fatal course **[f10.16]**. It would also seem difficult to distinguish this entity (if cCD3–) from AML, M0 with aberrant CD7 and CD56 expression **[f10.17]**.

Differentiation between AML and Malignant Lymphoma

Distinction of malignant lymphoma from a granulocytic or monocytic sarcoma is greatly aided by FCA, since the malignant cells of AML will variably express myelomonocytic markers in these disorders. Obviously, malignant lymphomas of B-cell origin will generally demonstrate a monoclonal or aberrant B-cell population, and those malignant lymphomas of T-cell origin will variably express T-cell antigens.

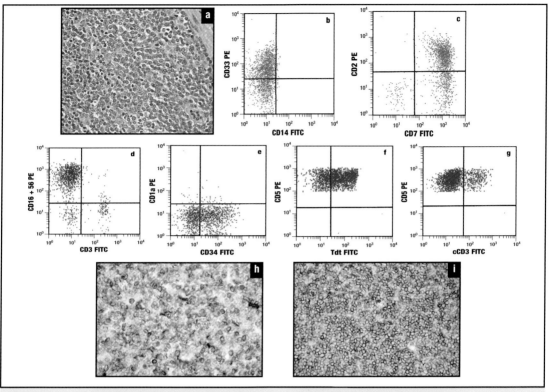

[f10.16] This case of myeloid/NK cell precursor acute leukemia presenting in lymph node is differentiated from a non-Hodgkin lymphoma and is fully characterized by flow cytometric analysis. The clinical history demonstrates a 35-year-old female with marked generalized lymphadenopathy associated with fatigue, but without associated weight loss, cough, or night sweats. The lymph node histology reveals sheets of blastic-appearing cells with fine nuclear chromatin and inconspicuous nucleoli **a**. The blasts express CD11b, CD13, CD33 **b**, CD2 **c**, CD5 (**f**, **g**), CD7 **c**, CD56 **d**, CD34 **e**, HLA-DR, and TdT **f** with dim, subset expression of cCD3 **g**. The blasts are negative for CD14, CD15, CD1a **e**, sCD3 **d**, CD4, CD8, CD57, and all B-cell antigens. The cytoplasmic expression of CD3 is better demonstrated by IHC **h**. CD56 by IHC shows strong immunoreactivity **i**. The cytogenetic results reveal del (7)(q22q32), t(10;12)(q22;p13), −10, add (18)(p11.2). A diagnosis of extramedullary involvement by myeloid/NK cell precursor acute leukemia is made.

Detection of Minimal Residual Disease and Relapse

Flow cytometric analysis is useful in defining a blast immunophenotype, which may be most useful in evaluating relapse/residual disease. An aberrant AML immunophenotype (eg, CD7+, CD19+) is particularly useful in detecting a residual or relapsing disease.

FCI Compared with Enzyme Cytochemical and IHC Techniques

Myeloperoxidase (MPO)

The subtyping of AML, M0 (vs AML, M1) is based on the negativity, or positivity within <3% of the blasts (in M0), with myeloperoxidase (MPO) and/or Sudan Black B by enzyme cytochemical methods. However, MPO may also be detected within the cytoplasm by flow cytometric (FC) and immunohistochemical (IHC) methods. Compared to the enzyme cytochemical method, detection of MPO within blasts by FC or IHC techniques appears to be more sensitive but less specific. Cases of precursor B-cell LL (up to 30%) and precursor T-cell LL (17%) were positive by the FC and IHC methods, although with dimmer intensities. There was no correlation of the flow cytometric MPO+ in these precursor LLs with myeloid antigen expression. The recommended cut-off for a positive MPO value remains at 3% for the enzyme cytochemical and FC methods [Nakase 1998, Peffault de Latour 2003, Kotylo 2000]. Absence of MPO staining by IHC staining may be useful in confirming the percentage of erythroid precursors, keeping in mind M0 blasts are often MPO-negative. These results stress the importance of interpreting MPO positivity in >3% of blasts and MPO negativity with additional immunophenotypic markers and the cytomorphology of the blasts.

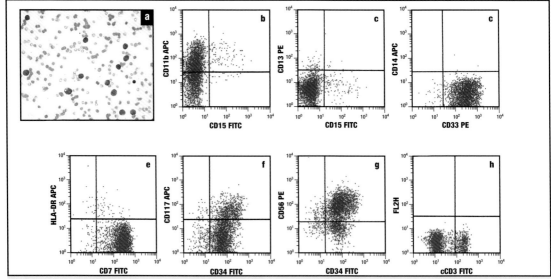

[f10.17] This case demonstrates the difficulty of distinguishing AML, M0 with aberrant CD7 and CD56 expressions from cCD3– myeloid/NK cell precursor acute leukemia. The clinical history reveals a 5-year-old female with a history of fever and leg pain associated with anemia, thrombocytopenia, and numerous blasts on the peripheral blood smear. The blasts in the peripheral blood are of varying size and show varying amounts of cytoplasm **a**. The blasts express CD11b **b**, CD33 **d** CD7 **e**, CD34 **f, g**, CD117 (partial expression, **f**), and CD56 **g**. The blasts are negative for CD15 **b,c**, CD13 **c**, CD14 **d**, and HLA-DR **e**, as well as all additional T-cell and B-cell antigens. They do not show significant expression of cCD3 **h**. The enzyme cytochemical stains for MPO, SBB, ANAE, ANBE, and CAE were all negative in the blasts. Cytogenetic results show 47, XX, del(1)(p21p31), add(2)(p23), del(11)(q21q23),t(12;13)(p13.1;q12), –15, –16, +22, +2,mar[10]. Diagnosis of AML, M0 vs myeloid/NK cell precursor acute leukemia is made.

Non-Specific Esterases

In contrast to the sensitive FC detection of MPO, FCA does not appear to be a sensitive method to detect monocytic cells (MCs) for the purpose of subtyping AMLs with a monocytic component. In a relatively recent study comparing non-specific esterase (NSE) staining with flow cytometry, there was an increased sensitivity of α naphthyl acetate esterase (ANAE) staining, but not alpha naphthyl butyrate esterase (ANBE) staining, to FCA in detecting MCs in AMML and AMoL. However, both NSE stains should be routinely performed, since there may be occasional to rare cases that reveal a higher percentage of monocytic cells, detected by ANBE staining rather than by ANAE staining [Dunphy 2004].

Immunohistochemical Markers and Recommended Panel

Although FCA is the preferred method of immunophenotypically differentiating acute leukemias, paraffin IHC staining may be useful in situations in which FCA cannot be performed. For example, when a BM aspirate is markedly hemodiluted or not able to be obtained for any reason, BM sections may be the only evaluable source to establish a diagnosis of MDS or AML and to distinguish these 2 entities from each other and from other possible hematolymphoid malignancies. As mentioned previously, it is important to interpret stains in light of other immunophenotypic markers (ie an IHC panel) and in combination with the morphologic features of each case.

There are IHC markers, for some of those antigens typically analyzed by FCA, that may be performed on BM sections to detect immature cells (ie, CD34, CD117, and TdT), to detect monocytic cells (ie, CD14), to distinguish erythroid from myeloid precursors (ie, CD33, MPO, and glycophorin A), and to detect megakaryoblasts (ie, CD61). Below follows a discussion of the comparisons of the detection of these above-mentioned antigens (for which there is data: CD34, CD117, and TdT) by these 2 techniques. There are no present publications describing the detection of CD14, CD33, and CD61 by FC vs IHC techniques. MPO has already been discussed previously.

CD34 and CD117

There are excellent studies reporting a high concordance rate of the sensitivity of immunodetection of

CD34 in AML by FC and IHC methods [Dunphy 2001, Manaloor 2000]. Only 1 study has reported CD34 expression to be more reliably determined by FCA [Arber 1996]. On the other hand, CD117 has been reported to have a higher sensitivity of immunodetection by FCA and to have a lesser sensitivity to immunodetection by IHC staining than CD34 [Dunphy 2001].

Due to the high sensitivity of CD34 immunodetection by IHC staining, it has been demonstrated that even in hemodiluted flow cytometry samples of bone marrow, the immunophenotypic data may be quite useful for subsequent IHC staining of the BM sections [Dunphy 2007]. It is important to remember that not all myeloblasts express CD34 and/ or CD117. However, if the blasts are CD34+ and/ or CD117+ by flow cytometry, IHC staining with CD34 and/or CD117 should be performed on the BM sections, since high-grade myelodysplasias or AMLs arising in the background of MDS may have small blasts (or "microblasts") that appear lymphoid by cytomorphological examination. In addition, there may be sampling differences between the BM aspirate material and the BM sections.

As mentioned above, CD34 appears to be significantly more reliable by IHC staining than CD117; however, in combination, they are most reliable and are complementary for an accurate quantitation of blasts. They should be performed on both BM clots and cores, due to their variable reactivity in paraffin-embedded and decalcified tissues. In the study referenced above, CD34 IHC staining was more intense in the BM core biopsy sections, whereas CD117 IHC staining was more intense in the BM clot sections. Thus, the decalcification process did not appear to have a uniform effect on the immunoreactivity of these markers.

Note that CD117 may also be expressed on mast cells, basophils, and promyelocytes, whereas CD34 is specific for non-erythroid blasts in BM sections [Dunphy 2007].

TdT

Terminal deoxynucleotidyl transferase (TdT) may be determined by both flow cytometry and IHC staining. Flow cytometry has been shown to be very sensitive in detecting as few as 2% blasts, and this technique further allows for multi-color analysis to confirm the presence of TdT on "T" vs "B" vs "myeloid" cells [Almasri 1991]. In contrast, TdT IHC staining does not necessarily correlate with the percentage of blasts in AML [Dunphy 2007].

This lack of significant correlation is due to the fact that TdT+ cells by IHC staining of BM tissue specimens most likely represent some myeloblasts expressing TdT (as it is a marker of immaturity and non-lineage specific) as well as other immature cells in the BM, such as hematogones. Hematogones are B-lymphocyte precursors commonly seen in children, but also may occur in marrows of adults and in regenerating marrows. They variably express B-cell precursor-associated antigens and TdT [McKenna 2004].

In addition, FCA detects quantitative differences between precursor T-cell or B-cell LL and AML and allows for determination of the definitive maturational stage of the precursor T-cell or B-cell LL [Farahat 1995].

PAX-5

Although PAX5 is not analyzed in routine practice by flow cytometry, this paraffin may serve as a surrogate marker for AML with t(8;21). Valbuena et al have shown that PAX 5 is expressed in every case of AML with t(8;21), and they confirmed this finding by Western blot methods [Valbuena 2006]. In addition, they showed that PAX5 expression is limited largely to AML with t(8;21), with only rare cases of AML, M0 (CD19–) and precursor T-cell lymphoblastic leukemia (CD19+) also expressing PAX5. The PAX5 expression correlated with the level of CD19 in the cases associated with t(8;21) and mostly showed weaker staining intensity than that of the mature B cells.

Recommended IHC Panel for Evaluation of AML and Differentiation from Other Hematolymphoid Malignancies

A recommended IHC panel for diagnosing AML (when there is no aspirable BM specimen for FCA or cytogenetic studies), and differentiating it from MDS and other hematolymphoid malignancies, includes CD3, CD14, CD20, CD33, CD34, CD79a, CD138, MPO, PAX5, and TdT [f10.18].

The study by Arber et al determined CD79a and TdT expression are the most frequently detected antigens in precursor-B-LL cases (89%, CD79a+; 100%, TdT+). However, CD79a may be detected in 11% of AML cases (most frequently of the APL subtype: 90% of APL cases are CD79a+) and TdT, in 13% of AML cases. However, CD20 was present on only 33% of precursor B-ALL cases. Nevertheless, 72% of precursor B-LL cases were identified by a CD79a+/ TdT+/MPO–/CD3– immunophenotype. All T-LL cases were either CD3+/CD79a–/MPO–/TdT+ or

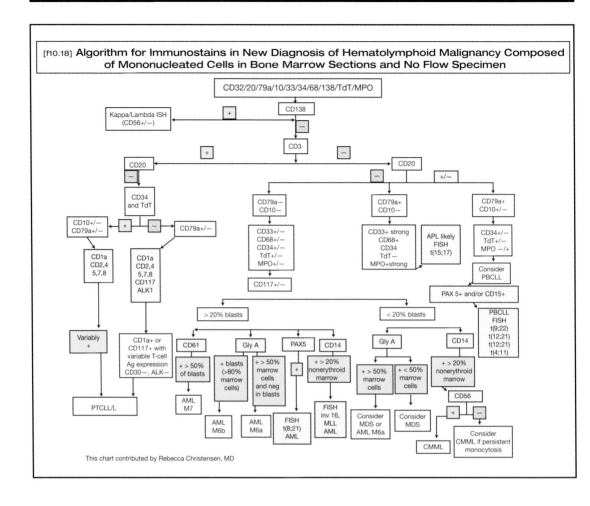

[f10.18] **Algorithm for Immunostains in New Diagnosis of Hematolymphoid Malignancy Composed of Mononucleated Cells in Bone Marrow Sections and No Flow Specimen**

This chart contributed by Rebecca Christensen, MD

CD3+/CD79a–/MPO–/TdT uninterpretable. Thus, this study recommended a panel of CD3, CD79a, MPO, and TdT as the most useful approach to paraffin immunophenotyping of acute leukemias [Arber 1996].

Due to the availability now of CD14 and CD33 for paraffin IHC, these antibodies may be considered in evaluating a monocytic component and recognizing an AML, M0 (in combination with the other immunophenotypic markers), respectively. In addition, PAX5 may be used as a surrogate marker for AML with t(8;21), when combined with the other immunophenotypic markers. PAX5 may also mark precursor B-cell LL and thus have a dual use in the IHC immunophenotyping of acute leukemias.

Lastly, the inv(16)(p13q22) or, less commonly, the t(16;16)(p13;q22) is characteristic of AMML with abnormal bone marrow eosinophils, also known as AML,M4Eo [Arthur 1983, Le Beau 1983, Liu 1995, Liu 1993]. This abnormality creates a fusion gene, 5′ core binding factor b (CBF-b) gene and the 3′ MYH11 gene, the latter encoding smooth muscle myosin heavy chain gene (SMMHC) [Liu 1993, Kundu 2002, Liu 1995]. Detection of this abnormality is important for diagnosis and is most commonly done by cytogenetic or molecular methods. A recent study by Zhao et al determined the utility of an IHC method, using a rabbit polyclonal antibody (AH107) against the C-terminus of the CBFb-SMMHC chimeric protein for a diagnosis of AML, M4Eo [Zhao 2006]. Immunohistochemical analysis of routinely processed paraffin-embedded BM sections showed that CBFb-SMMHC staining was predominantly nuclear in all cases of AML, M4Eo and was not nuclear in other AML types. Thus, this approach has been recommended as a specific, reliable, and convenient alternative to cytogenetic and molecular methods for the diagnosis of AML, M4Eo and may be particularly helpful in cases in which a BM aspirate is not available for cytogenetic and/or molecular studies.

When differentiating AML from MDS, or an acute leukemia from malignant lymphoma, CD34

t10.5 Immunohistochemical Immunophenotyping in Acute Leukemia with Markers Often Analyzed by Flow Cytometry, Enzyme Cytochemistry, or Cytogenetic/ Molecular Analyses

Type of Acute Leukemia	Markers	Reason	References
AML	MPO	96% of AMLs + Up to 30% of precursor B-LL and 17% of precursor T-LL may be MPO+ by IHC method, but with dimmer intensity	[Mann 1997], [Paietta 2004], [Sperling 1997], [Zhao 2006]
	CD14	Identify monocytic cells	
	CD33	Identify for diagnosis of AML, M0, when combined with morphology and other immunophenotypic markers	
	Glycorphorin A	AML, M6b	
	CD61	AML, M7	
	PAX5	Surrogate marker for t(8;21), when combined with morphology and other immunophenotypic markers	
	CBFβ-SMMHC Protein	Surrogate marker for inv(16)(p13q22) or t(16;16)(p13;q22), when combined with morphology and other immunophenotypic markers	
Precursor T-LL	CD3+/CD79a–/ MPO–/TdT+ or CD3+/CD79a–/ MPO–/TdT indeterminate	All cases with 1 of these 2 phenotypes; however, also reported that up to 60% of precursor T-cell LL may express cCD79a	[Paietta 2004], [Anon 1998]
Precursor B-LL	CD79a+/TdT+/ MPO–/CD3–	72% of cases identified with this phenotype; 89% of precursor B-LL are CD79a+; 100% of precursor B-LL are TdT+	[McKenna 2004]

may be particularly helpful in quantifying blasts, as previously discussed, and in excluding a mature B- or T-cell lymphoma, if expressed. CD138 is useful in distinguishing an acute leukemia from a plasma cell dyscrasia, since CD138 will be expressed in a plasma cell dyscrasia and negative in AML and precursor LLs.

A summary of IHC immunophenotyping of acute leukemias with markers often analyzed by flow cytometry and/or enzyme cytochemistry and molecular analyses is outlined in **[t10.5]**.

References

Almasri NM, Iturraspe JA, Benson NA, Chen MG, Braylan RC [1991] Flow cytometric analysis of terminal deoxynucleotidyl transferase. *Am J Clin Pathol* 95:376-380.

Anon [1998] The value of c-kit in the diagnosis of biphenotypic acute leukemia. EGIL (European Group for the Immunological Classification of Leukaemia). *Leukemia* 12:2038.

Arber DA, Jenkins KA [1996] Paraffin section immunophenotyping of acute leukemias in bone marrow specimens. *Am J Clin Pathol* 106:462-468.

Arthur DC, Bloomfield CD [1983] Partial deletion of the long arm of chromosome 16 and bone marrow eosinophilia in acute nonlymphocytic leukemia: A new association. *Blood* 61:994-998.

Brandt JT, Tisone JA, Bohman JE, Thiel KS [1997] Aberrant expression of CD19 as a marker of monocytic lineage in acute myelogenous leukemia. *Am J Clin Pathol* 107:283-291.

Carey JL, Hanson CA [1994] Flow cytometric analysis of leukemia and lymphoma. In: Keren DF, Hanson CA, Hurtubise PE, eds. *Flow Cytometry and Clinical Diagnosis.* 2nd ed. Chicago, IL: ASCP Press; 216-221.

De J, Zanjani R, Hibbard M, Davis BH [2007] Immunophenotypic profile predictive of KIT activating mutations in AML1-ETO leukemia. *Am J Clin Pathol* 128:550-557.

Dunphy CH [1999] Comprehensive review of adult acute myelogenous leukemia: Cytomorphological, enzyme cytochemical, flow cytometric immunophenotypic, and cytogenetic findings. *J Clin Lab Anal* 13:19-26.

Dunphy CH, Polski JM, Evans HL, Gardner LJ [2001] Evaluation of bone marrow specimens with acute myelogenous leukemia for CD34, CD15, CD117, and myeloperoxidase: comparison of flow cytometric and enzyme cytochemical vs immunohistochemical techniques. *Arch Path Lab Med* 125:1063-1069.

Dunphy CH, Orton SO, Mantell J [2004] Relative contributions of enzyme cytochemistry and flow cytometric immunophenotyping to the evaluation of acute myeloid leukemias with a monocytic component and the contribution of flow cytometric immunophenotyping to the evaluation of absolute monocytoses. *Am J Clin Pathol* 122:865-874.

Dunphy CH, O'Malley DP, Perkins SL, Chang CC [2007] Analysis of immunohistochemical markers in bone marrow sections to evaluate for myelodysplastic syndromes and acute myeloid leukemias. *Appl Immunohistochem Mol Morphol* 15:154-159.

Dunphy CH, Tang W [2007] The value of CD64 expression in distinguishing acute myeloid leukemia with monocytic differentiation from other subtypes of acute myeloid leukemia: a flow cytometric analysis of 64 cases. *Arch Pathol Lab Med* 131:748-754.

Eschoa C, Shidham V, Kouzova M, et al [1999] CD14 expression and nonspecific esterase staining in acute myeloid leukemia, AML, M4 and AML, M5. *Am J Clin Pathol* 112:88(Abstract);562.

Farahat N, Lens D, Morilla R, Matutes E, Catovsky D [1995] Differential TdT expression in acute leukemia by flow cytometry: A quantitative study. *Leukemia* 9:583-587.

Gassmann W, Loffler H [1995] Acute megakaryoblastic leukemia. *Leuk Lymphoma* 18 Suppl 1:69-73.

Jaffe E, Harris N, Stein H, et al [2001] *Tumours of Haematopoietic and Lymphoid Tissues.* Lyon, France: IARC Press; *World Health Organization Classification of Tumours.*

Käfer G, Willer A, Ludwig W, et al [1999] Intracellular expression of CD61 precedes surface expression. *Ann Hematol* 78:472-474.

Kaleem Z, Crawford E, Pathan MH, et al [2003] Flow cytometric analysis of acute leukemias. Diagnostic utility and critical analysis of data. *Arch Pathol Lab Med* 127:42-48.

Karandikar NJ, Aquino DB, McKenna RW, et al [2001] Transient myeloproliferative disorder and acute myeloid leukemia in Down syndrome: An immunophenotypic analysis. *Am J Clin Pathol* 116:204-210.

Kita K, Nakase K, Miwa H, et al [1992] Phenotypical characteristics of acute myelocytic leukemia associated with the t(8;21)(q22;q22) chromosome abnormality: frequent expression of immature B-cell antigen CD19 together with stem cell antigen CD34. *Blood* 80:470-477.

Kotylo PK, Seo I-S, Smith FO, et al [2000] Flow cytometric immunophenotypic characterization of pediatric and adult minimally differentiated acute myeloid leukemia (AML, M0). *Am J Clin Pathol* 113:193-200.

Krasinska AM, Wasik MA, Kamoun M, Scrhetzenmair R, Moore J, Salhany KE [1998] The usefulness of CD64, other monocyte-associated antigens, and CD45 gating in the subclassification of acute myeloid leukemias with monocytic differentiation. *Am J Clin Pathol* 110:797-805.

Kundu M, Chen A, Anderson S, et al [2002] Role of Cbfb in hematopoiesis and perturbations resulting from expression of the leukemogenic fusion gene Cbfb-MYH11. *Blood* 100:2449-2456.

Le Beau MM, Larson RA, Bitter MA, et al [1983] Association of an inversion of chromosome 16 with abnormal marrow eosinophils in acute myelomonocytic leukemia: a unique cytogenetic-clinicopathological association. *N Engl J Med* 309:630-636.

Lewis RE, Cruse JM, Sanders CM, et al [2006] The immunophenotype of pre-TALL/LBL revisited. *Exp Mol Pathol* 81:162-165.

Liu P, Tarle SA, Hajra A, et al [1993] Fusion between transcription factor CBF beta/PEBP2 beta and a myosin heavy chain in acute myeloid leukemia. *Science* 261:1041-1044.

Liu PP, Hajra A, Wijmenga C, et al [1995] Molecular pathogenesis of the chromosome 16 inversion in the M4Eo subtype of acute myeloid leukemia. *Blood* 85:2289-2302.

Liu PP, Hajra A, Wijmenga C, et al [1995] Molecular pathogenesis of the chromosome 16 inversion in the M4Eo subtype of acute myeloid leukemia. *Blood* 85:2289-2302.

Manaloor EJ, Neiman RS, Heilman DK, et al [2000] Immunohistochemistry can be used to subtype acute myeloid leukemia in routinely processed bone marrow biopsy specimens. Comparison with flow cytometry. *Am J Clin Pathol* 113:814-822.

Mann KP, DeCastro CM, Liu J, Moore Jo, Bigner SH, Traweek ST [1997] Neural cell adhesion molecule (CD56)-positive acute myelogenous leukemia and myelodysplastic and myeloproliferative syndromes. *Am J Clin Pathol* 107:653-660.

McKenna RW, Asplund SL, Kroft SH [2004] Immunophenotypic analysis of hematogones (B-lymphocyte precursors) and neoplastic lymphoblasts by 4-color flow cytometry. *Leukemia and Lymphoma* 45:277-285.

Nakase K, Sartor M, Bradstock K [1998] Detection of myeloperoxidase by flow cytometry in acute leukemia. *Cytometry (Communications in Clinical Cytometry)* 34:198-202.

Newell JO, Cessna MH, Greenwood J, Hartung L, Bahler DW [2003] Importance of CD117 in the evaluation of acute leukemias by flow cytometry. *Clin Cytometry* 52B:40-43.

Paietta E, Ferrando AA, Neuberg D, et al [2004] Activating FLT3 mutations in CD117/KIT(+) T-cell acute lymphoblastic leukemias. *Blood* 104:558-560.

Peffault de Latour R, Legrand O, Moreau D, et al [2003] Comparison of flow cytometry and enzyme cytochemistry for the detection of myeloperoxidase in acute myeloid leukaemia: Interests of a new positivity threshold. *Br J Haematol* 122:211-216.

Reuss-Borst MA, Steinke B, Waller HD, Buhring JH, Muller CA [1992] Phenotypic and clinical heterogeneity of CD56-positive acute nonlymphoblastic leukemia. *Ann Hematol* 64:78–82.

Scott AA, Head DR, Kopecky KJ, et al [1994] HLA-DR–, CD33+, CD56+, CD16– myeloid/natural killer cell acute leukemia: A previously unrecognized form of acute leukemia potentially misdiagnosed as French-American-British acute myeloid leukemia–M3. *Blood* 84:244-255.

Sperling C, Schwartz S, Buchner T, Thiel E, Ludwig WD [1997] Expression of the stem cell factor receptor C-KIT (CD117) in acute leukemias. *Haematologica* 82:617-621.

Suggs JL, Cruse JM, Lewis RE [2007] Aberrant myeloid marker expression in precursor B-cell and T-cell leukemias. *Exp Mol Pathol* 83:471-473.

Suzuki R, Yamamoto K, Seto M, et al [1997] CD7+ and CD56+ myeloid/natural killer cell precursor acute leukemia: A distinct hematolymphoid disease entity. *Blood* 90:2417-2428.

Thalhammer-Scherrer R, Mitterbauer G, Simonitsch I, et al [2002] The immunophenotype of 325 adult acute leukemias: Relationship to morphologic and molecular classification and proposal for a minimal screening program highly predictive for lineage discrimination. *Am J Clin Pathol* 117:380-389.

Valbuena JR, Medeiros LJ, Rassidakis GZ, et al [2006] Expression of B cell–specific activator protein/PAX5 in acute myeloid leukemia with t(8;21)(q22;q22). *Am J Clin Pathol* 126:235-240.

Villeneuve P, Kim DT, Xu W, Brandwein J, Chang H [2008] The morphological subcategories of acute monocytic leukemia (M5a and M5b) share similar immunophenotypic and cytogenetic features and clinical outcomes. *Leuk Res* 32:269-273.

Wells SJ, Bray RA, Stempora LL, et al [1996] CD117/CD34 expression in leukemic blasts. *Am J Clin Pathol* 106:192-195.

Zhao W, Claxton DF, Medeiros LJ, et al [2006] Immunohistochemical analysis of CBFβ-SMMHC protein reveals a unique nuclear localization in acute myeloid leukemia with inv(16)(p13q22). *AJSP* 30:1436-1444.

11 Precursor B-Cell Neoplasms

Chapter Contents

Classification

- ▶ Precursor B-lymphoblastic leukemia
- ▶ Precursor B-lymphoblastic lymphoma

Introduction

Precursor B-lymphoblastic leukemia/lymphoma (precursor B-LL/L) is a neoplasm of lymphoblasts committed to the B-cell lineage. The term "precursor B-lymphoblastic leukemia" applies if it is mainly marrow-based with >25% lymphoblasts in the bone marrow; "precursor B-lymphoblastic lymphoma" applies if it is mainly tissue-based with ≤25% lymphoblasts in the bone marrow. Prognosis in childhood precursor B-lymphoblastic leukemia depends on the following independent factors:

1. WBC ($>25 \times 10^3/mm^3$ [$>25 \times 10^9/L$])

2. age (<2 years and >10 years)

3. hypodiploidy, t(1;19)(q23;p13.3), t(9;22)(q34;q11.2), or t(v;11q23)

All 3 factors indicating a poor prognosis. Hyperdiploidy or t(12;21)(p13;q22) indicates a good prognosis.

The leukemic form of precursor B-lymphoblastic neoplasms is much more common than the lymphomatous presentation. When the lymphomatous form does occur, it is most often extranodal, commonly involving the skin or other extranodal site, and even presenting as lytic bone lesions. It less often involves lymph nodes and the mediastinum, as is frequently seen in precursor T-lymphoblastic lymphoma. with aggressive chemotherapy, localized precursor B-lymphoblastic lymphoma has a relatively good prognosis, and appears to have a better prognosis than precursor B-lymphoblastic leukemia [Lin 2000, Maitra 2001, Sander 1992, Nakamura 1991, Schmitt 1997, Iravani 1999].

Flow cytometric analysis is extremely useful in immunophenotyping and subtyping precursor B-LL/L, and is thus useful in diagnosis and prognostication of these neoplasms. The flow cytometric findings and correlation with subtype and particular cytogenetic abnormalities are further discussed below.

Diagnosis

Correlation of Specific Immunophenotype with Precursor B-Lymphoblastic Leukemia/Lymphoma Subtype, Stage of Differentiation, and Cytogenetic Abnormalities

The specific immunophenotypes of the 3 stages of precursor B-LL/L are outlined in [t11.1] and are demonstrated in [f10.8], [f11.1] and [f11.2], respectively. In addition, precursor B-lymphoblasts are almost always positive for cytoplasmic CD79a. CD45 may be absent, and cytoplasmic CD22 is considered lineage-specific. It is also important to recognize there may be occasional cases of precursor B-lymphoblastic leukemia with a mature immunophenotype (ie, with surface light chain expression) associated with L1 or L2 morphology and no evidence of a chromosomal translocation involving

t11.1 Immunophenotypes of B-Lineage Lymphoblastic Leukemias

Early Pre-B	Pre-B	Mature B (Burkitt)
CD19+, CD20–	CD19+, CD20+	CD19+, CD20–
CD24+	CD24+	CD24+
CD10±	CD10±	Intense CD10
Sig/light chain – TdT+	Sig/light chain – TdT+	Sig/light chain + TdT–

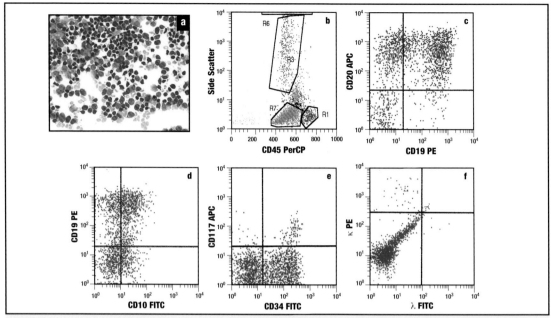

[f11.1] This case of precursor B-lymphoblastic leukemia occurred in a 69-year-old male with anemia, thrombocytopenia, and circulating blasts, and is characterized by variably sized lymphoblasts, with varying amounts of cytoplasm, observed in the BM aspirate smear **a**. Flow cytometric analysis of the bone marrow revealed the blasts had dim expression of CD45 **b** and a "pre-B" cell immunophenotype, in that they expressed CD19 (61%) **c, d**, CD20 (83%) **c**, CD10 **d**, CD34 **e**, and HLA-DR without expression of κ or λ surface light chains **f**, or any T or myelomonocytic markers analyzed. The cytogenetic results are normal. A diagnosis of precursor B lymphoblastic leukemia is made.

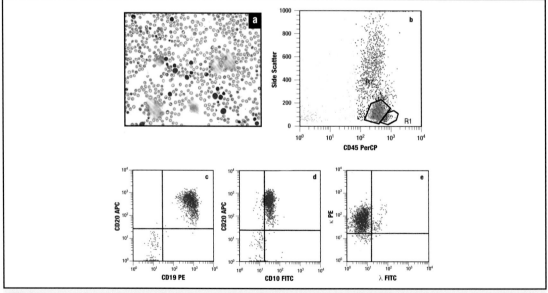

[f11.2] This case of B-cell leukemia/lymphoma also occurred in a 53-year-old female with a history of non-alcoholic fatty liver disease and a 3-week history of abdominal pain, nausea, fatigue, chin numbness, muscle aches, and a 6-pound weight loss. She is also thrombocytopenic and has occasional variably sized large abnormal lymphoid cells on the peripheral blood smear, and abnormal lymphoid cells, with cytoplasmic vacuoles, observed in a hemodiluted BM aspirate smear **a**. Flow cytometric analysis of the bone marrow revealed the abnormal lymphoid cells had moderate to strong expression of CD 45 **b** and a "mature-B" cell immunophenotype, in that they strongly expressed CD19 **c**, CD20 **c, d** with dimmer CD10 **d**, and HLA-DR with monoclonal expression of κ surface light chains **e** and no expression of CD34 or any T or myelomonocytic markers analyzed. The cytogenetic results demonstrate t(8;22). The diagnosis of Burkitt leukemia/lymphoma is made.

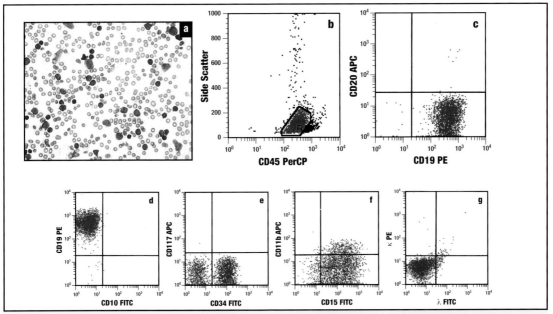

[f11.3] This case of precursor B-lymphoblastic leukemia occurred in a 4-month-old male, and was characterized by a marked leukocytosis (180 × 10³/mm³ [180 x 10⁹/L]), anemia, and thrombocytopenia associated with circulating blasts with a dimorphic blast population in the peripheral blood smear: smaller lymphoblasts and larger blasts with "monocytoid" features and abundant cytoplasm **a**. Flow cytometric analysis of the peripheral blood revealed the blasts had moderate to strong expression of CD45 **b** and an early "pre-B" cell immunophenotype, in that they expressed CD19 **c, d** without CD20 **c**, CD34 **e**, and HLA-DR. There was aberrant expression of CD15 **f**. The blasts did not express CD10 **d**, κ or λ surface light chains **g**, or any T or additional myelomonocytic markers analyzed. The cytogenetic results show t(4;11). Precursor B lymphoblastic leukemia associated with t(4;11) is diagnosed.

the *c-myc* gene **[f11.3]**. Such cases should not be considered Burkitt leukemia/lymphoma, but rather treated as precursor B-LL/L [Vasef 1998, Li 2003].

Flow cytometric analysis also allows for the detection of aberrant myeloid antigen expression (ie, CD13, CD33) in precursor B-lymphoblastic leukemia, which in adults is associated with a significantly lower complete remission rate and shorter survival. The distinction between precursor B-lymphoblastic leukemia with aberrant myeloid antigen expression **[f10.8]** and CD19+ AML **[f10.10]** may usually be made by the combination of markers expressed and review of the cytomorphology of the blasts in the peripheral blood and/or bone marrow (BM) aspirate smear. AML with aberrant CD19 expression is often associated with CD56 and CD34 expressions, with AML-M2 morphology, and with a t(8;21), as discussed in detail in the previous chapter on AML. Likewise, differentiation between precursor B-lymphoblastic leukemia with aberrant myeloid antigen expression and an acute leukemia of ambiguous lineage may be made by applying the criteria outlined in **[t11.3]**. Acute leukemia of ambiguous lineage is established when the score from 2 separate lineages is each >2 [Anon 1998].

In addition, flow cytometric analysis allows for the detection of a characteristic immunophenotype in precursor B-lymphoblastic leukemia associated with an *MLL* rearrangement: CD19+, CD15+, CD20–, CD10–, and HLA-DR+. The lymphoblasts in this leukemia are generally negative for all other myeloid antigens, as well as CD24 **[f11.4]**. It is important to recognize this subtype of precursor B-lymphoblastic leukemia, since it occurs in infants younger than 1 year of age and in adults and, as discussed above, is associated with a poor prognosis. In addition, rare cases of precursor B-lymphoblastic leukemia associated with an *MLL* rearrangement may demonstrate a mature immunophenotype (ie, λ sIg+, CD19+, CD10–, TdT–, and CD34–); these cases show no evidence of a *c-myc* rearrangement [Tsao 2004, Frater 2004].

Likewise, precursor B-lymphoblastic leukemia associated with t(1;19) has a characteristic immunophenotype: CD10+, CD34–, CD20– or dim, and usually cytoplasmic mu positive. This translocation, as discussed above, is also associated with a poor prognosis.

Precursor B-lymphoblastic leukemia associated with t(12;21) typically shows high-density expression of

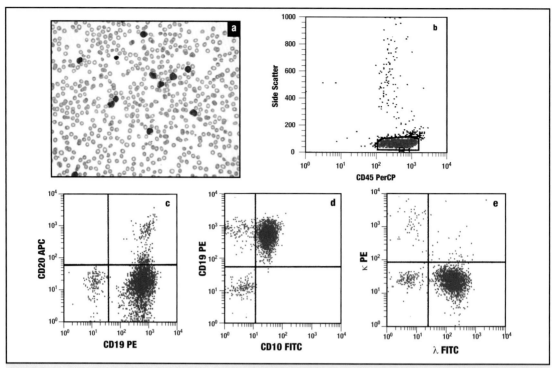

[f11.4] This case of precursor B lymphoblastic leukemia occurred in a 7-year-old female with a 1-week history of easy bruising, bleeding gums, and a petechial rash. She is also anemic, thrombocytopenic, and has an associated leukocytosis with numerous circulating variably sized lymphoblasts, with varying amounts of cytoplasm, observed in the peripheral blood smear a. Flow cytometric analysis of the peripheral blood revealed the blasts had strong expression of CD45 b and an aberrant "early pre-B" cell immunophenotype, in that they expressed CD19 c, d without CD20 c, and expressed CD10 d and HLA-DR with aberrant monoclonal expression of λ surface light chains e. They did not express CD34 or any T or myelomonocytic markers analyzed. The cytogenetic results were normal (FISH was negative for a *c-myc* translocation) and the diagnosis of precursor B lymphoblastic leukemia with an early pre-B immunophenotype and aberrant monoclonal λ light chain expression is made.

CD10 and HLA-DR with CD20-negativity. In contrast, this translocation, as discussed above, is associated with a good prognosis.

Differentiation between Precursor B-Lymphoblastic Leukemia and Reactive Conditions

As discussed in detail in Chapter 5, hematogones (B-lymphocyte precursors) may occur in large numbers in some healthy infants and young children and in a variety of diseases in both children and adults. In some instances, they may constitute 5% to more than 50% of cells in the bone marrow. In particular, increased numbers of hematogones may cause problems in diagnosis, due to the morphologic features they commonly share with neoplastic lymphoblasts. Their immunophenotype also has features in common with neoplastic B-lymphoblasts [t11.1] and [t11.2]. Although single- and 2-color flow cytometry do not reliably

differentiate hematogones from leukemic lymphoblasts, appropriately applied 3- and 4-color multiparametric flow cytometry are reported to distinguish between these cell populations in nearly all instances, as demonstrated in [f5.44] [f5.45] [f5.46]. Hematogones always exhibit a typical complex spectrum of antigen expression that defines the normal antigenic evolution of B-cell precursors and lacks aberrant expression. In contrast, neoplastic B-lymphoblasts show maturation arrest, according to their stage [t11.1], and exhibit varying numbers of immunophenotypic aberrancies (eg, expression of CD13, CD33). See [f11.1] [f11.2] [f11.3] [f11.4] [f11.5], demonstrating cases of precursor B-lymphoblastic leukemia and increased hematogones, respectively.

t11.2 Normal Maturational Sequence Bone Marrow Hematogones

Hematogones				Mature B-Cells
TdT				
CD34				
CD10 (brt)	CD10	CD10	CD10	
CD19	CD19	CD19	CD19	CD19
CD22 (dm)	CD22 (dm)	CD22 (dm)	CD22 (dm)	CD22
CD38 (brt)	CD38 (brt)	CD38 (brt)	CD38 (brt)	CD38 (brt/−)
		CD20 (dm)	CD20	CD20
		SIg	SIg	SIg

t11.3 Scoring System for the Definition of Acute Leukemias of Ambiguous Lineage*

Score	B-lymphoid	T-lymphoid	Myeloid
2	cCD79a[†]	cCD3 or sCD3	MPO
	cIgM	Anti-TCR	
	cCD22		
1	CD19	CD2	CD117
	CD20	CD5	CD13
	CD10	CD8	CD33
		CD10	CD65
0.5	TdT	TdT	CD14
	CD24	CD7	CD15
		CD1a	CD64

c, cytoplasmic; s, surface. *Acute leukemia of ambiguous lineage is established when the score from two separate lineages is each >2. [†]CD79a may also be expressed in some cases of precursor T lymphoblastic leukemia/lymphoma.

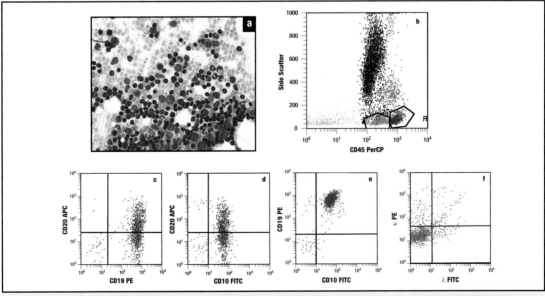

[f11.5] This 30-month-old male pediatric patient presents with thrombocytopenia and is being evaluated for ITP. Other CBC indices are essentially normal. There are increased lymphoid-appearing cells in the bone marrow aspirate smear **a** with smudged chromatin. Flow cytometric analysis of the bone marrow aspirate revealed that these lymphoid-appearing cells have dimmer expression of CD45 **b**, show expression of CD19 **c**, **d**, heterogeneous expression of CD20 **c**, **d**, expression of CD10 **d**, **e**, and expression of HLA-DR. They do not express κ or λ surface light chains **f**, CD34, or any T or myelomonocytic markers analyzed. The cytogenetic results are normal. Diagnosis of increased hematogones and increased megakaryocytes consistent with ITP is made.

Differentiation of Precursor B-Lymphoblastic Leukemia/Lymphoma from Mature B-Cell Lymphoma (Other Than Burkitt Lymphoma)

Since the early pre-B and pre-B stages of precursor B-LL/L lack light chain expression and various types of mature, or "peripheral" B-cell lymphoma may also show lack of light chain expression [Li 2002], one should keep in mind the distinction of these entities by morphologic and additional immunophenotypic features. The neoplastic cells of precursor B-LL/L should appear more "blastic" than the neoplastic cells of mature B-cell lymphoma. In addition, the neoplastic mature B cells will lack expressions of CD34 and TdT [f11.6].

Detection of Minimal Residual Disease and Relapse

By multiparameter flow cytometric analysis, minimal residual disease (MRD) may be reliably detected in precursor B-lymphoblastic leukemia [Dworzak 1999, Dworzak 2000]. The detection of MRD is based on comparing the aberrant phenotypes according to levels of expression of certain antigens (for example, CD10, CD19, CD34) in the neoplastic B-lymphoblasts to those of normal B-cell precursors. It is important to detect MRD, since early MRD detection may increase

the possibility to predict the risk for relapse and perhaps to select patients who would benefit from more intensified treatment or, even more interestingly, less intensive treatment. A relatively recent study by Bjorklund et al demonstrated that patients with MRD at a level of ≥0.01% of BM cells at follow-up time-points during and after first induction, and at the end of treatment had significantly lower disease-free survival in comparison to patients with MRD values <0.01% of BM cells [Bjorklund 2003]. It was suggested these patients with higher MRD values may benefit from upgrading therapy.

FCI vs IHC in Precursor B-Lymphoblastic Leukemia/Lymphoma

Since material may not always be available for flow cytometric analysis, the IHC findings in precursor B-LL/L are important for diagnosis and differentiation from reactive conditions (ie, hematogones), other hematolymphoid neoplasms (ie, AML, non-Hodgkin lymphomas), and non-hematolymphoid malignancies (ie, Ewing sarcoma).

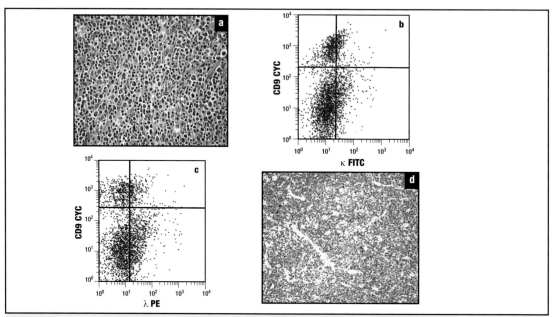

[f11.6] This case of diffuse large B-cell lymphoma lacks any surface light chain expression. The clinical history reveals a 31-year-old female with anemia, low-grade fever, weight loss, and systemic lymphadenopathy. A left axillary lymph node is biopsied. The histology of the involved lymph node **a** shows replacement of the nodal tissue by sheets of large cells. Flow cytograms of CD19 vs κ and CD19 vs λ show no light chain expression by the CD19+ cells **b, c**. The neoplastic cells intensely stain with CD20 by IHC **c** and BCL-2. The neoplastic B cells are negative for TdT, CD34, CD10, and BCL-6. The diagnosis of diffuse large B-cell lymphoma with lack of surface light chain expression by flow cytometry is made.

Differentiation of Precursor B-Lymphoblastic Leukemia/Lymphoma from Hematogones

Since multiparameter flow cytometric analysis is necessary for differentiation between neoplastic precursor B-lymphoblasts and hematogones, there are no well-described criteria for distinguishing between these cell types by IHC techniques.

Differentiation of Precursor B-Lymphoblastic Leukemia/Lymphoma from AML, Precursor T-Lymphoblastic Leukemia/Lymphoma, and Mature T-Cell and B-Cell Non-Hodgkin Lymphomas

AML

A large study by Arber et al addressed the usefulness of markers for immunophenotyping acute leukemias by paraffin IHC techniques, including CD3, CD20, CD34, CD43, CD68, CD79a, HLA-DR, myeloperoxidase (MPO), and terminal deoxynucleotidyl transferase (TdT) in predominantly Bouin-fixed, decalcified (s/p decal) bone marrow specimens [Arber 1996]. Myeloperoxidase and CD68 were the most specific myeloid markers (96% and 77% of AML cases positive, respectively). In fact, MPO+ AML cases even included all studied cases of M0 AML. However, 11% of precursor B-lymphoblastic leukemias were also MPO and CD68+ but generally weaker staining than in the AML cases. CD79a and TdT expression were the most frequently detected antigens in precursor B-lymphoblastic leukemias (89% CD79a+; 100% TdT+). However, CD79a was also detected in 11% of AML cases, most frequently of M3 subtype (90% of M3 cases CD79a+) and TdT in 13% of AML cases. A MPO+/CD79a+/HLA-DR– immunophenotype was only seen in M3 AML. In comparison to the flow cytometric results in this study, CD3 and CD20 were more reliably determined by paraffin IHC techniques; CD34 and HLA-DR were more reliably determined by flow cytometric analysis. However, CD20 was present in only 33% of precursor B-lymphoblastic leukemias. Nevertheless, 72% precursor B-lymphoblastic leukemias were identified by a CD79a+/TdT+/MPO–/CD3– immunophenotype. A simultaneous study by Chuang et al on B-5–, subsequently formalin-fixed, formic acid decalcified BM specimens supported the usefulness of these markers and the expected expression of CD20 in the more differentiated precursor B-LL/L cases (strongest in L3-Burkitt type) [Chuang 1997].

Other studies have also described the presence of MPO protein expression, as determined by IHC techniques in MPO enzyme-negative precursor B-lymphoblastic leukemia, in up to 56% of such cases [Austin 1998, Alvarado 1998]. There was no correlation of the MPO protein expression with other markers of myeloid differentiation, clinical or laboratory features, karyotypic patterns, or clinical outcome. It should also be kept in mind that MPO may also be detected by flow cytometric analysis. Results of MPO-positivity in precursor lymphoblastic leukemias by flow cytometry vary depending on the monoclonal antibody used [Leong 2004]. Anti-MPO (Dako, Denmark) has shown a high false positive result in 32% of precursor lymphoblastic leukemias, whereas anti-MPO (Becton Dickinson, California) has shown consistently negative results in precursor lymphoblastic leukemias. It has been suggested that the MPO positivity by these techniques in infant precursor B-lymphoblastic leukemia may be due to the derivation of the leukemic blasts from an immature hematopoietic precursor cell not fully committed to lymphoid differentiation [Austin 1998]. The importance lies in not interpreting MPO-positivity by an IHC technique or the flow cytometric technique using the DAKO antibody as an indicator of myeloid differentiation, or as a criterion to exclude a diagnosis of precursor B-lymphoblastic leukemia.

Another IHC marker, PAX5 (also known as B-cell-specific activator protein [BSAP]), is expressed in up to 98% of precursor B-lymphoblastic leukemias. However, as discussed in Chapter 10, Valbuena et al have shown that PAX5 is expressed in every case of AML with t(8;21) and largely limited to this AML subtype. In addition, rare cases of AML, M0 (CD19–) and precursor T-cell lymphoblastic leukemia (CD19+) may also express PAX5 [Valbuena 2006].

Based on this data, a recommended IHC panel for evaluating acute leukemias (when there is no aspirable BM specimen for flow cytometric analysis or cytogenetic studies), and differentiating it from other hematolymphoid malignancies, includes CD3, CD20, CD33, CD34, CD68, CD79a, CD138, myeloperoxidase (MPO), and terminal deoxynucleotidyl transferase (TdT). Additional markers that may be helpful include PAX5, CD14, CD117, additional T-cell antigens (including CD1a), CD61, and glycophorin A **[t10.4]**.

t11.4 Immunohistochemistry Panel Used to Distinguish between Precursor B-Lymphoblastic Leukemia/Lymphoma, DLBCL, and BL

IHC Marker	Precursor B-LL/L	DLBCL	BL
CD45RB (LCA)	Wk+ or –	Strong +	Strong +
CD20	– or wk+	Strong +	Strong+
CD10	±*	±*	Strong+
CD79a	+	+	+
PAX-5	+	+	+
BCL-2	–	±†	–†
BCL-6	–	±‡	+
CD34	+ (85%)	–	–
TdT	+ (95%)	–	–

BL, Burkitt lymphoma; DLBCL, diffuse large B-cell lymphoma; IHC, immunohistochemical; LCA, leukocyte common antigen; TdT, terminal deoxynucleotidyl transferase; wk weak.

*Early precursor B-LL/L may be CD10–. CD10 expression is seen in 80% of follicular lymphomas, and thus DLBCL of follicle center cell origin may variably express CD10.

†BCL-2 is expressed in most DLBCLs, but may occasionally be negative. BL may rarely express BCL-2 if associated with t(14;18) (ie, a "double-hit" lymphoma).

‡BCL-6 is expressed in DLBCLs of follicle center cell origin.

Precursor T-lymphoblastic leukemia/lymphoma

In the same study referred to previously by Arber et al, in comparison to precursor B-lymphoblastic leukemias, which have a CD79a+/TdT+/MPO–/CD3– immunophenotype in 72% of cases, all precursor T-lymphoblastic leukemias have a CD3+/CD79a–/MPO–/TdT+ or CD3+/CD79a–/MPO–/TdT uninterpretable immunophenotype [Arber 1996]. However, it should be kept in mind that CD79a has also been described as detected in 10%-50% of precursor T-LL/L [Pilozzi 1998]. One should also keep in mind that CD10 may be expressed in precursor T-LL/L, as previously discussed [f10.6].

Mature T-cell and B-cell non-Hodgkin lymphomas

As discussed above to some degree, precursor B-LL/L may need to be differentiated from a non-Hodgkin lymphoma (NHL). In general, precursor B-LL/L may be more easily distinguished from NHL of T-cell origin, since precursor B-LL/L does not express T-cell associated antigens that may be detected by IHC techniques (ie, CD1a, CD2, CD3, CD4, CD5, CD7, or CD8).

However, one should keep in mind that very rare cases of peripheral T-cell lymphomas (PTCLs) may express CD20 as well as CD79a; however, PTCLs are CD34– and TdT– and should have expression of other T-cell associated antigens [Yao 2001].

An important differential in the diagnosis of precursor B-LL/L is a mature B-cell NHL, especially Burkitt lymphoma (BL) and diffuse large B-cell lymphoma (DLBCL) [t11.4]. CD45 (leukocyte common antigen) may be weakly expressed or may be negative in precursor B-LL/L and is strongly expressed in B-cell NHL (DLBCL and BL). CD20 is typically strongly expressed in B-cell NHL (DLBCL and BL) but is variably expressed (negative to weakly expressed) in precursor B-LL/L, depending on the stage of differentiation, as discussed above. CD19 is not available for IHC staining in paraffin tissue. CD10 is variably expressed in precursor B-LL/L, again depending on the stage of differentiation, but it is also strongly expressed by BL and is expressed in up to 80% of follicle center cell lymphomas. Thus, DLBCL of follicle center cell origin may have variable expression of

CD10. PAX5 and CD79a are both positive in precursor B-LL/L and in mature B-cell NHLs (DLBCL and BL). BCL-2 protein expression by IHC techniques has been shown to be expressed in 38% of DLBCLs, 33% of high-grade B-cell Burkitt-like lymphomas, 0% of Burkitt lymphomas, and 0% of B-cell lymphoblastic lymphomas [Wheaton 1998]. BCL-2 positivity may rarely occur in BL and has been described when there is a coexistent t(14;18) and a Burkitt translocation. Thus, BCL-2 positivity may aid in excluding a precursor B-LL/L, when combined with morphology and additional immunophenotypic features, but will not distinguish between precursor B-LL/L and BL or a BCL-2-negative DLBCL. On the other hand, BCL-6 may help distinguish precursor B-LL/L from DLBCL of follicle center cell origin and BL, since BCL-6 is negative in precursor B-LL/L and positive in these other 2 entities. Lastly, CD34 and TdT are expressed in 85% and 95% of precursor B-LL/L cases, respectively, whereas all mature B-cell NHLs (DLBCL and BL) are both CD34- and TdT-negative.

Non-hematolymphoid malignancies

Diagnosing small round cell bone tumors in children may be problematic, especially in limited fixed tissue specimens. Distinguishing lymphoblastic lymphoma of bone and precursor lymphoblastic leukemia localized to the BM from intra-osseous Ewing sarcoma (ES) may be particularly difficult, due to overlapping morphologic and IHC features. Lymphoblastic lymphoma and ES are both CD99+, and lymphoblastic lymphoma is often non-reactive or only focally positive for "conventional" lymphoma markers. In addition, BCL-2 may be weakly positive in ES. As previously discussed, precursor B-lymphoblastic lymphoma may be weakly positive or negative for CD45, weakly positive or negative for CD20, and positive or negative for CD10. Vimentin may be demonstrated in both ES (88% of cases) and in 23% of lymphomas and leukemias [Ozdemirli 2001, Lucas 2001]. Thus, these conventional markers do not necessarily aid in distinguishing these entities. However, useful IHC markers for this differential diagnosis should include CD79a and PAX5, both positive in precursor B-lymphoblastic lymphoma and negative in ES. In addition, TdT-positivity (95% of precursor B-LL/L cases) and CD34-positivity (85% of precursor B-LL/L cases) should exclude ES.

References

Alvarado CS, Austin GE, Borowitz MJ, et al [1998] Myeloperoxidase gene expression in infant leukemia: A Pediatric Oncology Group Study. *Leuk Lymphoma* 29:145-160.

Anon [1998] The value of c-kit in the diagnosis of biphenotypic acute leukemia. EGIL (European Group for the Immunological Classification of Leukaemia). *Leukemia* 12:2038.

Arber DA, Jenkins KA [1996] Paraffin section immunophenotyping of acute leukemias in bone marrow specimens. *Am J Clin Pathol* 106:462-468.

Austin GE, Alvarado CS, Austin ED, et al [1998] Prevalence of myeloperoxidase gene expression in infant acute lymphocytic leukemia. *Am J Clin Pathol* 110:575-581.

Bjorklund E, Mazur J, Soderhall S, Porwit-MacDonald A [2003] Flow cytometric follow-up of minimal residual disease in bone marrow gives prognostic information in children with acute lymphoblastic leukemia. *Leukemia* 17:138-148.

Chuang SS, Li CY [1997] Useful panel of antibodies for the classification of acute leukemia by immunohistochemical methods in bone marrow trephine biopsy specimens. *Am J Clin Pathol* 107:410-418.

Dworzak MN, Stolz F, Froschl G, et al [1999] Detection of minimal residual disease in pediatric B-cell precursor acute lymphoblastic leukemia by comparative phenotype mapping: A study of five cases controlled by genetic methods. *Experimental Hematology* 27:673-681.

Dworzak MN, Fritsch G, Panzer-Grumayer ER, Mann G, Gadner H [2000] Detection of minimal residual disease in pediatric B-cell precursor acute lymphoblastic leukemia by comparative phenotype mapping: Method and significance. *Leuk Lymphoma* 38:295-308.

Frater JL, Batanian JR, O'Connor DM, Grosso LE [2004] Lymphoblastic leukemia with mature B-cell phenotype in infancy. *J Pediatr Hematol Oncol* 26:672-677.

Iravani S, Singleton TP, Ross CW, Schnitzer B [1999] Precursor B lymphoblastic lymphoma presenting as lytic bone lesions. *Am J Clin Pathol* 112:836-843.

Leong CF, Kalaichelvi AV, Cheong SK, Hamidah NH, Rahman J, Sivagengei K [2004] Comparison of myeloperoxidase detection by flow cytometry using two different clones of monoclonal antibodies. *Malays J Pathol* 26:111-116.

Li S, Eshleman JR, Borowitz MJ [2002] Lack of surface immunoglobulin light chain expression by flow cytometric immunophenotyping can help diagnose peripheral B-cell lymphoma. *Am J Clin Pathol* 118:229-234.

Li S, Lew G [2003] Is B-lineage acute lymphoblastic leukemia with a mature phenotype and L1 morphology a precursor B-lymphoblastic leukemia/lymphoma or Burkitt leukemia/lymphoma? *Arch Pathol Lab Med* 127:1340-1344.

Lin P, Jones D, Dorfman DM, Medeiros LJ [2000] Precursor B-cell lymphoblastic lymphoma: A predominantly extranodal tumor with low propensity for leukemic involvement. *AJSP* 24:1480-1490.

Lucas DR, Bentley G, Dan ME, Tabaczka P, Poulik JM, Mott MP [2001] Ewing sarcoma vs lymphoblastic lymphoma: A comparative immunohistochemical study. *Am J Clin Pathol* 115:11-17.

Maitra A, McKenna RW, Weinberg AG, Schneider N, Kroft SH [2001] Precursor B-cell lymphoblastic lymphoma: A study of nine cases lacking blood and bone marrow involvement and review of the literature. *Am J Clin Pathol* 115:868-875.

Nakamura N, Tominaga K, Abe M, Wakasa H [1991] A case of lymphoblastic lymphoma with pre-B cell phenotype. *Acta Haematol* 86:53-54.

Ozdemirli M, Fanburg-Smith JC, Hartmann D-P, Azumi N, Miettinen M [2001] Differentiating lymphoblastic lymphoma and Ewing's sarcoma: Lymphocyte markers and gene rearrangement. *Mod Pathol* 14:1175-1182.

Pilozzi E, Pulford K, Jones M, et al [1998] Co-expression of CD79a (JCB117) and CD3 by lymphoblastic lymphoma. *J Pathol* 186:140-143.

Sander CA, Jaffe ES, Gebhardt FC, Yano T, Medeiros LJ [1992] Mediastinal lymphoblastic lymphoma with an immature B-cell immunophenotype. *AJSP* 16:300-305.

Schmitt IM, Manente L, Di Matteo A, Felici F, Giangiacomi M, Chimenti S [1997] Lymphoblastic lymphoma of the pre-B phenotype with cutaneous presentation. *Dermatology* 195:289-292.

Tsao L, Draoua HY, Osunkwo I, et al [2004] Mature B-cell acute lymphoblastic leukemia with t(9;11) translocation: A distinct subset of B-cell acute lymphoblastic leukemia. *Mod Pathol* 17:832-839.

Valbuena JR, Medeiros LJ, Rassidakis GZ, et al [2006] Expression of B-cell-specific activator protein/PAX5 in acute myeloid leukemia with t(8;21)(q22;q22). *Am J Clin Pathol* 126:235-240.

Vasef MA, Brynes RK, Murata-Collins JL, Arber DA, Medeiros LJ [1998] Surface immunoglobulin light chain-positive acute lymphoblastic leukemia of FAB L1 or L2 type: A report of 6 cases in adults. *Am J Clin Pathol* 110:143-149.

Wheaton S, Netser J, Guinee D, Rahn M, Perkins S [1998] Bcl-2 and bax protein expression in indolent vs aggressive B-cell non-Hodgkin's lymphomas. *Hum Pathol* 29:820-825.

Yao X, Teruya-Feldstein J, Raffeld M, Sorbara L, Jaffe ES [2001] Peripheral T-cell lymphoma with aberrant expression of CD79a and CD20: a diagnostic pitfall. *Mod Pathol* 14:105-110.

12 Mature B-Cell Neoplasms

Chapter Contents

Classification

- Chronic lymphocytic leukemia/small lymphocytic lymphoma
- B-cell prolymphocytic leukemia
- Lymphoplasmacytic lymphoma/Waldenström macroglobulinemia
- Splenic B-cell marginal zone lymphoma (± villous lymphocytes)
- Hairy cell leukemia
- Plasma cell myeloma/plasmacytoma
- Extranodal marginal zone B-cell lymphoma of MALT type
- Nodal marginal zone B-cell lymphoma (± monocytoid B cells)
- Follicular lymphoma
- Mantle cell lymphoma
- Diffuse large B-cell lymphoma (DLBCL associated with chronic inflammation, 2008; large B-cell lymphoma arising in HHV8-associated multicentric Castleman disease, 2008)
  - Mediastinal (thymic) large B-cell lymphoma
  - Intravascular large B-cell lymphoma
  - (ALK+ large B-cell lymphoma, 2008)
  - (Plasmablastic lymphoma, 2008—also under lymphomas associated with HIV-infection; see below)
  - Primary effusion lymphoma
- Burkitt lymphoma/leukemia
- (B-cell lymphoma, unclassifiable, with features intermediate between DLBCL and Burkitt lymphoma, 2008)

- (B-cell lymphoma, unclassifiable, with features intermediate between DLBCL and classical Hodgkin lymphoma, 2008)
- Primary cutaneous B-cell lymphomas (WHO-EORTC classification)
  - Primary cutaneous marginal zone B-cell lymphoma
  - Primary cutaneous follicle center lymphoma
  - Primary cutaneous diffuse large B-cell lymphoma, leg type
  - Primary cutaneous diffuse large B-cell lymphoma, other

Introduction

Flow cytometric immunophenotyping (FCI) is particularly suited to the diagnosis and subclassification of mature B-cell neoplasms, primarily due to the ability of FCI to detect monoclonality and/or aberrancy of B cells. This chapter will first describe the applications of FCI to detect monoclonality/aberrancy of B cells, and then describe the immunophenotypes that may be detected by FCI in the various subtypes of mature B-cell neoplasms, as categorized by the WHO classification. The WHO classification is provided above, but the subtypes will be discussed in the order provided below, due to the logistics of comparing these entities in an efficient, practical manner.

Identification of Clonal/Aberrant B Cells and Distinguishing Follicular Hyperplasia from Follicular Lymphoma

FCI may be useful in differentiating florid follicular hyperplasia (FH) from follicular lymphoma (FL). This differentiation is most often accomplished by the detection of a monoclonal B-cell population by FCI. The normal range of the κ:λ ratio by FCI in reactive or benign lymphoid tissue has been reported to be 0.8 to 2.2 [Reichard 2003].

Although the reported normal range of the κ:λ ratio by FCI in reactive or benign lymphoid tissue is 0.8 to 2.2, there has been a recent report of "restricted κ:λ ratio" by FCI in the germinal center (GC) B-cells in Hashimoto thyroiditis (HT) [Chen 2006]. By 4-color FCI of 21 cases of HT, the CD10+ GC B-cells showed significantly higher mean κ:λ ratios than the CD10– B-cells (ie, 5.1 ± 3.3 vs 2.0 ± 0.8; P <.0001, Student t test). In 67% (18/21) of HT cases, the CD10+ GC B-cells had a κ:λ ratio >3.07 (the upper limit of the κ:λ ratio reported in reactive nodes; range, 3.2-14.4 in the 18 cases) ([f12.1], case with κ:λ ratio of 14.4). Cases tested by polymerase chain reaction (PCR) showed no evidence of a clonal proliferation, and none developed lymphoma during a 3-year clinical follow-up. This phenomenon is important to recognize in preventing a misdiagnosis of FL in patients with FH within HT.

In addition, there may be occasional cases of florid FH in which the clonality of the GC B cells is indeterminate by FCI. These cases may be distinguished by HLA-DO, a flow cytometric marker that is markedly down-regulated in CD10+ GC B cells of florid FH, in comparison to CD10– polytypic B cells and to CD10+ neoplastic cells of FL [Chen 2003]. In addition, multicolor FCI of expression of bcl-2, CD10, and CD20 may be useful in distinguishing FH from FL. In a recent study by Cook et al [2003], the presence of CD10+ cells with high bcl-2 expression predicted the presence of FL rather than FH with a positive predictive value of 100%. The analysis was performed on lymph node and bone marrow specimens [Cook 2003].

As detection of monoclonal B cells by FCI may be useful in establishing a diagnosis of B-cell NHL, it should also be noted that the lack of surface immunoglobulin (sIg) light chain expression by FCI helps identify peripheral B-cell lymphoma. In a recent study, Li et al [2002] studied cases with >25% B cells lacking sIg light chain expression all represented lymphoma. The lack of sIg light chain expression was not restricted to any particular subtype of B-cell lymphoma. By FCI, the identified sIg light chain-negative population was distinctly separate from the normal polytypic B cells. In 90% of cases, the identified population was larger by forward angle light scatter than the reactive T cells and polytypic B cells [f12.2]. In their review of reactive cases, no reactive case revealed >17% sIg– B cells. Such a case is demonstrated in [f12.3], with listmode output available on the accompanying disk.

Importance of Reviewing Dot Plots, Even with "Normal κ:λ Ratio"

Although most mature B-cell neoplasms exhibit monoclonal light chain or lack light-chain expression, there have been increasing numbers of reports that double light-chain gene rearrangements or dual light-chain expression

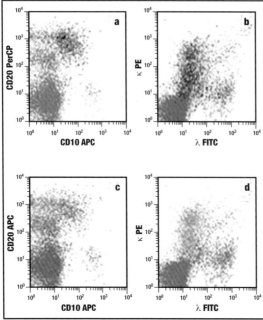

[f12.1] Flow cytometric histogram. **a,b**, CD10+/CD20+ germinal center (GC) B cells show significantly more expression of κ light chain (red, 4.45%) compared with λ (blue, 0.31%), resulting in a κ:λ ratio of 14.4. **c,d** In contrast, the CD10–/CD20+ non-GC B cells have a normal κ:λ ratio (κ, yellow, 11.25%; λ, green, 4.88%; ratio, 2.3). Note that the intensity of light chain expression in GC B cells is dimmer (weaker; ie, shifted to the left) than in non-GC B cells (comparison between **b** and **d**). *APC, allophycocyanin; FITC, fluorescein isothiocyanate; PE, phycoerythrin; PerCP, peridinin chlorophyll protein. Reprinted with permission from* [Chen 2006].

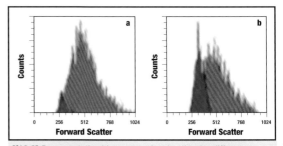

[f12.2] Representative histograms showing the size difference between surface immunoglobulin-negative B cells (red) and the background normal polytypic B cells (blue in **a**) or the reactive T lymphocytes (blue in **b**). *Reprinted with permission from* [Li 2002].

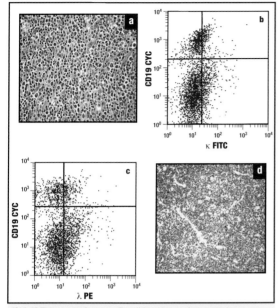

[f12.3] This case of mature B-cell lymphoma demonstrates significant lack of any light chain expression, indicating clonality. The clinical history reveals a 31-year-old female with anemia, low-grade fever, weight loss, and systemic lymphadenopathy. A left axillary lymph node is biopsied. The lymph node is effaced by a diffuse population of predominantly large abnormal lymphoid cells **a**. Flow cytometric analysis reveals a significant population of CD19+ cells with neither κ nor λ light chain expression (**b**, **c** upper left boxes, respectively). The CD20-positivity within the majority of lymphoid cells in the tissue section is confirmed by CD20 immunohistochemistry **c**, **d**. The diagnosis is made of diffuse large B-cell lymphoma with lack of surface light chain expression by flow cytometry.

by FCI may occur [del Senno 1987, Peltomaki 1988, Xu 2006]. In the presence of dual light-chain expression, the κ:λ ratio will likely show a polytypic pattern by FCI, depending on the percent of the dual-expressing B-cell population.

However, the κ+/CD19+ plus λ+/CD19+ B cells will exceed the total percent of CD19+ B cells. Therefore, visual inspection of the data plot histogram is critical, not only to evaluate the κ:λ ratio, but also to evaluate the sum of the κ+/CD19+ plus λ+/CD19+ expressing B cells **[f12.4]**. If this sum is 10% greater than the total percent of CD19+ B cells, or if the dual light-chain expressing B-cell populations comprise >10% of the total number of mature B cells, an IgH PCR study to look for clonality may be justified.

Order in Which Subtypes of Mature B-Cell Neoplasms Are Described

► Chronic lymphocytic leukemia/small lymphocytic lymphoma <EDIT OK?>
► B-cell prolymphocytic leukemia
► Mantle cell lymphoma
► Follicular lymphoma
► Lymphoplasmacytic lymphoma/Waldenström macroglobulinemia <EDIT OK?>
► Plasma cell myeloma/plasmacytoma
► Splenic marginal zone B-cell lymphoma (± villous lymphocytes)
► Extranodal marginal zone B-cell lymphoma of MALT type
► Nodal marginal zone B-cell lymphoma (± monocytoid B cells)
► Hairy cell leukemia
► Diffuse large B-cell lymphoma (including plasmablastic lymphoma and ALK+ DLBCL)
　► Mediastinal large B-cell lymphoma
　► Primary effusion lymphoma
► Burkitt lymphoma/Burkitt cell leukemia
► (B cell lymphoma, unclassifiable, with features intermediate between DLBCL and Burkitt lymphoma in differential diagnosis)

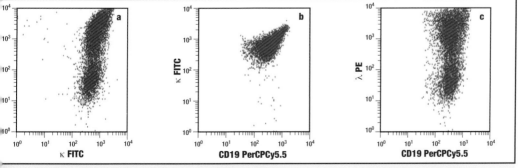

Four-color flow cytometric analysis shows a monotypic surface κ light-chain expression **b**. A significant number of the same cell ̄ion with κ:λ light-chain co-expression is also evident **a**. 64% of κ expressing cell population also expresses λ light chain **c**. *Reprinted ̄rmission from [Xu 2006].*

The flow

t12.1 Immunophenotypes of Small B-Cell Lymphomas/Leukemias

NHL	sIg	CD5	CD10	CD23	CD11c	CD103	CD25
CLL	wk	+	–	++/+	–	–	–
LPL	+	–	–	–	–	–	–
MCL	+	±	∓	∓	–	–	–
FL	+	∓	+	∓	–	–	–
MALT	+(IgM)	∓	–	–	+(wk)/–	–	–
NMZL	+(IgM/D)	–	–	–	+(wk)/–	–	–
SMZL	+(IgM/D)	–	–	–	+(wk)/–	+(wk)/–	–
HCL	+	–	–	–	++	++	++
HCL-V	+	–	–	–	+	∓	–

++, 90+% of cases antigen positive; +, 60%-89% of cases antigen positive; ±, 40%-59% of cases antigen positive; ∓, 10%-39% of cases antigen positive; –, <10% of cases antigen positive; CLL, chronic lymphocytic leukemia; FL, follicular lymphoma; HCL, hairy cell leukemia; HCL-V, hairy cell variant; LPL, lymphoplasmacytic lymphoma; MALT, mucosa-associated lymphoid tissue; MCL, mantle cell lymphoma; MZL, marginal zone lymphoma (MALT and nodal); NHL, non-Hodgkin lymphoma; NMZL, nodal marginal zone lymphoma; SMZL, splenic marginal zone lymphoma; wk, weak or dim staining, as compared to CD11c staining on normal monocytes, or CD11c and CD103 staining on HCL cells.

t12.2 Cytogenetic Abnormalities in Small B-cell Lymphomas/Leukemias

NHL	Cytogenetic Abnormalities
CLL	Trisomy 12; del(7q) (rare—plasmacytoid small lymphocytic lymphoma)
LPL	Trisomy 5, monosomy 8, del(6q)
MCL	t(11;14); trisomy 3(50%); del(7q)
FL	t(14;18) (80%)
MALT	t(11;18) (33%); t(1;14) (<5%); t(1;2) (<5%); trisomy 3 (85%); trisomy 12 (38%); trisomy 7 (15%)
NMZL	Trisomy 3 (50%); trisomy 12 (58%); trisomy 7 (33%); trisomy 18; del(6q); del(8q)
SMZL	Trisomy 3 (18%); del(7q) (40%); trisomy 12 (18%); trisomy 7 (12%); trisomy 18; del(6q); del(8q)
HCL and HCL-V	No characteristic abnormality

CLL, chronic lymphocytic leukemia; FL, follicular lymphoma; HCL, hairy cell leukemia; HCL-V, hairy cell variant LPL, lymphoplasmacytic lymphoma; MALT, mucosa-associated lymphoid tissue; MCL, mantle cell lymphoma; NHL, non-Hodgkin lymphoma; NMZL, nodal marginal zone lymphoma; SMZL, splenic marginal zone lymphoma.

cytometric immunophenotypic and cytogenetic features of the mature B-cell neoplasms, composed predominantly of small lymphocytes, are summarized in [t12.1] and [t12.2] for quick reference.

Chronic Lymphocytic Leukemia/ Small Lymphocytic Lymphoma

Definition

<EDIT OK?> Chronic lymphocytic leukemia/small lymphocytic lymphoma (CLL/SLL) is a neoplasm of monomorphic small, round B lymphocytes in the

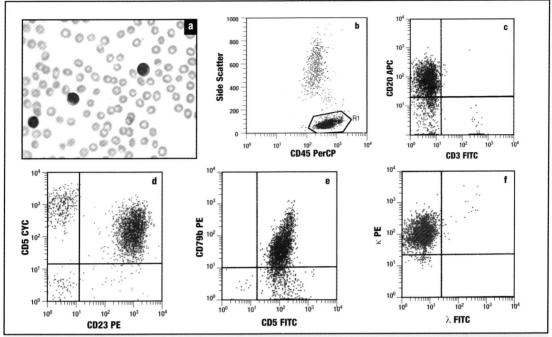

[f12.5] This case demonstrates the typical morphology and immunophenotypic features by flow cytometric analysis of CLL. The clinical history reveals a 54-year-old female with an absolute lymphocytosis ($54.3 \times 10^3/\mu L$) associated with thrombocytopenia. The peripheral blood smear reveals an increase in small, mature lymphocytes **a**. By flow cytometric analysis, there is an increase in cells in the lymphocyte region, characterized by low side light scatter and high expression of CD45 (**b**, increase in red dots). The cells within this region express CD20 (**c**, upper left box), co-express CD5 and CD23 (**d**, upper right box) as well as CD79b (**e**, upper right box), and reveal monoclonal κ surface light chain (**f**, upper left box). The diagnosis is made of chronic lymphocytic leukemia.

peripheral blood (PB), bone marrow (BM), and lymph nodes, admixed with prolymphocytes and paraimmunoblasts (pseudofollicles), usually expressing CD5 and CD23. The term SLL, consistent with CLL, is restricted to cases with the tissue morphology and immunophenotype of CLL, which are non-leukemic [Jaffe 2001].

Typical Immunophenotype

The tumor cells of SLL/CLL typically express weak or dim surface IgM or IgM and IgD, CD5, CD19, CD20 (weak), CD22 (weak), CD79a, CD23, CD43, CD11c (weak), and are CD10– and cyclin D1–. FMC7 and CD79b are, as a rule, negative or weakly expressed in typical CLL. A typical case is demonstrated in **[f12.5]** and the listmode output can be found on the accompanying disk.

Atypical CLL Variants

Morphologic variants

Cases of SLL/CLL with irregular nuclei and various morphologic variants of SLL may occur [Gupta 2000]. Atypical CLL, characterized by at least 10% lymphocytes with

clefted and folded nuclei in the PB, demonstrates significantly higher expression of CD23 than the expression seen in typical CLL. These patients generally have higher white blood cell counts and probability of disease progression [Frater 2001]. Such a case is demonstrated in **[f12.6]**; the listmode output can be found on the accompanying disk.

In addition, rare cases of CLL may be composed of neoplastic cells with morphologic features of "hairy cells," as demonstrated in a case example in **[f12.7]**; the listmode output may be found on the accompanying disk. The differentiation of CLL and hairy cell leukemia is discussed below under differential diagnoses.

Immunophenotypic variants

Some cases with typical CLL morphology may have a departure from the typical immunophenotype (ie, CD5– or CD23–, FMC7+ or CD11c+, or strong sIG, or CD79b+) [Matutes 1996, Criel 1999]. However, CD5– small B-cell leukemias are unlikely to represent CLL, and are classified more appropriately as NHL in the leukemic phase, based on a large study by Huang et al [1999]. This group found that, of only 3/192 cases classified as

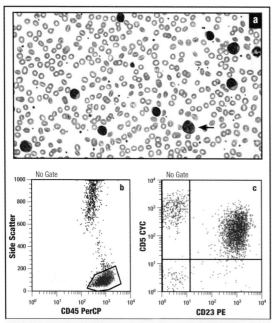

[f12.6] This case demonstrates atypical morphology for CLL. The clinical history reveals a 70-year-old female who presents with an absolute lymphocytosis (16.4 × 10³/μL). The peripheral blood smear reveals numerous cells with folded or "cleaved" nuclear borders (a, arrow). Again, by flow cytometric analysis there is an increase in cells with high CD45 expression and relatively low side light scatter. However, notice in comparison to [f12.15], the cells show a bulge with an increase in cells with somewhat higher side light scatter b. The cells within this region have a similar immunophenotype to typical CLL, with some cases showing increased intensity of CD23 expression (c, upper right box). The diagnosis is made of chronic lymphocytic leukemia with atypical morphology.

CD5– CLL, all 3 cases had features unusual for B-CLL, including bright sIg expression, bright CD20 expression, and absence of CD23 expression (2 cases) or Richter syndrome (1 case).

As mentioned earlier, higher intensity CD79b expression may occur in up to 20% of CLL cases. Of interest, this expression correlates with trisomy 12 and atypical immunophenotypic features; in turn, trisomy 12 in CLL correlates with a worse prognosis [Schlette 2003].

Detection of "Dual Light Chain Expression, Biclonality, and Bimodality" in CLL

As mentioned previously, there have been increasing numbers of reports that double light-chain gene rearrangements or dual light-chain expression by FCI can occur. This has been observed particularly in CLL [del Senno 1987, Peltomaki 1988, Xu 2006].

In addition, CLL may also be composed of 2 distinct clonal B-cell populations with different light chain restrictions, resulting in an apparent polytypic

pattern by FCI. This phenomenon may be deciphered by multi-color FCI, since the clones may have somewhat different immunophenotypes (ie, 1 population with dim CD19+, bright CD5+, moderate CD23+, and restricted κ, and the other population with moderate CD19+, bright CD5+, dim CD23+, and restricted λ). If not able to be deciphered by multi-color FCI, PCR may be indicated to determine the presence of 2 distinct clones [Chang 2006]. Such a case is demonstrated in [f12.8], with listmode output available on the accompanying disk.

Lastly, bimodal cell populations by multi-color FCI have been frequently observed in CLL [Cocco 2005]. In a study by Cocco et al, CD38 and CD13 were the most common antigens to demonstrate bimodality in CLL. However, CD20, CD11c, CD5, FMC-7, and sIg were also frequently bimodal in CLL [f12.9]. In particular, bimodality for CD38 trended toward a worse overall survival (OS).

Differential Diagnosis

Distinguishing CLL from the prolymphocytoid transformation of CLL (CLL/PLL) and B-prolymphocytic leukemia (B-PLL) arising in CLL

Since CLL, CLL/PLL, and PLL arising in CLL may have identical immunophenotypes by FCI, cytomorphological examination remains the mainstay in distinguishing these entities. CLL should have no more than 10% prolymphocytes identified within the PB; CLL/PLL has >10% but <55% prolymphocytes identified in the PB; and B-PLL arising in CLL has >55% prolymphocytes identified in the PB. In addition, FMC7 is typically strongly expressed in B-PLL arising in CLL [Delgado 2003].

Distinguishing CLL from mantle cell lymphoma with CD23 expression

Aberrant CD5 expression is characteristic of SLL/CLL and mantle cell lymphoma/leukemia (MCL/L). SLL/CLL may be reliably differentiated from MCL if CD23 is negative. However, dimly positive CD23 expression may be seen in SLL/CLL and MCL [f12.10]. In a study by Gong et al [2001], 12/22 MCLs were negative for CD23, and 10 showed dim CD23 expression. None of 25 CLL/SLLs were CD23–; 4 were dimly positive; and 21 were moderately or brightly positive. Thus, a significant proportion of MCL exhibited overlap of CD23 expression in the low-intensity range with CLL/SLL [Gong 2001]. Cases of CLL/SLL and MCL with dim expression of CD23 are demonstrated in [f12.11] and [f12.12], respectively, with the listmode output available

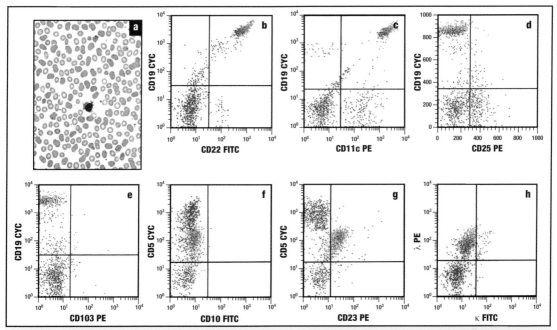

[f12.7] This case demonstrates "hairy cell" morphology in a case of CLL. The clinical history reveals an 83-year-old female with history of anemia and "hairy cells" seen by physician on review of peripheral blood smear. There is no evidence of splenomegaly. WBC $8.5 \times 10^3/$ mm^3 (8.5×10^9/L) with absolute lymphocyte count of 1.7×10^3/mm^3 (1.7×10^9/L) and absolute monocyte count of 700/µL; Hgb of 11.3 g/ dL; and platelet count of 195×10^3/mm^3 (195×10^9/L). The peripheral blood smear shows a "hairy cell" **a**. By flow cytometric analysis, 21% of cells fell within the lymphocyte region and there were 40% monoclonal B cells, which revealed expression of CD20 (not demonstrated) and CD19 **b-e** with CD22 (**b**, upper right box) and CD11c (**c**, upper right box), and no expression of CD25 **d** or CD103 **e**. In addition, there is co-expression of CD5 but not CD10 **f**, and co-expression of CD23 (**g**, upper right box), characteristic of CLL. There is λ light chain restriction **h**. The diagnosis is made of chronic lymphocytic leukemia with morphologic features of hairy cells.

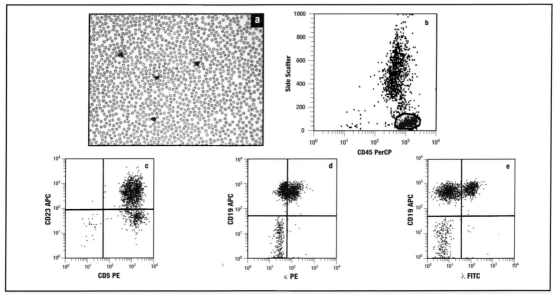

[f12.8] This case demonstrates a bi-clonal B-cell population in a case of CLL. The clinical history reveals a 77-year-old female with a history of squamous cell carcinoma, autoimmune hepatitis, and an absolute lymphocytosis (6.5×10^3/µL). The peripheral blood smear reveals an increase in small, round, mature lymphocytes **a**. By flow cytometric analysis, there is an increase in cells in the lymphocyte region, characterized by low side light scatter and high expression of CD45 (**b**, increase in red dots). The cells within this region are composed of 81% CD20+ cells with CD5 and CD23 being co-expressed **c**. Of interest, 45% of B cells express surface κ **d** and 29%, surface λ **e**, thus indicating 2 clones. The diagnosis is made of chronic lymphocytic leukemia with biclonal B-cells.

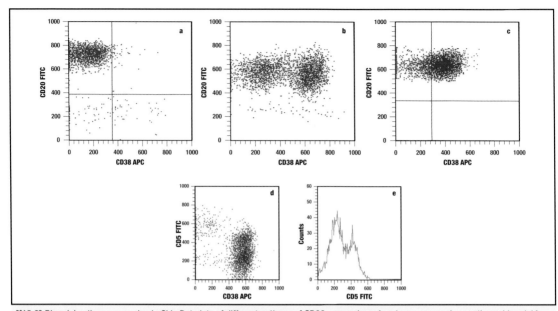

[f12.9] Bimodal antigen expression in CLL. Dot plots of different patterns of CD38 expression **a,b,c**: homogeneously negative **a**, bimodal **b** quadrant gates removed for clarity, and homogeneously positive **c**. Bimodal expression of CD5 **d,e**: dot plot **d**; **e** shows a histogram of the same specimen illustrated in **d**. *APC, allophycocyanin; FITC, fluorescein isothiocyanate. Reprinted with permission from [Cocco 2005].*

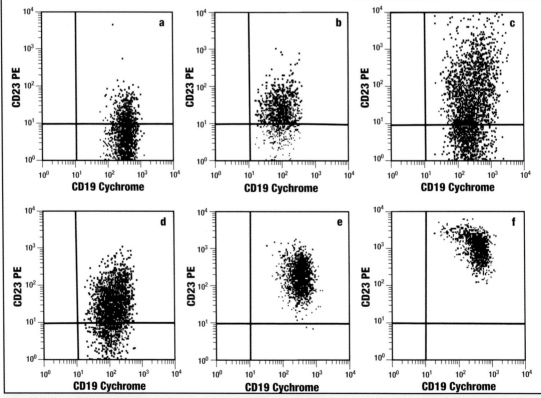

[f12.10] Patterns of CD23 expression in mantle cell lymphoma (MCL) and chronic lymphocytic leukemia/small lymphocytic lymphoma (CLL/SLL). MCL showing negative **a**, dimly positive **b**, and heterogeneous **c** CD23 expression; CLL/SLL with dimly positive **d**, moderately positive **e**, and brightly positive **f** CD23 expression. Overlap is present in the dimly positive category. *PE, phycoerythrin. Reprinted with permission from [Gong 2001].*

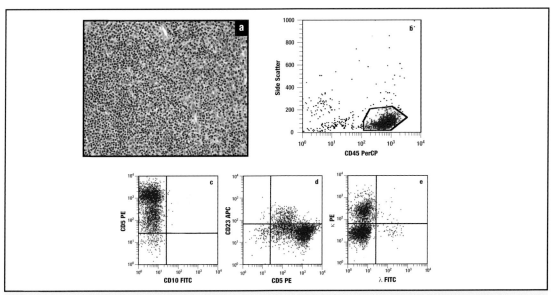

[f12.11] This case demonstrates small lymphocytic lymphoma (SLL)/CLL with dim CD23 expression. The clinical history reveals a 50-year-old female with lymphadenopathy. A right axillary lymph node is excised. The lymph node histology **a** reveals effacement of the lymph node by a diffuse population of predominantly small, round lymphocytes with scatter larger forms, characteristic of SLL. By flow cytometric analysis, there is an increase in cells within the lymphocyte region characterized by low side light scatter and high expression of CD45 (**b**, increase in red dots). Within the lymphocyte region, there are 31% monoclonal B cells with expression of CD19 and CD20 (not demonstrated) with co-expression of CD5 **c,d**, and CD23 (**d**, upper right box) with selective expression of surface κ **e**. Conventional cytogenetic and FISH [t(11;14)] studies are normal. The diagnosis is made of small lymphocytic lymphoma/CLL with dim CD23 expression.

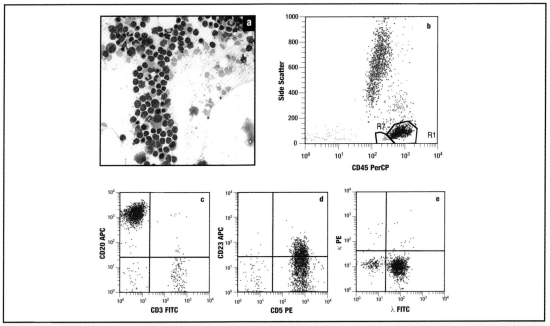

[f12.12] This case demonstrates mantle cell lymphoma with dim CD23 expression. The clinical history reveals a 50-year-old male with a history of mantle cell lymphoma with a recent peripheral blood study consistent with relapse. A bone marrow aspirate **a** reveals a marked increase in predominantly small, slightly irregular lymphocytes with scatter larger forms, characteristic of mantle cell lymphoma. By flow cytometric analysis, there is an increase in cells within the lymphocyte region characterized by low side light scatter and high expression of CD45 (**b**, increase in red dots). within the lymphocyte region, there are 89% monoclonal B cells with expression of CD19 and CD20 **c** with co-expression of CD5 and CD23 (**d**, upper right box) with selective expression of surface λ **e**. Conventional cytogenetic studies are normal, but the FISH [t(11;14)] study is abnormal. The diagnosis is made of involvement of bone marrow by mantle cell lymphoma with dim expression of CD23.

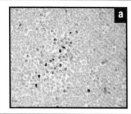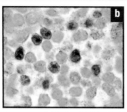

[f12.13] Focal cyclin D1 staining in CLL/SLL. **a** High magnification of cyclin D1 staining in proliferation center. Several positive cells are seen in a loose cluster. All proliferation centers had a similar staining pattern. Scattered positive large cells are rarely seen as well *(cyclin D1, original magnification, ×400).* **b** Cytologic detail of cyclin D1 staining inproliferation center. Note that the positive cells have prominent central nucleoli and are large *(cyclin D1, oil immersion, original magnification, ×1000). Reprinted with permission from* [O'Malley, 2005].

on the accompanying disk. Thus, immunohistochemical (IHC) and/or molecular analysis for cyclin D1 may be necessary in selected cases, keeping in mind focal cyclin D1 expression by immunohistochemistry may rarely occur in nodal CLL/SLL **[f12.13]**, in order to avoid a potential diagnostic pitfall [O'Malley 2005].

Another marker that may be useful in the differentiation of SLL/CLL from MCL is CD79b. This marker is characteristically absent or dimly expressed in SLL/CLL; CD79b expression in MCL is significantly higher [McCarron 2000]. However, as mentioned above, one should recognize that higher intensity CD79b expression may occur in up to 20% of CLL cases.

Distinguishing CLL from CD5+ MALT lymphoma

In addition, one should be aware that there are rare cases of CD5+ extranodal marginal zone B-cell lymphoma of mucosa-associated lymphoid tissue (MALT lymphoma) [Zaer 1998]. This differential diagnosis may be particularly difficult in small biopsy specimens. The recognition of pseudofollicles, prolymphocytes, and paraimmunoblasts would support SLL, whereas the findings of reactive follicles, marginal zone (centrocyte-like) cells, and plasma cells would support a CD5+ MALT lymphoma. If the biopsy is particularly small, cytogenetic results may aid in the differential diagnosis, since CD5+ MALT lymphoma may have associated abnormalities, including t(11;18), t(1;14), trisomy 3, or trisomy 7—abnormalities not associated with SLL. It is important to distinguish between SLL and CD5+ MALT lymphoma, since there has been a reported increased propensity for bone marrow involvement and relapse associated with these rare CD5+ MALT lymphoma cases [Ferry 1996].

Distinguishing CLL/SLL from hairy cell leukemia

Hairy cell leukemia (HCL) typically expresses pan-B-cell markers in association with CD103, CD11c, and CD25 [Chen 2006]. There have been no reports of CD5+ HCL; however, CD11c has been reported in up to 49% of CLL cases [Marotta 2000]. In addition, HCL may have atypical immunophenotypes with no expression of CD103 or CD25. Most often CLL may be distinguished from HCL by cytomorphology; however, in limited BM biopsy specimens, this differential diagnosis may be problematic. But the CD11c+ CLL cases were mainly seen in patients with early stage disease and no evidence of splenomegaly, as would be seen in HCL. In addition, careful examination of the fluorescence intensity of CD11c, calculated by mean fluorescence intensity (MFI), revealed significantly higher MFI of CD11c in HCL, compared to the values recorded in CLL.

Prognostic Markers in CLL: CD2, CD7, CD10, CD13, CD33, CD34, ZAP-70, CD38

Expression of aberrant markers by FCI, particularly CD2, CD7, CD10, CD13, CD33, and CD34, has been demonstrated to be associated with significantly shortened overall survival and increased aggressiveness [Kampalath 2003].

Expression of CD38 by >20%-30% of the neoplastic cells by FCI in CLL has been associated with an unfavorable prognosis [Ibrahim 2001, Del Poeta 2001]. Likewise, the expression of ZAP-70 as detected by FCI has been shown to correlate with immunoglobulin heavy-chain variable region (IgVH) mutational status (ie, unmutated immunoglobulin genes), more rapid disease progression, and poorer survival [Crespo 2003, Weistner 2003]. ZAP-70 detection by FCI has been somewhat problematic without high concordance rates [Chen 2007]. However, using >25% ZAP-70+ B cells as the cutoff, proper specimen processing, and the use of directly fluorescence-conjugated anti-ZAP-70 antibody have increased the usefulness of this method in estimating the ZAP-70 expression level in CLL **[f12.14]** [Slack 2007].

Comparison of FCI to Immunophenotyping by Paraffin Immunohistochemistry in CLL

It is extremely important to recognize that since CLL/SLL is characterized by dim expression of CD20 by FCI, this marker may appear negative by IHC staining. However, in such cases, a diagnosis of CLL/SLL may be reached by performing a panel of IHC stains, including CD3, CD5, and CD23; the neoplastic cells will typically be CD3– and CD5+/CD23+ by IHC staining.

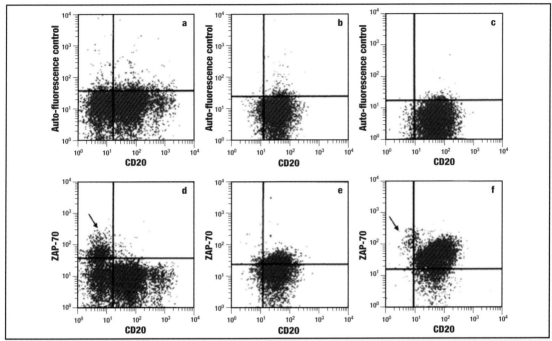

[f12.14] Flow cytometry dot plots illustrating ZAP-70 protein expression in the chronic lymphocytic leukemia cells from 3 newly diagnosed cases. The top panel (**a-c**) shows results of autofluorescence control vs CD20 in patients 1, 2, and 3, respectively. The bottom panel **d-f** shows results of ZAP-70 vs CD20 in the same 3 cases. Case 1 **a, d** shows 1% ZAP-70+ B cells, case 2 **b, e** shows 29% ZAP-70+ B cells, and case 3 **c, f** shows 80% ZAP-70+ B cells. Of note, the baseline thresholds were determined using the autofluorescence control (≤ 2%), and the actual levels of the baseline threshold varied from case to case. The T-cell population (denoted by arrows) also showed varying levels of ZAP-70 expression, as illustrated by comparing case 1 with case 3. In case 2, the T cells were too few to allow clear definition of this cell population. *Reprinted with permission from* [Slack 2007].

Of course, there may be cases in which the morphology and flow cytometric immunophenotype do not clearly distinguish between SLL/CLL and MCL. Such cases may require analysis of cyclin D1 by paraffin IHC staining. Cyclin D1 is a cell cycle protein that is over-expressed in MCL as a result of t(11;14) (q13;q32). Although FISH analysis for t(11;14) is much more sensitive than cyclin D1 by paraffin IHC staining (97% vs 69%), oftentimes the only material available for analysis is paraffin-embedded tissue. Real-time PCR analysis and routine cytogenetics do not offer increased sensitivity to paraffin IHC staining in detecting cyclin D1 [Belaud-Rotureau 2002]. Although cyclin D1 analysis by paraffin IHC staining is not highly sensitive, strong, diffuse reactivity of cyclin D1 in most monoclonal B cells has been shown to be extremely helpful in distinguishing MCL from CLL/SLL. However, recall that focal cyclin D1 expression by IHC may rarely occur in nodal CLL/SLL, in order to avoid a potential diagnostic pitfall [O'Malley 2005]. Other mature B-cell neoplasms that may express cyclin D1 by IHC staining include HCL and plasma cell myeloma [Miranda 2000, Troussard 2000]. The intensity of cyclin D1 by IHC staining in HCL is usually weak and in a subpopulation of the neoplastic cells.

The prognostic marker, ZAP-70, may be analyzed by FCI as well as by IHC staining. Of interest, the expression of ZAP-70 as detected by IHC staining in the BM biopsies has been related to the infiltration type. All samples with a diffuse infiltration pattern showed ZAP-70 staining, whereas cases with a nodular infiltration pattern were negative for ZAP-70. Those cases with mixed nodular and diffuse infiltration patterns showed variable ZAP-70 expression. In addition, the infiltration type was related to the mutation status in a subset of samples: mutation of the IgVH gene was restricted to the non-diffuse infiltration pattern and was not found in cases with diffuse infiltration of the bone marrow [Schade 2006]. In addition, Zanotti et al [2007] showed the concordance between ZAP-70 by IHC staining and ZAP-70 by FCI and IgVH mutational status was 89% (41/46) and 80% (41/49), respectively [Zanotti 2007]. Thus, detection of ZAP-70 expression by IHC staining on formalin-fixed BM biopsies at diagnosis may be useful in identifying patients with a poor prognosis in CLL.

B-Cell Prolymphocytic Leukemia

Definition

B-cell prolymphocytic leukemia (B-PLL) is a malignancy of B-prolymphocytes (medium-sized, round lymphoid cells with prominent nucleoli) affecting the PB, BM, and spleen. Prolymphocytes must exceed 55% of the PB lymphoid cells. Cases of transformed CLL and CLL with increased prolymphocytes are not included in this category of de-novo B-PLL.

Typical Immunophenotype

The cells of B-PLL strongly express surface IgM+/- IgD, as well as B-cell antigens (ie, CD19, CD20, CD22, CD79a, and CD79b) and FMC7. De-novo B-PLL may be distinguished from transformed cases of CLL, since the cells in the latter maintain the immunophenotype of CLL (ie, CD5+, CD23+), whereas the cells of de-novo B-PLL are CD5–. It is important to distinguish those cases arising in CLL, since CD5+ B-PLL has a longer median survival than CD5– B-PLL.

Differential Diagnosis

Prolymphocytic variant of mantle cell lymphoma

Leukemic manifestations of mantle cell lymphoma are seen in a minority of cases, usually associated with extensive tumors. Typically, the neoplastic cells in the PB resemble mantle cells with a mature chromatin pattern and irregular nuclear contours, or less frequently with a more "blastic" "chromatin pattern. However, cases of mantle cell leukemia with a prolymphocytic, or "prolymphocytoid," morphology have been described [Dunphy 2001, Ruchlemer 2004]. The cells of prolymphocytic mantle cell lymphoma/leukemia have the same immunophenotype as classical mantle cell lymphoma/leukemia, previously discussed above and also described in the section below regarding mantle cell lymphoma [Dunphy 2001]. Such a case is demonstrated in [f12.15] with the listmode output available on the accompanying disk.

Hairy Cell Variant

In addition, there is a variant of hairy cell leukemia with prolymphocytic morphology [termed hairy cell variant (HCL-V)], which typically presents with an elevated WBC count. Although HCL-V differs from classical HCL in clinical presentation, morphologic features, and response to therapy, it is termed HCL-V due to similar morphologic features (in BM and splenic tissue sections) and immunophenotypic features to classical HCL. Like classical HCL, the cells of HCL-V express pan B-cell antigens (ie, CD19, CD20, CD22, and CD79a) and CD11c, and are typically negative for CD5, CD10, and CD23. However, the immunophenotype of HCL-V differs somewhat from classical HCL (described previously above and also in the section below regarding hairy cell leukemia), in that there is variable expression of CD103 and lack of CD25. Such a case is demonstrated in [f12.16], with listmode output available on the accompanying disk. It is important to recognize this prolymphocytic variant of HCL since the response to treatment with agents effective in typical HCL is usually poor; median survival is significantly shorter in this variant, as compared to classical HCL.

Peripheralized paraimmunoblastic variant of SLL or large B-cell lymphoma

The paraimmunoblastic variant of SLL (SLL-PV) is characterized by a diffuse proliferation of cells normally comprising the pseudoproliferation centers (so-called paraimmunoblasts) and may be associated with an absolute lymphocytosis in approximately 13% of cases. When this variant peripheralizes, it may be difficult to distinguish from B-PLL [Pugh 1988]. The cells of SLL-PV will have the same immunophenotype as the cells of CLL/SLL. The differential diagnosis may occasionally be resolved by examination of lymph node pathology. Paraimmunoblasts are mitotically active, whereas prolymphocytes are not a mitotically active cell population. The lymph node morphology in SLL-PV is characterized by sheets of paraimmunoblasts mixed with prolymphocytes and infrequent collections of small lymphocytes; there is an associated pronounced mitotic activity. The lymph node morphology in CLL/PLL is more variable; however, there may be cases in which this differential diagnosis may not be resolved. A case of the paraimmunoblastic variant of SLL is demonstrated in [f12.17] of the accompanying disk.

T-cell prolymphocytic leukemia

B-PLL may be reliably distinguished from PLL of T-cell origin by FCI. In contrast to B-PLL, which has a mature B-cell immunophenotype, the cells of T-PLL express pan T-cell antigens (ie, CD2, CD3, CD5, and CD7) with CD4+/CD8– >CD4+/CD8+ >CD4–/CD8–.

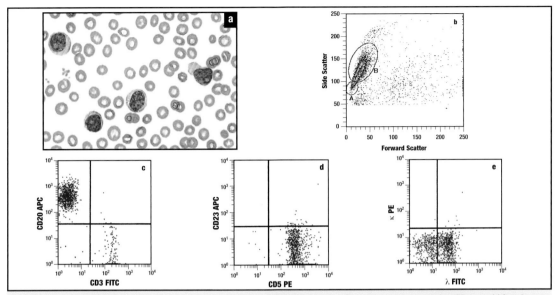

[f12.15] This case demonstrates the prolymphocytoid variant of mantle cell lymphoma. The clinical history reveals a 90-year-old female who presents with an elevated WBC count (89.7× 10³/μL) associated with anemia. The peripheral blood smear reveals the prolymphocytoid morphology **a**. The dot plot of side scatter vs forward scatter reveals an increase in cells within the "larger lymphoid" region **b**. These cells express CD20 (**c**, upper left box), aberrant CD5 (**d**, lower right box) without co-expression of CD23 **d**, and selective surface expression of κ light chain (**e**, lower right box). A subsequent bone marrow examination revealed cyclin D1 positivity by immunohistochemistry performed on the BM biopsy. The diagnosis is made of mantle cell leukemia/lymphoma with "prolymphocytoid" morphology.

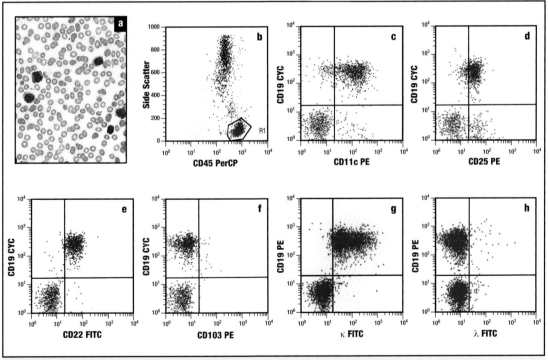

[f12.16] This case demonstrates the prolymphocytoid variant of hairy cell leukemia (ie, hairy cell variant—HCL-V) . The clinical history reveals an 82-year-old male who presents with an elevated WBC count (11.5 × 10³/μL). The peripheral blood smear reveals the prolymphocytoid morphology with occasional hairy cytoplasmic projections **a**. The dot plot of CD45 vs side scatter reveals an increase in side scatter, as compared to normal small lymphocytes **b**. These cells express CD19 **c-h**, CD11c **c**, CD25 **d**, CD22 **e**, and selective surface κ light chain **g**. They are negative for CD103 **f**. The diagnosis is made of hairy cell variant.

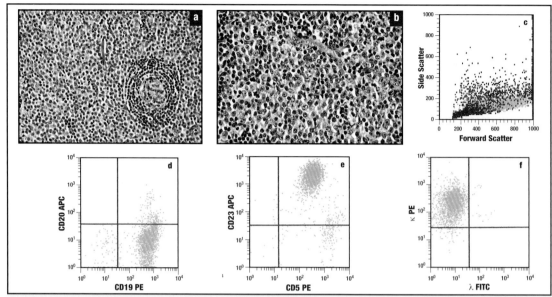

[f12.17] This case demonstrates the paraimmunoblastic variant of small lymphocytic lymphoma (PV-SLL). The clinical history reveals a 54-year-old male who presents with diffuse lymphadenopathy. A lymph node is biopsied. The histology of the lymph node reveals almost complete effacement of the lymph node by intermediate-sized to large cells; only a rare residual focus of small lymphocytes is observed **a**. Higher power reveals the characteristic morphology of paraimmunoblasts with varying numbers of inconspicuous nucleoli **b**. By flow cytometric analysis of the lymph node, the dot plot of forward scatter vs side scatter reveals an increase in cells with increased forward scatter (ie, larger sized cells; increase in pink dots) **c**. These cells express CD19 with loss of CD20 **c**, show co-expression of CD5 and CD23 (**d**, upper right box), and demonstrate selective surface expression of κ **f**. The diagnosis is made of paraimmunoblastic variant of small lymphocytic lymphoma.

Mantle Cell Lymphoma

Definition

Mantle cell lymphoma (MCL) is a B-cell neoplasm composed of neoplastic lymphocytes that are intermediate in morphology between those of B-CLL and FL. They have slightly irregular nuclear borders.

Typical Immunophenotype

The typical immunophenotype of MCL is co-expression of CD5 and CD20, no associated expression of CD23, expression of CD79b, and monoclonal light chain expression of an intermediate intensity. A typical case of MCL is demonstrated in **[f12.18]**, with the listmode output available on the accompanying disk. However, as discussed above, MCL may show dim expression of CD23, and a significant proportion of MCL exhibit overlap of CD23 expression in the low-intensity range with CLL/SLL. Such a case is demonstrated in **[f12.12]**, with the listmode output available on the accompanying disk.

Variants: Morphology and Immunophenotype

Morphologic variants that may be confused with other subtypes of mature B-cell neoplasms composed of predominantly small lymphocytes, including those with small, round lymphocytes with more clumped chromatin, resembling CLL/SLL and those with prominent foci of cells with abundant pale cytoplasm, resembling "monocytoid B cells."

In addition, occasional cases of classical MCL may demonstrate an associated clonal plasma cell population in the centers of neoplastic nodules and within reactive germinal centers [Young 2006]. Other morphologic variants of MCL (ie, blastoid variants—classic blastoid and pleomorphic) may be confused with mature B-cell neoplasms with large cell morphology (ie, diffuse large B-cell lymphoma-DLBCL or diffuse large cell lymphoma of T-cell origin), or even a granulocytic sarcoma. A case of blastoid variant of MCL is demonstrated in **[f12.19]**, with listmode output available on the accompanying disk.

Regarding variant immunophenotypes in MCL, in addition to the occasional occurrence of dim CD23 expression, there are also reports of CD5– MCL that are recognized based on the detection of BCL-1 by cytogenetic or molecular genetic techniques [Liu 2002]. Such a case of CD5– MCL is demonstrated in **[f12.20]**, with listmode output available on the accompanying disk.

Differential Diagnosis

CLL/SLL

This differential diagnosis was discussed above under CLL/SLL.

Follicular lymphoma

Mantle cell lymphoma may have a predominantly nodular pattern without a "mantle zone" pattern and without residual germinal centers, resembling FL. The neoplastic B cells of FL are typically CD5−, CD23±, and CD10+ with intense sIg light chain expression. In comparison, as described previously, the cells of MCL are typically CD5+ and CD10−. However, as also mentioned previously, MCL may occasionally be CD5−. In addition, the cells of MCL may rarely be CD10+ and the cells of FL may rarely be CD5+ [Dong 2003, Barry 2002]. In select cases, fluorescent in-situ hybridization (FISH) analysis for t(11;14) and/or t(14;18) may be necessary and useful in distinguishing these 2 subtypes of lymphoma.

Extranodal (MALT), nodal, and splenic marginal zone B-cell lymphoma

As mentioned, there is a morphologic variant of MCL characterized by prominent foci of cells with abundant pale cytoplasm, resembling "monocytoid B cells." Such cases may cause diagnostic confusion with marginal zone B-cell lymphoma. In addition, as discussed previously in the section about CLL/SLL, there are rare cases of CD5+ extranodal marginal zone B-cell (MALT) lymphoma [Zaer 1998]. This differential diagnosis may be particularly difficult in small biopsy specimens. The recognition of "pink histiocytes" would support MCL, whereas the findings of reactive follicles, marginal zone (centrocyte-like) cells, and plasma cells would support a CD5+ MALT lymphoma. However, as mentioned above, "monocytoid B cells" are characteristic of a morphologic variant of MCL, and occasional cases of MCL may show plasmacytic differentiation. If the biopsy is particularly small, cytogenetic results may aid in the differential diagnosis, since CD5+ MALT lymphoma may have associated abnormalities, including t(11;18), t(1;14), trisomy 3, or trisomy 7, whereas t(11;14) is characteristic of MCL. It is important to distinguish between MCL and MALT lymphoma, since MCL is considered an intermediate-grade lymphoma.

Lymphoplasmacytic lymphoma

Since occasional cases of MCL may demonstrate plasmacytic differentiation, diagnostic confusion with lymphoplasmacytic lymphoma may occur. The presence of "pink histiocytes" would favor MCL. Flow cytometric analysis in LPL cases typically detects a CD5−CD10− monoclonal B-cell population, which morphologically represents the small lymphocytes and plasmacytoid lymphocytes.

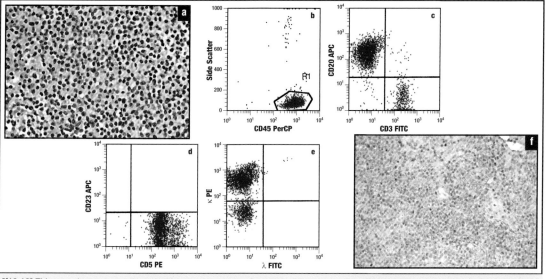

[f12.18] This case demonstrates the typical immunophenotype of mantle cell lymphoma. The clinical history reveals a 72-year-old male who presents with a large (9.5 × 7 × 5.7 cm) abdominal mass, which is biopsied. The histologic section of the abdominal mass reveals slightly irregular small to intermediate-sized lymphoid cells in a diffuse pattern **a**. By flow cytometric analysis, there is an increase in cells within the lymphocyte region characterized by low side light scatter and high expression of CD45 (**b**, increase in red dots). These cells express CD20 (**c**, upper left box), aberrant CD5 (**d**, lower right box) without co-expression of CD23 **d**, and selective surface expression of κ light chain (**e**, upper left box). Cyclin D1 immunohistochemistry demonstrates nuclear positivity **f**. The diagnosis is made of mantle cell lymphoma.

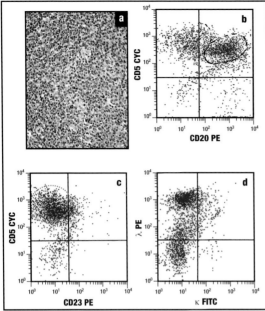

[f12.19] This case demonstrates a blastoid variant of mantle cell lymphoma. The clinical history reveals a 70-year-old male with lymphadenopathy. A right inguinal lymph node is biopsied. The histologic section of the lymph node reveals effacement of the normal lymph node architecture by a diffuse proliferation of predominantly large lymphoid cells associated with an increased mitotic rate **a**. By flow cytometric analysis, these large cells express CD20 with aberrant CD5 (**b**, upper right box), CD5 and CD23 (**c**, upper right box), and selective surface λ light chain (**b**, upper left box). The cytogenetic findings show 14 cells with 11;14 translocation and 7 of 14 cells, near-triploid. The diagnosis is made of blastoid variant of mantle cell lymphoma.

Small cell or "lymphoid" variant of plasma cell myeloma

This morphologic variant of plasma cell myeloma (PCM), as described below in the section of plasma cell myeloma/plasmacytoma, is characterized by small plasma cells with less abundant cytoplasm and a more "lymphoid" appearance. Such a case is demonstrated in **[f12.21]**, with the listmode output available on the accompanying disk. This morphologic variant is frequently associated with expression of CD20 as well as the t(11;14)(q13;32) and over-expression of cyclin D1, making distinction from MCL even more problematic [Young 2006, Robillard 2003]. A combination of other immunophenotypic features of plasma cell myeloma (ie, CD45−, CD5−, CD19−, CD138+, variable CD56+, monoclonal cytoplasmic light chain expression, and lack of surface light chain expression) are helpful in arriving at the correct diagnosis in these challenging cases. One should keep in mind that occasional cases of PCM may demonstrate CD45+ (although often dim in intensity), aberrant CD19+ (although not usually both CD19+ and CD20+), and monoclonal surface light chain expression (again, often dim in intensity).

Diffuse large B-cell or T-cell lymphoma and granulocytic sarcoma

As mentioned previously, the blastoid variants of MCL may cause diagnostic confusion with diffuse large cell

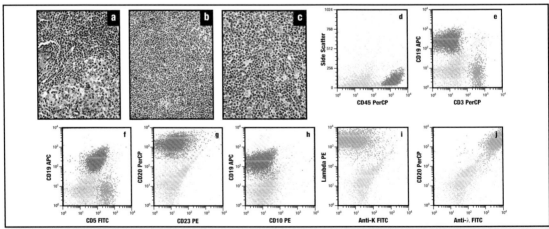

[f12.20] This case demonstrates mantle cell lymphoma with dim-negative expression of CD5. The clinical history reveals a 60-year-old male with left axillary lymphadenopathy, which is biopsied. The histologic sections of lymph node reveal an occasional residual germinal center (**a**, right side) with surrounding small to intermediate-sized lymphocytes with slightly irregular nuclear membranes (**b**, left side), with marked expansion in the interfollicular regions **b** and scattered pink histiocytes **c**, characteristic of mantle cell lymphoma. By flow cytometric analysis, there is an increase in cells within the lymphocyte region characterized by low side light scatter and high expression of CD45 (**d**, increase in red dots). These cells express CD19 **e, f, h**, CD20 **g**, and selective surface λ light chain **i, j**. They are clearly negative for CD23 **g** and CD10 **h** with equivocal expression (dim or no expression) of CD5 **f**. Cyclin-D1 IHC staining of the lymph node tissue revealed weak positivity. The diagnosis is made of mantle cell lymphoma with dim CD5 vs CD5-negativity.

lymphomas of B-cell or T-cell origin, as well as with granulocytic sarcoma. These may generally be distinguished from large cell lymphomas of T-cell origin, since T-cell lymphomas will typically show variable expression of T-cell associated antigens (ie, CD2, CD3, CD4, CD5, CD7, and CD8). Granulocytic sarcomas are typically distinguished by their variable expression of myelomonocytic markers, as AMLs and as described in Chapter 10. Distinction between the blastoid variants of MCL and DLBCL may be more problematic. The blastoid variants of MCL typically have a similar immunophenotype to classical MCL; however, there are occasional cases of CD5– MCL with blastoid morphology. In addition, there is a de-novo form of CD5+ DLBCL, with phenotypic and genotypic features different from MCL [Yamaguchi 2002]. The blastoid variants of MCL are important to recognize since these patients have a significantly worse prognosis than those with DLBCL. In such cases, the recognition of these morphologic variants of MCL relies on detection of the t(11;14) by IHC (cyclin D1), molecular [PCR analysis for t(11;14)], or cytogenetic [conventional cytogenetic or FISH analysis for t(11;14)] methods. Of further interest, de-novo CD5+ DLBCL is also characterized by a survival curve significantly inferior to that for patients with CD5– DLBCL (p= .0025) and may represent a unique subgroup of DLBCL [Yamaguchi 2002].

Immunohistochemical/Molecular/Cytogenetic Correlates

The t(11;14) may be detected by IHC, molecular, or cytogenetic techniques. By IHC methods, the cyclin D1 protein may be detected as a nuclear protein in approximately 69% of cases of MCL. Real-time PCR (RT-PCR) analysis and conventional cytogenetic analysis do not offer increased sensitivity to the paraffin IHC method in detecting cyclin D1. However, FISH analysis detects the t(11;14) in 97% of MCL cases and is the preferred method of detection [Belaud-Rotureau 2002]. Although cyclin D1 analysis by paraffin IHC is not highly sensitive, strong, diffuse reactivity of cyclin D1 in most monoclonal B cells has been shown to be highly specific for MCL. Hairy cell leukemia may also be cyclin D1+, but the staining has been described as usually weak and in a subpopulation of the tumor cells [Miranda 2000]. As discussed above, plasma-cell dyscrasias (particularly the small or "lymphoid" variant) may also show strong cyclin D1+ in tumor cells; however, the other immunophenotypic features should distinguish these entities, as described above. In addition, as

mentioned previously, cyclin D1 IHC staining may be focally observed in B-CLL/SLL [O'Malley 2005]. In fact, cyclins D1, D2, and D3 may all be expressed in CLL cells, as detected by a sensitive RNase protection assay. The order of expression in CLL cells by this technique is D3>D2>D1 [Meyerson 2008]. In fact by using high-resolution enzymatic amplification staining and flow cytometry, the D cyclins are shown to be differentially expressed in MCL and CLL with strong staining of cyclins D1 and D2 in MCL and low-level staining for both of these cyclins in CLL [Meyerson 2008].

Thus, it should not be surprising that cyclin D1– MCLs exist that may be identified by gene expression profiling (GEP) due to an "MCL signature." These cyclin D1– MCLs identified by this GEP signature may demonstrate over-expression of cyclin D2 or cyclin D3, indicating that overexpression of these proteins may functionally substitute for cyclin D1 and have a pathogenetic role in these MCL cases [Pan 2003].

Contribution of Paraffin Immunohistochemical Immunophenotyping

Obviously, paraffin IHC immunophenotyping is particularly useful when fresh tissue is not available or suitable for FCI. In addition, paraffin IHC staining is useful in detecting the cyclin D1 protein in up to ⅔ of MCL cases and may aid in establishing a diagnosis of classical MCL or of 1 of the morphologic variants of MCL. As discussed in detail above, one should also keep in mind that PCM and hairy cell leukemia may reveal IHC staining with cyclin D1. The immunophenotypic features of PCM were discussed in the differential diagnosis of the "lymphoid" variant above and are discussed in great detail in the PCM section below. Immunohistochemical staining with DBA.44 and TRAP may aid in distinguishing MCL from HCL. DBA.44 is positive in >90% of HCL cases. Dual DBA.44-positivity and TRAP-positivity in combination with the morphology is highly specific for an initial diagnosis of HCL [Hounieu 1992]. These markers are not expressed in MCL.

In regard to distinguishing MCL from LPL, cyclin D1 IHC staining is negative in LPL. In addition, the small lymphocytic and plasmacytoid lymphocytic population, detected by CD20 IHC staining, is intimately intermixed with the population of neoplastic mature-appearing plasma cells, detected by CD138 IHC staining. The clonality of the plasma cells may be demonstrated by IHC staining or in-situ hybridization staining with κ and λ.

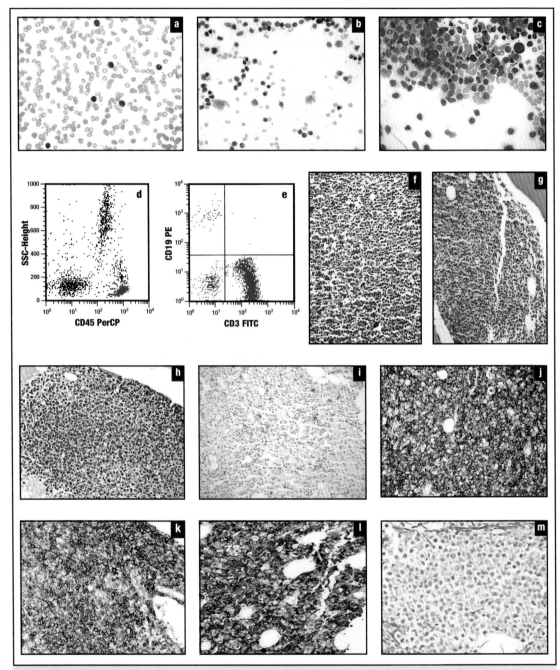

[f12.21] This case demonstrates a "lymphoid" or small cell variant of plasma cell myeloma. The clinical history reveals a 57-year-old female with history of thrombocytopenia, anemia, and atypical lymphocytes on peripheral blood smear. CBC results include WBC $14 \times 10^3/$mm^3 (14×10^9/L) with 20% LUC; absolute lymphocyte count 7.4×10^3/mm^3 (7.4×10^9/L); Hgb 7.9 g/dL; Plt 57×10^3/mm^3 (57×10^9/L). The peripheral blood smear reveals small lymphocytes with varying amounts of cytoplasm **a**. The bone marrow aspirate smears reveal an increase in small lymphoid cells, some with plasmacytoid features **b**, **c**. Flow cytometric analysis reveals a WBC count of 5.8×10^3/mm^3 (5.8×10^9/L) with 29% lymphocytes, 88% of which had a mature T-cell phenotype. They express CD2, CD3, CD5, and CD7; 40% express CD4 and 60% express CD8. There is no evidence of an aberrant or monoclonal B-cell population **d**. The bone marrow biopsy sections reveal a markedly hypercellular marrow with replacement of the marrow space by sheets of relatively lymphoid-appearing cells with areas of crush artifact **f-h**. Thus, the flow cytometry specimen was hemodiluted. CD3-IHC stain of the bone marrow core biopsy reveals rare, scattered positive cells **i**. On the other hand, CD20 **j** and CD138 **k** IHC stains of the bone marrow core biopsy reveal intense co-expression on the great majority of marrow cells. There is selective staining with κ by ISH of the bone marrow core biopsy **l**. λ by ISH is negative **m**. The diagnosis is made of lymphoid variant of multiple myeloma.

Follicular Lymphoma

Definition
Follicular lymphoma is a neoplasm of the B cells within the follicle center (FC) (ie, centrocytes/cleaved FC cells and centroblasts/noncleaved FC cells), with at least a partially follicular growth pattern.

Typical Immunophenotype
The neoplastic cells are usually CD19+, CD20+, CD5–, CD23±, CD10+, and intense surface light chain positive and sIg+. CD10 expression is encountered in approximately 80% of FL and is negative in up to 20% of FL. A typical case of FL is demonstrated in **[f12.22]**, with listmode output available on the accompanying disk.

Variants: Morphology and Immunophenotypes
Various morphologic variants of FL have been described, including a T-cell rich variant, a floral variant, a variant containing a prominent (>5%) component of monocytoid B cells, a variant with plasmacytic differentiation, and a variant with signet ring cell morphology [Dunphy 1998, Dunphy 1998, Sandhaus 1988, Abou-Elella 2000, Keith 1985]. In the T-cell rich variant and in the floral variant of FL, a monoclonal B-cell population may not be detected due to the extremely high content of

reactive T cells and/or to the presence of benign CD5+ mantle cells, which may obscure monoclonality. The floral variant may contain an increased number of reactive T cells or benign CD5+ mantle cells. These 2 variants may be difficult to morphologically distinguish from follicular hyperplasia (FH). Of further interest, there have also been reports of CD5+ monoclonal B cells in the floral variant [Tiesinga 2000]. Aberrant CD5 expression has also been described in grades 1-3 FL without morphologic features of the floral variant [Barry 2002]. These CD5+ FLs are important to recognize and distinguish from nodular variants of SLL and MCL. It is also important to recognize the morphologic variant of FL with a prominent MBC component, since this variant may be encountered in up to 9% of FLs and portends a significantly shorter survival than those with pure FL [Nathwani 1999].

Grading Follicular Lymphoma
Although histologic grading of FL continues to rely primarily on evaluating histological sections of excisional biopsy specimens, there have been findings suggesting the possible use of flow cytometry (ie, CD19/ forward scatter dot plot) in identifying centroblasts in FL, especially in small biopsies and fine needle aspirate (FNA) specimens [Mourad 2006]. However, flow cytometric analysis is not currently recommended for grading FLs, since evaluation of at least 10 neoplastic follicles

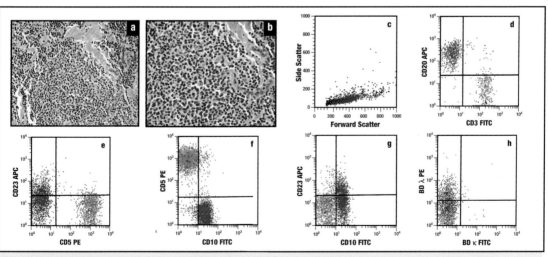

[f12.22] This case demonstrates a typical case of follicular lymphoma. The clinical history reveals a 63-year-old male with left neck lymphadenopathy, which is biopsied. The histologic sections reveal a malignant follicle **a**, which on higher power is composed of predominantly small, cleaved lymphocytes **b**. By flow cytometric analysis of the lymph node, there is an increase of cells in the small lymphocyte region, defined by low forward and side scatter **c**. These cells express CD20 **d**, CD19 (not demonstrated), variable CD23 **e, g**, dim CD10 **f, g**, and selective surface λ light chain (**h**, upper left). There is no co-expression of CD5 **e, f**. Conventional cytogenetic and FISH studies reveal a t(14;18). The diagnosis is made of follicular lymphoma, grade 1.

and evaluation of all tissue sections for a higher grade or diffuse area are currently recommended for grading FLs. For these reasons, a reliable grade of FL is not obtainable in limited biopsy or FNA specimens.

Differential Diagnosis

Follicular hyperplasia

This topic is discussed in detail in the introduction of this chapter.

CLL/SLL

CLL/SLL may have a "pseudofollicular" pattern and/or "cleaved" cell, resembling FL. The neoplastic B cells of CLL/SLL are typically CD5+, CD23+, and CD10– with dim light chain expression, whereas those of FL are CD5–, CD23±, and CD10+ with intense sIg light chain expression. In select cases, FISH analysis for t(14;18) (typically seen in low-grade FL) may be necessary and useful in distinguishing these 2 subtypes of lymphoma. However, one should keep in mind that rare cases of otherwise typical cases of CLL/SLL may harbor a t(14;18) [Dunphy 2008]. Such a case is demonstrated in [f12.23], with listmode output available on the accompanying disk.

Mantle cell lymphoma

This topic is discussed in detail in the section above on mantle cell lymphoma.

Hairy cell leukemia

This differential diagnosis may arise primarily because CD10-positivity may also be seen in HCL [Dunphy 1999, Jasionowski 2003]. Such a case is demonstrated in [f12.24], with listmode output available on the accompanying disk. These entities may usually be distinguished based on their differences in morphologic features and in the remainder of their immunophenotypic profiles (See the section below entitled, "Hairy Cell Leukemia" and [t12.1]). As mentioned previously, dual DBA.44-positivity and TRAP-positivity in combination with the characteristic morphology is highly specific for an initial diagnosis of HCL.

Lymphoplasmacytic Lymphoma

This differential diagnosis may arise primarily because plasmacytic differentiation may occur in up to 9% of FL cases [Keith 1985]. The plasmacytic differentiation in FL cases may be either polytypic or monotypic, and thus the possible diagnostic confusion with lymphoplasmacytic lymphoma. Cases of FL with polytypic plasma cells tend to have discretely follicular growth patterns with separation of the well-defined neoplastic follicles from the numerous plasma cells in the interfollicular regions. In those FLs with monotypic plasma cells, a proportion may also be associated with an IgM paraprotein. In such select cases, FISH analysis for t(14;18) may be necessary and useful in distinguishing these 2 subtypes of lymphoma.

Marginal zone B-cell lymphomas

Since FL may have a prominent component of monocytoid B cells, marginal zone B-cell lymphomas must also be considered in the differential diagnosis. As discussed below under the sections on marginal zone B-cell lymphomas, the neoplastic cells of MZLs are CD10– and may variably express CD11c and CD103. These immunophenotypic features and the lack of t(14;18) in these MZLs should aid in this differential diagnosis.

Contribution of Paraffin Immunohistochemical Immunophenotyping

Paraffin IHC staining may be helpful in subtyping B-cell lymphomas composed predominantly of small cells, such as FLs, particularly in cases where a nodular pattern is not readily apparent and also in cases where there is a consideration of a CLL/SLL with a nodular pattern or nodular MCL. As mentioned previously, CD10 is expressed by 80% of all types of FL and thus is not highly sensitive. Additional monoclonal antibodies available for paraffin IHC that may aid in establishing a diagnosis of FL include CDw75 and bcl-6. CDw75 and bcl-6 both stain normal germinal center cells. CDw75 variably stains B-cell lymphomas; most FL cases are positive, and most CLL/SLL and MCL cases are negative [Torlakovic 2002]. Bcl-6 is restricted to B cells of germinal center origin and 10%-15% of CD3/CD4+ intrafollicular T-cells [Butmarc 1998]. It is commonly expressed in low-grade FL and is rare in other indolent B-cell lymphoid malignancies [Ito 2002]. The combination of these 3 stains (CD10, CDw75, and bcl-6) in conjunction with CD5 are extremely useful in establishing a specific diagnosis of FL [Tsuboi 2000, Carbone 2002].

In addition, detection of the bcl-2 protein by IHC staining may be useful in distinguishing FH from FL. Bcl-2 is non-reactive in reactive germinal centers and is typically strongly reactive in the malignant nodules of FL. However, it should be noted that there are rare cases of FL which are composed of bcl-2– malignant nodules. The cutaneous variant of FL is most often bcl-2–, and its

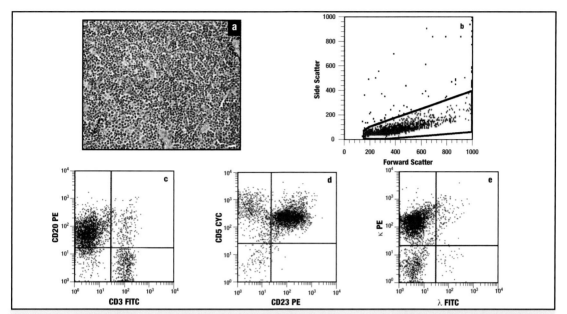

[f12.23] This case demonstrates a typical example of small lymphocytic lymphoma by morphology and flow cytometry associated with a t(14;18). The clinical history reveals a 67-year-old male with a history of hepatitis C infection and left axillary lymphadenopathy, which is biopsied. The histologic section of the lymph node reveals effacement of the normal lymph node architecture by a diffuse proliferation of predominantly small lymphocytes **a**. By flow cytometric analysis of the lymph node, there is an increase of cells in the small lymphocyte region, defined by low forward and side scatter **b**. These cells express CD19 (not demonstrated), CD20 **c**, CD23 with aberrant CD5 **d**, and selective surface λ light chain (**e**, upper left box). They did not express CD10. Conventional cytogenetic and FISH studies reveal a t(14;18) (q32;q31) (typical of follicular lymphoma). The diagnosis is made of small lymphocytic lymphoma with t(14;18).

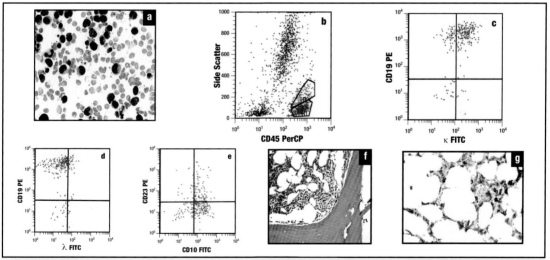

[f12.24] This case demonstrates expression of CD10 in a typical case of hairy cell leukemia. The clinical history reveals a 51-year-old male with previous submitted history of follicle center cell B-cell lymphoma, not responding to chemotherapy, and presently pancytopenic. Outside flow report of bone marrow indicates a population of 6% B-cells with expression of CD19, CD20, CD11c, HLA-DR, FMC-7, dim to moderate κ light chain, and dim CD10. No significant coexpression of CD5, CD23, or CD25 is identified. The coexpression of CD10 suggests a follicle center cell origin. The bone marrow aspirate reveals kidney-bean shaped lymphoid-appearing cells with abundant cytoplasm **a**. Flow cytometric analysis reveals a hypocellular marrow $8.15 \times 10^3/\text{mm}^3$ ($8.15 \times 10^9/\text{L}$) with 37% lymphocytes, composed of 88% T cells. There are 6% "larger" lymphoid cells by side scatter vs CD45 (**b**; green dots). These cells express CD19 **c**, **d** CD20 (not demonstrated), and CD10 **e** with no significant expression of CD23 **e** or CD5 (not demonstrated). There is selective surface κ light chain expression **c**. The subsequent histologic sections of the bone marrow core biopsy reveal the typical morphology of hairy cell leukemia **f**, with lymphoid-appearing cells with a "fried egg" appearance. DBA.44-IHC stain of the bone marrow core biopsy **g** confirmed the diagnosis of hairy cell leukemia with coexpression of CD10.

relationship to the other forms of FL is not clear at this time. Bcl-2+ reactive germinal centers have not been described [Ngan 1998].

One should also keep in mind that although expression of the bcl-2 protein is associated with the t(14;18) chromosome translocation and it is expressed on a significantly higher percentage of FLs associated with this translocation; expression of the bcl-2 oncogene protein is not specific for the t(14;18) chromosomal translocation [Skinnider 1999, Pezzella 1990, Wheaton 1998]. Bcl-2 protein expression may be detected in a substantial number of B-cell and T-cell lymphoproliferative disorders not associated with the t(14;18) [Wheaton 1998, Lai 1998].

Lastly, IHC staining may aid in grading FLs and predicting prognosis. Bcl-6 intranuclear IHC staining in FL tends to correlate with better prognosis [Bilalovic 2004]. In addition, IHC staining with CD20, PAX-5, and bcl-6 may more reliably determine the number of large transformed cells in neoplastic follicles [Martinez 2007]. Furthermore, Ki-67 staining by the IHC method seems to correlate with higher FL grades and International Prognostic Index (IPI) scores, even when not identified by routine histological grading [Wang 2005, Koster 2007].

Lymphoplasmacytic Lymphoma

Definition

Several mature B-cell neoplasms, including lymphoplasmacytic lymphoma (LPL), B-cell CLL, plasma cell myeloma, and marginal zone B-cell lymphoma may show maturation to plasmacytoid or plasma cells containing cytoplasmic immunoglobulin and clinically present with Waldenström macroglobulinemia (WM). Diagnosis of LPL is restricted to those lacking features of other lymphomas and thus is somewhat a diagnosis of exclusion in this regard. LPL is characterized by an intimate mixture of small B lymphocytes, plasmacytoid lymphocytes, and mature plasma cells, usually involving BM, lymph nodes, and spleen.

Typical Immunophenotype

Due to the spectrum of neoplastic cells involved in this lymphoma, the neoplastic cells have varying immunopenotypic features. The small B lymphocytes and plasmacytoid lymphocytes are typically CD19+, CD20+, CD22+, and CD79a+ with CD5–, CD10–, and CD23–. However, up to 40% of cases may show expression of CD23 [Lin 2005]. The small B lymphocytes have

monoclonal surface Ig, usually of IgM type (sometimes IgG and rarely IgA). The plasmacytoid lymphocytes typically have both surface and cytoplasmic monoclonal Ig. The population of neoplastic mature-appearing plasma cells typically also demonstrates cytoplasmic monoclonal Ig, is CD138+, and is negative for B-cell associated antigens. A typical case of LPL is demonstrated in [f12.25], with listmode output available on the accompanying disk.

Differential Diagnosis

Lymphoplasmacytic lymphoma may generally be differentiated from other types of B-cell lymphomas by applying the characteristic FCI findings outlined in [t12.1] and by identifying the presence of monoclonal plasma cells by IHC staining or in-situ hybridization. However, some small B-cell lymphomas may show plasmacytic differentiation, as previously discussed, and be diagnostically problematic.

Marginal zone lymphoma

Among the B-cell proliferative diseases, the differential diagnosis between MALT lymphoma and LPL may be particularly difficult, as there is considerable overlap in histological features and, occasionally, in clinical presentation. This is particularly true when the primary MALT lymphoma lesion is inconspicuous and not clinically recognizable. Even if it is recognized, the lymphoepithelial lesion and reactive lymphoid follicles, characteristic features of MALT lymphoma, may not be detectable in those presenting with primary macroglobulinemia. In such cases, it has been demonstrated that the detection of t(11;18)(q21;q21) and/or t(1;14)(p22;q32) is useful in differentiating these 2 lymphoma subtypes, since these 2 translocations are absent in LPL. Both t(11;18)(q21;q21) and t(1;14)(p22;q32) are significantly associated with advanced cases of MALT lymphoma. For example, t(11;18)(q21;q21) has been found in 78% of gastric MALT lymphomas at stage IIE or above [Liu 2002, Liu 2001]. MALT lymphoma associated with WM is usually at an advanced stage, typically showing bone marrow and peripheral blood involvement [Hirase 2000, Valdez 2002]. Thus, it is most likely that the incidence of these translocations in MALT lymphoma is associated with WM. In this regard, it is noteworthy that t(11;18)(q21;q21) has been observed in several MALT lymphomas associated with WM [Valdez 2002, Kobayashi 2001]. Thus, detection of these translocations by FISH analyses plays a significant role in the differential diagnosis between LPL and MALT lymphoma.

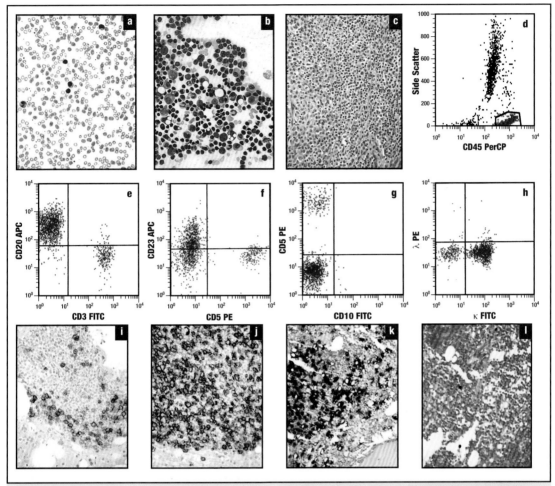

[f12.25] This case demonstrates a typical case of lymphoplasmacytic lymphoma. The clinical history reveals a 79-year-old male with a history of anemia, renal insufficiency, hypercalcemia, free κ light chains, and IgM κ monoclonal proteins detected by serum immunofixation. The peripheral blood smear reveals an occasional small lymphocyte with plasmacytoid features **a**. The bone marrow aspirate smear reveals an intimate mixture of small round lymphocytes, plasmacytoid lymphocytes, and mature plasma cells **b**. The histologic section of the bone marrow clot section reveals a hypercellular marrow with apparently increased plasma cells with intermixed small lymphoid cells **c**. By flow cytometric analysis, there is an increase in cells within the lymphocyte region characterized by low side light scatter and high expression of CD45 (**d**, increase in red dots). These cells express CD19 (not demonstrated), CD20 **e**, variable CD23 (**f**, upper left box) without CD5 (**f**, lower right box, and **g**), and selective surface κ light chain (**h**, lower right box). Subsequent CD138 IHC stain of the bone marrow histologic section highlights the increased plasma cells **i**. CD20-IHC stain of the bone marrow histologic section highlights even more positive cells **j** than identified by flow cytometric analysis, possibly due to sampling or a hemodiluted bone marrow sample submitted for flow cytometric analysis. κ and λ ISH performed on the bone marrow histologic sections reveal selective expression of κ in the plasma cells and small lymphoid cells **k,l**. Conventional cytogenetic and FISH (myeloma panel) studies are normal. The diagnosis is made of lymphoplasmacytic lymphoma.

Concomitant CLL/SLL and plasma cell dyscrasia

Relatively rare cases of coexistent (or concomitant) CLL/SLL and plasma cell myeloma (PCM) (or plasma cell dyscrasia) occur and may be confused diagnostically with LPL. However, the morphology typically differs in that there are discrete nodules, or infiltrates, of CLL/SLL and a separate population of monoclonal plasma cells in CLL/SLL. Such a case is demonstrated in **[f12.26]**, with listmode output available on the accompanying disk. In contrast, as previously demonstrated in **[f12.25]**, the characteristic morphology in LPL is a diffuse infiltrate, or nodules (in BM), composed of an intimate mixture of small, round lymphocytes, plasmacytoid lymphocytes, and mature plasma cells. "Pseudofollicles," as may be seen in CLL/SLL, are not seen. In addition, the immunophenotypic features of the small lymphocytes in LPL differ from those of CLL/SLL, in that the LPL small lymphocytes are CD5– and usually CD23–.

Mantle Cell Lymphoma with Monoclonal Plasma Cells

As previously discussed, occasional cases of MCL may demonstrate plasmacytic differentiation, causing diagnostic confusion with LPL. This differential diagnosis has been previously discussed above in the MCL section.

Follicular lymphoma with monoclonal plasma cells

Also as previously discussed, plasmacytic differentiation may occur in up to 9% of FL cases, causing diagnostic confusion with LPL. This differential diagnosis has been previously discussed above in the FL section.

"Lymphoid" or "small cell" variant of plasma cell myeloma

In general, LPL may be differentiated from PCM by the finding of a prominent population of monoclonal small B lymphocytes by FCI in LPL and a uniform population of monoclonal plasma cells in PCM. However, diagnostic confusion with the "small cell" or "lymphoid" morphological variant of PCM may occur due to the "lymphoid" morphology and CD20+, which are encountered in this variant. As discussed previously, the neoplastic cells of LPL include small lymphocytes, plasmacytoid lymphocytes, and plasma cells. The neoplastic cells of the "lymphoid" variant of PCM may show varying degrees of plasmacytic differentiation and are

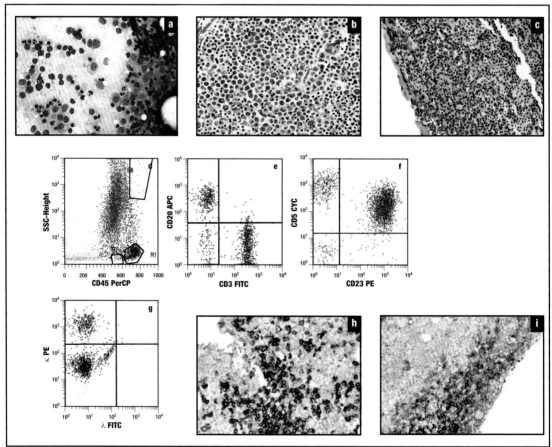

[f12.26] This case demonstrates a rare instance of coexistent CLL and plasma cell dyscrasia. The clinical history reveals a 30-year-old male with a history of B-cell non-Hodgkin lymphoma, with a good response to fludarabine, cytoxan, and rituximab. He currently has a prolonged, severe anemia, and thus a bone marrow examination is performed. The bone marrow aspirate reveals an increase in plasma cells **a**, which are also seen in the histologic section of the bone marrow clot section **b**. The histologic section of the bone marrow core biopsy also reveals an atypical lymphoid infiltrate (**c**, left side of image). By flow cytometric analysis, there is an increase in cells within the lymphocyte region characterized by low side light scatter and high expression of CD45 (**d**, increase in red dots). These cells express CD19 (not demonstrated), CD20 **e**, aberrant CD5 **f** with coexpression of CD20 (**e**, upper right box), with selective surface κ light chain (**g**, upper left box). The increase in plasma cells is confirmed by CD138-IHC staining of the bone marrow histologic section **h**. CD23-IHC stain of the bone marrow histologic section reveals intense expression in the atypical lymphoid infiltrate **i**. The diagnosis is made of coexistent CLL and plasma cell dyscrasia.

often CD20+, but otherwise immunophenotype as other cases of PCM (ie, CD45–, CD19–, CD138+, variable CD56+, monoclonal cytoplasmic light chain expression, and lack of surface light chain expression), as demonstrated previously in [f12.21]. In addition and as previously discussed, the "lymphoid" variant of PCM may be cyclin D1+. The neoplastic cells of LPL are cyclin D1–. These differences in immunophenotypic features are helpful in arriving at the correct diagnosis in these challenging cases.

Contribution of Paraffin Immunohistochemical Immunophenotyping

As previously discussed and demonstrated in [f12.25], LPL is composed of an intimate mixture of small, round lymphocytes, similar to those of B-CLL, plasmacytoid lymphocytes, and mature-appearing plasma cells. Due to the spectrum of neoplastic cells involved in this lymphoma, flow cytometric and IHC techniques are uniquely applied in establishing the diagnosis. Flow cytometric analysis typically detects a CD5–, CD10– monoclonal B-cell population, which morphologically represents the small lymphocytes and plasmacytoid lymphocytes. This population may also be detected by CD20 IHC staining. The population of neoplastic mature-appearing plasma cells is intimately associated with the small lymphocytes and plasmacytoid lymphocytes and is detected by CD138 IHC staining. The clonality of the plasma cells is demonstrated by IHC staining or in-situ hybridization with κ and λ light chains.

IHC staining may also be useful in distinguishing LPL and MALT lymphoma. The tumor cells with t(1;14)(p22;q32), as may be detected in MALT lymphoma and not in LPL, are characterized by strong uniform BCL10 nuclear staining [Ye 2003, Ye 2000]. Thus, BCL10 IHC staining may be used as a screening test for t(1;14)(p22;q32) or its variants. One should keep in mind that although LPL cases do not show strong BCL10 nuclear staining similar to that seen in t(1;14)(p22;q32) positive MALT lymphoma, up to 55% of LPL cases have been shown to demonstrate weak to moderate nuclear staining in >20% of the neoplastic cells. The significance of BCL10 nuclear expression in LPL is unknown. The nuclear BCL10 staining seen in LPL has not correlated with specific chromosomal abnormalities or MALT-associated translocations, or with NF-κB activation [Merzianu 2006].

Plasma Cell Neoplasms: Plasma Cell Myeloma

Definition

Plasma cell myeloma is a BM-based, multifocal neoplasm of plasma cells (PCs) associated with a serum monoclonal protein and skeletal destruction. Thus, the diagnosis is based on a combination of pathological, radiological, and clinical features.

Typical Immunophenotype

The neoplastic cells of PCM typically do not express the leukocyte common antigen (CD45), B-cell associated antigens (ie, CD19, CD20) or sIg and light chains, but do express CD38 and CD138, and demonstrate monoclonal cytoplasmic Ig (most commonly IgG, occasionally IgA, and rarely IgD, IgE, or IgM) and light chain. They may variably express CD56. In addition, occasional cases may demonstrate dim expression of CD45, expression of CD19 or CD20, or expression of dim monoclonal sIg or light chain expression (possibly due to the presence and non-specific sticking of the serum monoclonal protein) [Dunphy 1996]. A typical case of PCM is demonstrated in [f12.27], with listmode output available on the accompanying disk.

Variants: Morphology and Immunophenotypes

The neoplastic PCs in PCM may appear mature, appear blastic (ie, plasmablastic), appear dumbbell-shaped with pleomorphic and lobulated nuclei, or appear "lymphoid." In the "lymphoid" variant, the neoplastic PCs resemble small lymphocytes or plasmacytoid lymphocytes (see [f11.21], with listmode output available on the accompanying disk). Some studies have correlated the cells of this variant with expression of the mature B-cell antigen, CD20 [Fonseca 2002, Robillard 2003]. Recent studies have also demonstrated the relationship of this morphological phenotype with the recurrent chromosomal translocation, t(11;14)(q13;q32), commonly associated with mantle cell lymphoma (MCL) [Fonseca 2002, Robillard 2003, Hoyer 2000, Troussard 2000, Garand 2003, Matsuda 2005]. The diagnosis in these morphological variants with aberrant immunophenotypes is nevertheless established by the immunophenotypic recognition of a PC immunophenotype (ie, strong reactivity with CD138 and monoclonal cytoplasmic staining of the neoplastic PCs with κ or λ).

Prognostic Markers

The flow cytometric detection of myelomonocytic markers (ie, CD11b, CD13, CD14, CD15, and CD33) in PCM has been shown to correlate with a worse prognosis [Ruiz-Aruelles 1994]. Such a case is demonstrated in [f12.28], with listmode output available on the accompanying disk. Ely demonstrated that strong expression of CD56 by PCs of PCM correlated with the presence of lytic bone lesions [Ely 2002]. Indeed, others have shown the lack of or weak expression of CD56 by PCs in PCM characterized a special subset of myeloma associated with a lower osteolytic potential and a higher tendency for circulation of the malignant PCs in the PB. This subset was also characterized by more extensive BM infiltration and significantly decreased OS [Pellat-Deceunynck 1998, Rawstron 1999, Sahara 2002]. Chang et al also demonstrated recently the absence of CD56 on malignant PCs in cerebrospinal fluid is the hallmark of central nervous system involvement in PCM [Chang 2005].

Differential Diagnosis

Reactive plasmacytoses

Since cases of PCM may be composed of mature-appearing neoplastic cells, and high numbers of PCs may be encountered in reactive conditions, the distinction between PCM and a reactive plasmacytosis (RP) may rely on immunophenotypic features. Demonstration of monoclonal cytoplasmic light chain expression usually distinguishes PCM from RP, but in technically challenging cases, or in cases without demonstrable cytoplasmic light chain expression, the expression of CD56 aids in defining a clonal PC population. Although CD138 is expressed by both reactive and neoplastic PCs, CD56 expression by PCs has been shown to indicate clonality, not being identified in any cases of RP [Dunphy 2007].

Circulating low-grade B-cell neoplasms

Plasma cell leukemia (PCL) is a clinical variant of PCM, defined as a peripheral blood plasmacytosis of >20% or $2 \times 10^3/\text{mm}^3$ $(2 \times 10^9/\text{L})$ [Dunphy 1995]. The neoplastic cells in PCL often appear "lymphoid" and may express CD19 or CD20, causing diagnostic confusion with other

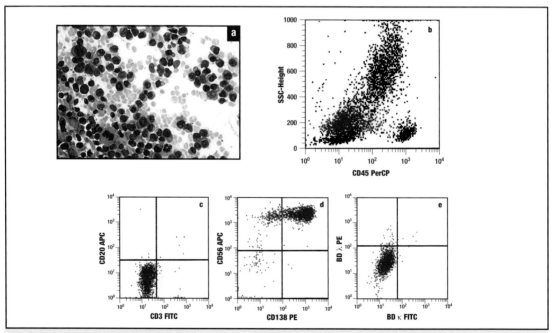

[f12.27] This case demonstrates the typical immunophenotype of a plasma cell myeloma by flow cytometric analysis. The clinical history reveals a 69-year-old female presenting with pancytopenia. The bone marrow aspirate smear reveals sheets of plasma cells **a**. By flow cytometric analysis, there is an increase in cells within the region characterized by low side light scatter and decreased expression of CD45 (**b**, increase in red dots). These cells are negative for CD20 and CD3 **c**. They co-express CD138 and CD56 (**d**, upper right box). They also do not demonstrate any light chain (κ or λ) expression **e**. Conventional cytogenetic studies reveal numerous abnormalities, including abnormalities of chromosome 11, and FISH studies reveal 3 cyclin-D1 hybridization signals. The diagnosis is made of plasma cell myeloma.

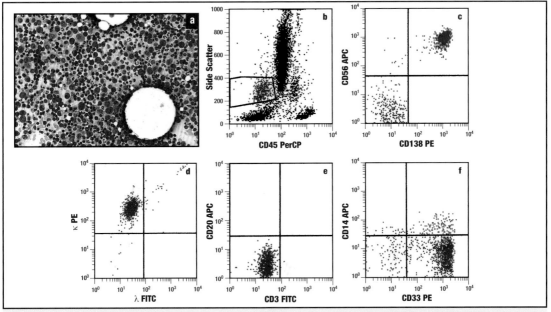

[f12.28] This case of plasma cell myeloma demonstrates aberrant selective surface light chain and myeloid antigen expressions. The clinical history reveals a 61-year-old female with a history of an IgA κ monoclonal serum protein and multiple soft tissue masses. A bone marrow aspirate reveals increased plasma cells **a**. By flow cytometric analysis, there is an increase in cells within the region characterized by moderate side light scatter and decreased expression of CD45 (**b**, increase in red dots). These cells reveal strong co-expression of CD56 and CD138 (**c**, upper right box), aberrant selective surface κ light chain (**d**, upper left box), no expression of CD20 **e**, and aberrant expression of CD33 (without CD14) (**f**, lower right box). Conventional cytogenetic studies reveal multiple structural and numerical abnormalities and FISH studies reveal 10% of cells positive for 3 p53 gene hybridization signals, and a *myc* gene rearrangement. The diagnosis is made of plasma cell myeloma with aberrant expression of selective surface κ light chain and CD33.

circulating chronic (low grade) B-cell neoplasms (eg, CLL, LPL). The distinction between these entities relies on the uniform, strong expression of CD138 and monoclonal cytoplasmic light chain expression by the neoplastic cells of PCL. Such a case is demonstrated in **[f12.29]**, with list mode output available on the accompanying disk.

Lymphoplasmacytic lymphoma

Lymphoplasmacytic lymphoma may be diagnostically confused with cases with concomitant SLL/CLL and plasma cell myeloma and with cases of the "small cell" or "lymphoid variant of PCM, as previously discussed above in the section of LPL

Contribution of Paraffin Immunohistochemical Immunophenotyping

Unfortunately, plasma cells (PCs) tend to strip in BM aspirate smear preparations. Based on this stripping artifact, and the occurrence of atypical morphologic forms, PCs may be difficult to recognize, and thus tend to be underestimated in BM aspirate differential counts. In addition, PCs often fall outside the gates of flow cytometric analysis. However, as previously discussed,

CD138 is an IHC marker of normal and neoplastic PCs that has been shown to be useful in quantitating PCs in paraffin sections of BM clots and cores [Dunphy 2007]. CD138 reliably detects PCs, and thus the diagnosis of PCM is greatly aided by IHC staining with CD138 and IHC staining or in-situ hybridization with κ and light chains. CD138 IHC staining of BM sections remains the standard for tumor burden in PCMs.

If a BM aspirate is not available for flow cytometric analysis or if establishing clonality by light chain restriction is problematic, CD56 may also be performed by IHC staining. CD56 IHC staining may aid in determining clonality of the PCs and also in determining prognosis, as previously discussed.

In addition, CD138 IHC staining may be useful in distinguishing LPL from PCM, since it is important to demonstrate the immunophenotypic features with intact morphology in this differential diagnosis. As mentioned and previously demonstrated in **[f12.25]**, LPL is characterized by the intimate mixture of small lymphocytes, plasmacytoid lymphocytes, and mature plasma cells with differing immunophenotypic profiles, as previously discussed in the section above on LPL.

Immunohistochemical staining for CD138 combined with IHC staining for κ and λ light chains or in situ hybridization for κ and λ light chain mRNA may be particularly useful in recognizing the "small cell" or "lymphoid" variant of PCM. As discussed previously, this morphological and immunophenotypic variant of PCM is often a diagnostic challenge. The morphology, combined with strong expression of CD20, especially when it occurs in the majority of the neoplastic cells, may present a diagnostic pitfall, mimicking other CD20+ mature B-cell lymphoproliferative disorders with lymphoplasmacytoid features [Young 2006, Yokote 2005, Davis 1992]. Chronic lymphocytic leukemia (CLL) [Evans 2000], mantle cell lymphoma [Young 2006], MZL [Davis 1992], FL [Frizzera 1986], and LPL may all demonstrate variable numbers of plasmacytic and lymphoplasmacytic cells. An extended IHC panel [including but not limited to CD19 and CD20 (pan B-cell antigens), CD10 and BCL6 (markers for GC cell differentiation), CD5 and CD23 (markers discriminatory for CLL and MCL), and κ and

λ light chains (for clonality detection)] is used to discriminate between these entities by their classical immunophenotypes. In general, strong membrane positivity with CD138 is demonstrated in >90% of the neoplastic cells in the "lymphoid" variant of PCM, and a greater percentage of PCs are identified by CD138 IHC immunostaining than appreciated on H&E stained sections. In addition, identification of specific chromosomal translocations by routine karyotyping, FISH, or IHC staining of the protein product, or mRNA is important in discriminating between the morphologically similar B-lymphoproliferative neoplasms. The t(11;14)(q13;q32), identified either by routine cytogenetics or by various molecular methods [Belaud-Rotureau 2002], is recognized as a key finding in mantle cell lymphoma [Yatabe 2000]. However, it is also the most common translocation found in PCM, albeit in a much lower frequency (reports varying from 2% to 4% of all PCM cases studied by routine cytogenetics, 10% to 25% of PCM cases with abnormal cytogenetics; and 15%-20% of all PCM cases by FISH

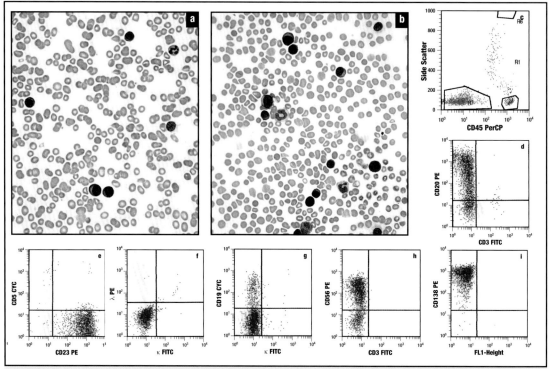

[f12.29] This case demonstrates an instance of plasma cell leukemia. The clinical history reveals a 62-year-old female with an elevated WBC count (34.9 × 10³/mm³ [34.9 × 10⁹/L]) associated with anemia and thrombocytopenia. The peripheral blood smear reveals an increase in lymphoid-appearing cells, some with plasmacytoid features **a,b**. By flow cytometric analysis, there is an increase in cells within the region characterized by low side light scatter and decreased expression of CD45 (**c**, increase in orange dots). These cells express CD20 heterogeneously **d**, partial CD23 without CD5 **e**, no surface light chain **f**, and partial expression of CD19 **g** associated with expressions of CD56 **h** and CD138 **i**. The diagnosis is made of plasma cell leukemia.

analysis) [Troussard 2000, Fonseca 2004]. Furthermore, several studies have demonstrated an association of the t(11;14)(q13;q32) with the oligosecretory variant of PCM, CD20 expression, and lymphoplasmacytic morphology [Fonseca 2002, Robillard 2003, Hoyer 2000, Garand 2003, Matsuda 2005]. In PCM cell lines, high levels of cyclin D1 expression are tightly linked to the presence of t(11;14)(q13;q32), but, interestingly, positivity by IHC may be detected in only up to 30% of patients [Troussard 2000, Pruneri 2000]. The frequent association of the "lymphoid" variant of PCM with t(11;14)(q13;32) and over-expression of cyclin D1 makes distinction from mantle cell lymphoma, which has a similar profile, even more problematic [Liu 2002]. A combination of immunohistochemistry (CD5–, CD138+, in situ hybridization for immunoglobulin light chains), and clinical and radiological data are helpful in arriving at the correct diagnosis in these challenging cases.

Plasma Cell Neoplasms: Plasmacytomas

Definition
Plasmacytomas are neoplasms of plasma cells, with the identical cytomorphological and immunophenotypic features of PCM, manifesting as localized osseous or extraosseous presentations.

Typical Immunophenotype
See the description above in the section of PCM.

Variants: Morphology and Immunophenotypes
See the description above in the section on PCM. In addition, plasmacytomas may present with an anaplastic morphology.

Differential Diagnosis

Extranodal marginal zone B-cell lymphoma (MALT lymphoma) with a prominent or predominant plasma cell component
Occasionally MALT lymphomas may have an extremely prominent monoclonal plasmacytic component, which may be diagnostically confused with an extraosseous plasmacytoma [Al-Marzooq 2004, Kokosadze 2004]. However, the MALT lymphomas with a prominent monoclonal plasmacytic component will often also contain a monoclonal small B-cell lymphocytic component, detectable by flow cytometric analysis. Such a case is demonstrated in [f12.30]. However, in some cases there will be no apparent centrocyte-like cells or monocytoid B cells. In the MALT lymphoma cases, reactive follicles are generally identified.

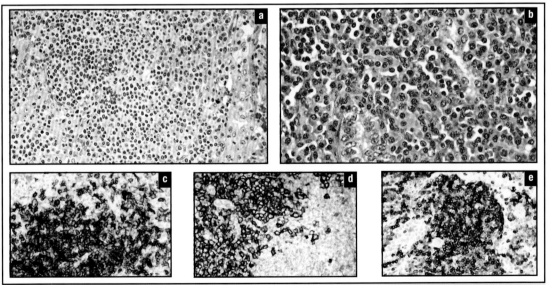

[f12.30] This case demonstrates a MALT lymphoma with a prominent plasmacytic component. The patient is a 57-year-old female with multiple bilateral pulmonary nodules, slightly increasing in size. The left lower lobe nodule is PET+, and is biopsied. The histologic sections reveal a monotonous proliferation of lymphoid appearing cells with abundant cytoplasm (monocytoid-appearing lymphoid cells) and admixed plasma cells **a**. In some areas, there are sheets of plasma cells **b**. The monocytoid lymphoid cells are CD20+ **c**, CD20-IHC stain), and the prominent plasma cell population is highlighted with a CD138-IHC stain **d**. A Bcl-2 IHC stain intensely stains the lymphoid cells and faintly stains the plasma cells **e**.

Nevertheless, the suggestion has been made that in mucosa-associated sites, plasmacytomas may actually represent MALT lymphomas that have undergone an extensive degree of plasmacytic differentiation [Hussong 1999].

Diffuse large B-cell or T-cell lymphoma and granulocytic sarcoma

Plasmablastic plasmacytoma may cause diagnostic confusion with diffuse large cell lymphomas of B-cell or T-cell origin, as well with granulocytic sarcoma. They may generally be distinguished from large cell lymphomas of T-cell origin, since T-cell lymphomas will typically show variable expression of T-cell associated antigens (ie, CD2, CD3, CD4, CD5, CD7, and CD8). Granulocytic sarcomas are typically distinguished by their variable expression of myelomonocytic markers, as AMLs and described in Chapter 10. Plasmablastic plasmacytomas generally are negative for B-cell associated antigens (ie, CD19 and CD20) and show strong expression of CD138 and monoclonal cytoplasmic light chain expression. Diffuse large B-cell lymphomas (DLBCLs) demonstrate expression of B-cell associated antigens (ie, CD19 and CD20) and are CD138–. However, 1 variant of DLBCL in the WHO classification, plasmablastic lymphoma (PBL), may pose a diagnostic dilemma with a plasmablastic plasmacytoma. This variant is further discussed below in the section on DLBCL and in Chapter 16. PBL is an uncommon, recently described B-cell-derived lymphoma displaying distinctive affinity for extranodal presentation in the oral cavity. Plasmablastic lymphoma is strongly associated with human immunodeficiency virus (HIV) infection but has been reported in HIV-negative individuals [Folk 2006]. Cases of PBL and plasmablastic PCM have been shown to have nearly identical immunophenotypes, being positive for CD138 and CD38 and negative for CD20, corresponding to a plasma cell immunophenotype. The only significant difference demonstrated between PBL and PCM is the presence of EBV-encoded RNA, being positive in all PBL cases tested and negative in all PCM cases. Representative cases of PBL and plasmablastic plasmacytoma are demonstrated in **[f12.31]** (with listmode output available on the accompanying disk) and **[f12.32]**, respectively. In conclusion, most cases of AIDS-related PBL have an immunophenotype and tumor suppressor gene expression profile virtually identical to plasmablastic PCM and unlike DLBCL [Vega 2005]. These results question the WHO classification of PBL as a variant of DLBCL.

Contribution of paraffin immunohistochemical immunophenotyping

Paraffin IHC staining for CD138 and IHC staining for κ and λ light chains or in situ hybridization for κ and λ light chain mRNA may be particularly useful in the differential diagnoses of plasmacytomas, discussed in the section above, since these techniques allow for the ideal detection of intracytoplasmic light chain clonality. In addition, IHC staining allows for the maintenance of the histologic architecture, which may be particularly important in distinguishing MALT lymphoma with a prominent monoclonal plasmacytic component from a plasmacytoma. EBV-encoded RNA may also be readily evaluated by in situ hybridization in the differential diagnosis of a plasmablastic plasmacytoma vs a PBL.

Splenic Marginal Zone B-Cell Lymphoma (± Villous Lymphocytes)

Definition

Splenic marginal zone lymphoma (SMZL) is defined by the WHO classification as a B-cell neoplasm composed of small lymphocytes that surround and replace the splenic white pulp germinal centers, effacing the follicle mantle and merging with a peripheral (marginal) zone of larger cells [Isaacson 2001]. Both small and larger cells may infiltrate the splenic red pulp. Splenic hilar lymph nodes and BM are often involved; lymphoma cells may be found in the PB as villous lymphocytes.

Typical Immunophenotype

The cells of SMZL have surface IgM and IgD, and are CD20+, CD79a+, CD22+, CD11c+, CD25–, CD103+(wk)/–, CD11c+(wk)/–, CD5–, CD10–, CD23–, CD43–, bcl-2+, and cyclin D1– (Table 1 in the Appendix) [Isaacson 2001, Savilo 1998, Wu 1996]. The intensity of pan-B antigens CD19, CD20 and CD22 are typically within the range seen on benign tissue B lymphocytes, as is the intensity of immunoglobulin light chain staining. A typical example of SMZL with circulating villous lymphocytes is demonstrated in **[f12.33]**, with listmode output available on the accompanying disk. Lastly, the neoplastic cells of extranodal MZL (MALT-type and SMZL) may have variable staining with DBA.44 and tartrate-resistant acid phosphatase (TRAP) [Dunphy 2008].

Differential Diagnosis

The differential diagnosis of primary SMZL predominantly includes other "small" B-cell non-Hodgkin lymphomas (NHLs), including secondary involvement by an extranodal or primary nodal MZL, hairy cell leukemia (HCL), CLL/SLL, MCL, and FL. These entities may usually be distinguished by cytomorphological and histopathological features, combined with immunophenotypic features, cytogenetic features, and/or molecular features.

Hairy cell leukemia and hairy cell variant

Hairy cell leukemia is usually easily differentiated from SMZL by morphology, since HCL has a leukemic pattern with obliteration of the white pulp and the formation red blood cell lakes. However, small samples, or a PB sample, provided as the initial diagnostic specimen may make this differential diagnosis more problematic. There are differences in the immunophenotypes of HCL and SMZL, as seen in [t12.1]. HCL is typically strongly positive for CD11c, CD103, and CD25, whereas SMZL is weakly positive or negative for CD11c as well as CD103 and negative for CD25. A typical case of HCL is demonstrated in [f12.34] on the accompanying disk. In addition, HCL may occasionally be CD10+ [Dunphy 1999]. Such a case was previously demonstrated in [f12.24] on the accompanying disk. The cytogenetic abnormalities described in SMZLs have not yet been identified in HCL.

Hairy cell variant (HCL-V) is another diagnostic consideration when small samples or peripheral blood samples are provided as the initial diagnostic specimen. The immunophenotype of HCL-V is best reviewed in comparison to the immunophenotype of the SMZL in [t12.1]. There is more immunophenotypic overlap between HCL-V and SMZL, in that CD11c is not as strongly positive as in HCL and CD103 may be negative or weakly positive, as in SMZL. A case of HCL-V was previously demonstrated in [f12.16] on the accompanying disk. Again, the cytogenetic abnormalities described in SMZL have not yet been identified in HCL-V.

Secondary involvement by extranodal or primary nodal MZLs

The spleen may be secondarily involved by extranodal (MALT) lymphomas; however, primary nodal MZL may only be diagnosed if there is no evidence of extranodal MALT site or splenic disease. Likewise, evidence of a primary MALT lymphoma would mitigate against a diagnosis of a primary SMZL. Yet, clinical history is not always available, and patients may present with coexistent involvement of the spleen and a MALT site

and/or a nodal site. All MZLs (extranodal and nodal) may present with similar morphology with or without varying degrees of plasmacytic differentiation. Of note, however, extensive plasma cell differentiation, resembling an extramedullary plasmacytoma, has primarily been described only in the nodal and extranodal MALT lymphomas [Hussong 1999]. Such a case was previously demonstrated in [f12.30]. In addition, there may be subtle differences in immunophenotypes and very useful differences in cytogenetic findings in these MZLs arising primarily as splenic, nodal, or MALT lymphomas, to help distinguish MZLs. These immunophenotypic features and cytogenetic findings may be reviewed in [t12.1] and [t12.2], respectively. CD103 may be weakly positive or negative in SMZL but is generally negative in nodal MZL and MALT lymphoma. In addition, CD5+ extranodal MALT lymphomas have been described with an increased propensity for bone marrow involvement and relapse [Ferry 1996]. CD5+ splenic MZL has not yet been described.

Large granular lymphocyte leukemia (LGLL)

Similar to HCL, LGLL may be morphologically considered in the differential diagnosis of SMZL. As later discussed in Chapter 14, LGLL may be of T-cell or true natural killer (NK)-cell origin. The immunophenotypes of NK-cell LGLL and T-cell LGLL are as follows: NK-LGL leukemia (CD2+, CD3–, CD4–, CD8+, CD16+, CD56+, CD57v) and T-LGL leukemia (CD2+, CD3+, CD4–, CD8+, CD16+/–, CD56–/+, CD57+). Thus, by flow cytometric analysis, LGLLs of T-cell or NK-cell origin should be clearly distinguished immunophenotypically from SMZL.

CLL/SLL

CLL/SLL should also be included in the differential diagnosis of SMZL. CLL/SLL typically shows variation when there is dominant infiltration of either the red or white pulp by a monotonous population of small lymphocytes. Marginal zones are not usually observed in CLL. The prolymphocytoid transformation of CLL may show increased numbers of prolymphocytes in the same distribution. Richter syndrome (large cell lymphoma transformation of CLL) may show splenic involvement. However, CLL/SLL and their related variants are usually easily distinguished from SMZL by their characteristic immunophenotype with CD5-positivity and CD23-positivity, as reviewed in [t12.1]. CD5-positivity has not been described in SMZL. Although del(7q) has also been described in a subset of

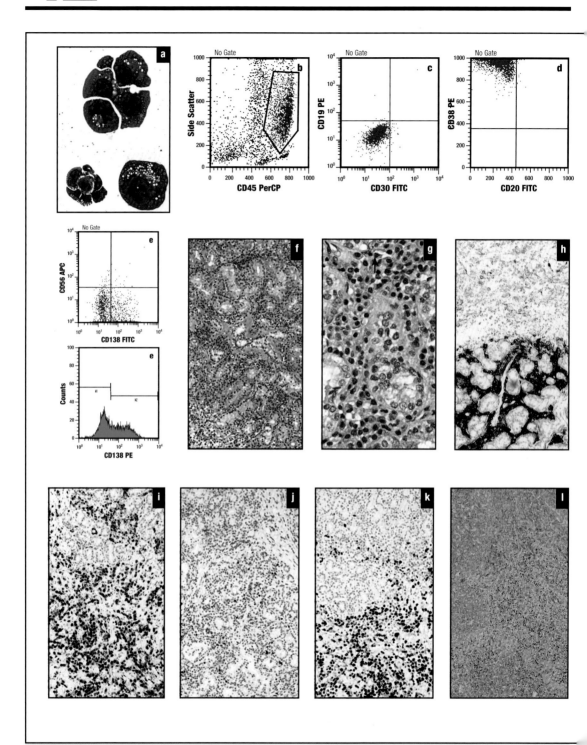

[f12.31] This case demonstrates a case of plasmablastic lymphoma. The clinical history reveals a 46-year-old HIV-positive male with left eye swelling and pain associated with abdominal discomfort and worsening distention. CT scan reveals mesenteric and retroperitoneal lymphadenopathy and splenomegaly with ascites. MRI shows bilateral lacrimal gland enlargement. EBV viral load is elevated (>2 million copies/mL), Paracentesis is performed, followed by a lacrimal gland biopsy and a bone marrow biopsy. The cytomorphology of the ascitic fluid reveals large, anaplastic cells with abundant, eccentric blue cytoplasm containing vacuoles **a**. By flow cytometric analysis, a population of 55% of cells is gated upon, characterized by bright CD45 expression and increased side scatter (**b**, gated red dots). These cells variably express CD38 **d**, CD138 **e**, and HLA-DR (not demonstrated).

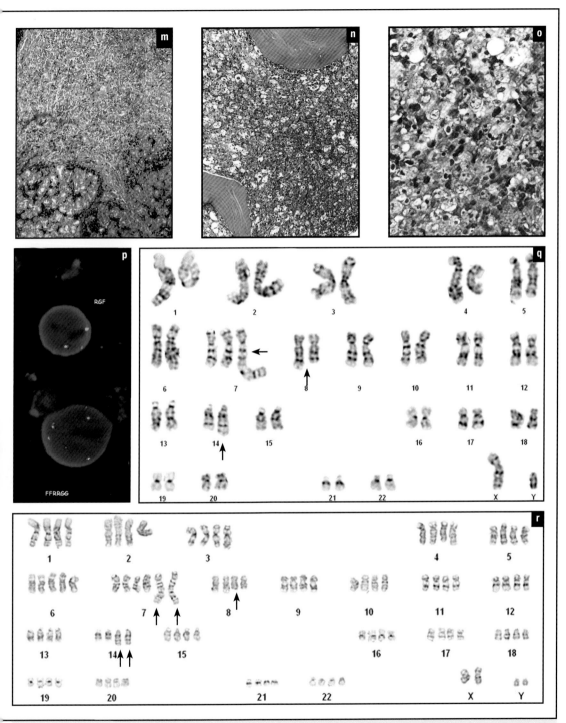

[f12.31 continued] They are negative for CD30 **c**, CD20 **d**, CD19 **c**, CD56 **e**, all myeloid antigens tested, as well as all T-cell antigens, and surface light chains (not demonstrated). Histologic sections of the lacrimal gland reveal infiltration by these large, abnormal plasmacytoid appearing cells (**f,g**, arrow). These cells are positive with the following IHC stains: CD138 **h**, MUM1 **i**, and Ki-67 **k**; they are negative with a PAX5 IHC stain **j**. In addition, these cells are EBER+ (**l**, ISH) and reveal monoclonal staining with κ (**m**, ISH). The bone marrow histologic sections reveal a markedly hypercellular marrow with infiltration by numerous large cells **n,o**. FISH (*c-myc*) results of the bone marrow and lacrimal gland specimens **p** and cytogenetic results from the peritoneal fluid **q** and bone marrow **r** are demonstrated. The diagnosis is made of plasmablastic lymphoma, involving lacrimal gland, peritoneal fluid, and bone marrow.

SLL with plasmacytoid features [Offit 1995], trisomy 3 in combination with del(7q) has not been described yet in CLL/SLL [Callet-Bauchu 2005]. In addition, by comparative genomic hybridization, the del(7q) in SMZL has been fine-mapped to a narrow region and has not been identified by this technique in CLL [Andersen 2004].

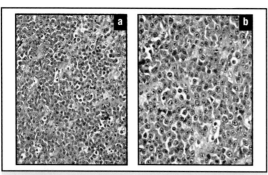

[f12.32] This case demonstrates the morphology of an anaplastic plasmacytoma. The patient is a 61-year-old female with an IgA κ monoclonal protein, an abdominal wall mass, and bone lesions. The abdominal mass is biopsied. Histologic sections of the abdominal mass reveal sheets of a relatively monotonous population of large cells with increased nuclear:cytoplasmic ratios with variable numbers of nucleoli and apoptotic cells in the background a, b.

Mantle cell lymphoma

Mantle cell lymphoma is a definite consideration in the differential diagnosis of SMZL, since MCL may present with splenomegaly and may show plasma cell differentiation as seen in MZL [Young 2006, Pittaluga 1996]. MCL typically shows white pulp expansion by a monotonous small lymphocytic infiltrate without diffuse red pulp infiltration. Cases of leukemic MCL may, however, show red pulp infiltration. The immunophenotype of MCL (with CD5+) should greatly aid in the distinction from SMZL, as reviewed in [t12.1]. In addition, although trisomy 3 may be encountered in up to 50% of MCL [Monni 1998], and del(7q) may also occur in MCL [Offit 1995], MCL is characteristically associated with t(11;14), and this translocation has not been identified in typical cases of SMZL.

Follicular Lymphoma

Follicular lymphoma should also be considered in the differential diagnosis of SMZL, since "marginal zones" may be observed in FL, and extracellular hyaline deposits may be common in both FL and SMZL. However, FL may be distinguished from SMZL by the presence of neoplastic follicles in FL. In addition, the

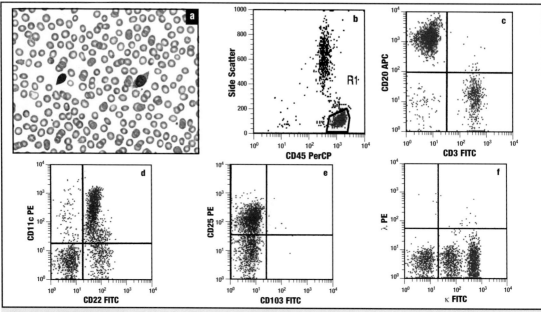

[f12.33] This case demonstrates a typical case of splenic marginal zone B-cell lymphoma with circulating villous lymphocytes. The clinical history reveals an 87-year-old male who presents with an absolute lymphocytosis associated with splenomegaly and thrombocytopenia. The peripheral blood smear reveals an increase in lymphoid-appearing cells, some with bipolar cytoplasmic projections a. By flow cytometric analysis, there is an increase in cells within a lymphoid region characterized by high CD45 expression and variable side scatter (low to moderate) (b, gated red dots). These cells express CD20 c, CD19 (not demonstrated), CD11c and CD22 (d, upper right box), as well as CD25 (e, upper left box) and selective surface κ (f, lower right box). There is no expression of CD5 (not demonstrated), CD10 (not demonstrated), CD23 (not demonstrated), nor CD103 e by the monoclonal B cells. The diagnosis is made of splenic marginal zone B-cell lymphoma with circulating villous lymphocytes.

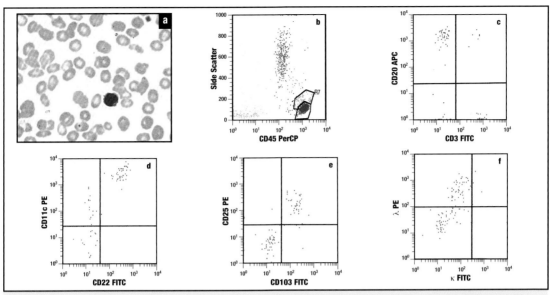

[f12.34] This case demonstrates a typical case of hairy cell leukemia. The clinical history reveals an 83-year-old male with pancytopenia and splenomegaly. The peripheral blood smear reveals a rare lymphoid-appearing cell with "hairy" projections **a**. By flow cytometric analysis, there is an increase in cells within a lymphoid region characterized by high CD45 expression and variable side scatter (low to moderate) (**b**, gated red dots). In addition, there is small population of cells with similar CD45 expression to the lymphocyte region, but higher side scatter (**b**, gated orange dots). These cells express CD20 **c**, CD19 (not demonstrated), CD11c and CD22 (**d**, upper right box), as well as CD25 and CD103 (**e**, upper right box) and selective surface κ (**f**, upper left box). There is no expression of CD5 (not demonstrated), CD10 (not demonstrated), nor CD23 (not demonstrated) by the monoclonal B cells. The diagnosis is made of hairy cell leukemia.

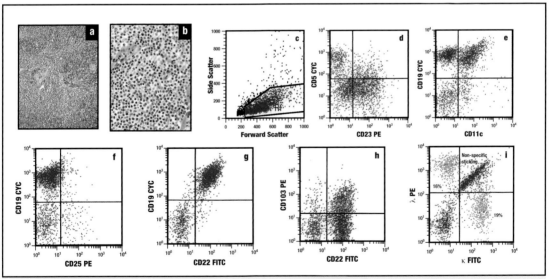

[f12.35] This case demonstrates a typical case of MALT lymphoma. The clinical history reveals a 64-year-old male with end stage liver disease secondary to cryptogenic cirrhosis and multiple pulmonary masses. A left lower lung wedge biopsy is performed. The histologic sections of the lung wedge biopsy reveal a proliferation of monotonous lymphoid-appearing cells with abundant cytoplasm **a,b**. By flow cytometric analysis of the tissue specimen, there is an increase in cells within the small to moderate-sized lymphocyte region, characterized by relatively low side scatter and increasing forward scatter (**c**, gated red dots). These cells express CD19 **e-g** CD20 (not demonstrated), and CD23 without co-expression of CD5 (**d**, lower right box). They demonstrate variable expression of CD11c on the CD19+ cells (**e**, upper left box demonstrates CD19+/CD11c-negative cells and upper right box reveals CD19+/CD11c+ cells), no expression of CD25 **f**, uniform expression of CD22 (**g**, upper right box and **h**), and variable, dim expression of CD103 (**h**, upper right box reveals dim expression of CD103 on the CD22+ cells, and **h**, lower right box reveals CD22+ cells with no expression of CD11c). There is no apparent restricted light chain restriction, but a significant number of the B cells (ie, 55%) have absolutely no associated light chain expression, indicating clonality **i**. The cytogenetic findings demonstrate trisomy 8, and the diagnosis is made of marginal zone B-cell lymphoma of MALT type.

immunophenotype of FL (with CD10+) should greatly aid in the distinction from SMZL, as reviewed in **[t12.1]**. Lastly, FL is often associated with a t(14;18), which has not been identified in SMZL.

Contribution of Paraffin Immunohistochemical Immunophenotyping

When fresh tissue is not available, IHC staining may aid in the above-described differential diagnoses. Although combined intense, diffuse TRAP+/DBA.44+ is highly sensitive for HCL, it is not entirely specific and may be observed in HCL-V and extranodal MZL [Dunphy 2008]. Nevertheless, negativity for 1 of these markers would certainly favor a SMZL rather than HCL or HCL-V. Cyclin D1+ would aid in distinguishing MCL and SMZL; combined bcl-6+, CD10+, and CD75+ would support a diagnosis of FL instead of SMZL.

Extranodal Marginal Zone B-Cell Lymphoma of MALT Type

Definition

This extranodal lymphoma is composed of small B cells, including marginal zone (centrocyte-like) cells, monocytoid-appearing cells, small lymphocytes, and scattered immunoblast- and centroblast-like cells. There is plasma cell differentiation in a proportion of the cases. The infiltrate is in the marginal zone of reactive B-cell follicles and extends into the interfollicular region. In epithelial tissues, the neoplastic cells from lymphoepithelial lesions.

Typical Immunophenotype

The neoplastic cells of MALT lymphoma typically express CD19, CD20, CD79a, and IgM (less often IgA or IgG) with demonstrable surface light chain restriction. They may be weakly positive or negative for CD11c. Associated plasma cells show monoclonal cytoplasmic light chain restriction in a third of the cases. The neoplastic small B cells are typically negative for CD5, CD10, CD23, CD103, and CD25. A typical case of MALT lymphoma is demonstrated in **[f12.35]**.

Variants: Morphology and Immunophenotypes

As previously discussed, MALT lymphomas may show extreme plasmacytic differentiation, being diagnostically confused with an extraosseous plasmacytoma. In addition, MALT lymphomas may aberrantly express CD5, and such cases have been associated with an increased propensity for BM involvement and relapse.

Differential Diagnosis

Splenic marginal zone B-cell lymphoma

This differential diagnosis has been discussed in the section above on SMZL.

Nodal marginal zone B-cell lymphoma

As discussed previously, nodal MZL may be diagnosed if there is no evidence of extranodal MALT site or splenic disease. Otherwise, their immunophenotypic features are quite similar, as may be seen in **[t12.1]**. There are some differences in their cytogenetic findings, as reviewed in **[t12.2]**.

CLL/SLL

As previously discussed in the section above on SMZL, CLL/SLL may generally be differentiated from MALT lymphoma by the CD5+ and CD23+ seen in CLL/SLL. However, occasional cases of CD5+ MALT lymphomas occur, as described previously. The finding of a t(11;18), t(1;14), trisomy 3, or trisomy 7 would favor a MALT lymphoma.

Mantle cell lymphoma

As previously discussed in the section of SMZL, the immunophenotype of MCL (with CD5+) should aid in the distinction from MALT lymphoma, as reviewed in **[t12.1]**. In addition, although trisomy 3 may be encountered in up to 50% of MCL [Monni 1998], and del(7q) may also occur in MCL [Dunphy 1999], MCL is characteristically associated with t(11;14), and this translocation has not been identified in MALT lymphoma.

Follicular lymphoma

Follicular lymphoma is another diagnostic consideration since "marginal zones" and monocytoid cells may be observed in FL. However, FL may be distinguished from MALT lymphoma by the presence of neoplastic follicles in FL. In addition, the immunophenotype of FL (with CD10+) should greatly aid in the distinction from SMZL, as reviewed in **[t12.1]**. Lastly, FL is often associated with a t(14;18), which has not been identified in MALT lymphoma.

Lymphoplasmacytic lymphoma

This differential diagnosis has been previously discussed in detail in the section above on LPL.

Plasmacytoma

This differential diagnosis has been previously discussed in detail in the section above on plasmacytoma.

Contribution of Paraffin Immunohistochemical Immunophenotyping

Paraffin IHC staining may be particularly helpful in evaluating small tissue biopsies for involvement by MALT lymphoma. In addition, the presence of monoclonal plasma cells and lymphoepithelial lesions, which may greatly aid in establishing a diagnosis of MALT lymphoma, may be detected ideally by this technique.

There is also an IHC marker, CD43, that is often touted as useful in establishing a diagnosis of MALT lymphoma in tissue sections. CD43 is a sialic acid-rich protein on the surface of lymphocytes that is important in T-cell activation, adhesion, and signal transduction. In addition to T cells, CD43 is also expressed by benign and malignant myeloid cells, histiocytes, and plasma cells [Farokhzad 2000, Rosenstein 1999, Cullinan 2002]. Expression of CD43 by B cells has been regarded as aberrant, because many B-cell lymphomas, including CLL/SLL, mantle cell lymphoma, Burkitt lymphoma (BL), and a subset of MZLs, co-express CD43 [Rosenstein 1999, Cullinan 2002, Lai 1999, Begueret 2002]. Benign follicle center, mantle, and marginal zone lymphocytes in lymph nodes, as well as most FLs, do not express CD43 [Lai 1999, Begueret 2002, Jung 2003, Treasure 1992]. However, a recent study has demonstrated that reactive B cells, chiefly in the perifollicular or mantle cell regions of the terminal ileum, often co-express CD43. Therefore, when using IHC staining to help distinguish reactive lymphoid infiltrates from malignant lymphoma in the distal small intestine, CD43 co-expression by B cells should not be used as a strict diagnostic criterion favoring MALT lymphoma [Lee 2005].

Nodal Marginal Zone B-Cell Lymphoma (± Monocytoid B Cells)

Definition

This primary nodal B-cell neoplasm is comprised of morphologically similar cells as those in SMZL and MALT lymphoma. As discussed previously, primary nodal MZL may be diagnosed if there is no evidence of extranodal MALT site or splenic disease.

Typical Immunophenotype

The typical immunophenotype of primary nodal MZL is identical to that of MALT lymphoma, as reviewed in **[t12.1]**; however, CD5+ has not been described in primary nodal MZL. A typical case of primary nodal MZL is demonstrated in **[f12.36]**.

Differential Diagnosis

Marginal zone hyperplasia

Marked marginal zone hyperplasia may be confused with primary nodal MZL. The presence of a monoclonal population of small B lymphocytes by flow cytometric analysis aids in establishing a diagnosis of MZL.

Secondary involvement of lymph node by extranodal marginal zone B-cell lymphoma (MALT) or splenic marginal zone B-cell lymphoma

As previously discussed, if a primary diagnosis of MALT lymphoma or SMZL has not been established, secondary involvement by 1 of these subtypes must be excluded in order to establish a diagnosis of primary nodal MZL. The immunophenotypes of MALT lymphoma and primary nodal MZL are identical, although CD5+ may be encountered in MALT lymphoma. The immunophenotypes of SMZL and primary nodal MZL may also be identical. However, there are some differences in their cytogenetic findings, as reviewed in **[t12.2]**, which may aid in the differential diagnosis. However, the primary issue is excluding the presence of primary splenic or MALT site disease.

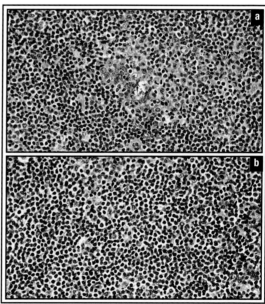

[f12.36] This case demonstrates the morphology of a typical case of primary nodal marginal zone B-cell lymphoma. The patient is a 67-year-old male with a history of prostate cancer and an enlarged left supraclavicular lymph node, which is biopsied. The histologic sections reveal a monotonous population of small to intermediate-sized lymphoid-appearing cells with abundant cytoplasm, so that the cells are clearly separated from each other **a**, **b**. κ and λ ISH reveals restricted κ expression (not demonstrated).

Follicular lymphoma

Since there is a morphologic variant of FL with a prominent component of monocytoid B cells, this variant should be considered in the differential diagnosis of a primary nodal MZL. This differential diagnosis is discussed above in the section regarding FL.

Hairy cell leukemia

Complete effacement of nodal tissue by MZL may histologically resemble leukemic infiltration of the lymph node by hairy cell leukemia. However, by flow cytometric analysis, the neoplastic cells of HCL typically have stronger expression of CD11c than the neoplastic cells of MZL, as well as strong, uniform expression of CD103 and CD25, as reviewed in **[t12.1]**.

Large granular lymphocyte leukemia

The differential diagnosis of LGLL from primary nodal MZL is similar to the differential diagnosis of LGLL from SMZL, as discussed in the section above regarding SMZL.

Systemic mastocytosis

The monocytoid B cells in primary nodal MZL may morphologically resemble mast cells in tissue sections. As described in Chapter 18, neoplastic mast cells do not express B-lineage or T-lineage associated antigens, but instead express CD2, CD117, and CD25 by flow cytometric analysis, greatly aiding in the distinction of these 2 entities.

Langerhans cell histiocytosis

The monocytoid B cells in primary nodal MZL may also morphologically resemble the neoplastic cells of Langerhans cell histiocytosis (LCH) in tissue sections. However, as described in Chapter 17, the neoplastic cells of LCH likewise do not express B-lineage associated antigens or most T-lineage associated antigens (except CD4), but rather express dim CD45 and CD1a. Again, the differences in immunophenotypes by flow cytometric analysis greatly aid in the distinction of these 2 entities.

Contribution of Paraffin Immunohistochemical Immunophenotyping

If fresh tissue is not available for the detection of monoclonal B cells by flow cytometric analysis in distinguishing marginal zone hyperplasia (MZH) from MZL, bcl-2 IHC staining may be helpful. However, one should keep in mind that bcl-2 has also been shown

to be consistently expressed by reactive marginal zone B cells of the spleen, abdominal lymph nodes, and ileal lymphoid tissue. Thus, bcl-2 expression should not be used as a criterion for discriminating between benign and malignant marginal zone B-cell proliferations involving these sites [Meda 2003].

Likewise, if fresh tissue is not available for distinguishing primary nodal MZL from HCL, IHC staining with DBA.44 and TRAP may aid in this differential diagnosis. One should keep in mind that although combined intense, diffuse TRAP+/DBA.44+ is highly sensitive for HCL, it is not entirely specific and may be observed in HC-V and extranodal MZL [Dunphy 2008]. However, DBA.44– and/or TRAP– would support a diagnosis of MZL rather than HCL in this differential diagnosis.

In the differential diagnosis of MZL and systemic mastocytosis, IHC staining with mast cell tryptase and toluidine blue may also aid in the differential diagnosis, since mast cells are positive for both of these markers, and the neoplastic cells of MZL are negative for both of these markers.

Hairy Cell Leukemia

Definition

Hairy cell leukemia is a neoplasm of small B-lymphoid cells with oval nuclei and abundant cytoplasm with "hairy" projections in BM and PB, diffusely infiltrating BM and splenic red pulp.

Typical Immunophenotype

The neoplastic cells of HCL typically are sIg+ (M±D, G, or A) and demonstrate expression of B-cell lineage associated antigens (ie, CD19, CD20, CD22, CD70a, but not CD79b) with associated strong expressions of CD11c, CD103, and CD25. They are typically negative for CD5, CD10, and CD23. A typical case of HCL has been previously demonstrated in **[f12.34]**, with list-mode output available on the accompanying disk.

Variant: Morphology and Immunophenotypes

HCL-variant (HCL-V) is a rare disease in which BM and splenic histology resemble HCL, but the patients present with a marked leukocytosis (instead of pancytopenia), and the circulating neoplastic cells resemble prolymphocytes. However, the immunophenotype of HCL-V differs somewhat from classical HCL, in that there is often IgG on the cell membrane, variable expression of CD103, and lack of CD25 expression. A case of HCL-V has been previously demonstrated in **[f12.16]**, with listmode output available on the accompanying disk. It is important to recognize this prolymphocytic variant of HCL, since the response to treatment with agents effective in typical HCL is usually poor and median survival is significantly shorter in this variant, as compared to classical HCL.

CD10+ may also be seen in HCL, as demonstrated previously in **[f12.24]**, with listmode output available on the accompanying disk. CD10+ HCL cases seem to be morphologically and clinically similar to CD10– HCL cases [Hounieu 1992, Dunphy 1999].

Rare cases of HCL may be negative for CD103 (6%) or CD25 (3%). However, there are no documented dual CD103–/CD25– cases of HCL [Chen 2006]. Again, these immunophenotypic variations do not appear to influence the clinical outcome in these patients.

Differential Diagnosis

Marginal zone lymphomas

Splenic MZL may present with circulating villous lymphocytes and BM involvement; primary nodal MZL and MALT lymphoma may show BM involvement. Although HCL has a leukemic pattern of involvement in BM sections, limited biopsy specimens may pose a diagnostic dilemma of HCL vs MZL. As previously discussed, the neoplastic cells of HCL typically show strong expression of CD11c, CD103, and CD25, whereas the neoplastic cells of the MZLs are negative for CD25, may show weak or no expression of CD11c, and possibly weak expression or no expression of CD103 in SMZL. Primary nodal MZL and MALT lymphoma are negative for CD103. However, as discussed previously, rare cases of HCL may be negative for CD103 (6%) or CD25 (3%), but there are no documented dual CD103–/CD25– cases of HCL. Thus, strong positivity for CD11c in combination with strong CD103 or CD25 would favor a diagnosis of HCL rather than MZL.

CLL/SLL

This differential diagnosis is discussed in detail in the section above on CLL/SLL.

Mantle cell lymphoma

Mantle cell lymphoma may present in the PB as mantle cell leukemia. The CD5+ and dual CD11c– and CD103– of the neoplastic cells of MCL should greatly aid in distinguishing it from HCL by flow cytometric analysis.

Follicular lymphoma

The differential diagnosis of FL and HCL may be somewhat problematic in cases of CD10+ HCL. However, the neoplastic cells of FL are negative for CD11c and CD103.

Large granular lymphocyte leukemia

In BM and splenic sections, the neoplastic cells of LGLL may strikingly resemble those of HCL. However, by flow cytometric analysis, these entities should be clearly distinguishable by their characteristic immunophenotypes: NK-LGL leukemia (CD2+, CD3–, CD4–, CD8+, CD16+, CD56+, CD57v) and T-LGL leukemia (CD2+, CD3+, CD4–, CD8+, CD16+/–, CD56–/+, CD57+).

Systemic mastocytosis

In BM and splenic sections, the neoplastic cells of systemic mastocytosis may also strikingly resemble those of HCL. As described in Chapter 18, neoplastic mast cells do not express B-lineage or T-lineage associated antigens, but instead express CD2, CD117, and CD25 by flow cytometric analysis, greatly aiding in the distinction of these 2 entities.

Langerhans cell histiocytosis

Lastly, in BM and splenic sections, the neoplastic cells of Langerhans cell histiocytosis (LCH) may strikingly resemble those of HCL. However, as described in Chapter 17, the neoplastic cells of LCH likewise do not express B-lineage associated antigens or most T-lineage associated antigens (except CD4), but rather express dim CD45 and CD1a. Again, the differences in immunophenotypes by flow cytometric analysis greatly aid in the distinction of these 2 entities.

Contribution of Paraffin Immunohistochemical Immunophenotyping

The neoplastic cells of HCL are often difficult to aspirate from the BM, and thus the diagnosis may often rely on immunophenotypic markers by paraffin IHC staining. As mentioned previously, although combined intense, diffuse TRAP+/DBA.44+ is highly sensitive for HCL, it is not entirely specific and may be observed in HC-V and extranodal MZL [Dunphy 2008]. However, DBA.44– or TRAP– would virtually exclude a diagnosis of HCL. Investigators in a subsequent study stained 500 B-cell tumors with antiannexin A1 and showed that antiannexin A1 protein expression was specific to HCL [Basso 2004]. This marker was especially useful in differentiating HCL from splenic lymphoma with villous lymphocytes and from HCL variant (2 entities that are sometimes in the differential diagnosis of HCL [Basso 2004, Falini 2004].

In distinguishing HCL and mantle cell lymphoma, one should keep in mind that the cyclin D1+ that may be encountered in HCL has been described as usually weak and in a subpopulation of the tumor cells.

In distinguishing CD10+ HCL from FL, the lack of DBA.44 and TRAP positivity and combined expressions of CD10, CDw75, and bcl-6 by IHC staining should greatly aid in distinguishing these 2 entities.

Immunohistochemical staining with CD117, mast cell tryptase, and toluidine blue may be used in distinguishing systemic mastocytosis from HCL.

Diffuse Large B-Cell Lymphoma

Definition

Diffuse large B-cell lymphoma (DLBCL) is defined as a diffuse proliferation of large neoplastic B-lymphoid cells (ie, approximately the size of or larger than a normal macrophage, or more than twice the size of a normal lymphocyte).

Immunophenotypes

Diffuse large B-cell lymphoma typically expresses various pan-B-cell markers, such as CD19, CD20, CD22, and CD79a, and demonstrates surface and/or cytoplasmic immunoglobulin (IgM>IgG>IgA) in 50%-75% of cases. DLBCL is generally divided into 3 immunophenoytpic expression patterns:

1. a germinal center B (GCB)-cell pattern expressing CD10 or bcl-6, but not expressing activation markers (MUM1/IRF4 and CD138)

2. an activated GCB-cell pattern expressing at least 1 of the GCB-cell markers (CD10 or bcl-6) and at least 1 of the activation markers (MUM1/IRF4 or CD138)

3. an activated non–GCB-cell pattern expressing MUM1/IRF4 or CD138 but not expressing GCB-cell markers.

Patients with pattern 1 have a much better OS when treated with CHOP chemotherapy than those with the other 2 patterns (P <.008) [Chang 2004]. The International Prognostic Index (IPI) scores and the expression patterns of these markers are independent prognostic markers. CD10 and CD138 may be determined by flow cytometric analysis, but bcl-6 and MUM1 are typically analyzed by IHC staining. In addition, one should keep in mind that when several of these markers have been more recently re-evaluated in the era of immunochemotherapy (eg, rituximab plus CHOP) for DLBCL, the prognostic advantage or disadvantage appears to be mitigated. For example, the unfavorable survival outcome in the non-GC subtype of DLBCL is alleviated [Farinha 2006, Mounier 2003]. Further discussion is provided in the subsection below regarding the contribution of paraffin IHC staining.

Variants: Morphology and Immunophenotypes

Morphologic variants include centroblastic, immunoblastic, T-cell/histiocyte-rich, and anaplastic. The centroblastic variant is composed of medium-sized to large cells with vesicular nuclei and 2-4 membrane-bound nucleoli. The immunoblastic variant is composed of immunoblasts with the characteristic centrally-located nucleolus and abundant basophilic cytoplasm. The T-cell/histiocyte-rich [also referred to as T-cell rich (TCR) or lymphohistiocytic-rich (LHR)] variant is characterized by a background rich in reactive T cells and variable numbers of histiocytes. In this variant, flow cytometric analysis may fail to reveal a monoclonal or aberrant B-cell population, due to the large number of reactive T cells and histiocytes in the tissue. The anaplastic variant is morphologically similar, but not biologically related, to anaplastic CD30+ large cell lymphoma of cytotoxic T-cell origin (ALCL). The cells of the anaplastic variant of DLBCL are also generally CD30+. Such a case is demonstrated in **[f12.37]**.

Additional rare variants that have been included in the DLBCL subtype in the WHO classification are plasmablastic lymphoma (PBL) (also included under lymphomas associated with HIV infection) and DLBCL with expression of full-length ALK (or ALK+ DLBCL).

As discussed previously in the section above entitled "Plasmacytomas," PBL typically presents in the oral cavity in the setting of HIV infection; however, PBL has also been encountered in non-HIV patients. Cases of PBL are positive for CD138 and CD38 and negative for CD20, corresponding to a plasma cell immunophenotype. EBV-encoded RNA has been demonstrated in all PBL cases tested. A representative case of PBL has been demonstrated in **[f12.31]**, with listmode output available on the accompanying disk. Since most cases of AIDS-

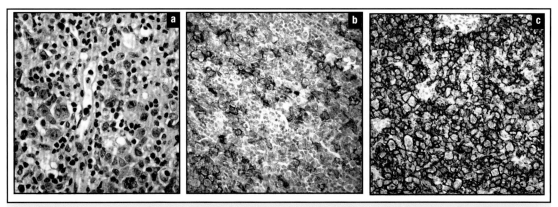

[f12.37] This case demonstrates a case of the relatively unusual anaplastic variant of diffuse large B-cell lymphoma. The patient is a 31-year-old male with left cervical lymphadenopathy, which is biopsied. Histologic section of the lymph node reveals the anaplastic cells, occasionally with Reed-Sternberg-like features **a**. Immunostains reveal intense, uniform reactivity with CD30 (**b**, CD30), as typically seen in ALCL, but also with CD20 (**c**, CD20). The cells are negative for CD3, CD15, and ALK-1 *(courtesy Dr Peter Banks, Carolinas Medical Center, Charlotte, NC)*.

related PBL have an immunophenotype and tumor suppressor gene expression profile virtually identical to anaplastic (or plasmablastic) plasma cell myeloma, and unlike DLBCL, the question arises as to the validity of the WHO classification of PBL as a variant of DLBCL [Vega 2005]. PBL is also discussed in Chapter 16.

The other rare variant mentioned above, ALK1+ DLBCL (also referred to as DLBCL of plasmablastic type), is composed of monomorphic large immunoblast-like cells with round, pale nuclei containing large central nucleoli and associated with abundant amphophilic cytoplasm, sometimes with plasmacytic differentiation. These neoplastic cells are CD30–, CD20–, weakly CD45+, and CD138+, and express monoclonal intracytoplasmic IgA. In addition, they are EMA+ and ALK+ (showing a granular cytoplasmic and dot-like positivity with ALK protein in the Golgi area by IHC staining). ALK+ DLBCL is associated with the following 2 characteristic types of ALK gene rearrangements: the CLTC–ALK fusion caused by a t(2;17)(p23;q23) translocation and the NPM1–ALK fusion caused by a t(2;5)(p23;q35) translocation. However, in contrast to ALCL, most reported cases of ALK+ DLBCL have the former translocation, and only 3 cases have shown the latter translocation. Such a case is demonstrated in **[f12.38]**.

In addition, as mentioned earlier in the section of mantle cell lymphoma, there is a de-novo form of CD5+ DLBCL (negative for cyclin D1). Of further interest, de-novo CD5+ DLBCL is also characterized by a survival curve significantly inferior to that for patients with CD5– DLBCL (p= .0025) and may represent a

unique subgroup of DLBCL [Yamaguchi 2002]. Such a case is demonstrated in **[f12.39]**.

Differential Diagnosis

Blastoid variants of mantle cell lymphoma
The major differential diagnosis with the blastoid variant of mantle cell lymphoma is CD5+ de-novo DLBCL, as discussed in the section above regarding mantle cell lymphoma.

Richter syndrome and paraimmunoblastic variant of SLL
Richter syndrome and the paraimmunoblastic variant of SLL may be differentiated from DLBCL and CD5+ de-novo DLBCL, since they typically retain their immunophenotype (ie, CD5+, CD23+) [Dunphy 1997]. CD5+ de-novo DLBCL is typically CD23–.

Large cell transformation of MALT lymphoma
Transformed centroblast- or immunoblast-like cells may be present in variable numbers in MALT lymphoma, but when solid or sheet-like proliferations of trans-formed cells are encountered, a diagnosis of DLBCL and the presence of accompanying MALT lymphoma should be noted. without a previous diagnosis of MALT lymphoma, or in limited biopsy specimens without a demonstrable coexisting MALT lymphoma, the differential diagnosis of de-novo DLBCL vs a DLBCL aris-ing in the setting of a MALT lymphoma occurs. CD10 may be expressed in up to 67% of DLBCL cases associated with MALT lymphoma. Therefore, in some cases,

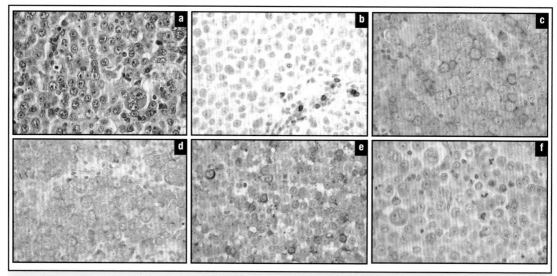

[f12.38] This case demonstrates an ALK+ diffuse large B-cell lymphoma (DLBCL) (DLBCL-plasmablastic variant). The patient is a 13-year-old female with multiple enlarged lymph nodes in the neck. The H&E section **a** reveals sheets of anaplastic-appearing cells with plasmacytoid features. The neoplastic cells are negative for CD20, CD79a **b**, CD2, CD3, CD5, CD4, CD8, CD30 (**c**, occasional cell positive), and CD45. They are positive for ALK-1 **d**, CD138 **e**, IgG, and λ **f**. Molecular analysis reveals a clonal rearrangement for IgH and λ. Conventional cytogenetic studies demonstrate a complex karyotype including t(2;17). FISH studies confirm that this represents CLTC-ALK fusion. *(This case was included in the cases of the 2003 Society for Hematopathology/European Association for Haematopathology Workshop in Memphis, entitled "Reactive and Neoplastic Disorders in Pediatric Hematopathology: Impact of Molecular, Cytogenetic, and Flow Cytometric Methodologies on Diagnosis and Treatment," which Dr Dunphy attended in Memphis in 2003; a CD with case histories and images was provided to her as a participant and contributor).*

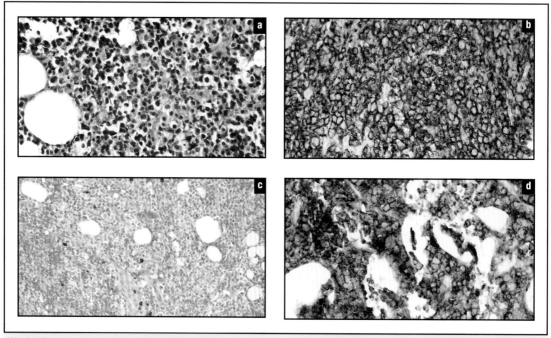

[f12.39] This case demonstrates a CD5+ de-novo diffuse large B-cell lymphoma. The patient is a 55-year-old female with left inguinal lymphadenopathy, which is biopsied. The histologic section of lymph node reveals complete effacement of the lymph node architecture by a diffuse proliferation of predominantly large abnormal lymphoid-appearing cells **a**. Immunostains reveal intense, uniform staining of the large cells with CD20 **b**. CD3 stains scattered small lymphocytes in the background **c**. However, CD5 is co-expressed on the large B cells **d**. CD23 and cyclin D1 immunostains (not demonstrated) are negative. FISH analysis for t(11;14) is negative.

the distinction may rely on the differential characteristic translocations encountered in MALT-associated lymphomas, DLBCLs of follicle center cell origin, etc. A representative case is demonstrated in [f12.40].

Mediastinal (thymic) large B-cell lymphoma

This lymphoma is described in detail in the next section regarding primary mediastinal B-cell lymphoma. Please see that section for its differentiation from de-novo DLBCL as defined by the WHO classification.

Burkitt lymphoma and atypical variant of Burkitt lymphoma

Burkitt lymphoma (BL), as will be discussed in that section below, typically has a very characteristic morphology and immunophenotype (CD19+, CD20+, CD22+, CD10+, and monoclonal sIg). with such classical morphology, the differential diagnosis with DLBCL is usually straightforward; however, when the atypical variant of BL is encountered, the differential diagnosis with DLBCL is more problematic. The atypical variant of BL is composed of a more pleomorphic neoplastic population than that encountered in classical BL. The differential diagnosis between these entities will be further and primarily discussed in the subsection below regarding the contribution of paraffin IHC immunophenotyping. In such cases, the differential diagnosis also often relies on the demonstration of a translocation of *c-myc*, which is characteristic of BL. However, one should keep in mind that DLBCLs with morphological high-grade features may also harbor a *c-myc* rearrangement or *c-myc* amplification, have a poor prognosis, and be treated similarly to BL and its atypical variant [McClure 2005, Mossafa 2006]. In addition, there are "double hit" DLBCLs that have coexistence of a t(14;18) and a *c-myc* translocation (ie, B-cell lymphoma, unclassifiable, with features intermediate between DLBCL and Burkitt lymphoma). Their immunophenotypic profile will again be further and primarily discussed in the subsection below regarding the contribution of paraffin IHC immunophenotyping. These "double hit" lymphomas are associated with a particularly poor prognosis— worse than BL [Kanungo 2006, Le Gouill 2007].

Precursor B- and T-cell lymphoblastic lymphoma/ leukemia

Precursor B- and T-cell lymphoblastic lymphomas/leukemias are also high-grade lymphoid neoplasms that must be distinguished from DLBCL with high-grade features. By flow cytometric analysis, precursor B-cell lymphoblastic neoplasms do not typically express surface

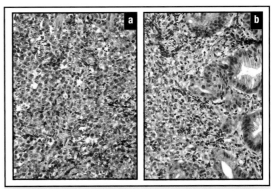

[f12.40] This case demonstrates a diffuse large B-cell lymphoma (DLBCL) arising in MALT, although there is no evidence of a low-grade MALT component. The patient is a 60-year-old female with a history of DLBCL of the breast, now with abnormal PET imaging noted in the stomach. Histologic sections of the stomach biopsy reveal a diffuse proliferation by large abnormal lymphoid-appearing cells a. There are adjacent glands in areas, with no evidence of a low-grade MALT component b. Cytogenetic studies reveal trisomy 3.

Ig or light chains and do express TdT, in contrast to DLBCL. In addition, a proportion of these precursor neoplasms express CD34, whereas the neoplastic cells of DLBCL are uniformly CD34–. The neoplastic cells of DLBCL generally demonstrate stronger CD45 and CD20 expression than precursor B-cell neoplasms. It is also important to recognize that there may be occasional cases of precursor B-lymphoblastic leukemia with a mature immunophenotype (ie, with surface light chain expression) associated with L1 or L2 morphology and no evidence of a chromosomal translocation involving the *c-myc* gene [f11.3]. This entity is further discussed below in the section regarding Burkitt lymphoma/leukemia. Precursor T-cell neoplasms will have variable expression of T-cell antigens, depending on their stage of maturation (ie, CD1a, CD2, cCD3, sCD3, CD4, CD5, CD7, and CD8) and are discussed in Chapter 13.

Granulocytic sarcoma

Granulocytic sarcomas are typically distinguished by their variable expression of myelomonocytic markers, as AMLs, and described in Chapter 10. One should keep in mind that AMLs associated with t(8;21) are also associated with PAX-5 nuclear positivity by IHC staining.

Large cell lymphomas of mature T-cell origin

Large cell lymphomas of mature T-cell origin are usually distinguished from DLBCL by their variable expression of T-cell markers (ie, CD2, CD3, CD4, CD5, CD7, and CD8) and lack of B-cell markers.

Distinguishing T-cell rich/histiocytic-rich variant of DLBCL (TCR/LHR-DLBCL) from lymphocyte-predominant Hodgkin lymphoma (LPHL), classical Hodgkin lymphoma (cHL), and the lymphohistiocytic-rich variant of anaplastic CD30+ large cell lymphoma

The variant of T-cell rich DLBCL may be difficult, if not impossible, to distinguish from a pure, diffuse type of LPHL, and has been a matter of controversy [McBride 1996, Rudiger 1998, Schmidt 1990]. This differential diagnosis is further and primarily discussed in the subsection below regarding the contribution of paraffin IHC immunophenotyping. Likewise, distinguishing TCR/LHR-DLBCL from cHL and the lymphohistiocytic-rich variant of ALCL is also discussed in the same subsection below.

Anaplastic CD30+ large cell lymphoma (ALCL)

Other variants of DLBCL that must be distinguished from ALCL include the anaplastic CD30+ variant of DLBCL and DLBCL with expression of full-length ALK (or ALK+ DLBCL of plasmablastic type). The anaplastic CD30+ variant of DLBCL shows similar anaplastic morphology to classical ALCL and is generally CD30+, as may be encountered in ALCL; however, the neoplastic cells express B-cell surface antigens, as other DLBCLs, and are negative for all T-cell associated antigens. The ALK+ DLBCL of plasmablastic type on the other hand is CD30– and does not express B-cell or T-cell surface antigens but rather expresses CD138 in association with ALK-positivity.

Plasmablastic myeloma/plasmacytoma

The differential diagnosis between PBL and plasmablastic myeloma/plasmacytoma has been discussed in detail in the section above regarding plasma cell neoplasms.

Contribution of Paraffin Immunohistochemical Immunophenotyping

Paraffin IHC staining may be applied to immunophenotyping B-cells composed of intermediate-sized to large cells, to determine their cell of origin and biologic potential. As was previously discussed, MUM1 expression, in combination with the evaluations of CD10, bcl-6, and CD138, may allow for the distinction of the following 3 immunophenotypic profiles in DLBCLs [Chang 2004]:

1. a germinal center B (GCB)-cell pattern expressing CD10 or bcl-6, but not expressing activation markers (MUM1/IRF4 and CD138)

2. an activated GCB-cell pattern expressing at least 1 of the GCB-cell markers (CD10 or bcl-6) and at least 1 of the activation markers (MUM1/IRF4 or CD138),

3. an activated non–GCB-cell pattern expressing MUM1/IRF4 or CD138 but not expressing GCB-cell markers.

Diffuse large B-cell lymphomas of GC cell origin (DLBCLs-GC) generally have a similar immunophenotype to that of FL, which has previously been described; DLBCLs-GC more frequently have an absence of CD10. In addition, it has been demonstrated that CD10+ DLBCLs-GC, particularly those cases with low IPI scores, have a better prognosis [Chang 2002]. Subsequent studies have supported the association of CD10-positivity, bcl-6-positivity, and MUM1-negativity in DLBCLs-GC with increased OS and event-free survival (EFS) [Hans 2003]. However, when several of these markers have been more recently re-evaluated in the era of immunochemotherapy for DLBCL [ie, rituximab plus CHOP (R-CHOP)], the prognostic advantage or disadvantage appears to be mitigated. For example, the unfavorable survival outcome of the non-GC subtype of DLBCL is alleviated [Farinha 2006, Mounier 2003]. Likewise, Winter et al reported that by administering R-CHOP, the difference between bcl-6+ and bcl-6– cases was essentially eliminated [Winter 2006].

Of interest, bcl-6 protein expression has also been observed in DLBCL of the stomach and small intestine [Kevon 2003]. In a study by Kevon et al, 2 distinct patterns of bcl-6 expression were recognized in this group of lymphomas: diffusely dense (>75% cells+), seen in those of GC-cell derivation, and sporadic (<75% cells positive with lack of consistently dense positivity), seen in non-GC-cell DLBCL, including those associated with MALT lymphoma. In addition, as previously mentioned, CD10 may be expressed in up to 67% of DLBCL cases associated with MALT lymphoma. Thus, bcl-6 and CD10 may be expressed in DLBCL of non-GC origin; however, the pattern of bcl-6 protein expression is distinctly different. This pattern of expression may be helpful in distinguishing de-novo DLBCL from DLBCL arising in MALT lymphoma, when there is no previously established diagnosis of MALT lymphoma, when limited tissue is available for evaluation, or when no remaining MALT lymphoma is identifiable.

Immunohistochemical staining may also be useful in evaluating primary central nervous system (CNS) DLBCLs among immunocompetent individuals. In a study by Chang et al, expression of p53, *c-myc*, and bcl-6 correlated with poorer overall survival and an increased mortality rate [Chang 2003]. MUM1 was not analyzed in this study. In addition, this same group of authors reported that expression of p53 or *c-myc* in non-CNS DLBCLs correlated with an adverse clinical outcome [Chang 2000]. Another recent study by Braaten et al of non-HIV associated primary CNS lymphomas revealed that bcl-6 expression predicted longer OS [Braaten 2003].

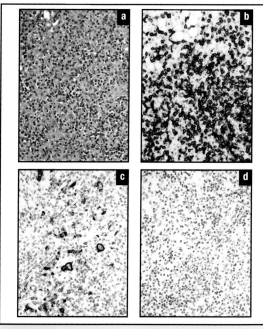

[f12.41] This case demonstrates the typical histology and immunophenotype of pure, diffuse lymphocyte-predominant Hodgkin lymphoma. The patient is a 15-year-old male with a history of nausea, vomiting, abdominal pain, and an 11-pound weight loss associated with multiple liver and splenic masses and extensive lymphadenopathy. A liver mass is biopsied. Histologic sections of the liver biopsy reveal a diffuse infiltrate with numerous small lymphocytes in the background intermixed with scattered larger lymphoid forms and numerous apoptotic cells **a**. By flow cytometric analysis of the liver tissue, 34% of cells are within the lymphocyte region. within this region, there are 80% T cells (CD4:CD8 ratio is 3.4) and only 1% B cells (not demonstrated). Immunohistochemical stains reveal numerous T cells in the background (**b**, CD3) with scattered clearly identifiable large B cells (**c**, CD20), which are ringed by CD57+ cells (**d**, CD57).

This group was also associated with MUM1 expression, indicating an activated GC-cell immunophenotype.

In addition to determining the immunophenotypic profile of DLBCLs and a prognosis, paraffin IHC immunophenotyping may be widely applied in recognizing the various morphologic and immunophenotypic variants of DLBCL, as described previously. T-cell-rich or lymphohistiocytic-rich DLBCL (TCR-DLBCL or LHR-DLBCL) may be better defined by paraffin IHC staining, since these lymphomas typically do not reveal a monoclonal B-cell population by FCI due to the low number of malignant cells relative to the background cells. These DLBCLs are characterized by a background rich (>80% background cells) in lymphocytes, with or without a histiocytic component. This group of DLBCLs represents a heterogeneous group and by paraffin IHC staining, the scattered large malignant B cells have the following immunophenotype: CD20+, CD10−/+ (25%-50%), CD5 (10%), bcl-2+ (30%-50%), and bcl-6+ (majority of cases). The distinction of TCR-DLBCL from a pure, diffuse type of lymphocyte-predominant Hodgkin lymphoma (LPHL) may not be possible and has been a matter of controversy [McBride 1996, Rudiger 1998, Schmidt 1990]. As discussed later in Chapter 15, the L&H cells are typically ringed by CD3+ and/or CD57+ lymphocytes by paraffin IHC staining. A representative case of pure, diffuse LPHL is demonstrated in **[f12.41]**. However, areas within nodular LPHL (NLPHL) may have a diffuse pattern, characterized by scattered L&H cells set in a diffuse background of reactive T cells with a loss of CD57+ T cells, as well as a loss of the follicular dendritic cell meshwork. So unless the characteristic ringing of L&H cells by CD3 or CD57 is clearly demonstrated, the distinction of LPHL with a diffuse pattern from TCR-DLBCL primarily relies on the presence of a nodular component of LPHL existing in association with the diffuse areas in the same biopsy. In the absence of a nodular component of LPHL, a purely diffuse pattern would be regarded as TCR-DLBCL. In the report on NLPHL by Fan et al [2003], the diffuse pattern of LPHL (TCR-DLBCL-like) was significantly more common in recurring cases than in those without recurrence, and the predominance of a diffuse pattern was even a stronger prediction of recurrence [Fan 2003]. Thus, although the distinction between TCR-DLBCL and pure, diffuse LPHL has been controversial, a predominant diffuse pattern is important to recognize.

The TCR- and LHR-DLBCL variants may be distinguished from cHL and the lymphohistiocytic-rich variant of ALCL primarily by IHC staining. The neoplastic cells of cHL are CD45–, intensely CD30+, and typically CD15+ with CD20-positivity in up to 37% of cases. However, the CD20-positivity is less intense and not as uniform as seen in the TCR– and LHR-rich variants of DLBCL. The neoplastic cells of the lymphohistiocytic-rich variant of ALCL are uniformly and intensely positive for CD30, may variably express T-cell antigens, and are uniformly negative for all B-cell markers.

The anaplastic variant of DLBCL is a CD30+ diffuse anaplastic lymphoma of B-cell origin [Maes 2001], which may be morphologically difficult to differentiate from ALCL. The distinction is based on the B-cell immunophenotype in the variant of DLBCL and the T-cell or "null" cell immunophenotype characteristic of ALCL in the WHO classification.

The anaplastic variant of DLBCL may also be diagnostically confused with ALK+ DLBCL (also referred to as DLBCL of plasmablastic type). However, these entities should be distinguished by differences in their IHC staining patterns. The ALK+ DLBCL (also referred to as DLBCL of plasmablastic type) is characterized by the following immunophenotype by IHC staining: ALK+, CD30–, CD20–, EMA+, and CD138+, and monoclonal cytoplasmic Ig or light chain, best demonstrated by ISH staining. As mentioned previously, ALK+ DLBCL is associated with 2 characteristic types of ALK gene rearrangements: the CLTC–ALK fusion caused by a t(2;17)(p23;q23) translocation and the NPM1–ALK fusion caused by a t(2;5)(p23;q35) translocation [Chen 2006, Chen 2003, Cook 2003, Li 2002, del Senno 1987, Peltomaki 2988]. However, in contrast to ALCL, most reported cases of ALK+ DLBCL have the former translocation and only 3 cases have shown the latter translocation [Adam 2003, Chikatsu 2003]. To further complicate these differential diagnoses, plasmablastic lymphoma (PBL) is another variant of DLBCL, according to the WHO classification. A representative case was demonstrated in [f12.31], with listmode output available on the accompanying disk. As discussed, this type of lymphoma typically presents in the oral cavity and occurs in an immunocompromised setting (eg, human immunodeficiency virus syndrome) and has the following immunophenotype: CD45 (LCA)–, CD20–, CD138+, EMA+, and monoclonal cytoplasmic Ig or light chain. Although cases of ALK+ DLBCL (or DLBCL of plasmacytic type) have not

been reportedly HIV+, PBL may also occur in HIV-patients. The main immunophenotypic difference between these 2 entities is the ALK-positivity in the DLBCL of plasmacytic type and ALK-negativity in PBL. Plasmablastic plasmacytoma has an identical immunophenotype to the ALK+ DLBCL (or DLBCL of plasmablastic type) but is ALK–. A representative case was demonstrated in [f12.32]. As discussed in the section above regarding plasmacytoma, plasmablastic plasmacytoma is most often distinguished from PBL by the presence of EBV-encoded RNA, being positive in all PBL cases tested and negative in all plasmacytoma cases. The immunophenotypic features of ALCL, the anaplastic variant of DLBLC, DLBCL of plasmablastic type (ALK+ DLBCL), PBL, and plasmablastic plasmacytoma, as well as another entity to be discussed later (ie, primary effusion lymphoma-PEL) are compared in [t12.3].

De-novo CD5+ DBLCL may be distinguished from a blastoid variant of MCL based on the association of t(11;14) in the large cell variants of MCL. Cyclin D1 may thus be evaluated by paraffin IHC staining, although as discussed previously, the sensitivity is not particularly high. Nevertheless, this distinction may not be clinically relevant since the general group of de-novo CD5+ DLBCLs have an aggressive clinical course, characterized by very poor treatment outcome associated with frequent relapses.

Burkitt lymphoma is also of GC cell origin and typically reveals strong expression of CD10 (90% of BL cases) and bcl-6 (100% of BL cases). Such a case is demonstrated in [f12.44], with listmode output available on the accompanying disk. However, in contrast to DLBCL-GC, bcl-2 is typically not expressed in BL. As discussed previously, the differential diagnosis of BL includes DLBCL with morphological high-grade features, including those with a *c-myc* rearrangement or amplification. Ki-67 (MIB-1) has been claimed as a useful marker by paraffin IHC to distinguish BL from DLBCL with morphological high-grade features. The MIB-1 index should be >98% and not <95% in BL. In contrast, the MIB-1 index in DLBCL with *c-myc* rearrangement is typically <95%. However, atypical variants of BL may have a MIB index <95%, and DLBCLs with a *c-myc* rearrangement or amplification may have a MIB index >95%. Another immunophenotypic difference is the presence of bcl-2 in a higher percentage (75%) of the DLBCL cases [Nakamura 2002]. However, as mentioned previously, DLBCLs with a *c-myc* rearrangement or amplification have a poor prognosis and should be treated similarly to BL and its atypical variant.

As mentioned previously, "double hit" lymphomas are those that have a co-existent t(14;18) and *c-myc* translocation and have an extremely poor prognosis. In contrast to BL, they are most often bcl-2+ by paraffin IHC staining and typically have a MIB index <95%.

Mediastinal (Thymic) Large B-Cell Lymphoma

Definition
Primary mediastinal (thymic) large B-cell lymphoma (PMBCL) is a subtype of DLBCL arising in the mediastinum of putative B-cell origin with distinctive clinical, morphologic, immunophenotypic, and genotypic features. It tends to affect females in their third to fifth decades who present with a large mediastinal mass. Histologically, there is a diffuse infiltrate of centroblasts, immunoblasts, multilobated cells, and/or Reed-Sternberg-like cells, often associated with delicate packeting sclerosis or with coarse sclerosis. Oftentimes, the malignant cells often have a distinctive clear cytoplasm.

Typical Immunophenotype
The neoplastic cells of PMBCL typically express CD45, CD19, and CD20; however, they often lack surface Ig and light chain expression by flow cytometric analysis. They are also typically CD5– and CD10–. Due to the marked degree of fibrosis in some cases, flow cytometric analysis may not even detect an aberrant B-cell population. By paraffin IHC staining, there is generally weak CD30 expression, which may be either focal or extensive. A representative case is demonstrated in **[f12.42]**.

Differential Diagnosis

Diffuse large B-cell lymphoma
The distinction between PMBCL and DLBCL lies primarily in the distinctive clinical and morphologic features of PMBCL. However, there may be clinical and morphologic overlapping features which may make this differential diagnosis more problematic. In addition, although lack of sIg and light chain expression is typical of PMBCL, this finding is clearly not specific to this lymphoma and may be encountered in various types of mature B-cell lymphomas. In such cases, paraffin IHC staining may be helpful in defining the genotypic differences between PMBCL and DLBCL, as will be

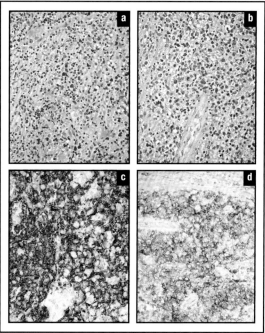

[f12.42] This case demonstrates a typical case of primary mediastinal large B-cell lymphoma (PMBCL). The patient is a 53-year-old female with a large anterior mediastinal mass (6 × 8 cms), which is biopsied. Histologic sections of the anterior mediastinal biopsy reveal a diffuse proliferation of predominantly large cells in a background with increased fibrosis **a**. In some areas, the sheets of large cells have clear, abundant cytoplasm **b**. By flow cytometric analysis, there are 16% of cells within the lymphocyte region with only 5% polyclonal B cells detected (not demonstrated). Immunostaining reveals uniform, intense positivity of the large cells with CD20 **c**. There is more variable but definite staining with CD30 **d**. The neoplastic B cells are negative for CD5, CD10, bcl-2, MUM1, CD138, and CD15. A subset of the neoplastic B cells also stains with bcl-6 (not demonstrated).

discussed in the subsection below regarding the contribution of paraffin IHC immunophenotyping. In addition, it is important to recognize PMBCL as a distinct entity, distinguishable from DLBCL, since PMBCL represents a clinically favorable subgroup of DLBCL (ie, better 5-year survival rate, 64%, than all DLBCLs after therapy, 46%) [Jaffe 2001, Savage 2003].

Classical Hodgkin lymphoma
Since the clinical presentation of classical Hodgkin lymphoma (cHL) and PMBCL may be quite similar, and PMBCL may show coarse sclerosis, the syncytial variant of nodular sclerosing cHL should be considered in the differential diagnosis. By flow cytometric analysis, cHL will not demonstrate a CD20+ aberrant population; although occasional cases of PMBCL will also not reveal an aberrant B-cell population by flow cytometric

t12.3 Immunophenotypes of Anaplastic/Plasmablastic Hematolymphoid Neoplasms

Marker	ALCL	DLBCL, Anaplastic Variant	ALK+ DLBCL (Plasmablastic Type)	Anaplastic Plasmacytoma*	Plasmablastic Lymphoma*	Primary Effusion Lymphoma
CD45 (LCA)	±	+	NR	–	–	+
CD20	–	+	–	–	–	–
T-cell markers	±	–	–	–	–	cCD3, CD7†
CD30	+	+	–	–/+	–/+	+
CD138	–	–	+	+	+	+
VS38C	–	–	+	+	+	NR
EMA	+	+	+	+	+	NR
cIg	–	+	+	+	+	–
ALK	±	–	+	–	–	–

*Plasmablastic plasmacytoma may be differentiated from plasmablastic lymphoma by the detection of EBER-ISH positivity in PBL.

†Aberrant cytoplasmic CD3 expression, CD7, and CD56 may be encountered in primary effusion lymphomas (PEL). In addition, HHV8-KSHV-associated latent nuclear protein may be detected by immunohistochemistry in PEL.

NR, not reported.

analysis, due to the marked degree of fibrosis. The distinction between these 2 entities is further and primarily discussed in the subsection below regarding the contribution of paraffin IHC immunophenotyping.

Anaplastic large cell lymphoma

The morphology and CD30 positivity in PMBCL may raise the differential diagnosis of an ALCL. By flow cytometric analysis, ALCL will not demonstrate a CD20+ aberrant population, as seen in cHL and occasionally seen in markedly fibrotic cases of PMBCL. The distinction between these 2 entities is further and primarily discussed in the subsection below regarding the contribution of paraffin IHC immunophenotyping.

Contribution of Paraffin Immunohistochemical Immunophenotyping

Paraffin IHC staining may be quite helpful in establishing a diagnosis of PMBCL. PMBCL is typically associated with a moderate to marked degree of tumoral sclerosis, often yielding too few cells for flow cytometric analysis, or a relatively low number of tumoral cells in the sample for flow cytometric analysis. In addition, by flow cytometric analysis, the malignant B cells not only are few in number but also, as mentioned above,

typically lack any sIg or light chain expression. Although the *bcl-2*, *bcl-6*, and *c-myc* genes are usually germline by paraffin IHC staining, PMBCL typically has the following immunophenotype: CD45 (LCA)+, CD20+, CD79a+, CD5–, CD10–/+ (32% of cases), CD30+ (weak-strong, focal-extensive), CD15–, ALK1–, PAX5/BSAP+, BOB.1+, Oct-2+, bcl-2+, bcl-6±, MAL protein± (70% of cases), MUM1/IR4±, and CD138–. Igs are typically negative both by IHC and ISH. As mentioned previously, thymic B cells have been proposed as the putative normal counterpart of PMBCL and is supported by the identification of MAL protein expression in 70% of PMBCL [Copie-Bergman 2002]. This study also supports the concept that a sizable fraction of PMBCL is from activated germinal center or post-germinal center cells. The demonstration of MAL protein helps distinguish this subtype of DLBCL. In addition, recent studies suggest PMBCL may be distinguished immunohistochemically from DLBCL by the co-expression of c-Rel and TRAF1, seen in 53% of PMBCLs, but in only 2% of DLBCLs [Rodig 2007]. However, the findings of bcl-6 positivity and variable CD10 positivity in this group also suggests evidence for derivation from germinal center B cells, at least in a subset of these lymphomas [Copie-Bergman 2002, de Leval 2001]. In select cases, identification of this subtype may rely on distinctive genetic features in PMBCL, including hyperdiploidy, additional chromosomal material from 9p, and REL gene amplification.

Paraffin IHC staining is thus useful in differentiating PMBCL from nodular sclerosis cHL, since CD45 (LCA) is expressed in PMBCL and negative in cHL, and CD15 is negative in PMBCL and typically expressed in cHL.

Paraffin IHC staining is also useful in differentiating PMBCL from ALCL, since PMBCL expresses CD20, weakly expresses CD30, either focally or extensively, and is ALK–, whereas ALCL is CD20–, variably expresses T-cell antigens, is extensively, strongly positive for CD30, and variably expresses ALK.

Intravascular Large B-Cell Lymphoma

Definition

Intravascular large B-cell lymphoma (also referred to as angiotropic lymphoma) is a rare subtype of extranodal DLBCL, characterized by the presence of large lymphoma cells (centroblasts or immunoblasts) only present in the lumina of small blood vessels, particularly capillaries, and often causing occlusion/thrombosis. The most common sites are the skin and central nervous system.

Typical Immunophenotype

Most cases of intravascular LBCL are of B-cell origin and typically express B-cell associated antigens (ie, CD19, CD20, CD22, CD79a) with CD5 expression in some cases [Carroll 1986, Domizio 1989, Sheibani 1986, Theaker 1986]. Rare intravascular lymphomas of T-cell origin have been reported [Theaker 1986, Sepp 1990].

Differential Diagnosis

Diffuse large B-cell lymphoma

The primary distinction of this subtype of DLBCL is its characteristic primary localization to the lumina of small blood vessels.

T-cell lymphoma

Since rare cases of intravascular lymphomas may be of T-cell origin, this distinction is based on variable expression of T-cell markers by the neoplastic cells, rather than B-cell markers, as seen most commonly in intravascular lymphomas.

Metastatic carcinoma

Since metastatic carcinoma may show vascular invasion and spread, it should be considered in the differential diagnosis of an intravascular LCL.

Contribution of paraffin immunohistochemical immunophenotyping

Paraffin IHC staining may be useful in differentiating intravascular LCL from a metastatic carcinoma, since the intravascular LBCL is CD45+, CD20+, EMA–, and cytokeratin–.

Primary Effusion Lymphoma

Definition

Primary effusion lymphoma (PEL) is a neoplasm of large B cells usually presenting as serous effusions without detectable tumor masses. By definition, there is no discrete contiguous lymphomatous mass associated with the effusion. The WHO classification states that PEL is universally associated with human herpes virus 8 (HHV-8)/Kaposi sarcoma herpes virus (KSHV), most often occurring in the setting of immunodeficiency (eg, HIV infection, post-transplantation). EBV genome is also detected in the majority of cases [Sepp 1990]. The neoplastic cells may exhibit a range of appearances, from large immunoblastic or plasmablastic cells to more anaplastic morphology. Some neoplastic cells may even resemble Reed-Sternberg cells.

Typical Immunophenotype

The neoplastic cells of PEL typically express CD45 but are negative for pan-B-cell markers (ie, CD19, CD20, and CD79a) as well as sIg, cIg, and most T-cell markers. Activation and plasma cell-related markers, such as CD30, CD38, and CD138 are usually expressed. A case of PEL is demonstrated in [f12.43], with listmode output available on the accompanying disk.

Variant Immunophenotype

Aberrant expression of cCD3, as well as CD7 and CD56, has been reported in PEL [Polski 2000, Beaty 1997].

Differential Diagnosis

Diffuse large B-cell lymphoma with high-grade features and Burkitt lymphoma

The distinction between PEL and involvement of a body fluid by a DLBCL with high-grade features or a BL primarily relies on the absence of a contiguous or other

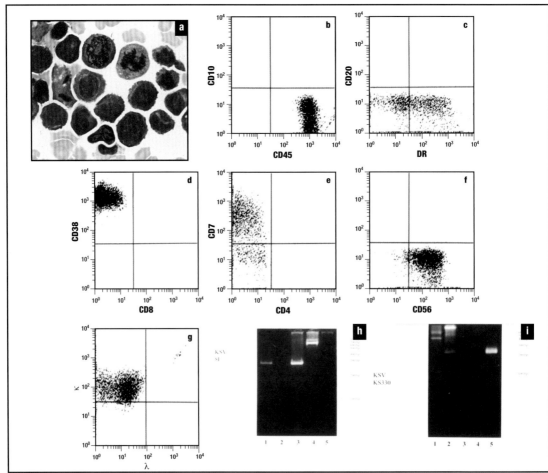

[f12.43] This case demonstrates a primary effusion lymphoma in a non-HIV patient with aberrant expression of CD7 and CD56 [Sheibani 1986]. The clinical history reveals an 80-year-old man with a history of multiple medical problems (including hypertension, ischemic heart disease, chronic obstructive pulmonary disease, peripheral vascular disease, renal insufficiency, and status-post cerebrovascular accident with a residual left-sided weakness), recently presented with progressive shortness of breath. Bilateral pleural effusions were identified. There was no peripheral lymphadenopathy or evidence of tumor by computed tomography scan. The patient underwent a thoracocenthesis; over 2 L of fluid was removed from the left pleural space. The cytomorphology of the pleural fluid reveals numerous large abnormal lymphoid-appearing cells with varying amounts of dark blue cytoplasm **a**. Shown are the following: **b-g** Gating: large cell region (high-forward scatter and low-side scatter) containing the majority of neoplastic cells. The neoplastic cells are positive for CD45 **b**, HLA-DR **c**, CD38 **d**, CD7 **e**, CD56 **f**, and selective surface κ light chain **g**. Axis Y: FITC; axis X: PE. Total indicates number of events. **h** Identification of HHV8 genome. A single band corresponding to HHV-8 in the original PCR reaction (8E primer pair; line 3: patient, line 1: positive control, line 2: master mix control, lines 4 and 5: negative control). **i** Identification of HHV8 genome. A single band corresponding to HHV-8 in the nested PCR reaction (KS330 primer pair; line 2: patient, lines 1 and 3: negative control, line 4: master mix control, line 5: positive control). The diagnosis is made of primary effusion lymphoma.

primary site of lymphomatous involvement. In addition, DLBCL with high-grade features and BL both have a mature B-cell immunophenotype with expression of surface B-cell antigens and are typically negative for CD30, CD138, and T-cell antigens.

Anaplastic large B-cell lymphoma

Due to the anaplastic features of (and expression of CD30 by) the neoplastic cells of PEL, ALCL should be considered in the differential diagnosis. However, the neoplastic cells of PEL typically express CD138 (not encountered in anaplastic CD30+ LCL) and are uniformly ALK–. Although some cases of PEL may demonstrate an aberrant rearrangement of T-cell receptor (TCR) genes, cases of PEL typically demonstrate rearranged and mutated Ig genes. ALCLs typically demonstrate a rearrangement of TCR but do not demonstrate an Ig gene rearrangement or mutation.

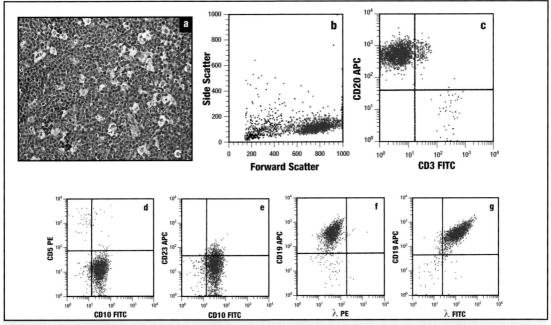

[f12.44] This case demonstrates a classical Burkitt lymphoma. The clinical history reveals an 11-year-old male who presents with a small bowel mass, which is biopsied. Histologic section of the mass reveals a monomorphic population of intermediate-sized lymphocytes associated with a starry-sky appearance in the background **a**. By flow cytometric analysis of the mass, there is an increase in cells within the intermediate-sized to large-cell lymphocyte region, characterized by relatively low side scatter and increased forward scatter **b**. These cells express CD19 **f**, CD20 **c**, CD10 **d, e**, and selective surface λ light chain **f**. There is no co-expression of CD5 **d** or CD23 **e**. The cytogenetic findings demonstrate t(8;14). Diagnosis of Burkitt lymphoma is made.

Plasmablastic lymphoma and plasmablastic plasmacytoma (see [t12.3])

Since the neoplastic cells of PEL may appear plasmablastic and express CD138, differential diagnoses should also include PBL and plasmablastic plasmacytoma. This distinction again is primarily based on sole body cavity involvement with no contiguous mass or other site of disease. In addition, although the neoplastic cells of PEL may appear plasmablastic and express CD138, they typically do not demonstrate cytoplasmic expression of Ig or light chains, as seen in PBL and plasmablastic plasmacytoma.

Contribution of Paraffin Immunohistochemical Immunophenotyping

Although PEL is a primary lymphoma arising within a body cavity as an effusion, cell blocks may be prepared for IHC staining. The nuclei of the neoplastic cells are positive for the HHV8/KSHV-associated latent protein by IHC staining [Dupin 1999]. In addition, EBER positivity by in-situ hybridization may also be demonstrated in PEL. Other lymphomas that may be included in the differential diagnosis of PEL are negative for HHV8.

Burkitt Lymphoma/Burkitt Cell Leukemia

Definition

Burkitt lymphoma (BL) is a highly aggressive lymphoma, typically composed of a monomorphic population of intermediate-sized neoplastic B cells with associated dark blue cytoplasm containing numerous cytoplasmic vacuoles (in Wright-stained preparations), numerous mitotic figures, and a starry-sky appearance in tissue sections. It is constantly associated with a translocation involving MYC, and variably associated with EBV.

Typical Immunophenotype

The neoplastic cells of BL typically express membrane IgM with light chain restriction, B-cell associated antigens (ie, CD19, CD20, and CD22), and CD10. They are typically negative for CD5, CD23 and TdT, although rare cases of CD5+ BL have been reported [Lin 1999]. A representative case of classical BL is demonstrated in **[f12.44]**, with listmode output available on the accompanying disk.

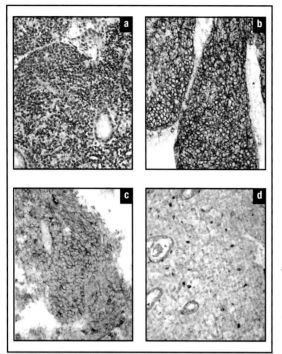

[f12.45] This case demonstrates an "atypical" variant of Burkitt lymphoma. The patient is a 57-year-old male with a large abdominal mass involving the gastric antrum and pancreas. A gastric biopsy is performed. Histologic section of the gastric antral mass reveals a diffuse proliferation of large abnormal lymphoid-appearing cells **a**. The infiltrate appears more pleomorphic than that encountered in classical Burkitt lymphoma. Immunostains reveal uniform, strong reactivity for CD20 **b**, definitive staining with CD10 **c**, uniform, strong nuclear staining with bcl-6 (not demonstrated), and no staining of the neoplastic B cells with bcl-2 **d**, MUM1, CD5, or CD138 (not demonstrated). FISH reveals a *c-myc* rearrangement.

Variants: Morphology and Immunophenotype

Morphologic variants of BL include atypical Burkitt (ie, Burkitt-like) and BL with plasmacytoid differentiation. The atypical Burkitt variant is characterized by a more pleomorphic population of neoplastic cells than classical BL. Like classical BL, this variant shows a high proliferative index, and it is reserved for cases with a proven or strong presumptive evidence of a *c-myc* translocation. A representative case is demonstrated in [f12.45]. The variant of BL with plasmacytoid differentiation is characterized by some neoplastic cells demonstrating eccentric basophilic cytoplasm with a single, prominent nucleolus and associated with monoclonal intracytoplasmic Ig.

Differential Diagnosis

Diffuse large B-cell lymphoma and plasmablastic lymphoma

Diffuse large B-cell lymphoma with high-grade features may be difficult to distinguish from BL, particularly the atypical Burkitt variant. This differential diagnosis has been discussed in detail in the section above regarding DLBCL. A representative case of DLBCL with c-myc rearrangement is demonstrated in [f12.46]. Plasmablastic lymphoma should also be considered in the differential diagnosis of BL with plasmacytoid differentiation. However, in this variant of BL, only some cells typically show plasmacytoid differentiation.

"Double hit" lymphomas

"Double hit" lymphomas are DLBCLs with high-grade features and a co-existent t(14;18) and *c-myc* rearrangement. A representative case is demonstrated in [f12.46]. They have also been discussed in the differential diagnosis of BL in the section above regarding DLBCL.

Blastoid variants of mantle cell lymphoma and CD5+ de-novo DBLCL

Rare cases of CD5+ BL may cause diagnostic confusion with blastoid variants of mantle cell lymphoma and CD5+ de-novo DLBLC, since all of these entities are CD23–. However, CD5+ BL is associated with a *c-myc* translocation and blastoid variants of MCL are associated with the t(11;14).

Precursor B- and T-cell lymphoblastic lymphoma/ leukemia

Precursor B- and T-cell lymphoblastic lymphoma/leukemia are also high-grade lymphoid neoplasms that must be distinguished from BL. By flow cytometric analysis, they do not typically express surface Ig or light chains, but they do express TdT, in contrast to BL. In addition, a proportion of these precursor neoplasms express CD34, whereas the neoplastic cells of BL are uniformly CD34–. The neoplastic cells of BL generally demonstrate stronger CD45 and CD20 expression than precursor B-cell neoplasms. It is also important to recognize there may be occasional cases of precursor B-lymphoblastic leukemia with a mature immunophenotype (ie, with surface light chain expression) associated with L1 or L2 morphology and no evidence of a chromosomal translocation involving the *c-myc* gene [f11.3]. Such cases should not be considered Burkitt leukemia/lymphoma but rather treated as

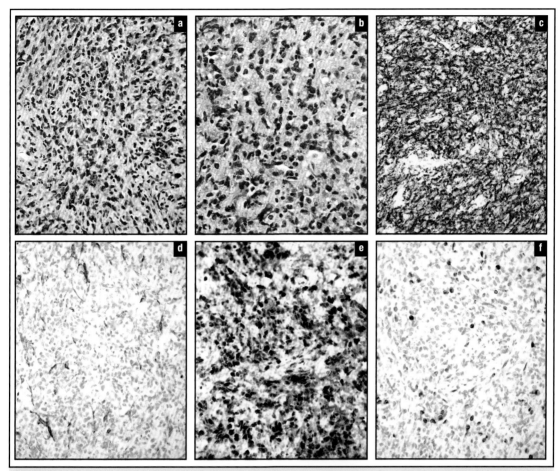

[f12.46] This case demonstrates a diffuse large B-cell lymphoma with a *c-myc* rearrangement. The patient is a 48-year-old female presenting with nausea, vomiting, and pelvic pain. A pelvic mass is detected, obstructing bilateral ureters, and is biopsied. Histologic sections of the pelvic mass reveal a diffuse proliferation of large, pleomorphic lymphoid-appearing cells associated with crush artifact **a**, **b**. Immunostains reveal uniform strong reactivity for CD20 **c** and bcl-6 **e**. The neoplastic B-cells are negative for CD5 (not demonstrated), CD10 **d**, MUM1 and CD138 (not demonstrated), as well as bcl-2 **f**. FISH reveals a *c-myc* rearrangement.

precursor B-lymphoblastic leukemia [Vasef 1998, Li 2003]. Precursor T-cell neoplasms will have variable expression of T-cell antigens depending on their stage of maturation (ie, CD1a, CD2, cCD3, sCD3, CD4, CD5, CD7, and CD8).

Contribution of Paraffin Immunohistochemical Immunophenotyping

Since BL is a malignant lymphoma of GC-cell origin, bcl-6 positivity may be demonstrated by IHC staining. In addition, bcl-2 is negative by IHC staining in BL and may be helpful diagnostically. Ki-67, or the MIB index, may also be evaluated by IHC staining. As discussed previously, the MIB-1 index should be >98% and not <95% in BL. In contrast, the MIB-1 index in DLBCL with *c-myc* rearrangement is typically <95%. However, atypical variants of BL may have a MIB index <95%, and DLBCLs with a *c-myc* rearrangement or amplification may have a MIB index >95%. In addition, DLBCLs with a *c-myc* rearrangement or amplification have a poor prognosis and should be treated similarly to BL and its atypical variant. Lastly, as mentioned previously, "double hit" lymphomas are those that have a co-existent t(14;18) and *c-myc* translocation and have an extremely poor prognosis **[f12.47]**. In contrast to BL, they are most often bcl-2+ by paraffin IHC staining and typically have a MIB index <95%.

Primary Cutaneous Marginal Zone B-Cell Lymphoma

Definition

Primary cutaneous marginal zone B-cell lymphoma (PCMZL) is an indolent lymphoma with a nodular to diffuse growth pattern composed of small B cells including marginal zone (centrocyte-like) cells, lymphoplasmacytoid cells, and plasma cells admixed with small numbers of centroblast- or immunoblast-like cells and many reactive T cells. Reactive germinal centers are frequently observed and may be surrounded by a population of small to medium-sized cells with irregular nuclei, inconspicuous nucleoli, and abundant pale cytoplasm (marginal zone B-cells). PCMZLs rarely show transformation into a diffuse large B-cell lymphoma, but a relative increase in large transformed cells may be seen in some cases. This category includes cases previously designated as primary cutaneous immunocytoma and cases of cutaneous follicular lymphoid hyperplasia with monotypic plasma cells [Rijlaarsdam 1993, Schmid 1995]. Exceptional cases of primary cutaneous plasmacytoma without an underlying plasma cell dyscrasia show considerable overlap with PCMZL, and such cases are included in this category [Torne 1990]. PCMZL is considered part of the broad group of MALT lymphomas, as discussed previously.

Typical Immunophenotype

The immunophenotype of PCMZL is similar to that discussed previously in the section entitled, "Extranodal Marginal Zone B-Cell Lymphoma of MALT Type." The neoplastic cells are negative for CD5 in all cases of PCMZL described. Monotypic plasma cells are often located at the periphery of the infiltrates and in the superficial dermis beneath the epidermis [Rijlaarsdam 1993, Schmid 1995, Cerroni 1997, Bailey 1996]. Immunoglobulin heavy chains (IgH) are clonally rearranged. Recent studies suggest the presence of the t(14;18)(q32;q21) involving the IGH gene on chromosome 14 and the MLT gene on chromosome 18 in a proportion of PCMZL [Streubel 2003]. However, other translocations observed in gastric MALT lymphomas, such as t(11;18)(q21;q21) and t(1;14)(p22;q32) have not been found in PCMZL [Hallermann 2004, Ye 2003, Gronbaek 2003].

Differential Diagnosis

The primary differential diagnoses of PCMZL include systemic involvement by MZL, small lymphocytic lymphoma (SLL), mantle cell lymphoma (MCL) or follicular lymphoma (FL), and primary cutaneous follicle center lymphoma (PCFCL). These other subtypes (excluding PCFCL) have been discussed previously in the appropriate sections. PCFCL is discussed in the next section, and this differential diagnosis will be addressed in that section as well.

Comparison of FCI to Immunophenotyping by Paraffin Immunohistochemistry

FCI allows for the detection of monoclonal small B cells in PCMZL, whereas paraffin IHC staining allows for the detection of monoclonal plasma cells and the presence of bcl-2 protein in the neoplastic cells.

Primary Cutaneous Follicle Center Lymphoma

Definition

Primary cutaneous follicle center lymphoma (PCFCL) is defined as a tumor of neoplastic follicle center cells, usually a mixture of centrocytes (small and large cleaved follicle center cells) and variable numbers of centroblasts (large non-cleaved follicle center cells with prominent nucleoli). Large centrocytes, often multilobated, are a common feature of PCFCL. In addition, the large neoplastic B cells may have a fibroblast-like appearance. This lymphoma may demonstrate a follicular, a follicular and diffuse, or a diffuse growth pattern and almost always spares the epidermis. Small and early lesions contain a mixture of centrocytes, relatively few centroblasts, and many reactive T cells, and they may demonstrate follicular growth pattern or, more often, remnants of a follicular growth pattern. The follicles are ill-defined, lack tangible-body macrophages, and generally have reduced or absent mantle zones [Cerroni 2000, Goodlad 2002]. with progression to tumorous lesions, the neoplastic B cells increase both in number and size, whereas the number of reactive T cells steadily decreases [Santucci 1991, Willemze 1987]. Tumorous skin lesions generally show a monotonous population of large follicle center cells, generally large centrocytes and multilobated cells, and, in rare cases, spindle-shaped cells with a variable admixture of centroblasts and immunoblasts [Santucci 1991, Willemze 1987, Berti 1988, Grange 2001, Cerroni 2000]. However, it should be noted that lymphomas with a diffuse growth pattern and a monotonous proliferation of centroblasts and immunoblasts are excluded and, if primary to the skin, are classified as primary cutaneous large B-cell lymphoma (PCLBCL), discussed in the corresponding section below.

Typical Immunophenotype

The neoplastic cells express the B-cell associated antigens (ie, CD19, CD20, and CD79a), are bcl-6+, generally show monotypic sIg, and are negative for CD5, CD43, and MUM1 [Goodlad 2002, de Leval 2001, Hoefnagel 2003, Hoefnagel 2005]. Absence of detectable sIg is frequent in tumorous lesions showing a diffuse population of large follicle center cells. CD10 expression is frequently observed in cases with a follicular growth pattern but is uncommon in PCFCL with a diffuse growth pattern [Hoefnagel 2003, Hoefnagel 2005, Kim 2003]. Of interest, unlike nodal and secondary cutaneous follicular lymphomas, PCFCL does not express bcl-2 protein or only show faint bcl-2 staining in a minority of neoplastic B cells [Cerroni 2000, Cerroni 1994, Geelen 1998]. In most studies, PCFCL (including cases with a follicular growth pattern) does not show the t(14;18), which is characteristically found in systemic follicular lymphomas and a proportion of systemic diffuse large B-cell lymphomas [Goodlad 2002, Kim 2003, Child 2001]. 201-201 PCFCL has the gene expression profile of germinal center-like large B-cell lymphomas [Hoefnagel 2005]. Although recent studies report the presence of t(14;18) and/or bcl-2 expression in a significant minority of PCFCL, there are no differences in clinical presentation and behavior between bcl-2 and/or t(14;18) positive and negative cases [Cerroni 2000, Kim 2003, Cerroni 1994, Goodlad 2003, Aguilera 2001, Mirza 2002, Bergman 2001]. On the other hand, recent studies suggest that expression of bcl-2 protein by >50% of the neoplastic B cells in PCFCL with a diffuse proliferation of large centrocytes (observed in approximately 15% of cases) is associated with a more unfavorable prognosis [Grange 2004]. Further studies are warranted to define the clinical and biological significance of bcl-2 expression and/or the presence of t(14;18) observed in some cases of PCFCL. Nevertheless, demonstration of bcl-2 expression and/or t(14;18) should always raise the suspicion of systemic involvement by a lymphoma, secondarily involving the skin.

Differential Diagnosis

The primary differential diagnosis of PCFCL includes systemic involvement by FL or DLBCL, or primary cutaneous involvement by DLBCL (PCLBCL) or MZL (PCMZL). PCFCL is usually distinguished from systemic FL by the exclusion of a primary FL at a non-cutaneous site, as well as by bcl-2 negativity and the absence of the t(14;18) in PCFCL. This issue has been discussed above in the immunophenotypic features of PCFCL. As also mentioned previously, lymphomas with a diffuse growth pattern and a monotonous proliferation of centroblasts and immunoblasts are excluded from being classified as PCFCL. If primary to the skin, they are best classified as primary cutaneous diffuse large B-cell lymphoma (PCLBCL). These will be discussed in the sections to follow below. PCFCL may be distinguished from PCMZL by the presence of CD10 and bcl-6 in PCFCL; these are both negative in the neoplastic cells of PCMZL.

Comparison of FCI to Immunophenotyping by Paraffin Immunohistochemistry

FCI allows for the detection of monoclonal B cells with co-expression of CD10 (in those with a follicular growth pattern). Paraffin IHC staining allows for the detection of bcl-6 protein in the neoplastic cells and generally shows negativity for bcl-2 protein and MUM1.

Primary Cutaneous Diffuse Large B-Cell Lymphoma, Leg Type

Definition

PCLBCL characteristically presents with skin lesions on the (lower) legs. Histologically, there are diffuse infiltrates, which often extend into the subcutaneous tissue. These infiltrates generally show a monotonous, predominant population or confluent sheets of centroblasts and immunoblasts [Grange 2001, Vermeer 1996]. Mitotic figures are frequently observed. Small B cells are lacking and reactive T cells are relatively few, often confined to perivascular areas. Uncommonly, skin lesions with a similar morphology and phenotype can arise at sites other than the legs.

Typical Immunophenotype

The neoplastic B cells express B-cell associated antigens (ie, CD19, CD20, CD79a), show monotypic sIg and/or cIg, show strong bcl-2 protein expression, usually express bcl-6 and MUM-1, and are generally CD10- [Hoefnagel 2003, Hoefnagel 2005, Paulli 2002]. The t(14;18) is not found in PCLBCL. Chromosomal imbalances have been identified in up to 85% of PCLBCL, with gains in 18q and 7p and loss of 6q as the most common findings [Hallermann 2004, Mao 2002].

Differential Diagnosis

The primary diagnostic considerations in the differential diagnosis of PCLBCL-leg type include systemic LBCL,

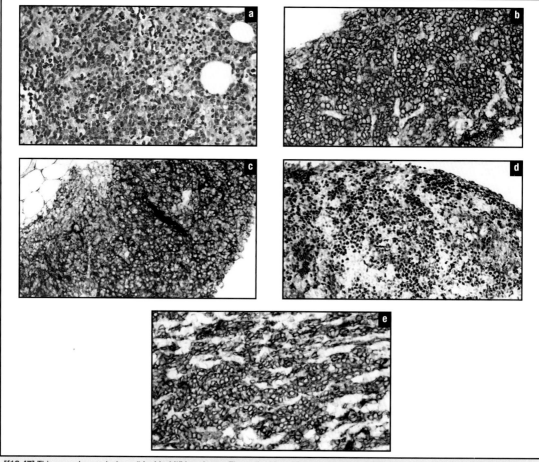

[f12.47] This case demonstrates a "double-hit" lymphoma. The patient is a 63-year-old male with a right pelvic mass, which is biopsied. Histologic section of the pelvic mass reveals a diffuse proliferation of intermediate to large lymphoid appearing cells with numerous apoptotic cells **a**. Immunostains reveal uniform, strong reactivity with CD20 **b**, CD10 **c**, bcl-6 **d**, and bcl-2 **e**. They are negative for MUM1, CD5, and CD138 (not demonstrated). FISH studies reveal both a t(14;18) and a *c-myc* rearrangement.

PCFCL with a diffuse infiltration of large centrocytes, and PCLBCL, other (discussed in the next section). Systemic LBCL predominantly relies on a primary diagnosis of LBCL at a non-cutaneous site. Unlike PCLBCL-leg type, PCFCL with a diffuse infiltration of large centrocytes is generally bcl-2–. In addition, recent studies have demonstrated translocations involving myc, bcl-6 and IgH genes in 11 of 14 PCLBCL-leg, but not in patients with PCFCL with a diffuse infiltration of large centrocytes [Hallermann 2004]. PCLBCL-leg type may be distinguished from PCLBCL, other (as described below) based on the activated germinal center immunophenotype in PCLBCL-leg type. It is important to recognize PCLBCL-leg type since it has an inferior prognosis compared to PCLBCL presenting at other sites [Grange 2001].

Comparison of FCI to Immunophenotyping by Paraffin Immunohistochemistry

FCI aids in detecting a monoclonal B-cell population and demonstrates absence for CD10. IHC staining is useful in demonstrating strong bcl-2 protein expression in the neoplastic cells and in usually demonstrating bcl-6 and MUM1 expressions: typical of an activated germinal center cell immunophenotype.

Primary Cutaneous Diffuse Large B-Cell Lymphoma, Other

The term PCLBCL, other, refers to rare cases of large B-cell lymphomas arising in the skin, which do not belong to the group of PCLBCL, leg type, or the group of PCFCL. These cases include morphological variants of DLBCL already discussed, such as anaplastic or plasmablastic subtypes or T-cell/histiocyte-rich large B-cell lymphomas. PCLBCL, other, excludes cases representing a skin manifestation of a systemic lymphoma. The same immunophenotypic features apply as previously discussed, but unlike their nodal counterparts, they appear to have an excellent prognosis [Sander 1996, Li 2001]. In addition, rare cases of primary cutaneous intravascular large B-cell lymphoma may be included in the category PCLBCL, other. The same immunophenotypic features again apply. Patients presenting with only skin lesions in intravascular large B-cell lymphoma appear to have a significantly better survival than patients with other clinical presentations (3-year overall survival 56% vs 22%) [Ferreri 2004].

Evaluating for Relapse, Composite Lymphomas, and Bone Marrow Staging

Flow cytometric immunophenotyping is not only useful in subtyping the various subtypes of mature B-cell neoplasms, as discussed in detail already in this chapter, but is also useful for detecting a mature B-cell neoplasm when co-existent with a classical Hodgkin lymphoma or T-cell NHL (ie, composite lymphoma) or AML, in evaluating sites for relapse, and in staging BM specimens for lymphomatous involvement. One should keep in mind that after therapy, mature B-cell neoplasms may lose light chain expression or lose marker expression (ie, CD10 may not be expressed in cases of relapsed follicular lymphoma). In addition, when treated with rituximab, B-cell lymphomas will often lack CD20 expression, and thus additional B-cell markers by flow cytometry (eg, CD19) or by IHC staining (ie, PAX-5) may be required to evaluate for lymphomatous involvement.

In a large retrospective study, evaluating the contribution of flow cytometric analysis to staging of bone marrow specimens for B-cell malignant neoplasms, 81% of cases showed complete concordance between the morphologic and FCI findings. In 11% of cases, the morphologic examination alone detected involvement and in 5% of cases, the FCI data detected involvement in a morphologically negative or "suggestive" bone marrow core. Combining these modalities is considered essential to evaluating bone marrow specimens for involvement by B-cell malignant neoplasms [Dunphy 1998].

References

Abou-Elella A, Shafer MT, Wan XY, et al [2000] Lymphomas with follicular and monocytoid B-cell components: Evidence for a common clonal origin from follicle center cells. *Am J Clin Pathol* 114:516-522.

Adam P, Katzenberger T, Seeberger H, et al [2003] A case of a diffuse large B-cell lymphoma of plasmablastic type associated with the t(2;5)(p23;q35) chromosome translocation. *Am J Surg Pathol* 27:1473-1476.

Aguilera NS, Tomaszewski MM, Moad JC, Bauer FA, Taubenberger JK, Abbondanzo SL [2001] Cutaneous follicle center lymphoma: A clinicopathologic study of 19 cases. *Mod Pathol* 14:828-835.

Al-Marzooq YM, Chopra R, Younis M, Al-Mulhim AS, Al-Mommatten MI, Al-Omran SH [2004] Thyroid low-grade B-cell lymphoma (MALT type) with extreme plasmacytic differentiation: Report of a case diagnosed by fine-needle aspiration and flow cytometric study. *Diagn Cytopathol* 31:52-56.

Andersen CL, Gruszka-Westwood A, Ostergaard M, et al [2004] A narrow deletion of 7q is common to HCL, and SMZL, but not CLL. *Eur J Haematol* 72:390-402.

Bailey EM, Ferry JA, Harris NL, Mihm MC, Jacobson JO, Duncan LM [1996] Marginal zone lymphoma (low-grade B-cell lymphoma of mucosa-associated lymphoid tissue type) of skin and subcutaneous tissue: A study of 15 patients. *Am J Surg Pathol* 20:1011-1023.

Barry TS, Jaffe ES, Kingma DW, et al [2002] CD5+ follicular lymphoma: A clinicopathologic study of three cases. *Am J Clin Pathol* 118:589-598.

Basso K, Liso A, Tiacci E, et al [2004] Gene expression profiling of hairy cell leukemia reveals a phenotype related to memory B cells with altered expression of chemokine and adhesion receptors. *J Exp Med* 199:59-68.

Beaty MW, Kumar S, Sorbara L, Miller K, Raffeld M, Jaffe ES [1997] A biophenotypic human herpesvirus 8-associated primary bowel lymphoma. *Am J Surg Pathol* 21:719-724.

Begueret H, Vergier B, Parrens M, et al [2002] Primary lung small B-cell lymphoma vs lymphoid hyperplasia: Evaluation of diagnostic criteria in 26 cases. *Am J Surg Pathol* 26:76-81.

Belaud-Rotureau MA, Parrens M, Dubus P, Garroste JC, de Mascarel A, Merlio JP [2002] A comparative analysis of FISH, RT-PCR, PCR, and immunohistochemistry for the diagnosis of mantle cell lymphomas. *Mod Pathol* 15:517-525.

Bergman R, Kurtin PJ, Gibson LE, Hull PR, Kimlinger TK, Schroeter AL [2001] Clinicopathologic, immunophenotypic, and molecular characterization of primary cutaneous follicular B-cell lymphoma. *Arch Dermatol* 137:432-439.

Berti E, Alessi E, Caputo R, Gianotti R, Delia D, Vezzoni P [1988] Reticulohistiocytoma of the dorsum. *J Am Acad Dermatol* 19:259-272.

Bilalovic N, Blystad AK, Golouh R, et al [2004] Expression of bcl-6 and CD10 protein is associated with longer overall survival and time to treatment failure in follicular lymphoma. *Am J Clin Pathol* 121:34-42.

Braaten KM, Betensky RA, de Leval L [2003] Bcl-6 expression predicts improved survival in patients with primary central nervous system lymphoma. *Clin Cancer Research* 9:1063-1069.

Butmarc JR, Kourea HP, Levi E, Kadin ME [1998] Improved detection of CD5 epitope in formalin-fixed paraffin-embedded sections of benign and neoplastic lymphoid tissues by using biotinylated tyramine enhancement after antigen retrieval. *Am J Clin Pathol* 109:682-688.

Callet-Bauchu E, Baseggio L, Felman P, et al [2005] Cytogenetic analysis delineates a spectrum of chromosomal changes that can distinguish non-MALT marginal zone B-cell lymphomas among mature B-cell entities: A description of 103 cases. *Leukemia* 19:1818-1823.

Carbone A, Gloghini A, Aldinucci D, Gattel V, Dalla-Favera R, Gaidano G [2002] Expression pattern of MUM1/IRF4 in the spectrum of pathology of Hodgkin's disease. *Br J Haematol* 117:336-372.

Carroll TJ, Schelper RL, Goeken JA, Kemp JD [1986] Neoplastic angioendotheliomatosis: Immunopathologic and morphologic evidence for intravascular malignant lymphomatosis. *Am J Clin Pathol* 10:169-175.

Cerroni L, Volkenandt M, Rieger E, Soyer HP, Kerl H [1994] Bcl-2 protein expression and correlation with the interchromosomal (14;18) translocation in cutaneous lymphomas and pseudolymphomas. *J Invest Dermatol* 102:231-235.

Cerroni L, Signoretti S, Höfler G, et al [1997] Primary cutaneous marginal zone B-cell lymphoma: A recently described entity of low-grade malignant cutaneous B-cell lymphoma. *Am J Surg Pathol* 21:1307-1315.

Cerroni L, Arzberger E, Pütz B, et al [2000] Primary cutaneous follicular center cell lymphoma with follicular growth pattern. *Blood* 95:3922-3928.

Cerroni L, El-Shabrawi-Caelen L, Pink-Fuches R, LeBoit PE, Kerl H [2000] Cutaneous spindle-cell lymphoma: A morphologic variant of cutaneous large B-cell lymphoma. *Am J Dermato Pathol* 22: 299-309

Chang C, Liu Y, Cleveland RP, Perkins SL [2000] Expression of *c-Myc* and p53 correlates with clinical outcome in diffuse large B-cell lymphomas. *Am J Clin Pathol* 113:512-518.

Chang CC, Cleveland RP, Perkins SL [2002] CD10 expression and survival. *Am J Clin Pathol* 117:660-661.

Chang CC, Kampalath B, Schultz C, et al [2003] Expression of p53, c-Myc, or Bcl-6 suggests a poor prognosis in primary central nervous system diffuse large B-cell lymphoma among immunocompetent individuals. *Arch Pathol Lab Med* 127:208-212.

Chang CC, McClintock S, Cleveland RP, et al [2004] Immunohistochemical expression patterns of germinal center and activation B-cell markers correlate with prognosis in diffuse large B-cell lymphoma. *Am J Surg Pathol* 28:464-470.

Chang H, Bartlett E, Patterson B, et al [2005] The absence of CD56 on malignant plasma cells in the cerebrospinal fluid is the hallmark of multiple myeloma involving central nervous system. *Br J Haematol* 129:539-541.

Chang H, Cerny J [2006] Molecular characterization of chronic lymphocytic leukemia with two distinct cell populations. *Am J Clin Pathol* 126:23-28.

Chen HI, Akpolat I, Mody DR, et al [2006] Restricted κ/λ light chain ration by flow cytometry in germinal center B cells in Hashimoto thyroiditis. *Am J Clin Pathol* 125:42-48.

Chen X, Jensen PE, Li S [2003] HLA-DO. A useful marker to distinguish florid follicular hyperplasia from follicular lymphoma by flow cytometry. *Am J Clin Pathol* 119:842-851.

Chen YH, Tallman MS, Goolsby C, Peterson L [2006] Immunophenotypic variations in hairy cell leukemia. *Am J Clin Pathol* 125:251-259.

Chen YH, Peterson LC, Dittmann D, et al [2007] Comparative analysis of flow cytometric techniques in assessment of ZAP-70 expression in relation to IgVH mutational status in chronic lymphocytic leukemia. *Am J Clin Pathol* 127:182-191.

Chikatsu N, Kojima H, Suzukawa K, et al [2003] ALK+, CD30−, CD20− large B-cell lymphoma containing anaplastic lymphoma kinase (ALK) fused to clathrin heavy chain gene (CLTC). *Mod Pathol* 16:828-832.

Child FJ, Russell-Jones R, Woolford AJ, et al [2001] Absence of the t(14;18) chromosomal translocation in primary cutaneous B-cell lymphoma. *Br J Dermatol* 144:735-744.

Cocco AE, Osei ES, Thut DM, et al [2005] Bimodal cell populations are common in chronic lymphocytic leukemia but do not impact overall survival. *Am J Clin Pathol* 123:818-825.

Cook JR, Craig FE, Swerdlow SH [2003] Bcl-2 expression by multicolor flow cytometric analysis assists in the diagnosis of follicular lymphoma in lymph node and bone marrow. *Am J Clin Pathol* 119:145-151.

Copie-Bergman C, Plonquet A, Alonso MA, et al [2002] MAL expression in lymphoid cells: Further evidence for MAL as a distinct molecular marker of primary mediastinal large B-cell lymphomas. *Mod Pathol* 15:1172-1180.

Crespo M, Bosch F, Villamor N, Bellosilla B, et al [2003] ZAP-70 expression as a surrogate for immunoglobulin-variable-region mutations in chronic lymphocytic leukemia. *N Engl J Med* 348:1767-1775.

Criel A, Michaux L, Wolf-Peeters C [1999] The concept of typical and atypical chronic lymphocytic leukaemia. *Leuk Lymphoma* 33:33-45.

Cullinan P. Sperling AI, Burkhardt JK [2002] The distal pole complex: A novel membrane domain distal to the immunological synapse. *Immunol Rev* 189:111-122.

Davis GG, York JC, Glick AD, McCurley TL, Collins RD, Cousar JB [1992] Plasmacytic differentiation in parafollicular (monocytoid) B-cell lymphoma. A study of 12 cases. *Am J Surg Pathol* 16:1066-1074.

de Leval L, Harris NL, Longtine J, Ferry JA, Duncan LM [2001] Cutaneous B-cell lymphomas of follicular and marginal zone types. Use of Bcl-6, CD10, Bcl-2, and CD21 in differential diagnosis and classification. *Am J Surg Pathol* 25:732-741.

de Leval L, Ferry JA, Falini B, Shipp M, Harris NL [2001] Expression of bcl-6 and CD10 in primary mediastinal large B-cell lymphoma: Evidence for derivation from germinal center B-cells. *Am J Surg Pathol* 25:1277-1282.

Del Poeta G, Maurillo L, Venditti A, et al [2001] Clinical significance of CD38 expression in chronic lymphocytic leukemia. *Blood* 98:2633-2639.

del Senno L, Gandini D, Gambari R, Lanza F, Tomasi P, Castoldi G [1987] Monoclonal origin of B cells producing κ, lambda and κ lambda immunoglobulin light chains in a patient with chronic lymphocytic leukemia. *Leuk Res* 11:1093-1098.

Delgado J, Matutes E, Morilla AM, et al [2003] Diagnostic significance of CD20 and FMC7 expression in B-cell disorders. *Am J Clin Pathol* 120:754-759.

Domizio P, Hall PA, Cotter F, et al [1989] Angiotropic large cell lymphoma (ALCL): Morphological, immunohistochemical, and genotypic studies with analysis of previous reports. *Hematol Oncol* 7:195-206.

Dong HY, Gorczyca W, Liu Z, et al [2003] B-cell lymphomas with coexpression of CD5 and CD10. *Am J Clin Pathol* 119:218-230.

Dunphy CH, Petruska PJ, Janney C, et al [1995] Plasma cell leukemia presenting with striking number of circulating cells. *Cell Vision* 2:214-217.

Dunphy CH, Galindo LM, Velasquez WS [1996] Multiple myeloma with monoclonal surface immunoglobulin expression: A case report. *Acta Cytol* 40:358-362.

Dunphy CH, Wheaton SE, Perkins SL [1997] CD23 expression in transformed small lymphocytic lymphomas/chronic lymphocytic leukemias and blastic transformations of mantle cell lymphoma. *Mod Pathol* 10:818-822.

Dunphy CH, Lattuada LP Jr [1998] Follicular center cell lymphoma with an extremely high content of T cells: Case report with useful diagnostic techniques. *Arch Pathol Lab Med* 122:936-938.

Dunphy CH, Wolaniuk JW, Turgeon RP [1998] Flow cytometric findings in the floral variant of follicular lymphoma. *J Clin Lab Anal* 12:310-314.

Dunphy CH [1998] Combining morphology and flow cytometric immunophenotyping to evaluate bone marrow specimens for B-cell malignant neoplasms. *Am J Clin Pathol* 109:625-630.

Dunphy CH, Oza YU, Skelly ME [1999] An otherwise typical case of non-Japanese hairy cell leukemia with CD10 and CDw75 expression: Response to cladaribine phosphate therapy. *J of Clin Lab Anal* 13:141-144.

Dunphy CH, Perkins SL [2001] Large cell variants of CD5+, CD23- B-cell lymphoma/leukemia. *Arch Pathol Lab Med* 125:513-518.

Dunphy CH, Perkins SL [2001] Mantle cell leukemia, prolymphocytoid type: A rarely described form. *Leuk Lymphoma* 41:683-687.

Dunphy CH; Nies MK, Gabriel DA [2007] Correlation of plasma cell percentages by CD138 immunohistochemistry, cyclin D1 status, and CD56 expression with clinical parameters and overall survival in plasma cell myeloma. *Appl Immunohistochem Mol Morphol* 15:248-254.

Dunphy CH, Tang W [2008] Usefulness of routine conventional cytogenetic analysis in tissues submitted or "lymphoma work-up." *Leuk Lymphoma* 49:75-80.

Dunphy CH [2008] Reaction patterns of TRAP and DBA.44 in hairy cell leukemia, hairy cell variant, and nodal and extranodal marginal zone B-cell lymphomas. *Appl Immunohistochem Mol Morphol* 2008 Jan 25 [Epub ahead of print].

Dupin N, Fisher C, Kellam P, et al [1999] Distribution of human herpesvirus-B latently infected cells in Kaposi's sarcoma, multicentric Castleman's disease, and primary effusion lymphoma. *Proc Natl Acad Sci USA* 96:4546-4551.

Ely SA, Knowles DM [2002] Expression of CD56/neural cell adhesion molecule correlates with the presence of lytic bone lesions in multiple myeloma and distinguishes myeloma from monoclonal gammopathy of undetermined significance and lymphomas with plasmacytoid differentiation. *Am J Pathol* 160:1293–1299.

Evans HL, Polski JM, Deshpande V, Dunphy CH [2000] CD5+ true SLL/CLL with plasmacytic differentiation and an unusual 1p36 translocation: Case report and review of the literature. *Leuk Lymphoma* 39:625-632.

Falini B, Tiacci E, Liso A, et al [2004] Simple diagnostic assay for hairy cell leukaemia by immunocytochemical detection of annexin 1 (ANXA1). *Lancet* 363:2194.

Fan Z, Natkunam Y, Bair E, Tibshirani R, Warnke RA [2003] Characterization of variant patterns of nodular lymphocyte predominant Hodgkin lymphoma with immunohistologic and clinical correlation. *Am J Surg Pathol* 27:1346-1356.

Farinha P, Sehn L, Skinnider B, Connors JM, Gascoyne RD [2006] Addition of rituximab to CHOP improves survival in the non-GCB subtype of diffuse large B-cell lymphoma. *Blood* 108:275-282.

Farokhzad OC, Teodoridis JM, Park H, et al [2000] CD43 gene expression is mediated by a nuclear factor which binds pyrimidine-rich single strand DNA. *Nuclei Acids Res* 28:2256-2267.

Ferreri AJM, Campo E, Seymour JF, et al [2004] Intravascular lymphoma: Clinical presentation, natural history, management and prognostic factors in a series of 38 cases with special emphasis on the "cutaneous variant." *Br J Haematol* 127:173-183.

Ferry JA, Yang W-I, Zukerberg LR, Wotherspoon AC, Arnold A, Harris NL [1996] CD5+ extranodal marginal zone B-cell (MALT) lymphoma. A low grade neoplasm with a propensity for bone marrow involvement and relapse. *Am J Clin Pathol* 105:31-37.

Folk GS, Abbondanzo SL, Childers EL, Foss RD [2006] Plasmablastic lymphoma: A clinicopathologic correlation. *Ann Diagn Pathol* 10:8-12.

Fonseca R, Blood EA, Oken MM, et al [2002] Myeloma and the t(11;14)(q13;q32); Evidence for a biologically defined unique subset of patients. *Blood* 99:3735-3741.

Fonseca R, Barlogie B, Bataille R, et al [2004] Genetics and cytogenetics of multiple myeloma: A workshop report. *Cancer Res* 64:1546-1558.

Frater JL, McCarron KF, Hammel JP, et al [2001] Typical and atypical chronic lymphocytic leukemia differ clinically and immunophenotypically. *Am J Clin Pathol* 116:655-664.

Frizzera G, Anaya JS, Banks PM [1986] Neoplastic plasma cells in follicular lymphomas. Clinical and pathologic findings in six cases. *Virchows Arch A Pathol Anat Histopathol* 409:149-162.

Garand R, Avet-Loiseau H, Accard F, Moreau P, Harousseau JL, Bataille R [2003] t(11;14) and t(4;14) translocations correlated with mature lymphoplasmacytoid and immature morphology, respectively, in multiple myeloma. *Leukemia* 17:2032-2035.

Geelen FAMJ, Vermeer MH, Meijer CJLM, et al [1998] Bcl-2 expression in primary cutaneous large B-cell lymphoma is site-related. *J Clin Oncol* 16:2080-2085.

Gong JZ, Lagoo AS, Peters D, et al [2001] Value of CD23 determination by flow cytometry in differentiating mantle cell lymphoma from chronic lymphocytic leukemia/small lymphocytic lymphoma. *Am J Clin Pathol* 116:893-897.

Goodlad JR, Krajewski AS, Batstone PJ, et al [2002] Primary cutaneous follicular lymphoma. A clinicopathologic and molecular study of 16 cases in support of a distinct entity. *Am J Surg Pathol* 26:733-741.

Goodlad JR, Krajewski AS, Batstone PJ, et al [2003] Primary cutaneous diffuse large B-cell lymphoma: Prognostic significance and clinicopathologic subtypes. *Am J Surg Pathol* 27:1538-1545.

Grange F, Bekkenk MW, Wechsler J, et al [2001] Prognostic factors in primary cutaneous large B-cell lymphomas: A European multicenter study. *J Clin Oncol* 19:3602-3610.

Grange F, Petrella T, Beylot-Barry M, et al [2004] Bcl-2 protein expression is the strongest independent prognostic factor of survival in primary cutaneous large B-cell lymphomas. *Blood* 103:3662-3668.

Gronbaek K, Ralfkiaer E, Kalla J, Skovgaard GL, Guldberg P [2003] Infrequent somatic Fas mutations but no evidence of Bcl-10 mutations or t(11;18) in primary cutaneous MALT-type lymphoma. *J Pathol* 201:134-140.

Gupta D, Lim MS, Medeiros LJ, Elenitoba-Johnson KSJ [2000] Small lymphocytic lymphoma with perifollicular, marginal zone, or interfollicular distribution. *Mod Pathol* 13:1161-1166.

Hallermann C, Kaune K, Siebert R, et al [2004] Cytogenetic aberration patterns differ in subtypes of primary cutaneous B-cell lymphomas. *J Invest Dermatol* 122:1495-1502.

Hallermann C, Kaune KM, Gesk S, et al [2004] Molecular cytogenetic analysis of chromosomal breakpoints in the IGH, MYC, BCL6 and MALT1 gene loci in primary cutaneous B-cell lymphomas. *J Invest Dermatol* 123:213-219.

Hans CP, Weisenburger DD, Greiner TC [2003] Confirmation of the molecular classification of diffuse large B-cell lymphoma by immunohistochemistry using a tissue microarray. *Blood* 2003; Sept. 22 (Epub).

Hirase N, Yufu Y, Abe Y, et al [2000] Primary macroglobulinemia with t(11;18)(q21;q21). *Cancer Genet Cytogenet* 117:113–117.

Hoefnagel JJ, Vermeer MH, Janssen PM, Fleuren GJ, Meijer CJLM, Willemze R [2003] Bcl-2, Bcl-6 and CD10 expression in cutaneous B-cell lymphoma: Further support for a follicle centre cell origin and differential diagnostic significance. *Br J Dermatol* 149:1183-1191.

Hoefnagel JJ, Dijkman R, Basso K, et al [2005] Distinct types of primary cutaneous large B-cell lymphoma identified by gene expression profiling. *Blood* 105:3671-3678.

Horenstein MG, Nador RG, Chadburn A, et al [1997] Epstein-Barr virus latent gene expression in primary effusion lymphomas containing Kaposi's sarcoma-associated herpesvirus/human herpesvirus-8. *Blood* 90:1186-1191.

Hounieu M, Chittal SM, al Saati T [1992] Hairy cell leukemia. Diagnosis of bone marrow involvement in paraffin-embedded sections with monoclonal antibody DBA.44. *Am J Clin Pathol* 98:26-33.

Hoyer JD, Hanson CA, Fonseca R, Greipp PR, Dewald GW, Kurtin PJ [2000] The (11;14)(q13;q32) translocation in Multiple Myeloma. A morphological and immunohistochemical study. *Am J Clin Pathol* 113:831-837.

Huang JC, Finn WG, Goolsby CL, et al [1999] CD5– small B-cell leukemias are rarely classifiable as chronic lymphocytic leukemia. *Am J Clin Pathol* 111:123-130.

Hussong JW, Perkins SL, Schnitzer B, Hargreaves H, Frizzera G [1999] Extramedullary plasmacytoma. A form of marginal zone cell lymphoma? *Am J Clin Pathol* 111:111-116.

Ibrahim S, Keating M, Kim-Anh D, et al [2001] CD38 expression as an important prognostic factor in B-cell chronic lymphocytic leukemia. *Blood* 98:181-186.

Isaacson PG, Piris MA, Catovsky D, et al [2001] Splenic marginal zone lymphoma. In: Jaffe ES, Harris NL, Stein H, Vardiman JW, eds. *World Health Organization Classification of Tumors: Pathology and Genetics of Tumours of Haematopoietic and Lymphoid Tissues*. Lyon, France: IARC Press; 132-134.

Ito M, Iida S, Inagaki H, et al [2002] MUM1/IRF4 expression is an unfavorable prognostic marker in B-cell chronic lymphocytic leukemia (CLL)/small lymphocytic lymphoma (SLL). *Jpn J Cancer Res* 93:685-694.

Jaffe ES, Harris NL, Stein H, Vardiman JW, eds [2001] *World Health Organization Classification of Tumours. Pathology and Genetics of Tumours of Haematopoietic and Lymphoid Tissues*. Lyon, France: IARC Press.

Jasionawski TM, Hartung L, Greenwood JH, Perkins SL, Bahler DW [2003] Analysis of CD10+ hairy cell leukemia. *Am J Clin Pathol* 120:228-235.

Jung G, Eisenmann JC, Thiebault S, et al [2003] Cell surface CD43 determination improves diagnostic precision in late B-cell diseases. *Br J Haematol* 120:496-499.

Kampalath B, Barcos MP, Stewart C [2003] Phenotypic heterogeneity of B cells in patients with chronic lymphocytic leukemia/small lymphocytic lymphoma. *Am J Clin Pathol* 119:824-832.

Kanungo A, Medeiros LJ, Abruzzo LV, Lin P [2006] Lymphoid neoplasms associated with concurrent t(14;18) and 8q24-c-MYC translocation generally have a poor prognosis. *Mod Pathol* 19:25-33.

Keith TA, Cousar JB, Glick AD, Vogler LB, Collins RD [1985] Plasmacytic differentiation in follicular center cell (FCC) lymphomas. *Am J Clin Pathol* 84:283-290.

Kevon MS, Go JH, Choi JS, et al [2003] Critical evaluation of bcl-6 protein expression in diffuse large B-cell lymphoma of the stomach and small intestine. *Am J Surg Pathol* 27:790-798.

Kim BK, Surti U, Pandya AG, Swerdlow SH [2003] Primary and secondary cutaneous diffuse large B-cell lymphomas. *Am J Surg Pathol* 27:356-364.

Kobayashi Y, Nakata M, Maekawa M, et al [2001] Detection of t(11;18) in MALT-type lymphoma with dual-color fluorescence in situ hybridization and reverse transcriptase-polymerase chain reaction analysis. *Diagn Mol Pathol* 10:207-213.

Kokosadze NV, Kovrigina AM, Probatova NA [2004] Stomach MALT-lymphoma with marked plasmocytic differentiation: A variant of Mott's cell tumor. *Arkh Patol* 66:40-42.

Koster A, Tromp HA, Raemaekers JMM, et al [2007] The prognostic significance of the intra-follicular tumor cell proliferative rate in follicular lymphoma. *Haematologica* 92:184-190.

Lai R, Arber DA, Chang KL, Wilson CS, Weiss LM [1998] Frequency of bcl-2 expression in non-Hodgkin's lymphoma: A study of 778 cases with comparison of marginal zone lymphoma and monocytoid B-cell hyperplasia. *Mod Pathol* 11:864-869.

Lai R, Weiss LM, Chang KL, et al [1999] Frequency of CD43 expression in non-Hodgkin lymphoma. A survey of 742 cases and further characterization of rare CD43+ follicular lymphomas. *Am J Clin Pathol* 111:488-494.

Le Gouill S, Talmant P, Touzeau C, et al [2007] The clinical presentation and prognosis of diffuse large B-cell lymphoma with t(14;18) and 8q24/c-MYC rearrangement. *Haematologica* 92:1335-1342.

Lee PS, Beneck D, Weisberger J, Gorczyca W [2005] Coexpression of CD43 by benign B cells in the terminal ileum. *Appl Immunohistochem Mol Morphol* 13:138-141.

Li S, Griffin CA, Mann RB, Borowitz MJ [2001] Primary cutaneous T-cell rich B-cell lymphoma: Clinically distinct from its nodal counterpart? *Mod Pathol* 14:10-13.

Li S, Eshleman JR, Borowitz MJ [2002] Lack of surface immunoglobulin light chain expression by flow cytometric immunophenotyping can help diagnose peripheral B-cell lymphoma. *Am J Clin Pathol* 118:229-234.

Li S, Lew G [2003] Is B-lineage acute lymphoblastic leukemia with a mature phenotype and L1 morphology a precursor B-lymphoblastic leukemia/lymphoma or Burkitt leukemia/lymphoma? *Arch Pathol Lab Med* 127:1340-1344.

Lin CW, O'Brien S, Faber J, et al [1999] De-novo CD5+ Burkitt lymphoma/leukemia. *Am J Clin Pathol* 112:828-835.

Lin P, Medeiros LJ [2005] Lymphoplasmacytic lymphoma/Waldenström macroglobulinemia: an evolving concept. *Adv Anat Pathol* 12:246-255.

Liu H, Ye H, Dogan A, et al [2001] T(11;18)(q21;q21) is associated with advanced mucosa-associated lymphoid tissue lymphoma that expresses nuclear BCL10. *Blood* 98:1182–1187.

Liu H, Ye H, Ruskone-Fourmestraux A, et al [2002] T(11;18) is a marker for all stage gastric MALT lymphomas that will not respond to H. pylori eradication. *Gastroenterology* 122:1286–1294.

Liu Z, Dong HY, Gorczyca W, et al [2002] CD5-mantle cell lymphoma. *Am J Clin Pathol* 118:216-224.

Maes B, Anastasopoulou A, Kluin-Nelemans JC, et al [2001] Among diffuse large B-cell lymphomas, T-cell-rich/histiocyte-rich BCL and CD30+ anaplastic B-cell subtypes exhibit distinct clinical features. *Ann Oncol* 12:853-858.

Mao X, Lillington D, Child FJ, Russell-Jones R, Young B, Whittaker S [2002] Comparative genomic hybridization analysis of primary cutaneous B-cell lymphomas: Identification of common genomic alterations in disease pathogenesis. *Genes Chromosomes Cancer* 35:144-155.

Marotta G, Raspadori D, Sestigiani C, Scalia G, Bigazzi C, Lauria F [2000] Expression of the CD11c antigen in B-cell chronic lymphoproliferative disorders. *Leuk Lymphoma* 37:145-149.

Martinez AE, Dunphy CH [2007] Grading of follicular lymphoma: Comparison of routine histology with immunohistochemistry. *Arch Pathol Lab Med* 131:1084-1088.

Matsuda I, Mori Y, Nakagawa Y, Sawanobori M, Uemura N, Suzuki K [2005] Close correlations between CD20 expression, a small mature plasma cell morphology, and t(11 ; 14) in multiple myeloma. *Rinsho Ketsueki* 46:1293-1297.

Matutes E, Oscier D, Garcia-Marco J, et al [1996] Trisomy 12 defines a group of CLL with atypical morphology: Correlation between cytogenetic, clinical and laboratory features in 544 patients. *Br J Haematol* 92:382-388.

McBride JA, Rodriguez J, Luthra R, et al [1996] T-cell-rich B-cell lymphoma simulating lymphocyte-rich Hodgkin disease. *Am J Surg Pathol* 20:193-201.

McCarron KF, Hammel JP, Hsi ED [2000] Usefulness of CD79b expression in the diagnosis of B-cell chronic lymphoproliferative disorders. *Am J Clin Pathol* 113:805-813.

McClure RF, Remstein ED, Macon WR, et al [2005] Adult B-cell lymphomas with Burkitt-like morphology are phenotypically and genotypically heterogeneous with aggressive clinical behavior. *Am J Surg Pathol* 29:1652-1660.

Meda BA, Frost M, Newell J, et al [2003] Bcl-2 is consistently expressed in hyperplastic marginal zones of the spleen, abdominal lymph nodes, ileal lymphoid tissue. *Am J Surg Pathol* 27:888-894.

Merzianu M, Jiang L, Lin P, et al [2006] Nuclear BCL10-expression is common in lymphoplasmacytic lymphoma/Waldenström macroglobulinemia and does not correlate with p65 NF-κB activation. *Mod Pathol* 19:891-898.

Meyerson HJ, MacLennan G, Husel W, Tse W, Lazarus H, Kaplan D [2008] D cyclins in CD5+ B-cell lymphoproliferative disorders: Cyclin D1 and cyclin D2 identify diagnostic groups and cyclin D1 correlates with ZAP-70 expression in chronic lymphocytic leukemia. *Am J Clin Pathol* 125:241-250.

Miranda RN, Briggs RC, Kinney MC, Veno PA, Hammer RD, Cousar JB [2000] Immunohistochemical detection of cyclin D1 using optimized conditions is highly specific for mantle cell lymphoma and hairy cell leukemia. *Mod Pathol* 13:1308-1314.

Mirza I, Macpherson S, Paproski S, et al [2002] Primary cutaneous follicular lymphoma: An assessment of clinical, histopathologic, immunophenotypic, and molecular features. *J Clin Oncol* 20:647-655.

Monni O, Oinonen R, Elonen E, et al [1998] Gain of 3q and deletion of 11q22 are frequent aberrations in mantle cell lymphoma. *Genes Chromosomes Cancer* 21:298-307.

Mossafa H, Damotte D, Jenabian A, et al [2006] Non-Hodgkin's lymphomas with Burkitt-like cells are associated with c-Myc amplification and poor prognosis. *Leukemia & Lymphoma* 47:1885-1893.

Mounier N, Brier J, Gisselbrecht C, et al [2003] Rituximab plus CHOP (R-CHOP) overcomes bcl-2-associated resistance to chemotherapy in elderly patients with diffuse large B-cell lymphoma (DLBCL). *Blood* 101:4279-4284.

Mourad WA, Rawas F, Shoukri M, et al [2006] Grading of follicular lymphoma using flow cytometry. *Ann Saudi Med* 26:205-210.

Nakamura N, Nakamine H, Tamaru J-I, et al [2002] The distinction between Burkitt lymphoma and diffuse large B-cell lymphoma with c-myc rearrangement. *Mod Pathol* 15:771-776.

Nathwani BN, Anderson JR, Armitage JO, et al [1999] Clinical significance of follicular lymphoma with monocytoid B cells. *Human Pathol* 30:263-268.

Ngan B-Y, Chen-Levy Z, Weiss LM, Warnke RA, Cleary ML [1998] Expression in non-Hodgkin's lymphoma of the bcl-2 protein associated with the t(14;18) chromosomal translocation. *N Engl J Med* 318:638-644.

O'Malley DP, Vance GH, Orazi A [2005] Chronic lymphocytic leukemia/small lymphocytic lymphoma with trisomy 12 and focal cyclin D1 expression: A potential diagnostic pitfall. *Arch Path Lab Med* 129:92-95.

Offit K, Louie DC, Parsa NZ, Noy A, Chaganti RS [1995] Del(7)(q32) is associated with a subset of small lymphocytic lymphoma with plasmacytoid features. *Blood* 86:2365-2370.

Pan Z, Shen Y, Du C, et al [2003] Two newly characterized germinal center B cell-associated genes, GCET1 and GCET2, have differential expression in normal and neoplastic B cells. *Am J Pathol* 163:135-144.

Paul JT, Henson ES, Mai S, et al [2005] Cyclin D expression in chronic lymphocytic leukemia. *Leuk Lymphoma* 46:1275-1285.

Paulli M, Viglio A, Vivenza D, et al [2002] Primary cutaneous large B-cell lymphoma of the leg: Histogenetic analysis of a controversial clinicopathologic entity. *Hum Pathol* 33:937-943.

Pellat-Deceunynck C, Barille S, Jego G, et al [1998] The absence of CD56(NCAM) on malignant plasma cells is a hallmark of plasma cell leukemia and of a special subset of multiple myeloma. *Leukemia* 12:1977-1982.

Peltomaki P, Bianchi NO, Knuutila S, et al [1988] Immunoglobulin kappa and lambda light-chain dual genotype rearrangement in a patient with kappa-secreting B-CLL. *Eur J Cancer Clin Oncol* 24:1233-1238.

Pezzella F, Tse GD, Cordell JL, Pulford KAF, Gatter KC, Mason DY [1990] Expression of the bcl-2 oncogene protein is not specific for the 14;18 chromosomal translocation. *Am J Pathol* 137:225-232.

Pittaluga S, Verhoef G, Criel A, et al [1996] "Small" B-cell non-Hodgkin's lymphomas with splenomegaly at presentation are either mantle cell lymphoma or marginal zone cell lymphoma. A study based on histology, cytology, immunohistochemistry, and cytogenetic analysis. *Am J Surg Pathol* 20:211-223.

Polski JM, Evans HL, Grosso LE, Popovic WJ, Taylor L, Dunphy CH [2000] CD7 and CD56-positive primary effusion lymphoma in a human immunodeficiency virus-negative host. *Leuk Lymphoma* 39:633-639.

Pruneri G, Fabris S, Baldini L, et al [2000] Immunohistochemical analysis of cyclin D1 shows deregulated expression in multiple myeloma with the t(11;14). *Am J Pathol* 156:1505-1513.

Pugh WC, Manning JT, Butler JJ [1988] Paraimmunoblastic variant of small lymphocytic lymphoma/leukemia. *Am J Surg Pathol* 12:907-917.

Rawstron A, Barrans S, Blythe D, et al [1999] Distribution of myeloma plasma cells in peripheral blood and bone marrow correlates with CD56 expression. *Br J Haematol* 104:138–143.

Reichard KK, McKenna RW, Kroft SH [2003] Comparative analysis of light chain expression in germinal center cells and mantle cells of reactive lymphoid tissues. *Am J Clin Pathol* 119:130-136.

Rijlaarsdam JU, van der Putte SCJ, Berti E, et al [1993] Cutaneous immunocytomas: A clinicopathologic study of 26 cases. *Histopathology* 23:119-125.

Robillard N, Avet-Loiseau H, Garand R, et al [2003] CD20 is associated with a small mature plasma cell morphology and t(11;14) in multiple myeloma. *Blood* 102:1070-1071.

Rodig S, Savage K, LaCasce A, et al [2007] Expression of TRAF1 and nuclear c-Rel distinguishes primary mediastinal large cell lymphoma from other types of diffuse large B-cell lymphoma. *Am J Surg Pathol* 31:106-112.

Rosenstein Y, Santana A, Pedraza-Alva G [1999] CD43, a molecule with multiple functions. *Immunol Res* 20:89-99.

Ruchlemer R, Parry-Jones N, Brito-BabapulleV, et al [2004] B-prolymphocytic leukemia with t(11;14) revisited: A splenomegalic form of mantle cell lymphoma evolving with leukaemia. *Br J Haematol* 125:330-336.

Rudiger T, Jaffe ES, Delsol G, et al [1998] Workshop report on Hodgkin disease and related disease ('gray zone' lymphoma). *Ann Oncol* 9(suppl):31-38.

Ruiz-Aruelles GJ, San Miguel JF [1994] Cell surface markers in multiple myeloma. *May Clin Proc* 69:684-690.

Sahara N, Takeshita A, Shigeno K, et al [2002] Clinicopathological and prognostic characteristics of CD56-negative multiple myeloma. *Br J Haematol* 117:882–885.

Sander CA, Kaudewitz P, Kutzner H, et al [1996] T-cell rich B-cell lymphoma presenting in the skin. A clinicopathologic analysis of six cases. *J Cutan Pathol* 23:101-108.

Sandhaus LM, Voelkerding K, Raska K [1988] Follicular lymphoma mimicking transformation of germinal centers: Immunologic analysis of a case. *Am J Clin Pathol* 90:518-519.

Santucci M, Pimpinelli N, Arganini L [1991] Primary cutaneous B-cell lymphoma: A unique type of low-grade lymphoma. *Cancer* 67:2311-2326.

Savage KJ, Monti S, Kutok JL [2003] The molecular signature of mediastinal large B-cell lymphoma differs from that of other diffuse large B-cell lymphomas and shares features with classical Hodgkin lymphoma. *Blood* 102:3871-3879.

Savilo E, Campo E, Mollejo M, et al [1998] Absence of cyclin D1 protein expression in splenic marginal zone lymphoma. *Mod Pathol* 11:601-606.

Schade U, Bock O, Vornhusen S, et al [2006] Bone marrow infiltration pattern in B-cell chronic lymphocytic leukemia is related to immunoglobulin heavy-chain variable region mutation status and expression of 70-kd ζ-associated protein (ZAP-70). *Hum Pathol* 37:1153-1161.

Schlette E, Medeiros LJ, Keating M, Lai R [2003] CD79b expression in chronic lymphocytic leukemia. Association with trisomy 12 and atypical immunophenotype. *Arch Pathol Lab Med* 127:561-566.

Schmidt U, Metz KA, Leder LD, et al [1990] T-cell-rich B-cell lymphoma and lymphocyte predominant Hodgkin disease: Two closely related entities? *Br J Haematol* 2:398-403.

Schmid U, Eckert F, Griesser H, et al [1995] Cutaneous follicular lymphoid hyperplasia with monotypic plasma cells. A clinicopathologic study of 18 patients. *Am J Surg Pathol* 19:12-20.

Sepp N, Schuler G, Romani N, et al [1990] "Intravascular lymphomatosis" (angioendotheliomatosis): Evidence for a T-cell origin in two cases. *Hum Pathol* 21:1051-1058.

Sheibani K, Battifora H, Winberg CD, et al [1986] Further evidence that "malignant angioendotheliomatosis" is an angiotropic large-cell lymphoma. *N Engl J Med* 314:943-948.

Skinnider BF, Horsman DE, Dupuis B, Gascoyne RD [1999] Bcl-6 and Bcl-2 protein expression in diffuse large B-cell lymphoma and follicular lymphoma: Correlation with 3q27 and 18q21 chromosomal abnormalities. *Hum Pathol* 30:803-808.

Slack GW, Wizniak J, Dabbagh L, Shi X, Gelebart P, Lai R [2007] Flow cytometric detection of ZAP-70 in chronic lymphocytic leukemia: Correlation with immunocytochemistry and Western blot analysis. *Arch Path Lab Med* 131:50-56.

Streubel B, Lamprecht A, Dierlamm J, et al [2003] T(14;18) (q32;q21) involving IGH and MALT1 is a frequent chromosomal aberration in MALT lymphoma. *Blood* 101:2335-2339.

Theaker JM, Gatter KC, Esiri MM, Esterbrook P [1986] Neoplastic angioendotheliomatosis: further evidence supporting a lymphoid origin. *Histopathology* 10:1261-1270.

Tiesinga JJ, Wu CD, Inghirami G [2000] CD5+ follicle center lymphoma. Immunophenotyping detects a unique subset of "floral" follicular lymphoma. *Am J Clin Pathol* 114:912-921.

Torlakovic E, Torlakovic G, Nguyen PL, Brunning RD, Delabie J [2002] The value of anti-Pax-5 immunostaining in routinely fixed and paraffin-embedded sections. A novel pan pre-B and B-cell marker. *Am J Surg Pathol* 26:1343-1350.

Torne R, Su WPD, Winkelmann RK, Smolle J, Kerl H [1990] Clinicopathologic study of cutaneous plasmacytoma. *Int J Dermatol* 29:562-566.

Treasure J, Lane A, Jones DB, et al [1992] CD43 expression in B-cell lymphoma. *J Clin Pathol* 45:1018-1022.

Troussard X, Avet-Loiseau H, Macro M, Mellerin MP, Malet M, Roussel M, Sola B [2000] Cyclin D1 expression in patients with multiple myeloma. *Hematol J* 1:181-185.

Tsuboi K, Inagaki H, Kato M [2000] MUM1/IRF4 expression as a frequent event in mature lymphoid malignancies. *Leukemia* 14:449-456.

Valdez R, Finn WG, Ross CW, et al [2002] Waldenström macroglobulinemia caused by extranodal marginal zone B-cell lymphoma: A report of six cases. *Am J Clin Pathol* 116:495-496.

Vasef MA, Brynes RK, Murata-Collins JL, Arber DA, Medeiros LJ [1998] Surface immunoglobulin light chain-positive acute lymphoblastic leukemia of FAB L1 or L2 type: A report of 6 cases in adults. *Am J Clin Pathol* 110:143-149.

Vega F, Chang CC, Medeiros LJ, et al [2005] Plasmablastic lymphomas and plasmablastic plasma cell myelomas had nearly identical immunophenotypic profiles. *Mod Pathol* 18:806-815.

Vermeer MH, Geelen FAMJ, van Haselen CW, et al [1996] Primary cutaneous large B-cell lymphomas of the legs: A distinct type of cutaneous B-cell lymphoma with an intermediate prognosis. *Arch Dermatol* 132:1304-1308.

Wang SA, Wang L, Hochberg E, Muzihansky A, Harris NL, Hasserjian RP [2005] Low histologic grade follicular lymphoma with high proliferation index: Morphologic and clinical features. *Am J Surg Pathol* 29:1490-1496.

Weistner A, Rosenwald A, Barry TS, et al [2003] ZAP-70 expression identifies a chronic lymphocytic leukemia subtype with unmutated immunoglobulin genes, inferior clinical outcome, and distinct gene expression profile. *Blood* 101:4944-4951.

Wheaton S, Netser J, Guinee D, Rahn M, Perkins S [1998] Bcl-2 and bax protein expression in indolent vs aggressive B-cell non-Hodgkin's lymphomas. *Hum Pathol* 29:820-825.

Willemze R, Meijer CJLM, Scheffer E, et al [1987] Diffuse large cell lymphomas of follicle center cell origin presenting in the skin: A clinicopathologic and immunologic study of 16 patients. *Am J Pathol* 126:325-333.[

Winter JN, Weller EA, Horning SJ, et al [2006] Prognostic significance of Bcl-6 protein expression in DLBCL treated with CHOP or R-CHOP: A prospective correlative study. *Blood* 107:4207-4213.

Wu CD, Jackson CL, Medeiros LJ [1996] Splenic marginal zone cell lymphoma: An immunophenotypic and molecular study of five cases. *Am J Clin Pathol* 105:277-285.

Xu D [2006] Dual surface immunoglobulin light-chain expression in B-cell lymphoproliferative disorders. *Arch Path Lab Med* 130:853-856.

Yamaguchi M, Seto M, Okamoto M, et al [2002] w CD5+ diffuse large B-cell lymphoma: A clinicopathologic study of 109 patients. *Blood* 99:815-821.

Yatabe Y, Suzuki R, Tobinai K, et al [2000] Significance of cyclin D1 overexpression for the diagnosis of mantle cell lymphoma: A clinicopathologic comparison of cyclin D1-positive MCL and cyclin D1-negative MCL-like B-cell lymphoma. *Blood* 95:2253-2261.

Ye H, Dogan A, Karran L, et al [2000] BCL10 expression in normal and neoplastic lymphoid tissue: Nuclear localization in MALT lymphoma. *Am J Pathol* 157:1147-1154.

Ye H, Liu H, Attygalle A, et al [2003] Variable frequencies of t(11;18)(q21;q21) in MALT lymphomas of different sites: Significant association with CagA strains of H. pylori in gastric MALT lymphoma. *Blood* 102:1012-1018.

Yokote T, Akioka T, Miyamoto H, et al [2005] Pulmonary parenchymal infiltrates in a patient with CD20-positive multiple myeloma. *Eur J Haematol* 74:61-65.

Young KH, Chan WC, Fu K, et al [2006] Mantle cell lymphoma with plasma cell differentiation. *Am J Surg Pathol* 30:954-961.

Zaer FS, Braylan RC, Zander DS, Iturraspe MT, Almasri NM [1998] Multiparametric flow cytometry in the diagnosis and characterization of low-grade pulmonary mucosa-associated lymphoid tissue lymphomas. *Mod Pathol* 11:525-532.

Zanotti R, Ambrosetti A, Lestani M, et al [2007] ZAP-70 expression, as detected by immunohistochemistry on bone marrow biopsies from early-phase CLL patients, is a strong adverse prognostic factor. *Leukemia* 21:102-109.

13 Precursor T-Cell Neoplasms

Chapter Contents

Classification

- ▸ Precursor T-lymphoblastic leukemia
- ▸ Precursor T-lymphoblastic lymphoma

Introduction

Precursor T-lymphoblastic leukemia (T-ALL)/lymphoma (T-LBL) is a neoplasm of lymphoblasts committed to the T-cell lineage. It is typically composed of small to intermediate-sized blasts with scant cytoplasm, involving bone marrow (BM) and peripheral blood (PB) in T-ALL, and not infrequently presenting with primary nodal or extranodal involvement in T-LBL. When the process is confined to a mass lesion without any or only minimal PB or BM involvement, the diagnosis is T-LBL. When there is extensive PB and BM involvement, T-ALL is the appropriate diagnosis. However, in some patients there may be a mass lesion and up to 25% lymphoblasts in the BM. In this situation, the preferred designation is T-LBL and arbitrary, since T-ALL and T-LBL are biologically unified.

Diagnosis

Correlation of Specific Immunophenotype with Precursor T-Lymphoblastic Leukemia/Lymphoma Subtype and Stage of Differentiation

The immunophenotypes of T-cell ALL are outlined in **[t13.1]** and are best evaluated by FCI [Keren 1994]. These immunophenotypic subtypes correspond to stages of normal thymocyte development: the early pre-thymocyte and prothymocyte stages are CD4– and CD8–; the common (or cortical) thymocyte stage is the only stage that is CD4+ and CD8+; and the mature thymocyte stage is single positive for CD4 (T-helper) or CD8 (T-suppressor). In addition to being negative for CD4 and CD8, the early subtype is negative for surface CD3 (sCD3) but positive for cytoplasmic CD3 (cCD3). The more differentiated, common thymocyte subtype is positive for cCD3, may show variable positivity for sCD3, and is dual positive for CD4 and CD8. The mature subtype is positive for surface CD3 (negative for cCD3), negative for CD1a, and positive for either CD4 or CD8. Case examples of precursor T-cell lymphoblastic leukemia at the various stages of T-cell differentiation are demonstrated in **[f13.1]**-**[f13.6]**. The most sensitive antigens for T-ALL include CD7, CD5, and CD2 in combination, and they are expressed in virtually all cases of T-ALL. In isolation, they may be aberrantly expressed in acute myeloid leukemia (AML).

T-LBL most often has an immunophenotype corresponding to the common thymocyte stage of differentiation. In addition, it should be recognized that precursor T-cell lymphoblastic neoplasms may also aberrantly express CD10 **[f10.6]**. Of interest, there is also a unique subset of de-novo adult T-ALL that co-expresses CD117 **[f10.7]** and cCD3 and is associated with activating mutations in the FLT3 RTK gene. Activating FLT3 mutations are the most common genetic aberrations in AML, resulting in the constitutive activation of this receptor tyrosine kinase (RTK), but such mutations are have been rarely found in ALL. This unique subset of T-ALL indicates the need for clinical trials to test the efficacy of drugs inhibiting the FLT3 RTK in this subset of patients [Paietta 2004].

Differentiation between T-ALL and Reactive Conditions

As discussed in detail in Chapter 5, hematogones (B-lymphocyte precursors) may occur in large numbers in some healthy infants and young children and in a variety of diseases in both children and adults. In some instances, they may constitute 5% to >50% of cells in the bone marrow. In particular, increased numbers of hematogones may cause problems in diagnosis, due to the morphologic features they commonly share with neoplastic lymphoblasts. However, the immunophenotype of hematogones has features in common with

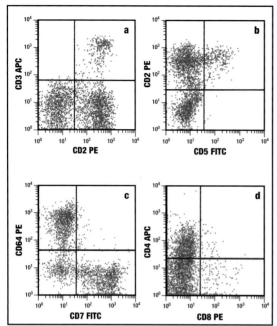

[f13.1] This case with a previous history of precursor T-cell lymphoblastic leukemia demonstrates minimal residual disease with an early thymocyte stage. The clinical history reveals a 15-year-old male with a history of relapsed precursor T-cell lymphoblastic leukemia with CNS involvement, status post systemic and intrathecal chemotherapy, for BM evaluation. By morphology, only 2% blasts are detected on the BM aspirate smears. Flow cytometric analysis reveals 1% of cells within the "immature cell" region. Cells within this region variably express CD2 **a**, **b** CD7 **c**, CD10, CD13, CD33 (all not demonstrated) and are negative for CD3 **a**, CD5 **b**, and CD4 and CD8 **d** (CD4 reveals nonspecific staining), as well as all myelomonocytic markers (CD64, **c**; others, not demonstrated) and HLA-DR, CD56, and CD34 (all, not demonstrated). The cytogenetic results show numerous structural and numerical abnormalities, including a homozygous deletion of the p16/p15 locus on 9p2. Diagnosis is made of minimal residual precursor T-cell lymphoblastic leukemia, early thymocyte stage.

neoplastic B-lymphoblasts. Although T-ALL may show aberrant expression of CD10, the immunophenotype of hematogones is usually easily distinguished from the immunophenotypes discussed previously in T-ALL.

Differentiation from Langerhans Cell Histiocytosis

Although the common thymocyte stage of T-ALL/LBL shows expression of CD1a and Langerhans cells are CD1a+, these 2 entities are usually easily distinguished by combining cytomorphology, the pattern of involvement, and their additional, unique immunophenotypic features. Langerhans cells are characterized by their grooved, folded, indented, or lobulated nuclei with moderately abundant and slightly eosinophilic

cytoplasm. In Langerhans cell histiocytosis (LCH), they are characteristically accompanied by variable numbers of eosinophils, histiocytes, neutrophils, and small lymphocytes and infiltrate as focal lesions in BM (often associated with fibrosis) or adjacent to or within a malignant lymphoma. In addition, the cells of LCH do not express any additional T-cell antigens and are CD34– and TdT–.

Differentiation between T-ALL/LBL and Mature T-Cell Leukemias/Lymphomas

Since the mature thymocyte stage of T-ALL may show expression of either CD4 or CD8 in association with expression of CD2, CD5, CD7, and sCD3 (without expression of cCD3, CD1a, or CD34), there may be immunophenotypic overlap between this stage of T-ALL and mature T-cell leukemias/lymphomas. However, these entities may usually be distinguished by the blastic morphology in T-ALL/LBL and the lack of TdT-positivity in mature T-cell disorders. However, one should keep in mind the mature stage of T-ALL/LBL may also lack TdT-positivity. In some cases, cytogenetic findings may be helpful in distinguishing such entities. [t13.2] summarizes the cytogenetic findings in precursor T-ALL/LBL [Han 2007].

Differentiation between T-LBL and Thymoma

As discussed previously, T-LBL most often has an immunophenotype that corresponds to the common thymocyte stage of differentiation. The immunophenotype of thymoma is identical to this stage. In addition, as T-LBL may aberrantly express CD10, so may thymoma [Nakajima 2000]. However, flow cytometric analysis allows for the distinction between thymoma and T-LBL. Flow cytometric immunophenotypic features characteristic of thymoma include a smear pattern of CD4/CD8 co-expression [f13.7a], a smear pattern of CD3 and TdT expression [f13.7b], and lack of T-cell antigen deletion (with the exception of partial CD3). In contrast, T-LBL shows much more variability in expression patterns and is characterized by a tight pattern of CD4/CD8 expression [f13.7c], significant T-cell antigen deletion, and absence of the CD3 or TdT smear pattern [f13.1d] [Cessna 2002]. Another subsequent 4-color flow cytometric study of lymphocyte-rich thymomas and precursor T-cell lymphoblastic neoplasms demonstrates the thymocytes in all of the thymoma cases contain 3 distinct subpopulations:

t13.1 Immunophenotypes of Precursor T-Cell Lymphoblastic Neoplasms

Antigen	Pre-Thymocytes	Pre-T ALL (I) Prothymocytes	Pre-T ALL (II) Common Thymocytes	T-ALL (III) Mature Thymocytes	
				T-H	T-S
CD1a	–	–	+	–	–
CD2	±	±	±	+	+
cCD3	±	+	±	–	–
sCD3	–	–	–/+	+	+
CD5	–/+	+	+	+	+
CD7	+	+	+	+	+
CD4	–	–	+	+	–
CD8	–	–	+	–	+
HLA-DR	±	–	–	–	–
CD34	±	–	–	–	–
TdT	+	+	+	+	+

cCD3, cytoplasmic CD3; sCD3, surface CD3.

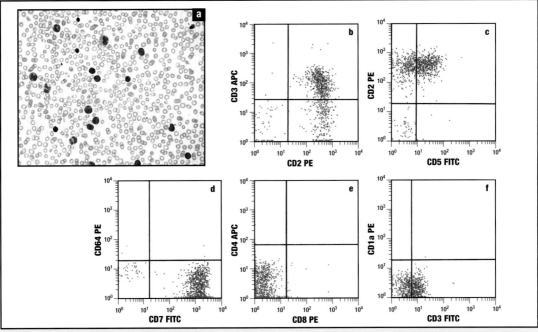

[f13.2] This case of precursor T-cell lymphoblastic leukemia demonstrates an even earlier thymocyte stage than the case demonstrated in [f13.1]. The clinical history reveals a 14-year-old male with a 7-month history of "EBV infection" and splenetomy due to a ruptured spleen presents with an unresolving increased WBC count and thrombocytopenia. CBC data show WBC 60 × 10³/mm³ (60 × 10⁹/L), Hgb 10.9 g/dL, Plt 36 × 10³/mm³ (36 × 10⁹/L). The peripheral blood smear morphology **a** reveals numerous blasts (23%). By flow cytometric analysis, the blasts variably express CD3 **b, f**, CD2 **b, c**, CD5 **c**, CD7 **d**, CD10, CD13, CD56, and CD45. They do not express additional myelomonocytic markers (CD64, **d**; others, not demonstrated), CD4 or CD8 **e**, CD1a **f**, or HLA-DR (not demonstrated). The cytogenetic results show numerous structural and numerical abnormalities, including a homozygous deletion of the p16/q5 locus at 9p21. A diagnosis is made of precursor T-cell lymphoblastic leukemia (earlier stage due to lack of CD1a, CD4, and CD8).

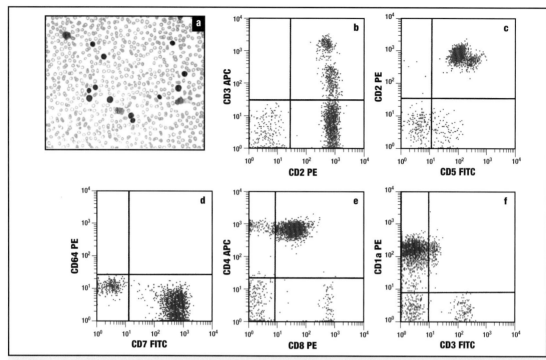

[f13.3] This case of precursor T-cell lymphoblastic leukemia demonstrates a common thymocyte stage of differentiation. The clinical history reveals a 4-year-old male presenting with a large anterior mediastinal mass and a markedly elevated WBC count. CBC data include WBC 81.4 × 10³/mm³ (81.4 × 10⁹/L), Hgb 11.2 g/dL, Plt 59 × 10³/mm³ (59 × 10⁹/L) are provided. The peripheral blood smear morphology **a** reveals numerous blasts (48%). By flow cytometric analysis, the blasts express CD2 **b, c**, partial subset CD3 **b, f**, CD5 **c**, CD7 **d**, dual CD4 and CD8 **e**, CD1a **f**, and dim subset expression of CD15 (not demonstrated). They do not express other myelomonocytic antigens (CD64, **d**; others, not demonstrated), CD34, or CD10 (both, not demonstrated). The diagnosis is made of precursor T-cell lymphoblastic leukemia, common thymocyte immunophenotype.

t13.2 Reported Genetic Abnomalities in T-ALL/LBL

Abnormality	Estimated Frequency
Translocations of 14q11* with various partners: t(10;14)(q24;q11) t(5;14)† t(11;14)(p15;q11) t(11;14)(p13;q11)	Most common recurrent abnormality 5%-10%
Deletion of chromosome 6	15%-18%
Chromosome 9p21 abnormality	15%
Deletion of p16INK4 α	80% by FISH
Duplication of chromosome 9q34	33%
Amplification of ABL gene	3% by FISH
11q23 abns including t(11;19)(q23;q13.3)	rare
t(8;13)(p11;q12)‡	rare

T-ALL/LBL has been reported with a normal karyotype in 30%-40% of cases.
*14q11 is the site of the TCRα and TCRδ genes.
†t(5;14)/HOX11L2+ T-ALL shows higher CD1a+/CD10+/cCD3+.‡t(8;13)(p11;q12) has been demonstrated in T-ALL associated with eosinophilia and a high risk of subsequent myeloid malignancy.
FISH, fluorescent in situ hybridization

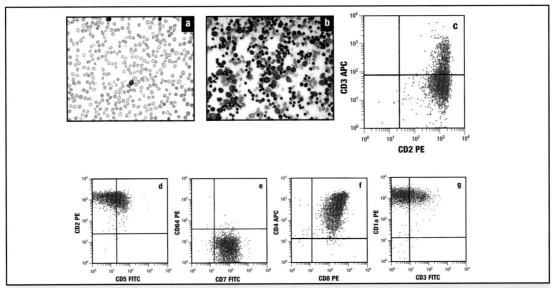

[f13.4] This case of precursor T-cell lymphoblastic leukemia demonstrates a common thymocyte stage of differentiation with loss of CD5 expression. The clinical history reveals a 38-year-old male with diffuse lymphadenopathy, night sweats, and lower extremity edema. A bone marrow biopsy is performed to rule out lymphoma. CBC data include WBC $6.5 \times 10^3/mm^3$ ($6.5 \times 10^9/L$), Hgb 7.9 g/dL, Plt $41 \times 10^3/mm^3$ ($41 \times 10^9/L$). The peripheral blood smear morphology **a** reveals a few scattered blasts. The BM touch preparation **b** reveals numerous blasts. A suspension of the BM core biopsy is analyzed by flow cytometric analysis. The blasts express CD2 **c, d**, partial subset CD3 **c, g**, CD7 **e**, dual CD4 and CD8 **f**, and CD1a **g**. They do not express CD5 **d**, myelomonocytic antigens (CD64, **e**; others, not demonstrated), CD34, or CD10 (both, not demonstrated). The cytogenetic results demonstrate numerous structural and numerical abnormalities, including loss of copies of chromosome 14. Diagnosis is made of precursor T-cell lymphoblastic leukemia/lymphoma, common thymocyte immunophenotype with some loss of expression of CD5.

1. the least mature cells (double-negative) expressed low-density CD45, CD2, and CD5, high-density CD7, CD10, CD34, and heterogeneous CD4 and CD8, and were sCD3−

2. the immature cells (double-positive) expressed CD2, CD5, CD7, CD4, CD8, heterogeneous sCD3, and intermediate-density CD45, and were CD10− and CD34-

3. the mature cells (single-positive) expressed CD2, sCD3, CD5, CD7, and CD4 or CD8

The heterogeneous expression of sCD3, CD4, and CD8, as demonstrated in these 3 distinct subpopulations, created a characteristic smearing pattern for these antigens as discussed previously. There was no loss of T-cell associated antigens in any of the thymoma cases studied. In all precursor T-ALL/LBL cases, the lymphoblasts showed slightly increased light scatter properties compared with those of thymocytes, indicating relatively larger size and more complex cytoplasm. In addition, the T-lymphoblasts formed a tight cluster without discrete subpopulations or a smearing pattern. Of 5 double-negative cases, 4 demonstrated loss of CD2, CD10, or CD34 expression. Of 7 double-positive cases, 5 showed complete loss of sCD3, CD2, and/or CD5; 4 were CD10+; and 2 were CD34+. Of 3 single-positive cases, 2 showed loss of CD2 and/or aberrant expression of CD34. Thus, this study concluded the analysis of antigen expression pattern, the presence or absence of T cell-associated antigen deletion, and the expression of CD10 and CD34 by 4-color flow cytometry can help differentiate thymoma from T-ALL/LBL [Li 2004]. Lastly, distinguishing between thymoma and T-LBL must always also rely on correlation of the flow cytometric immunophenotypic data with the morphology.

A case example of lymphocyte-rich thymoma is demonstrated in **[f13.8]**.

Differentiation between T-LBL and mature B-cell lymphomas

In lymph nodes and extranodal tissues, the major differential diagnosis of T-LBL in children is Burkitt lymphoma (BL); in adults, the differential diagnosis also includes the blastoid variant of mantle cell lymphoma (MCL-BV). Although T-LBL may show aberrant

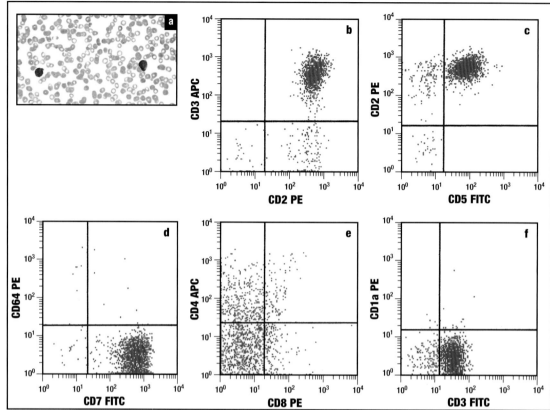

[f13.5] This case of precursor T-cell lymphoblastic leukemia demonstrates a helper T-cell immunophenotype. The clinical history reveals a 23-year-old male who presents with a history of precursor T-cell lymphoblastic leukemia and recent involvement of the peripheral blood (PB). A follow-up PB specimen is sent for flow cytometric analysis. CBC data include WBC $0.6 \times 10^3/mm^3$ (0.6×10^9/L), Hgb: 10.3 g/dL, Plt $8 \times 10^3/mm^3$ (8×10^9/L). The PB smear morphology **a** reveals numerous blasts (50%). By flow cytometric analysis, the blasts express CD2 **b, c**, CD3 **b, f**, CD5 **c**, CD7 **d**, CD4 **e**, and dim subset expression of CD15 (not demonstrated). They do not express CD8 **e**, CD1a **f**, other myelomonocytic antigens (CD64, **d**; others, not demonstrated), CD34, or CD10 (both, not demonstrated). The diagnosis is made of relapsing/persistent precursor T-cell lymphoblastic leukemia, helper immunophenotype with heterogeneous expression of CD4.

CD10 expression, the mature B-cell immunophenotype (ie, TdT–) in BL (with CD10+) and in MCL-BV (with aberrant CD5+), by flow cytometric analysis, easily distinguishes these lymphomas from T-LBL.

Differentiation between T-ALL with Aberrant Myeloid Antigen Expression from AML with Aberrant T-Cell Antigen Expression and Acute Leukemia of Ambiguous Lineage

The distinction between T-ALL with aberrant myeloid antigen expression and AML with aberrant T-cell antigen expression may usually be made by the combination of markers expressed and review of the cytomorphology of the blasts in the PB and/or BM aspirate smear. AML with aberrant T-cell antigen expression (ie, CD2, CD7, or CD5 but not CD3) is HLA-DR+, whereas T-ALL is generally HLA-DR– **[f10.2]**. However, one should

keep in mind that occasional cases of AML may also be HLA-DR– **[f10.4]** and thus must be distinguished from T-ALL with aberrant myeloid antigen expression, which occasionally may also express HLA-DR **[f10.5]**. Among AMLs, CD2 co-expression is almost exclusively restricted to 2 AML subtypes, M3 variant (AML, M3v) and M4-eos, and their related molecular aberrations. The most valuable markers to differentiate between myeloperoxidase (MPO)-negative AML (subtype M0) and T-ALL including CD13, CD33, and CD117, typical of M0, and intracytoplasmic CD3 (cCD3), CD2, and CD10, which may be aberrantly expressed in T-ALL **[f10.6]** [Thalhammer-Scherrer 2002].

One should also keep in mind that although CD117 has previously been considered an extremely useful marker of AML by flow cytometric analysis, subsequent reports have demonstrated CD117

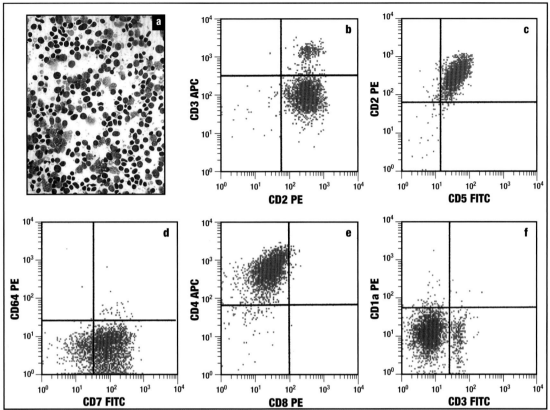

[f13.6] This case of precursor T-cell lymphoblastic leukemia demonstrates a helper T-cell immunophenotype with loss of CD3 expression. The clinical history reveals a 6-year-old male with an elevated WBC count. CBC data include WBC 82 × 10³/mm3 (82 × 10⁹/L), Hgb 5.1 g/dL, Plt 25 × 10³/mm³ (25 × 10⁹/L). A bone marrow aspirate smear morphology **a** reveals numerous blasts (95%). By flow cytometric analysis, the blasts express CD2 **b, c**, CD5 **c**, CD7 **d**, and CD4 **e**. They do not express CD3 **b, f**, CD8 **e**, CD1a **f**, any myelomonocytic antigens (CD64, **d**; others, not demonstrated), CD34, or CD10 (both, not demonstrated). The cytogenetic analysis detected a heterozygous deletion of the p16/p15 locus on 9p21. The diagnosis was made of precursor T-cell lymphoblastic leukemia, helper immunophenotype with loss of CD3 expression.

expression in a small proportion of T-ALL (9%), mainly consisting of those of immature pro-T/pre-T-cell origin **[f10.7]** [Paietta 2004].

Flow cytometric analysis is useful in distinguishing T-ALL with aberrant antigen expression from acute leukemias of ambiguous lineage **[f10.15]**, which generally have a poor prognosis. This distinction is based on a scoring system as demonstrated in **[t13.3]**. Acute leukemia of ambiguous lineage is established when the score from 2 separate lineages is each >2 [Anon 1998].

Differentiation between T-ALL and Precursor B-ALL

Since T-ALL and precursor B-ALL may have morphologic similarities and be CD34+/TdT+, these entities may cause diagnostic confusion. In addition, although cCD79a and CD10 are characteristically expressed

in precursor B-ALL, up to 60% of T-ALL may also express cCD79a, and up to 47% of T-ALL, CD10 **[f10.6]** [Lewis 2006, Pilozzi 1998]. Nevertheless, they may usually be easily distinguished by flow cytometric analysis, which reveals expression of CD19, variable expression of CD20, and no expression of T-cell markers in precursor B-ALL, whereas T-ALL reveals the combined expression of CD7, CD5, and CD2 in virtually all cases with variable expressions of CD4, CD8, cCD3, and sCD3. In addition, although CD117 expression may be seen in up to 9% of T-ALL, CD117 expression is particularly rare in precursor B-ALL and occurs in <3%-5% of cases [Newell 2003, Suggs 2007, Sperling 1997].

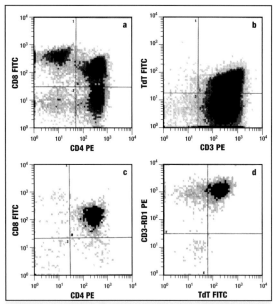

[f13.7] a Smear pattern of CD4 (x-axis)/CD8 (y-axis) characteristic of thymoma. **b** Smear pattern of TdT (y-axis)/CD3 (x-axis) characteristic of thymoma. **c** Tight pattern of CD4 (x-axis)/CD8 (y-axis) characteristic of T-lymphoblastic lymphoma. **d** Tight pattern of TdT (x-axis)/CD3 (y-axis) characteristic of T-lymphoblastic lymphoma.

t13.3 Scoring System for the Definition of Acute Leukemias of Ambiguous Lineage*

Score	B-Lymphoid	T-Lymphoid	Myeloid
2	cCD79a †	cCD3 or sCD3	MPO
	cIgM	Anti-TCR	
	cCD22		
1	CD19	CD2	CD117
	CD20	CD5	CD13
	CD10	CD8	CD33
		CD10	CD65
0.5	TdT	TdT	CD14
	CD24	CD7	CD15
		CD1a	CD64

c, cytoplasmic; s, surface.

*Acute leukemia of ambiguous lineage is established when the score from 2 separate lineages is each >2.

†CD79a may also be expressed in some cases of precursor T lymphoblastic leukemia/lymphoma.

Detection of Minimal Residual Disease and Relapse

The unique immunophenotypes of T-ALL are particularly helpful in distinguishing between relapse of T-ALL and hematogones (as previously discussed with an early B-cell immunophenotype) or recovery myeloblasts by flow cytometric analysis.

FCI vs IHC in Precursor T-Lymphoblastic Leukemia/Lymphoma

Since material may not always be available for flow cytometric analysis, the immunohistochemical (IHC) findings in T-ALL/LBL are important for diagnosis and differentiation from reactive conditions (ie, hematogones), other hematolymphoid neoplasms (ie, AML, non-Hodgkin lymphomas), and non-hematolymphoid malignancies (ie, Ewing sarcoma).

Differentiation of T-ALL from Hematogones and Precursor B-ALL

The most useful markers for differentiating T-ALL from hematogones and precursor B-ALL include T-cell markers (ie, CD1a, CD2, CD3, CD4, CD5, CD7, and CD8), which will be variably expressed in T-ALL and negative in hematogones, since CD10, CD79a, and TdT may all be expressed in T-ALL, hematogones, and precursor B-ALL. PAX-5 may also be useful in distinguishing T-ALL from hematogones and precursor B-ALL, since PAX-5 is not expressed in T-ALL but is expressed by hematogones and precursor B-ALL.

Differentiation of T-ALL from AML and Mature T-Cell and B-Cell Non-Hodgkin Lymphomas

AML

As discussed in Chapter 10, a recommended IHC panel for evaluating acute leukemias (when there is no aspirable BM specimen for flow cytometric analysis or cytogenetic studies) and differentiating it from other hematolymphoid malignancies, including CD3, CD20, CD33, CD34, CD68, CD79a, CD138, myeloperoxidase (MPO), and terminal deoxynucleotidyl transferase (TdT). Additional markers that may be helpful include PAX5, CD14, CD117, additional T-cell antigens (including CD1a), CD61, and Glycophorin A **[t10.4]**.

Myeloperoxidase and CD68 are the most specific myeloid markers. However, CD79a may be detected in up to 11% of AML cases, most frequently of M3

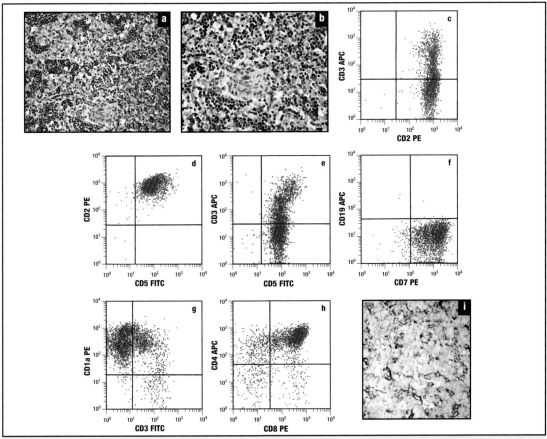

[f13.8] This case demonstrates a lymphocyte-rich thymoma. The clinical history reveals a 6-year-old male with a mediastinal mass, which is subsequently biopsied. H&E sections reveal a background rich in small lymphocytes intermixed with larger, spindle-shaped cells and an apparent Hassell corpuscle **a, b**. By flow cytometric analysis, the lymphocytes heterogeneously express CD3 **c, e, g**, uniformly express CD2 **c, d**, CD5 **d, e**, CD7 **f**, CD1a **g**, and dually express CD4 and CD8 **h**. The cytokeratin stain **i** highlights the epithelial component. The cytogenetic results are normal. The diagnosis is made of lymphocyte-rich thymoma.

subtype (90% of M3 cases are CD79a+) and TdT, in up to 13% of AML cases. A MPO+/CD79a+/HLA-DR– immunophenotype was only seen in AML, M3. In comparison to the flow cytometric results in this study, CD3 and CD20 were more reliably determined by paraffin IHC techniques; and CD34 and HLA-DR were more reliably determined by flow cytometric analysis. In the same study referred to previously by Arber et al, all precursor T-ALLs had either a CD3+/CD79a–/MPO–/TdT+ or CD3+/CD79a–/MPO–/TdT uninterpretable immunophenotype [Arber 1996]. However, as previously discussed, it should be kept in mind that CD79a may be detected in 10%-50% of precursor T-ALL [Pilozzi 1998], and CD10 may also be expressed in precursor T-ALL **[f10.6]**.

Mature B-cell and T-cell non-Hodgkin lymphomas

As discussed previously, T-LBL may need to be differentiated from BL and MCL-BV. These entities are usually easily distinguished, since the mature B-cell lymphomas express CD20 and PAX-5 by paraffin IHC staining and are negative for TdT and CD34. BL does not typically express any T-cell antigens, although rare cases of CD5+ BL have been reported [Lin 1999]. The blastic variant of MCL typically shows aberrant expression of CD5 but is negative for all other T-cell antigens.

Mature T-cell non-Hodgkin lymphomas may usually be distinguished from T-LBL by the blastic morphology in T-LBL and the lack of TdT-positivity in mature T-cell disorders. However, one should keep in mind the mature stage of T-LBL may also lack TdT-positivity. In some cases, cytogenetic findings may be helpful in distinguishing such entities.

Non-hematolymphoid malignancies

Diagnosing small round cell bone tumors in children may be problematic, especially in limited fixed-tissue specimens. Distinguishing T-LBL from intraosseous Ewing sarcoma (ES) may be particularly difficult due to overlapping morphologic and IHC features. CD99 (MIC2) is characteristically expressed in precursor B- and T-cell lymphoblastic lymphomas/leukemias, as well as in Ewing sarcoma/primitive neuroectodermal tumors (ES/PNET). Vimentin may be demonstrated in both ES (88% of cases) and in 23% of lymphomas and leukemias [Ozdemirli 2001, Lucas 2001]. However, useful IHC markers for the differential diagnosis of T-LBL and ES include T-cell antigens (ie, CD1a, CD2, CD3, CD4, CD5, CD7, and CD8), TdT, CD34, C-kit, and CD10, which all may show variable positivity in T-LBL, but are all negative in ES.

References

No authors listed [1998] The value of *c-kit* in the diagnosis of biphenotypic acute leukemia. EGIL (European Group for the Immunological Classification of Leukaemia). *Leukemia* 12:2038.

Arber DA, Jenkins KA [1996] Paraffin section immunophenotyping of acute leukemias in bone marrow specimens. *Am J Clin Pathol* 106:462-468.

Cessna MH, Dunphy C, Brown M, et al [2002] Differentiation of thymoma from T-lymphoblastic lymphoma by flow cytometry. *Mod Pathol* 15:234A(981).

Han X, Bueso-Ramos CE [2007] Precursor T-cell acute lymphoblastic leukemia/lymphoblastic lymphoma and acute biphenotypic leukemias. *Am J Clin Pathol* 127:528-544.

Keren DF, Hanson CA, Hurtubise PE, eds [1994] *Flow Cytometry and Clinical Diagnosis.* Chicago: ASCP Press; 214.

Lewis RE, Cruse JM, Sanders CM, et al [2006] The immunophenotype of pre-T-ALL/LBL revisited. *Exp Mol Pathol* 81:162-165.

Li S, Juco J, Mann KP, Holden JT [2004] Flow cytometry in the differential diagnosis of lymphocyte-rich thymoma from precursor T-cell acute lymphoblastic leukemia/lymphoblastic lymphoma. *Am J Clin Pathol* 121:268-74.

Lin CW, O'Brien S, Faber J, et al [1999] De-novo CD5+ Burkitt lymphoma/leukemia. *Am J Clin Pathol* 112:828-835.

Lucas DR, Bentley G, Dan ME, Tabaczka P, Poulik JM, Mott MP [2001] Ewing sarcoma vs lymphoblastic lymphoma: A comparative immunohistochemical study. *Am J Clin Pathol* 115:11-17.

Nakajima J, Takamoto S, Oka T, Tanaka M, Takeuchi E, Murakawa T [2000] Flow cytometric analysis of lymphoid cells in thymic epithelial neoplasms. *Eur J Cardiothorac Surg* 18:287-292.

Newell JO, Cessna MH, Greenwood J, Hartung L, Bahler DW [2003] Importance of CD117 in the evaluation of acute leukemias by flow cytometry. *Clin Cytometry* 52B:40-43.

Ozdemirli M, Fanburg-Smith JC, Hartmann D-P, Azumi N, Miettinen M [2001] Differentiating lymphoblastic lymphoma and Ewing's sarcoma: Lymphocyte markers and gene rearrangement. *Mod Pathol* 14:1175-1182.

Paietta E, Ferrando AA, Neuberg D, et al [2004] Activating FLT3 mutations in CD117/KIT(+) T-cell acute lymphoblastic leukemias. *Blood* 104:558-560.

Pilozzi E, Pulford K, Jones M, et al [1998] Co-expression of CD79a (JCB117) and CD3 by lymphoblastic lymphoma. *J Pathol* 186:140-143.

Sperling C, Schwartz S, Buchner T, Thiel E, Ludwig WD [1997] Expression of the stem cell factor receptor C-KIT (CD117) in acute leukemias. *Haematologica* 82:617-621.

Suggs JL, Cruse JM, Lewis RE [2007] Aberrant myeloid marker expression in precursor B-cell and T-cell leukemias. *Exp Mol Pathol* 83:471-473.

Thalhammer-Scherrer R, Mitterbauer G, Simonitsch I, et al [2002] The immunophenotype of 325 adult acute leukemias: Relationship to morphologic and molecular classification and proposal for a minimal screening program highly predictive for lineage discrimination. *Am J Clin Pathol* 117:380-389.

14 Mature T-Cell and Natural Killer (NK)-Cell Neoplasms

Chapter Contents

Classification

- Leukemic/disseminated
  - T-cell prolymphocytic leukemia
  - T-cell large granular lymphocytic leukemia
  - (Chronic lymphoproliferative disoreders of NK cells, 2008)
  - Aggressive NK cell leukemia
  - (Systemic EBV+ T-cell lymphoproliferative disease of childhood, 2008)
  - Adult T-cell leukemia/lymphoma
- Primary cutaneous (WHO-EORTC classification)
  - Mycosis fungoides (indolent)
  - Sézary syndrome (aggressive)
  - Primary cutaneous CD30+ T-cell lymphoproliferative disorders (indolent)
  - (Hydroa vacciniforme-like lymphoma, 2008)
    - Primary cutaneous anaplastic large cell lymphoma
    - Lymphomatoid papulosis
- Subcutaneous panniculitis-like T-cell lymphoma (indolent)
- Provisional entities (No longer provisional, 2008)
  - Primary cutaneous CD4+ small/medium-sized pleomorphic T-cell lymphoma (indolent)
  - Primary cutaneous aggressive epidermotropic CD8+ cytotoxic T-cell lymphoma (aggressive)
  - Primary cutaneous γδ T-cell lymphoma (aggressive)
  - Primary cutaneous NK/T-cell lymphoma, nasal type (aggressive)
  - Primary cutaneous peripheral T-cell lymphoma, unspecified (aggressive)
- Other extranodal
  - Extranodal NK/T-cell lymphoma, nasal type
  - Enteropathy-type T-cell lymphoma (Enteropathy-associated T-cell lymphoma, 2008)
  - Hepatosplenic γδ T-cell lymphoma (Hepatosplenic T-cell lymphoma, 2008)
  - Primary extranodal peripheral T-cell lymphoma, unspecified
- Nodal
  - Angioimmunoblastic T-cell lymphoma
  - Peripheral T-cell lymphoma, unspecified
  - Anaplastic large cell lymphoma (ALK+ and ALK−, 2008)
- Neoplasm of uncertain lineage and stage of differentiation
  - Blastic NK cell lymphoma (ie, CD4+CD56+ hematodermic tumor) (Blastic plasmacytoid dendritic cell neoplasm, 2008)

Introduction

Techniques to differentiate between reactive T-cell and natural killer (NK)-cell processes, and mature T-cell and NK-cell neoplasms, respectively, based on determination of clonality will be discussed, followed by discussions of the specific disease entities.

Differentiation between Mature T-Cell Neoplasms and Reactive Conditions

Detection of aberrant immunophenotype and significance

Unlike the more common mature B-cell neoplasms, in which clonality is often easily established by flow cytometric immunophenotyping (FCI) and detection of restricted light chain expression, there is no entirely specific, diagnostic FCI signature of a clonal T-cell population. Mature T-cell lymphomas may have variable immunophenotypes by FCI. There may be variable loss of a pan T-cell antigen (ie, CD2, CD3, CD5, or CD7); however, not all clonal populations demonstrate loss of a T-cell antigen. Most cases are CD4+; some are CD8+, CD4-/CD8-, or CD4+/CD8+. A representative case of a mature T-cell neoplasm [ie, Sézary syndrome (SS)] with dual loss of both CD4 and CD8 expressions is demonstrated in [f14.1], with the listmode output available on the accompanying disk. Immunophenotypic features that may be detected by FCA and helpful in establishing a diagnosis of a T-cell neoplasm include the following: deletion or decreased expression of 1 of the pan T-cell antigens, anomalous T-cell subset antigen expression (ie, expression not expected according to normal T-cell development, as discussed in detail in Chapter 13), T-cell subset antigen restriction (CD4 vs CD8), a precursor T-cell immunophenotype (as discussed in detail in Chapter 13), aberrant expression of non-T-cell-lineage antigens (ie, CD20 or major myeloid antigens: CD13 or CD33), blastic markers (ie, CD34 or TdT), additional markers not normally expected (ie, CD16, CD30, CD56, or CD57), or T-cell receptors (TCRs), as discussed in more detail below. In addition, review of the inherent forward and side light scatter (FSC and SSC, respectively) properties of the cells may also provide important diagnostic clues. Although most T-cell neoplasms display normal SSC properties (similar to normal T lymphocytes), approximately 25% of cases may demonstrate increased or markedly increased SSC. FSC is typically normal (similar to normal lymphocytes) in over half of T-cell neoplasms, and increased or markedly increased in the remaining cases [Gorczyca 2002].

However, none of these features described above is 100% specific, since aberrant expression of pan-T antigens may be seen in viral infections (particularly loss of CD7), B-cell malignancies (aberrant co-expression of CD5 in chronic lymphocytic leukemia/small lymphocytic lymphoma and mantle cell lymphoma), or in reactive changes following administration of certain medications. An increased CD4:CD8 ratio is often observed in Hodgkin lymphoma. Flow cytometric features that are most suspicious for a mature T-cell neoplasm include the complete loss of 1 or more pan-T antigens, diminished expression of more than 2 pan-T-cell antigens in conjunction with altered light scatter properties, and CD4/CD8 dual-positive or dual-negative expression (except thymic lesions). Of course, correlation with the cytomorphologic features of each case is also critical for an accurate interpretation of the FC data.

Detection of clonality by T-cell receptor Vβ analysis

The TCR is a cell surface molecule responsible for recognizing antigens bound to major histocompatibility complex (MHC) molecules. They are transmembrane heterodimers composed of 2 polypeptide chains (α/β or γ/δ). The majority of T cells express the TCR α/β, while up to 15% of T cells may express the γ and δ chains [Ciccone 1988, Esin 1996]. The TCR is also associated with the CD3 protein complex possessing multiple polypeptide chains, and the CD3 complex together with the TCR forms the TCR complex. The TCR polypeptides are members of the immunoglobulin superfamily, and the receptor molecule possesses 1 N-terminal variable domain, 1 constant domain, a transmembrane/cell membrane-spanning region, and a short cytoplasmic tail at the C-terminal end. The TCR gene locus comprises many segments of genes, including the variable (V), diversity (D), joint (J), and constant (C) genes. The variable domains of TCR α and γ chains are generated by VJ recombination, while those of the β and δ chains are generated by VDJ recombination. It is the unique combination of the segments, along with palindromic and random nucleotide additions and deletions at the junctional sites, that accounts for the great diversity of specific TCRs for processed antigen. The hypervariable or complementarity-determining regions (CDRs) encoded in TCR-variable domains are responsible for recognizing processed antigens.

FCI of the T-cell repertoire with monoclonal antibodies directed against V domains of TCR-Vβ molecules was adopted after many monoclonal antibodies against V domains of TCR-Vβ molecules

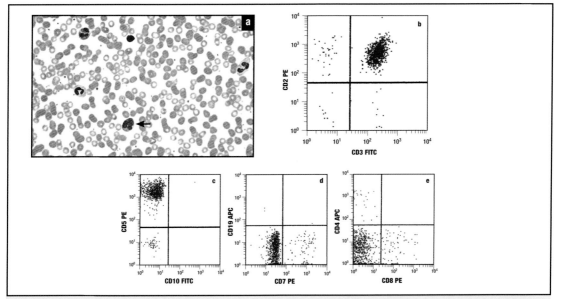

[f14.1] This case of Sézary syndrome demonstrates a rare CD4–/CD8– immunophenotype. The clinical history reveals a 58-year-old male with a history of Sézary syndrome who presents with continued fevers and a concern for sepsis. A peripheral blood specimen is submitted for flow cytometric analysis. CBC data include WBC 10.9 × 10³/mm³ (10.9 × 10⁹/L), Hgb 10.3 g/dL, Plt 356 × 10³/mm³ (356 × 10⁹/L) absolute lymphocyte count: 2.3 × 10³/mm³ (2.3 × 10⁹/L). The peripheral blood smear morphology **a** demonstrates a convoluted lymphocyte (arrow). By flow cytometric analysis, the lymphocyte region (19% of the peripheral WBCs) is composed of 95% T cells with an aberrant immunophenotype. The aberrant T cells express CD3 **b**, CD2 **b**, and CD5 **c** with loss of CD7 **d**, CD4 **e**, and CD8 **e**. The diagnosis is made of Sézary syndrome, lacking CD4 and CD8 expressions.

were developed [Van den Beemd 2000, McCoy 1996]. Based on the sequence identity at the nucleotide level, the TCRβ variable protein classification system, established by the World Health Organization, has resulted in the identification of 25 different functional Vβ families (with 91 subfamily and allele members in total) [Kazatchkine 1995]. Because of this diversity, each individual TCR-Vβ segment is expressed in only a small percentage of T cells [Rosenberg 1992]. Therefore, a panel of antibodies against different TCR-Vβ segments may be applied to determine the presence of an expanded usage of a single Vβ domain and thus, the presence of a clonally rearranged TCR-Vβ segment. Such a case is demonstrated in **[f14.2]**, with the listmode output available on the accompanying disk. As such, the FCI-based detection of the TCR β-chain, using a panel of monoclonal antibodies that recognize individual TCR β-chain V regions, is an attractive alternative approach to polymerase chain reaction (PCR) studies, since it easily and rapidly provides precise quantitative information regarding T-cell clonality. Furthermore, it is possible to combine Vβ domain monoclonal antibodies with other markers to selectively analyze different T-cell subsets [McCoy 1996].

It should be noted that the 24 different anti-TCR-Vβ antibodies in the IOTest Beta Mark kit recognize approximately 70% of the normal human TCR-Vβ repertoire. However, this does not infer it may be useful in detecting only 70% of cases with clonal T-cell populations. In fact, if the selected target T cells express CD3 and the α/β receptor, and none of the 24 anti- TCR-Vβ antibodies binds to them, it may also be assumed these cells represent a clone of T cells that are not recognized by the available 24 antibodies Indeed, most of these cases will demonstrate clonal TCR gene rearrangements by molecular analysis [Lima 2001, Beck 2003, Morice 2004, Morice 2006].

Although peripheral blood has been the type of specimen most often studied by TCR-Vβ testing, body fluid specimens, bone marrow aspirates, and cell suspensions of lymphoid tissue biopsies (from lymph nodes and extranodal sites) may also be similarly analyzed. The overall patterns of polyclonal TCR-Vβ expression of T cells in peripheral blood, bone marrows, and lymphoid tissues are all very similar [Li 2007].

At what levels should one define an expanded T-cell subset as a monoclonal T-cell population? Some authors have used a cutoff >3 standard deviations above the

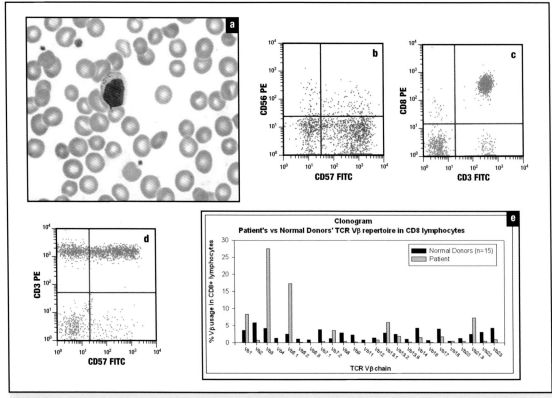

[f14.2] This case demonstrates the application of T-cell receptor Vβ testing in a typical T-cell large granular lymphocytic leukemia. The clinical history reveals a 66-year-old man with persistent chest pain. Studies showed widespread lymphadenopathy, diagnosed as mantle cell, with BM involvement. He received R-CHOP ×6, BEAM conditioning, and autologous bone marrow transplant (au-BMT). Six weeks post-au-BMT, a 2 cm left axillary lymph node was associated with a peripheral blood lymphocytosis (8,100 × 10³/mm³ (8,100 × 10⁹/L) with abnormal lymphocytes). The peripheral blood smear morphology **a** demonstrates a typical large granular lymphocyte. By flow cytometric analysis **b-d**, these cells express CD2, CD3 **c, d**, CD5, CD7, CD8 **c**, and CD57 **b, d** and do not express CD4, CD16, or CD56 **b**. No monoclonal B-cell population is detected. Flow cytometric studies for the T-cell receptor β chain showed clonal expansion of the Vb3 chain **e**. The diagnosis is made of T-cell large granular lymphocytic leukemia following au-BMT for mantle cell lymphoma.

mean percentage of control Vβ values, or they have used reference data provided by the antibody manufacturer that contain the mean, standard deviation, and minimum and maximum values for each Vβ family as a percentage of total CD3+ cells [Beck 2003, Fitzgerald 1995, van den Beemd 2000]. In other publications, clonality has been defined as the expression of a single TCR-Vβ, either 10-fold above its normal maximum or by >50% of the T cells in any analyzed population [Morice 2004]. Cases have been considered suggestive of containing clonal T cells by TCR-Vβ FCI if, in any analyzed population, a single TCR-Vβ is expressed by 40%-49% of the cells, or if >70% of the cells fail to react with any of the TCR-Vβ antibodies tested. Cases failing to meet any of the aforementioned criteria have been considered non-clonal [Morice 2004].

It should be emphasized that the presence of clonal T cells does not necessarily imply T-cell malignancy. It is well known that clonal T cells detected by PCR analysis of TCR gene rearrangements may be seen in some cases without evidence of T-cell neoplasia, such as in the elderly or in patients with reactive inflammatory processes or autoimmune disorders [Lamberson 2001, Masuko-Hongo 1998, Posnett 1994]. Likewise, TCR-Vβ restrictions may be observed in non-neoplastic conditions, and therefore, the finding of an abnormal expansion of TCR-Vβ clone must always be interpreted in combination with morphology, the clinical context, and other laboratory findings. To address these equivocal cases, one should also look at other phenotypic features of the putative abnormal cells, such as size and aberrant antigen expression. These informative features cannot be obtained by molecular analysis of TCR gene arrangements alone.

Compared with the PCR assay for TCR gene rearrangements, FCI is faster and, more importantly, can accurately quantitate the number of clonal T cells, enabling follow-up studies and detection of residual disease. The recent report by Beck et al describes a sensitivity of 89% for direct detection of pathogenic Vβ restriction and a specificity of 88% by this technique [Beck 2003]. with increasing numbers of anti-TCR antibodies and the availability of 6- to 8-color flow cytometers, FCI should become even more efficient and a standard practice in the clinical laboratory for the evaluation of T-cell clonality.

Differentiation between Mature NK-Cell Neoplasms and Reactive Conditions

Immunophenotypic attributes of NK cells, traditional NK-cell-associated antigens, and their role in diagnosing NK-cell proliferative disorders

Natural killer (NK) cells are a distinct lymphocyte subset that, like cytotoxic T cells, recognize and destroy abnormal self-cells. The defining features of a true NK cell include large granular lymphocyte (LGL) cytology, the absence of TCR gene rearrangements (ie, TCR genes in germline configuration) or a fully assembled TCR-CD3 complex, and the expressions of CD16 and CD56 [Lotzova 1989, Lanier 1986]. Large granular lymphocytes derive from 2 major cell lines: natural killer cells and T cells. Clonal expansions of large granular lymphocytes may be categorized based on a combination of clinical features, cytomorphology, FC immunophenotype, and clonality analysis into the following: chronic NK cell expansion (chronic NK cell lymphocytosis), NK large granular lymphocytic (LGL) leukemia (also termed aggressive NK cell leukemia), and T-LGL leukemia. Clonality may be defined by the detection of a single band for the joined termini of the EBV genome or by the analyses of NK antigens (ie, EB6 and GL183) or killer cell immunoglobulin receptors (KIRs) (both analyses discussed in further detail in the next subsection) in those of NK-cell origin, and by the detection of a TCR gene rearrangement in those of T-cell origin.

Mature NK-cell neoplasms must be differentiated from secondary or "reactive" LGL expansions (in which the absolute NK cell count rarely exceeds 2×10^9/L). The causes of secondary LGL expansions include malignancies (ie, leukemia, lymphoma, solid tumors, and myelodysplastic syndromes), immune thrombocytopenia purpura, a host of viral infections (ie, EBV, CMV, Hep B virus, Hep C virus, and HIV), connective tissue diseases,

as well as post-chemotherapy and post-bone marrow transplantation settings. Because NK cells, unlike T cells, lack a uniquely rearranged antigen receptor gene that may be used for clonality assessment, establishing the presence of an immunophenotypically distinct cell population is a central element in diagnosing NK-cell lymphoproliferative disorders.

Traditional NK-cell--associated antigens include CD16, [a receptor for the Fc portion of IgG (FcγRIII)], CD56 (a neural cell adhesion molecule) and CD57. Mature NK cells are virtually all CD16+, and they may be subdivided into 2 distinct subsets. One subset has bright CD16 and dim CD56 expression (approximately 90% of NK cells), and the other has dim surface CD16 and bright surface CD56 expression (the remaining 10% of NK cells). As with most, if not all, NK-cell antigens, CD16 is also present on a small proportion (<5%) of normal cytotoxic T cells [Farag 2006]. There are no currently available antibodies to CD16 that are reactive in paraffin-embedded material. Although CD56 is commonly associated with NK-cell lineage, it is expressed on a wide variety of hematopoietic and nonhematopoietic cells, including T cells. CD57 is a cell-surface glycoprotein expressed by approximately two-thirds of NK cells and was first identified in this cell type [Abo 1981]. CD57 is also expressed by a number of other cell types, including memory cytotoxic T cells [Tarazona 2000], and may have some value in defining the aberrant immunophenotype of clonally expanded NK-cell populations.

By FCI, normal NK cells are CD2+/CD5–, CD7+/CD3–, typically show partial co-expression of CD8 (with a staining intensity that is approximately half that seen on the CD8+ T cells) [Trinchieri 1989], and are CD16+ or CD16+/CD56+. In normal NK cells, a range of CD16 expression should be observed.

Aberrant NK-cell populations may have diminished expression of CD2 or CD7 and demonstrate an abnormal gain of expression of CD5. In NK-cell lymphoproliferative disorders, the cells may be uniformly CD8+, a finding that is sufficiently distinctive to be considered aberrant. Given that normal NK cells are weakly CD8+, the absence of this antigen on NK cells is not sufficient to reliably distinguish them as abnormal. The pattern of CD16 expression by NK cells may be useful in identifying abnormal NK-cell populations. In NK-cell large granular lymphocytic leukemia (NK-LGLL), the cells often exhibit uniform bright CD16 expression [Morice 2003]. It is interesting that this bright expression of CD16 in NK-LGLL tends to be associated with diminished to absent staining for CD56 and CD57. Even with these described aberrancies, the usefulness of FCI is somewhat limited. Abnormal NK cells may show normal patterns of expression of CD2, CD7, CD16, and CD56, and, conversely, normal NK cells may show altered expression of these antigens [Zambello 1993]. Thus, determination of NK cell "clonality" would be helpful in these situations.

Detection of NK cell subsets and NK cell clonality [t14.1]
Reactive or secondary NK-cell expansions may be differentiated from chronic NK-cell lymphocytosis of clonal origin (ie, chronic lymphoproliferative disorders of NK cells) and from NK-LGLL by analysis of NK antigens, EB6 and GL183. Normal NK cells express these antigens as 4 subsets (EB6+/GL183+, EB6+/GL183–, EB6–/GL183–, and EB6–/GL183+). However, clonality is defined by expression of a restricted phenotype [Lanier 1998]. More recently, new classes of NK-associated major histocompatibility complex receptors have been described that may be of value in evaluating NK-cell and cytotoxic T-cell populations. These receptors are now known to be encoded by at least 2 distinct families of genes and gene products, including KIRs, which are members of the immunoglobulin gene superfamily, and the CD94/NKG2 complexes, which are members of the C-type lectin superfamily [Leibson 1998]. They are now broadly referred to as NK-cell receptors, or NKRs,

There are multiple KIR isoforms, each of which is encoded by a single gene and contains 2 or 3 extracellular immunoglobulin-like domains. These structurally distinct KIRs each recognize a specific group of MHC-I alleles. In contrast, the ligands for the CD94/NKG2 complexes are a group of MHC-I-related antigens with limited polymorphism such as HLA-E [Hoffmann 2000]. From a diagnostic perspective, the KIRs are of particular interest because they are stably expressed over multiple cell generations and, therefore, can serve as a marker of clonal cellular expansion. In contrast, the CD94/NKG2 complexes are not clonally expressed. The usefulness of KIR expression patterns in detecting clonal cellular expansions has been established, in large part, through FC studies of T-LGLL. In this disorder of memory T cells, the uniform expression of a single (or multiple) KIR isoform has been found to be highly correlated with the presence of clonal TCR gene rearrangements [Morice 2003, Pascal 2004]. Paraffin-reactive antibody reagents to the KIR antigens are not currently available.

In NK-LGLL, approximately one third of cases exhibit restricted expression of a single (or multiple)

---

t14.1 Methods for Establishing NK Cell Clonality

1. Detection of a single band for the joined termini of the EBV genome

2. Detetion of a restricted NK phenotype (ie, EB6+/GL183+, EB6+/GL183–, EB6–/GL183+, or EB6–/GL183–)

3. Detection of the uniform expression of a single (or multiple) KIR isoform

EBV, Epstein-Barr virus; KIR, killer cell immunoglobulin receptor; NK, natural killer.

KIR isoform strongly associated with clonality in T-LGL [Morice 2003, Epling-Burnette 2004, Warren 2003]. The remaining NK-LGLL cases lack detectable expression of the 3 ubiquitously expressed KIRs (ie CD158a, CD158b, and CD158e). The uniform absence of these KIRs on NK cells is aberrant because in normal NK-cell populations, there are subsets positive for each.

As mentioned previously, unlike the KIRs, CD94/NKG2 heterodimers and similar receptors (such as CD161) cannot serve as surrogate markers of clonality. Nevertheless, these antigens are still helpful in evaluating NK-cell populations. In NK-LGLL, the abnormal cells often show uniform bright expression of CD94 exclusively paired with NKG2A to form an inhibitory receptor complex [Morice 2003, Herling 2004a]. This is in contrast to normal NK cells, in which there is variable staining intensity for CD94 with a mixture of CD94/NKG2A and CD94/NKG2C heterodimers present. Abnormal loss of CD161 expression is also frequent in NK-LGL. These patterns of CD94/NKG2A heterodimers and CD161 expression can serve as additional features to distinguish NK-LGL from reactive NK-cell expansions. Thus, a comprehensive approach to NK cell immunophenotyping, including evaluation of NKRs, can enable the distinction of abnormal NK-cell expansions from cytotoxic T cells and reactive NK-cell populations.

Leukemic/Disseminated T-Cell Prolymphocytic Leukemia (T-PLL)

Definition

T-cell prolymphocytic leukemia (T-PLL) is an aggressive T-cell leukemia characterized by the proliferation of small to medium-sized prolymphocytes with a mature post-thymic T-cell phenotype involving the peripheral blood (PB), bone marrow (BM), lymph nodes, liver, spleen, and skin.

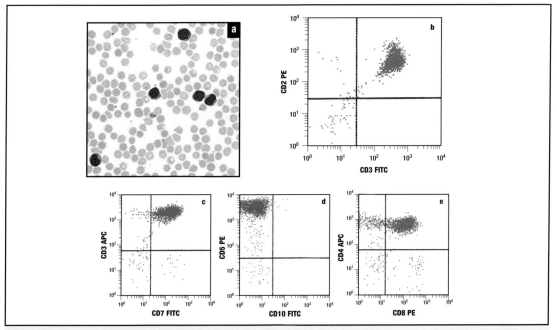

[f14.3] This case demonstrates a typical T-cell prolymphocytic leukemia. The clinical history reveals a 57-year-old female with a history of T-cell prolymphocytic leukemia who presents with an elevated WBC count. A peripheral blood specimen is submitted for flow cytometric analysis. CBC data include WBC 35.5 × 10³/mm³ (35.5 × 10⁹/L), Hgb 14.5 g/dL, Plt 95 × 10³/mm³ (95 × 10⁹/L), absolute lymphocyte count 28.6 × 10³/mm³ (28.6 × 10⁹/L). The peripheral blood smear morphology **a** demonstrates lymphocytes with a prominent nucleolus. By flow cytometric analysis, the lymphocyte region (80% of the peripheral WBCs) is composed of 97% T cells with an aberrant immunophenotype. The aberrant T cells express CD3 **b, c**, CD2 **b**, CD7 **c**, CD5 **d**, CD25 (not demonstrated), and dual expressions of CD4 **e** and CD8 **e**. The diagnosis is made of T-cell prolymphocytic leukemia, with coexpression of CD4 and CD8.

Typical Immunophenotype

T-PLL expresses pan-T-cell antigens (CD2, CD3, CD5, CD7) with CD4+/CD8− >CD4+/CD8+ (up to a third of cases) >CD4−/CD8+ (approximately 15% of cases). Other markers of immaturity (ie, CD34, CD1a, and TdT) are absent [Herling 2004b, Catovsky 2001].

Morphologic Variants

Although nuclear chromatin condensation is typically present, characteristic of a mature cell disorder, the nuclear contours and prevalence of distinctive central nucleoli are quite variable in T-PLL. Some cases exhibit a single, prominent central nucleolus (like B-PLL), whereas others exhibit nuclear irregularity with inconspicuous nucleoli and some, round nuclear contours with highly condensed nuclear chromatin and inconspicuous nucleoli (ie, small-cell variant, like CLL). Representative cases of T-PLL and the small-cell variant are demonstrated in **[f14.3]** and **[f14.4]** (with the list-mode output available on the accompanying disk), respectively.

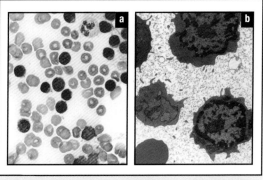

[f14.4] This case demonstrates the morphology of the small cell variant of T-cell prolymphcotyic leukemia. The peripheral blood smear morphology **a** demonstrates the small round lymphocytes without a recognizable nucleolus by light microscopy. However, by electron microscopy **b**, the nucleolus is demonstrated.

Differential Diagnosis

CLL

The morphology of T-CLL and the small cell variant of T-PLL are indistinguishable based on light microscopy alone. They are composed of small lymphocytes with morphology similar to B-CLL. It is important to distinguish B-CLL from T-CLL and the small-cell variant of T-PLL due to a more aggressive clinical course associated with T-CLL and T-PLL [Dunphy 1995]. The small cell variant of T-PLL and T-CLL may be distinguished from B-CLL by the differences in immunophenotype (see Chapter 12 for the detailed immunophenotypic features of B-CLL). On the other hand, the distinction between T-CLL and the small cell variant of T-PLL must be based on electron microscopic examination. The cells of T-CLL do not possess nucleoli by ultrastructure, whereas the cells of the small cell variant of T-PLL all contain a single nucleolus by EM. However, the distinction between T-CLL and the small-cell variant of T-PLL seems less important, since both of these entities have a similar aggressive clinical course.

B-PLL
T-PLL may be distinguished from B-PLL by the differences in their immunophenotypes (see Chapter 12 for the detailed immunophenotypic features of B-PLL).

Mycosis fungoides (MF)/Sézary syndrome (SS), adult T-cell leukemia/lymphoma (ATLL), and peripheralized T-cell lymphoma
The cases of T-PLL exhibiting nuclear irregularity with inconspicuous nucleoli may morphologically mimic MF/SS or ATLL. The immunophenotypic features are compared in [t14.2]. Cases of MF/SS and ATLL characteristically have extremely folded nuclear contours and lack expression of CD7. ATLL characteristically also expresses CD25. The distinction of T-PLL from a peripheralizing T-cell lymphoma would likely depend on a prior diagnostic lymphoid tissue biopsy. If the clinical history, morphology, and immunophenotypic features do not allow distinction of these entities, the demonstration of TCL-1 oncoprotein expression by immunohistochemical (IHC) staining may be reasonably specific for T-PLL [Herling 2004a, Valbuena 2005]. A diagnosis of T-PLL should be strongly considered in cases with prototypic clinical and hematologic features even when neither TCL-1 IHC staining nor the cytogenetic rearrangement involving the TCL-1 locus is detected. Since conventional karyotyping often misses detection of TCL-1 locus rearrangements, fluorescent in-situ hybridization (FISH) studies are routinely recommended in cases negative by conventional cytogenetic analysis. However, one should keep in mind that TCL-1 expression is well-documented in many other neoplasms, including B-cell leukemias and lymphomas, and non-neoplastic cells [Valbuena 2005, Herling 2006, Teitell 2005].

Precursor T-cell lymphoblastic leukemia/lymphoma
T-PLL may be distinguished from precursor T-cell lymphoblastic neoplasms by the lack of expressions of CD34, CD1a, and TdT in T-PLL.

T-Cell Large Granular Lymphocytic Leukemia (LGLL)

Definition
T-cell large granular lymphocytic leukemia (T-LGLL) is defined as a chronic clonal proliferation of large granular lymphocytes ($>2 \times 10^3/mm^3$ [$>2 \times 10^9/L$]) for at least 6 months duration. The morphology of a typical large granular lymphocyte is characterized by a copious amount of light bluish cytoplasm and fine azurophilic granules. As mentioned previously, they may be of T-cell or true NK-cell origin. T-LGLLs are usually indolent and associated with neutropenia, recurrent infection, rheumatoid arthritis, and splenomegaly.

Typical Immunophenotype and Variants
The immunophenotype of T-LGLL is outlined in [t14.2]. By FCI, the neoplastic cells of T-LGLL reveal expression of CD8 and abnormal expression of 2 or more pan-T-cell antigens in 80% of cases. CD5 and CD7 are most commonly abnormal, with dim or absent expression the most common, although abnormal bright expression may be seen as well [Morice 2003, Lundell 2005, Gorczyca 2002]. Abnormal, diminished expression of CD2, CD3, or other T-cell antigens may also rarely be demonstrated. Normal T-LGLL cells are CD16- and CD56-. The neoplastic cells of T-LGLL express CD16 in approximately 80% of cases and CD57 in almost all cases. They reveal a T-cell gene rearrangement, most often of the αβ type. A representative case is demonstrated in [f14.5].

There are 3 notable variants of T-LGLL, based primarily on immunophenotypic differences. These are rare, and it is unclear whether they have significantly different clinical findings to justify being classified as distinct entities. They are described as follows:

1. CD4+ T-LGLL differs from typical T-LGLL in that 80% of patients have normal physical examination findings with only rare splenomegaly, somewhat more frequent lymphadenopathy, and lacking neutropenia and anemia, in contrast with CD8+ T-LGLL [Herling 2004b, Lima 2003]. There is no apparent association with rheumatoid arthritis or other rheumatologic diseases.

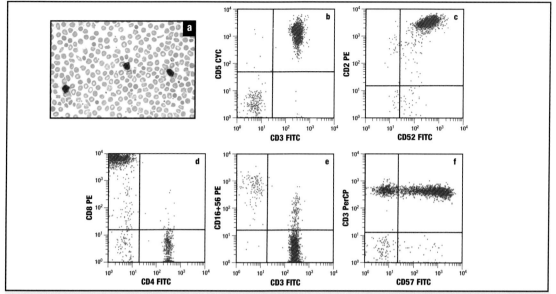

[f14.5] This case demonstrates the typical morphology and immunophenotype of T-cell large granular lymphocytic leukemia. The clinical history reveals a 71-year-old male with a previous clinical history of colorectal cancer and subsequent blastic mantle cell leukemia (treated with an autologous stem cell transplant 6 weeks previously) who now presents with an absolute lymphocytosis. A peripheral blood specimen is submitted for flow cytometric analysis. CBC data include WBC $18.3 \times 10^3/mm^3$ ($18.3 \times 10^9/L$), Hgb 13.8 g/dL, Plt $266 \times 10^3/mm^3$ ($266 \times 10^9/L$), absolute lymphocyte count $13.4 \times 10^3/mm^3$ ($13.4 \times 10^9/L$). The peripheral blood smear morphology **a** demonstrates large granular lymphocytes. By flow cytometric analysis, the lymphocyte region (73% of the peripheral WBCs) is composed of 93% of cells expressing CD3 **b, e, f**, CD5 **b**, CD2 **c**, intense CD8 **d**, and CD57 **f** without CD16 or CD56 **e**. The PCR molecular analysis reveal TCR γ gene rearrangement. Diagnosis is made of T-cell large granular lymphocytic leukemia.

2. CD8+ T-LGLLs co-expressing CD56 may have a more aggressive clinical behavior [Gentile 1998]. Although large studies do not exist, cases of T-LGLL expressing CD56 may require closer follow-up to evaluate for an aggressive clinical course.

3. Cases of γδ T-LGLL (CD8+) exist but are rare in comparison with αβ T-LGLLs. The immunophenotype of γδ T-LGLL varies somewhat from that of the typical αβ type: CD3+, CD2+, CD4–, CD8 variable (38%), CD5 variable (60%), CD7 variable (100%), CD16+ in most cases (86%), CD56 variable (38%), and CD57 variable (57%) [Herling 2004b, Kondo 2001, Saito 2002, Makishima 2003, Shichishima 2004, Ahmad 2005]. In comparison with other γδ lymphoproliferative disorders, γδ T-LGL leukemias have an excellent prognosis and are considered an indolent disease. However, studies directly comparing αβ T-LGL leukemia have not been reported [O'Malley 2007].

Differential Diagnosis

Reactive T-cell LGL

As mentioned previously, reactive large granular lymphocytoses may occur secondary to many causes. A reactive T-cell LGL is differentiated from a T-cell LGLL primarily by the demonstration of a clonal T-cell population in T-cell LGLL.

Reactive NK-cell LGL, chronic NK-cell lymphocytosis, and NK-LGLL

Large granular lymphocytes, as discussed previously, may be of NK-cell or T-cell lineage [Loughran 1993]. Neoplastic entities associated with this proliferation include the following: NK-cell expansion (or chronic NK cell lymphocytosis), NK-LGLL (or aggressive NK-cell leukemia), and T-LGLL (all discussed above) [Zambello 1993, Semenzato 1997]. Chronic NK-cell lymphocytosis and T-LGLL have a more chronic, indolent course than NK-LGLL. Patients with NK-LGL leukemia present at a younger age and have an acute clinical course with systemic disease. T-LGLL may be distinguished from reactive NK-LGL, chronic NK-cell lymphocytosis, and NK-LGLL most often by its distinctive flow cytometric immunophenoypes, as outlined in **[t14.2]**.

t14.2 NK- and T-Cell Neoplasms: Surface Antigens and Associated Cytogenetic Abnormalities

Disease Entity	CD2	CD3	CD4	CD5	CD7	CD8	CD16	CD56	CD57	Additional FC, IHC, Molecular, and Cytogenetic Abnormalities (Abns)
T-PLL	+	+	±	+	+	±	–	–	–	TCL1 +; 36 TCR gene rearrangements detected; abns of chromosomes 8 or 14 [Dunphy 1995]; most distinctive: inv(14)(q11q32)
T-CLL	+	+	±	+	+	±	–	–	–	TCR gene rearrangements detected; abns of chromosome 14 [Witzig 1986]
T-LGLL (3 phenotypic variants; see text for further details)	var+	var+	±	+	+	±	+(80% of cases)	±	+	TCR gene rearrangements detected, most often αβ; trisomies 8 and 14 [Loughran 1985]
Chronic NK-cell lymphocytosis	var+, dim	–	–	±	var+, dim	±	+, uniform and bright	–/wk+	–/wk+	*
NK-LGLL (ie aggressive NK-cell leukemia) and Extranodal NK/T-cell lymphoma, nasal type	+	–‡	–	–	–	–	Usually –	Usually – +	Usually –	TCR and Ig genes germline in majority of cases; EBV + (EBER-ISH); cytotoxic granule-associated proteins (ie, perforin granzyme B, and TIA-1) +; del(6q) and chromosome X copy gain [Wong 2000]
ATLL‡	+	var+	±	+	–	±	–	–	–	TCR gene rearrangements detected; HTLV-1 +; large transformed cells may be CD30+; cytotoxic granule-associated proteins –; trisomies 3, 7, or 21, del(14q), and loss of X [Naeim 2001]
MF and SS†	±	+/rare–	+	±	–	Rare+	–	–	–	TCR gene rearrangements detected; cytotoxic granule-associated proteins + in a fraction of neoplastic cells in advanced MF lesions; abnormal 2p, 6q, isochromosome 17q, and del(13q14) [Brito-Babapulle 2001]
SPTCL	ND	+	–	ND	ND	+	ND	ND	Focal, rare+	TCR gene rearrangement detected, αβ type only; cytotoxic granule-associated proteins +; EBV–
Primary cutaneous CD4+ small/medium sized pleomorphic TCL	ND	+	+	ND	ND	–	ND	ND	ND	TCR gene rearrangements detected; cytotoxic granule-associated proteins–; no consistent cytogenetic abns
Primary cutaneous aggressive epidermotropic CD8+ cytotoxic TCL	–	+	–	–	±	+	ND	ND	ND	TCR gene rearrangements detected; cytotoxic granule-associated proteins +; EBV–; no specific cytogenetic abns

Entity	Comments
aggressive epidermotropic CD8+ cytotoxic TCL	TCR gene rearrangements detected; cytotoxic granule-associated proteins +; EBV–; no specific cytogenetic abns
ETL	CD103+; TCR β and γ gene rearrangements detected; cytotoxic granule-associated proteins+; EBV–; CD30+ in varying proportion of neoplastic cells; EBV–; recurrent chromosomal gains of 9q, 7q, 5q, and 1q and recurrent losses of 8p, 13q, and 9p; most eminent chromosomal abn is gain of 9q33-q34, only rarely detectable in other types of PTCL [Zettl 2002, Deleeuw 2007]
γδ TCL	CD25–; CD30–; EBV–; TCR gene rearrangements detected, most often γδ type, but also αβ type—same features; hepatosplenic form: TIA-1+, granzyme B and perforin–; mucosal and cutaneous forms: TIA-1, granzyme B, and perforin+; isochromosome 7q: consistent abn of hepatosplenic TCL51;145-147; trisomy 8 and loss of Y also reported
AITL	Neoplastic cells are CD4+, CD10+, CXCL13+; generally normal CD4:CD8 ratio (background non-neoplastic CD8+ cells); increased CD21+ FDCs; interfollicular CD20+ large cells are typically EBV+ and clonal; TCR gene rearrangement detected (up to 80% of cases); most common cytogenetic abns: trisomies 3 and 5, an extra X
ALCL	CD25+; CD30 uniformly and intensely +; CD45 variably + (negative more often by IHC staining); CD13, CD15, and CD33 may be aberrantly expressed; cytotoxic granule-associated proteins+; EBV generally–; CD44v marks systemic (not primary cutaneous) ALCL [Liang 2002]; ALK (NPM/ALK)+ in 60%-85% of primary systemic cases; TCR gene rearrangements detected
PTCL, NOS	EBV generally–; CD30 may be variably + in large cell variants, not as strongly/uniformly as ALCL; TCR gene rearrangements detected; cytotoxic granule-associated proteins–; variable cytogenetic abns [Brito-Babapulle 2001]
HDT	CD45+, CD43+, HLA-DR+, CD45RA+, TCL1+, BCAD2+, MxA+, CD123+, CD68+, EBV–, MPO–; no TCR gene rearrangements detected; no single defining genetic abn; complex structural chromosomal abns, most frequent abn: del 5q (up to 72% of cases), followed (decreasing frequency): abns of 13q, 12p, and 6q and losses of 15 and 9. [Brody 1995, Kameoka 1998, Petrella 1999, DiGiuseppe 1997, Leroux 2002]

AITL, angioimmunoblastic TCL; ALCL, anaplastic large cell lymphoma; ATLL, adult T-cell leukemia/lymphoma; BCAD, blood dendritic cell antigen; CLL, chronic lymphocytic leukemia; EBV, Epstein Barr virus; ETL, enteropathy-associated TCL; FC, flow cytometric; FDCs, follicular dendritic cells; HDT, CD4+CD56+ hematodermic tumor; Ig, immunoglobulin; IHC, immunohistochemical; LGLL, large granular lymphocytic leukemia; MF, mycosis fungoides; MPO, myeloperoxidase; MxA, myxovirus A; ND, not described; NK, natural killer; PLL, prolymphocytic leukemia; PTCL, NOS, peripheral TCL, not otherwise specified; SPTCL, subcutaneous panniculitis-like T-cell lymphoma; SS, Sézary syndrome; TCL, T-cell lymphoma; TCR, T-cell receptor; var, variable; wk, weak;

*Chromosomal abnormalities have not been well-defined in NK-cell expansions.

†CD25 is characteristically expressed in ATLL, and may be variably expressed in SS. In addition, CD26 negativity combined with CD4 positivity and CD7 negativity is useful in following patients with a known diagnosis of SS

‡cCD3 may be demonstrated in these cases.

§Pleomorphic-anaplastic ETL is usually associated with a history of celiac disease and is usually CD56–; monomorphic ETL most often occurs without a history of celiac disease and is usually CD56+/CD8+.

Mastocytosis

Systemic mastocytosis may mimic T-LGLL involving the spleen, BM, and nodal sites. As described in Chapter 18, neoplastic mast cells do not express B-lineage or T-lineage associated antigens but instead express CD2, CD117, and CD25 by FCI, greatly aiding in the distinction of these 2 entities.

CLL

T-LGLL may easily be differentiated from B-CLL by the differences in their flow cytometric immunophenotypes (see Chapter 12 for the detailed immunophenotypic features of B-CLL).

T-PLL

T-PLL is usually associated with a relatively rapid onset and an aggressive clinical course. Rare cases of T-PLL may be CD8+ (15%), but most cases are CD4+ or CD4+/CD8+. As discussed previously, cytogenetic abnormalities are seen in most cases, and TCL1 staining is positive, in contrast with T-LGLL.

Hepatosplenic T-cell lymphoma

Hepatosplenic T-cell lymphoma may have similar sites of involvement (PB, BM, and spleen) but is more frequent in younger patients and has a more aggressive clinical course than T-LGLL. Also, it differs from T-LGLL in immunophenotype (most cases are CD4–/CD8–) and by the presence of isochromosome 7q [Alonsozana 1997].

Extranodal NK/T-cell lymphoma, nasal type

There is considerable overlap in the immunophenotype of T-LGLL and extranodal nasal-type NK/T lymphoma, although a leukemic form of the latter entity exists. Significantly different findings in extranodal nasal-type NK/T lymphoma include the abnormal, slightly larger granular lymphocytes, frequent presence of CD56, lack of CD8 expression, and EBV positivity. It is thought that the entity, described below as aggressive NK-cell leukemia, may actually correspond to a leukemic form of extranodal NK/T lymphoma of the nasal type, and would have comparable differences with T-LGLL, both morphologically and immunophenotypically.

Aggressive NK-Cell Leukemia

Definition

Aggressive NK-cell leukemia is characterized by a systemic proliferation of NK cells with an aggressive clinical course.

Typical Immunophenotype

The neoplastic cells are CD2+, sCD3–, cCD3+, CD56+ and positive for cytotoxic granule-associated proteins (ie, perforin, TIA-1, and granzyme B), which are identical to the immunophenotype of extranodal NK/T-cell lymphoma, nasal type. CD16 may be expressed, but CD57 is usually negative. CD11b may also be expressed. The great majority of cases harbor EBV in a clonal episomal form. A representative case is demonstrated in [f14.6], with the listmode output available on the accompanying disk.

Differential Diagnosis

Acute leukemia, myeloid/natural killer precursor acute leukemia, and CD4+/CD56+ hematodermic tumor (alias blastoid natural killer cell lymphoma)

Since these cells are larger than normal LGLs and have cytoplasmic granules, the consideration of an AML, a CD56+ precursor T-cell lymphoblastic leukemia, or a myeloid/NK precursor acute leukemia may arise. Myeloid/NK cell precursor acute leukemia is characterized by co-expression of myeloid and natural killer cell antigens (ie, expression of CD7, CD33, CD34, CD56, and frequently HLA-DR but not other NK, T-cell, or B-cell markers) and an aggressive clinical course. On the other hand, the cells of aggressive NK-cell leukemia lack all markers of immaturity (ie, CD34, CD1a, and TdT) and do not express myelomonocytic markers, other than CD11b. Lastly the neoplastic cells of CD4+/CD56+ hematodermic tumor (HDT) are tumors of plasmacytoid dendritic cell lineage and express CD4 and CD56 in the absence of lineage-specific markers of T cells, B cells, or myelomonocytic markers. Expression of EBV antigens actually excludes a diagnosis of HDT and aids in distinguishing these entities [Suzuki 1997].

Peripheralized large cell lymphoma, including peripheralized NK/T-cell lymphoma, nasal type

Due to the immunophenotypic features, the main consideration is whether aggressive NK-cell leukemia actually represents the peripheralized form of extranodal NK/T-cell lymphoma, nasal type.

Systemic EBV+ T-Cell Lymphoproliferative Disease of Childhood

Definition

Systemic EBV+ T-cell LPD of childhood is a rapidly progressive, life-threatening childhood (and young adulthood) illness with multisystem organ failure, sepsis, and

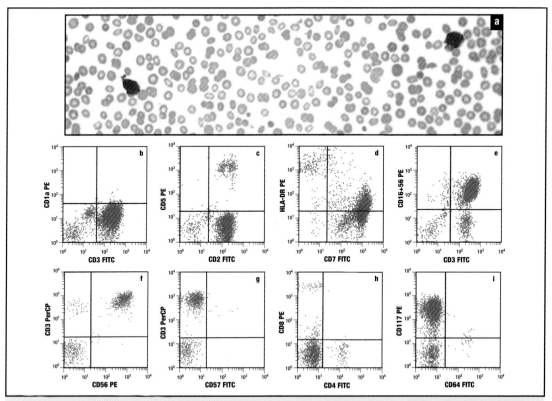

[f14.6] This case demonstrates an aggressive NK-cell leukemia. The clinical history reveals a 63-year-old male who presents with a history of cirrhosis associated with increased swelling, fatigue, and worsening jaundice over the previous 2 weeks. He has an associated anemia and thrombocytopenia. A peripheral blood specimen is submitted for flow cytometric analysis. CBC data include WBC $4.9 \times 10^3/mm^3$ (4.9×10^9/L), Hgb 10 g/dL, Plt $45 \times 10^3/mm^3$ (45×10^9/L). The peripheral blood smear morphology **a** reveals large lymphoid cells with predominantly clumped nuclear chromatin. By flow cytometric analysis, the "expanded" (ie, increased number of cells within a "lymphoid" region composed of a mixture of small to large lymphoid cells) lymphocyte region is composed of 94% T cells with an aberrant immunophenotype. The aberrant T cells express CD3 **b,e-g**, CD2 **c**, CD7 **d**, variable HLA-DR **d**, and CD56 **e, f**. They do not express CD1a **b**, CD5 **c**, CD57 **g**, CD4 **h**, or CD8 **h**. There is aberrant expression of CD117 **i**. The diagnosis is made of aggressive NK-cell leukemia.

The neoplastic (EBV-infected) T-cells have the following immunophenotype: CD2+, CD3+, CD56-, and TIA-1+ (CD8+ in the setting of primary acute EBV infection; CD4+ in the setting of chronic, active EBV infection; and rarely, CD4+/CD8+).

Contribution of In-Situ Hybridization

In-situ hybridization for EBER shows that the majority of the infiltrating lymphoid cells are positive.

Adult T-Cell Leukemia/Lymphoma (ATLL)

Definition

Adult T-cell leukemia/lymphoma (ATLL) is a peripheral T-cell neoplasm most often composed of highly pleomorphic lymphoid cells. The disease is usually widely disseminated and is caused by the human T-cell leukemia virus type 1 (HTLV-1).

acteristically expressed in all cases of ATLL and may be variably expressed in MF/SS. Large transformed cells may be CD30+, while ALK, TIA-1, and granzyme B are all negative. A representative case is demonstrated in [f14.7], with the listmode output available on the accompanying disk.

Differential Diagnosis

Reactive T-cell lymphocytosis

In endemic areas, there may be cases in which a reactive T-cell lymphocytosis may cause diagnostic confusion with ATLL. However, dim CD3 expression in ATLL is a useful feature to distinguish ATLL cells from non-neoplastic T cells, in addition to the morphologic features.

T-PLL

The small cell variant of T-PLL with nuclear irregularities may cause diagnostic confusion with ATLL. Cases

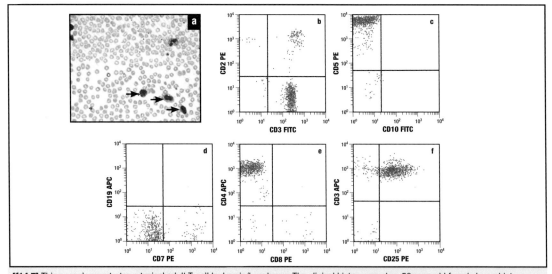

[f14.7] This case demonstrates a typical adult T-cell leukemia/lymphoma. The clinical history reveals a 59-year-old female has a history of HTLV-associated adult T-cell leukemia/lymphoma, acute variant and a follow-up BM biopsy is performed. CBC data include WBC 9.2 × 10³/mm³ (9.2 × 10⁹/L), Hgb 8.6 g/dL, Plt 490 × 10³/mm³ (490 × 10⁹/L). The peripheral blood smear morphology **a** reveals convoluted lymphoid cells (arrow). The bone marrow aspirate smear reveals approximately 5% of cells with similar morphology. By flow cytometric analysis of the bone marrow aspirate, cells within the lymphocyte region (13% of marrow cells) are composed of 97% T cells with an aberrant immunophenotype. The aberrant T cells express CD3 **b, f** and CD5 **c** with loss of CD2 **b** and CD7 **d**. The aberrant T cells express CD4 **e** but not CD8 **e**, and express CD25 **f**. The cytogenetic results reveal numerous structural and numerical abnormalities, including abnormalities of chromosomes 1, 3, and 14. The diagnosis of adult T-cell leukemia/lymphoma is made.

of T-PLL, however, are HTLV-1− and express TCL1 oncoprotein by IHC staining. As mentioned previously, a diagnosis of T-PLL should be strongly considered in cases with prototypic clinical and hematologic features, even when neither TCL1 IHC staining nor the cytogenetic rearrangement involving the TCL-1 locus is detected. Since conventional karyotyping often misses detection of TCL1 locus rearrangements, FISH studies are routinely recommended in cases negative by conventional cytogenetic analysis.

Mycosis fungoides/Sézary syndrome

The cells of adult T-cell leukemia/lymphoma (ATLL) have nuclei with marked irregularities and foldings; some have a "floret" appearance. The cells of MF/SS are also characterized by their folded nuclei. These 2 entities may generally be differentiated by their respective immunophenotypes. In general, ATLL expresses a CD4+/CD8− phenotype with common loss of CD7 expression; however, additional T-cell antigens are generally not lost. CD25 is characteristically expressed in ATLL. In general, SS expresses a CD4+/CD8− phenotype with a common loss of CD7 expression. In addition, other T-cell antigens, particularly CD2, may rarely be lost in SS. In contrast to ATLL, CD25 is generally not expressed in SS.

Peripheralized T-cell lymphoma

The distinction of T-PLL from a peripheralizing T-cell lymphoma would likely depend on a prior diagnostic lymphoid tissue biopsy. If the clinical history, morphology, and immunophenotypic features do not allow distinction of these entities, the demonstration of HTLV-1 is specific for ATLL.

Primary Cutaneous Mycosis Fungoides (Indolent)

Definition

MF is a mature T-cell lymphoma presenting in the skin with plaques/patches and characterized by epidermal and dermal infiltration of small to medium-sized T-cells with cerebriform nuclei.

Typical Immunophenotype and Variations

The characteristic immunophenotype of MF (outlined in **[t14.2]**) is CD4+/CD8− with CD7 commonly lost and variable expression of CD2. Loss of pan T-cell antigens, including CD2, CD3, and CD5, may occur and is usually a feature of disease progression [Kinney 2007]. In rare cases of otherwise classical MF, a CD4−/CD8+ mature T-cell immunophenotype may be demonstrated

[Petrella 2002, Berti 1999, Ralfkiaer 1994, Whittam 2000]. Such a case is demonstrated in **[f14.8]**, with the listmode output available on the accompanying disk. In addition, although not absolutely specific, a low CD8/CD3 ratio in the epidermal component of a lymphocytic infiltrate supports the diagnosis of MF [Ortonne 2003]. CD25 is generally negative in MF. Cytotoxic granule-associated proteins are not expressed in the early patch/plaque lesions but may be positive in a fraction of neoplastic cells in more advanced lesions.

Contribution of FCI

Since skin biopsies are often small or limited in their yield of cells in a suspension for FCI, immunophenotyping often relies primarily on IHC staining in MF cases.

Differential Diagnosis

Benign cutaneous lymphoid lesions

The distinction between MF and benign cutaneous lymphoid lesions by morphologic features is beyond the scope of this discussion. However, immunophenotypic features that would favor a diagnosis of MF vs a benign cutaneous lymphoid lesion with equivocal morphologic features include loss of more than 1 pan-T-cell antigen. Although CD7 is characteristically lost by the cells of MF, a lack of CD7 expression is not infrequently also demonstrated in benign cutaneous lesions [Ralfkiaer 1991].

ATLL with skin involvement

This differential diagnosis is primarily discussed above in the section regarding ATLL. Note that CD4 expression and epidermotropism are also features of ATLL. Differentiating MF from ATLL relies primarily on the marked nuclear irregularity and typically uniform expression of CD25 by the majority of neoplastic cells in ATLL. A majority of United States patients with MF have antibodies to tax but not to the structural proteins of HTLV-1, as demonstrated in ATLL [Pancake 1996, Pancake 1995].

Secondary skin involvement by a nodal/extranodal T-cell lymphoma

MF is a primary cutaneous T-cell lymphoma and thus should be diagnosed in the absence of a prior diagnosis of a nodal/extranodal T-cell lymphoma. In addition, lack of epidermal involvement, as generally seen in secondary involvement, would not be expected in MF. The immunophenotypic features of the nodal/extranodal T-cell lymphomas are discussed in the corresponding sections below.

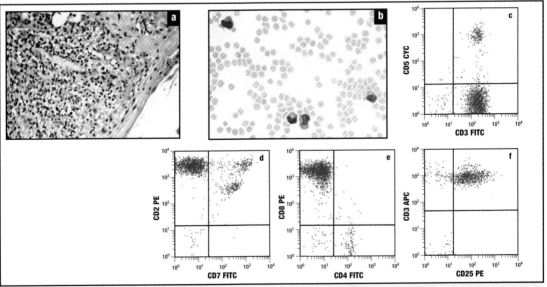

[f14.8] This case demonstrates a rare CD8+ mycosis fungoides. The clinical history reveals a 30-year-old male who presents with a 5-year history of a psoriasiform dermatitis, a necrotic plaque on the scalp associated with infiltrative plaques and tumors on the extremities and trunk, and cervical lymphadenopathy. A scalp punch biopsy and cervical lymph node FNA are performed. The H&E section of skin **a** reveals the atypical lymphoid infiltrate. The FNA cytomorphology of the lymph node **b** reveals the abnormal lymphoid cells. By flow cytometric analysis of the FNA specimen, the lymphocyte region is composed of 97% T cells with an aberrant immunophenotype. The aberrant T cells express CD3 **c, f**, CD2 **d**, CD8 **e**, and dim CD25 **f**. They do not express CD5 **c**, CD7 **d**, or CD4 **e**. The diagnosis of CD8+ mycosis fungoides is made.

Comparison of FCI to Immunophenotyping by Paraffin Immunohistochemistry

As mentioned previously, immunophenotyping may often rely primarily on IHC staining in MF cases. In addition, IHC staining may be particularly useful to correlate the immunophenotypic features with the histologic findings, since a low CD8/CD3 ratio in the epidermal component of a lymphocytic infiltrate may be useful in establishing a diagnosis of MF.

Sézary Syndrome (Aggressive)

Definition

Traditionally SS is considered a variant of MF, which is much more aggressive with generalized involvement, characterized by the presence of erythroderma, lymphadenopathy, and peripheralization. A recent study has demonstrated that a significant proportion of skin biopsies from SS patients do not demonstrate epidermotropism, indicating a high proportion of primary SS, correlating with a more aggressive disease course [Vonderheid 2002].

Typical Immunophenotype

As in MF and outlined in [t14.2].

Differential Diagnosis

Reactive T-cell lymphocytosis vs involvement of peripheral blood by MF/SS

Cells of MF/SS in the peripheral blood usually show more nuclear irregularities than reactive T lymphocytes; however, there will be morphologic overlap. And although loss of CD7 is characteristic of MF/SS, CD7 is not infrequently lost in benign T-cell lymphoid processes in the peripheral blood and skin. However, loss of more than 1 T-cell antigen supports a neoplastic T-cell process. Another flow cytometric marker that may be useful in this regard is CD26. This marker is variably expressed by normal peripheral blood T-cells and initially was considered absent or dim in most, if not all, cases of MF/SS [Jones 2001]. In fact, the absence of both CD7 and CD26 with CD4-positivity has been considered highly specific for SS cells in the peripheral blood [Sokolowska-Wojdylo 2005]. However, a most recent study has determined CD26-negativity is not highly specific in differentiating SS/MF from benign T lymphoid processes [Kelemen 2008]. In this study, CD26-negativity was found in 59% of SS cases, 33% of MF cases, and 14% of benign T-lymphoid processes. Even so, in addition to the findings of major T-cell antigen loss, CD26-negativity may

improve the sensitivity of FCI in patients with SS. An increased sensitivity (ie, 86%) may be achieved by combining the diagnostic power of the 2 approaches. Based on these results, a threshold of >30% CD4+/CD7–/CD26– cells in the peripheral blood by FCI has been recommended for a specific diagnosis of SS. In addition, the finding of a CD4+/CD7–/CD26– population may be more helpful in following patients with a known diagnosis of SS, rather than in establishing an initial diagnosis. In equivocal cases, T-cell clonality studies may also be useful in establishing a diagnosis and follow-up testing in cases of SS. The International Society for Cutaneous Lymphomas recommends a combination of increased lymphocytes with evidence of a T-cell clone in the blood as a criterion for SS [Vonderheid 1985].

T-PLL

The small cell variant of T-PLL with nuclear irregularities may cause diagnostic confusion with primary SS. Virtually all cases of SS lack CD7 expression and may show loss of other pan T-cell antigens, which is not typical of T-PLL. In addition, cases of T-PLL typically express TCL-1 oncoprotein by IHC staining. However, in equivocal cases, FISH studies for detection of TCL-1 locus rearrangements are recommended.

ATLL (as discussed above in the section regarding ATLL and MF) peripheralized T-cell lymphoma

The distinction of SS from a peripheralizing T-cell lymphoma would likely depend on a prior diagnostic skin biopsy of MF or a lymphoid tissue biopsy of a primary nodal/extranodal T-cell lymphoma. If there is no prior documented diagnosis of MF or a primary nodal/extranodal T-cell lymphoma, then primary SS is the recommended diagnosis.

Contribution of FCI

Since SS is defined as peripheral blood involvement by these neoplastic T-cells, FCI is the preferred method to establish a diagnosis and follow patients for residual disease, based on the immunophentoypic markers previously discussed.

Primary Cutaneous CD30+ T-Cell Lymphoproliferative Disorders (Indolent)

Three types of primary cutaneous CD30+ T-cell lymphoproliferative disorders are recognized, as follows:

1. Primary cutaneous anaplastic large cell lymphoma (C-ALCL)

2. Lymphomatoid papulosis (LyP)

3. Borderline lesions.

C-ALCL and LyP represent approximately 30% of primary cutaneous lymphoid neoplasms. C-ALCL and LyP form a spectrum of disease, and histologic criteria alone are often insufficient to differentiate between the 2 ends of this spectrum [Willemze 1993]. The clinical appearance and course are used as criteria for a definitive diagnosis and treatment choice. The term "borderline lesion" refers to cases in which, despite careful clinicopathologic correlation, a definitive distinction between C-ALCL and LyP cannot be made. Close clinical follow-up will generally disclose whether the patient has C-ALCL or LyP [Bekkenk 2000].

Primary Cutaneous Anaplastic Large Cell Lymphoma

Definition
Primary cutaneous anaplastic large cell lymphoma. (C-ALCL) is composed of large cells with an anaplastic, pleomorphic, or immunoblastic cytomorphology and expression of the CD30 antigen by the majority (more than 75%) of tumor cells [Willemze 1993].

There is no clinical evidence or history of LyP, MF, or another type of cutaneous T-cell lymphoma.

Typical Immunophenotype and Variations
The neoplastic cells generally show an activated CD4+ T-cell phenotype with variable loss of CD2, CD5, and/ or CD3, and frequent expression of cytotoxic granule-associated proteins (granzyme B, TIA-1, perforin) [Kaudewitz 1989, Kummer 1997]. Some cases (<5%) have a CD8+ T-cell phenotype. CD30 must be expressed by the majority (more than 75%) of the neoplastic T cells [Beljaards 1989],[Unlike systemic CD30+ ALCLs, most C-ALCLs express the cutaneous lymphocyte antigen (CLA) but do not express epithelial membrane antigen (EMA) and anaplastic lymphoma kinase (ALK), indicative of the 2;5 translocation or its variants [Willemze 1997, de Bruin 1993, DeCouteau 1996]. Unlike Hodgkin lymphoma cells, staining for CD15 is generally negative. Co-expression of CD56 is observed in rare cases but does not appear to be associated with an unfavorable prognosis [Natkunam 2000]. A representative case is demonstrated in [f14.9], with the listmode output available on the accompanying disk.

Contribution of FCI
FCI may detect CD30 expression on the cell surface, and the great majority of cases express 1 or more T-cell antigens. Some may show a "null cell" immunophenotype (ie, lacking any T-cell, B-cell, histiocytic, or plasmacytic antigens) but typically reveal a TCR gene rearrangement. More interestingly, there may be aberrant expression of myelomonocytic markers (ie, CD13, CD33, and CD15) by anaplastic large cell lymphomas presenting in the skin [Juco 2003, Dunphy 2000]. The expression of CD30 and variable expression of T-cell markers aid in differentiating an ALCL in the skin from a granulocytic sarcoma.

Differential Diagnosis

Lymphomatoid papulosis
Since histologic criteria alone are often insufficient to differentiate between C-ALCL and LyP, a discussion of clinical and pathologic features is warranted. LyP and C-ALCL have distinct but sometimes overlapping clinical features. Clinical features supporting the diagnosis of C-ALCL over LyP are a size >2 cm and a duration of any single lesion for more than 3 months without regression. C-ALCL lesions are typically solitary or clustered. Less frequently, there may be multiple nodules or tumors that are often ulcerated and occur, in decreasing order, on the extremities, head and neck, and trunk. On the other hand, LyP lesions are always regressing and present initially in young to middle-aged adults (median age, 45 years) and less often in children [Nijsten 2004]. LyP lesions proceed through a 6- to 8-week cycle of papular to papulonecrotic lesions that are usually smaller than 1 cm and heal with a scar. In classic cases, the course of LyP is chronic, with numerous recurrences of lesions over several months to years.

In most cases, LyP and C-ALCL may also be distinguished by the density and distribution of the large CD30+ tumor cells. In C-ALCL, tumor cells are typically present in large clusters and sheets and extend into the subcutaneous tissue. Tumor cells may surround, infiltrate, and expand blood vessel walls, but overt vascular destruction is usually not present [Sioutos 1992, Macgrogan 1996]. Tumor cytomorphologic features are predominantly anaplastic with indented folded nuclei (hallmark) or embryoid nuclei, but approximately 20% of C-ALCL cases show irregular hyperchromatic or immunoblastic nuclear features.

On the other hand, the histologic picture of LyP is extremely variable and in part correlates with the age of the biopsied skin lesion. Three histologic subtypes of LyP

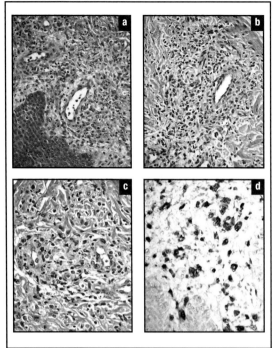

[f14.9] This case demonstrates a primary cutaneous CD30+ anaplastic large cell lymphoma (ALCL). The clinical history reveals a 81-year-old male who presents with erythematous, well circumscribed papules on the abdomen, and a punch biopsy of the abdominal skin is performed. H&E sections **a-c** reveal the characteristic morphology. Although most primary cutaneous ALCLs are ALK–, this case demonstrates ALK-positivity **d** and helps in differentiating it from lymphomatoid papulosis. The diagnosis of primary cutaneous CD30+ anaplastic large cell lymphoma is made.

Types A and C of LyP have the same immunophenotype as C-ALCL. Molecular studies may be more useful in differentiating LyP and C-ALCL. As expected, given the higher density of tumor cells, clonal TCR gene rearrangements are more frequently detected in ALCL than in LyP [Basarab 1998, Steinhoff 2002, Kadin 1987, Chott 1996, Gellrich 2004].

Systemic ALCL

In differentiating C-ALCL from systemic ALCL involving the skin, C-ALCL arises in older patients (median age, 40-67 years) but rarely in children (<2% of C-ALCL) [Bekkenk 2000, Kumar 2005, Fink-Puches 2004]. In pediatric patients, CD30+ skin lesions are much more likely to be secondary to systemic ALK+ ALCL. Immunostaining may be helpful for excluding cutaneous involvement by systemic ALCL. ALK expression is highly associated with systemic disease and is only rarely present in C-ALCL [ten Berge 2000, DeCoteau 1996, Sasaki 2004]. Loss of pan-T-cell antigens is common in C-ALCL and LyP (ie, CD3 loss in 70% of C-ALCL cases) but is not as frequent as in systemic ALK+ ALCL [Bonzheim 2004]. Nevertheless, most markers will not distinguish between types of CD30+ tumors. As mentioned previously, C-ALCL cases frequently express 1 or more cytotoxic granule-associated proteins (ie, TIA-1 or granzyme B), and approximately 20% to 30% express epithelial membrane antigen (EMA); therefore, the presence of EMA cannot be taken as evidence of systemic disease [Vergier 1998, Felgar 1999, Boulland 2000]. Clusterin is also expressed in most cases of systemic and C-ALCL [Nascimento 2004, Saffer 2002, Lae 2002]. On the other hand, CD44v6 (a variant form of CD44, which is a multifunctional cell surface adhesion molecule) has been shown to be an independent marker of the systemic form of ALCL [Liang 2002].

Granulocytic sarcoma

As mentioned previously, ALCL may express myelomonocytic markers, but the expression of CD30, variable expression of T-cell markers, and lack of immature markers should distinguish ALCL from granulocytic sarcoma.

Contribution of Paraffin Immunophenotyping to Diagnosis

Paraffin IHC staining offers the ability to detect ALK expression, which helps differentiate C-ALCL from systemic ALCL. In addition, paraffin IHC staining may be particularly useful in differentiating LyP from C-ALCL,

(types A, B, and C) have been described that represent a spectrum with overlapping features [Willemze 1993, Bekkenk 2000, El Shabrawi-Caelen 2004]. In LyP type A lesions, scattered or small clusters of large, sometimes multinucleated or Reed-Sternberg–like, CD30+ cells are intermingled with numerous inflammatory cells, such as histiocytes, small lymphocytes, neutrophils, and/or eosinophils. LyP type B is uncommon (<10%) and is characterized by an epidermotropic infiltrate of small atypical cells with cerebriform nuclei, similar to that observed in MF. LyP type C lesions demonstrate a monotonous population of numerous large CD30+ T cells, in clusters with relatively few admixed inflammatory cells. Type C is difficult to distinguish histologically from ALCL, except by clinical history and depth of tumor invasion. LyP has minimal (if any) involvement of subcutaneous tissue.

There are no immunophenotypic features yet identified that clearly distinguish C-ALCL from LyP.

so that histopathologic correlation with the pattern of IHC staining may be assessed.

Lymphomatoid Papulosis

Definition
Lymphomatoid papulosis is defined as a chronic, recurrent, self-healing papulonecrotic or papulonodular skin disease with histologic features suggestive of a (CD30+) malignant lymphoma.

Typical Immunophenotype
The large atypical cells in the LyP type A and type C lesions have the same phenotype as the tumor cells in C-ALCL [Kadin 1985]. The atypical cells with cerebriform nuclei in the LyP type B lesions have a CD3+, CD4+, CD8− phenotype and do not express CD30 antigen.

Differential Diagnosis

Primary cutaneous ALCL and systemic ALCL
As discussed above in the section regarding C-ALCL.

Subcutaneous Panniculitis-Like T-Cell Lymphoma (Indolent)

Definition
Subcutaneous panniculitis-like T-cell lymphoma (SPTCL) is defined as a cytotoxic T-cell lymphoma characterized by the presence of primarily subcutaneous infiltrates of small, medium-sized, or large pleomorphic T cells associated with numerous macrophages and often with marked tumor necrosis and karyorrhexis.

Typical Immunophenotype and Variations
These lymphomas show a $\alpha/\beta+$, CD3+, CD4−, CD8+ T-cell phenotype, with expression of cytotoxic granule-associated proteins (ie, TIA-1, granzyme B, and perforin) [Salhany 1998, Santucci 2003, Hoque 2003, Massone 2004]. CD30 and CD56 (focal) are rarely, if ever, expressed. They demonstrate clonal TCR gene rearrangements, and the Epstein-Barr virus (EBV) is absent. There is another group of "SPTCL" with γ/δ T-cell phenotype that is typically CD4−, CD8−, often co-expresses CD56, and has a more aggressive clinical course. In the WHO-EORTC classification, the term "SPTCL" is reserved for cases with an $\alpha/\beta+$ T-cell phenotype, whereas cases with a $\gamma/\delta+$ T-cell phenotype are included in the category of cutaneous γ/δ T-cell lymphomas, described in more detail below [Massone 2004].

Differential Diagnosis

Primary cutaneous $\gamma\delta$ T-cell lymphoma
"SPTCL" as defined in the WHO classification with an $\alpha/\beta+$ T-cell phenotype is usually CD8-, is restricted to the subcutaneous tissue (no dermal or epidermal involvement), and often runs an indolent clinical course [Salhany 1998, Santucci 2003, Hoque 2003, Massone 2004]. In contrast, SPTCL with a $\gamma/\delta+$ T-cell phenotype is typically CD4−, CD8−, and often co-expresses CD56. The neoplastic infiltrates in this variant are not confined to the subcutaneous tissue but may involve the epidermis and/or dermis as well, and it invariably has a very poor prognosis [Salhany 1998, Santucci 2003, Hoque 2003, Burg 1991]. This subtype is grouped under primary cutaneous γ/δ T-cell lymphoma.

Extranodal NK/T-cell lymphoma, nasal type
"SPTCL" as defined by the WHO classification can usually be distinguished from extranodal NK/T-cell lymphoma primarily by immunophenotypic features, since SPTCL is rarely CD56+ and EBV−. As described below in the section regarding other extranodal lymphomas, extranodal NK/T-cell lymphoma of the nasal type is most often sCD3−, CD2+, CD56+, and EBV+. The TCR is usually in germline configuration, but it may be rearranged in rare cases with a cytotoxic T-cell phenotype.

Comparison of FCI to Immunophenotyping by Paraffin Immunohistochemistry
FCI is often helpful in these cases by demonstrating the characteristic T-cell immunophenotype and by distinguishing sCD3 vs cCD3. However, paraffin IHC staining is also helpful in determining the presence of cytotoxic granule-associated proteins (ie, TIA-1, granzyme B, and perforin) and the absence of EBV by EBER-in-situ hybridization (EBER-ISH). In addition, limited tissue specimens may be better evaluated by paraffin IHC staining.

Hydroa Vacciniforme-Like Lymphoma

Definition
Hydroa vacciniforme-like lymphoma is an EBV-positive cutaneous T-cell lymphoma occurring in children and associated with sun sensitivity. The neoplastic cells may also be of NK-cell origin, when associated with mosquito bite hypersensitivity.

Typical immunophenotype

The neoplastic cells have a cytotoxic T-cell, or less often, NK-cell immunophenotype with expression of CD56.

Contribution of In-situ Hybridization

In-situ hybridization for EBER shows positivity in all of the neoplastic cells. LMP1 is generally negative.

Primary Cutaneous Small-Medium CD4+ TCL (Indolent)

Definition

Primary cutaneous CD4+ small/medium-sized pleomorphic T-cell lymphoma is a CTCL defined by a predominance of small- to medium-sized CD4+ pleomorphic T cells without (a history of) patches and plaques typical of MF, and in most cases, a favorable clinical course [Willemze 1997]. In the WHO-EORTC classification, the term "small/medium-sized pleomorphic CTCL" is restricted to cases with a CD4+ T-cell phenotype. Cases with a CD3+, CD4–, CD8+ phenotype usually have a more aggressive clinical course and are included in the group of aggressive epidermotropic CD8+ CTCLs described below [Bekkenk 2003].

Typical Immunophenotype

By definition these lymphomas have a CD3+, CD4+, CD8–, CD30– phenotype, sometimes with loss of pan-T-cell markers. Cytotoxic granule-associated proteins are generally not expressed [Burg 1991], and the TCR genes are clonally rearranged [von den Driesch 2002, Friedmann 1995].

Differential Diagnosis

MF

Since this lymphoma is composed of CD4+ small/medium-sized pleomorphic T-cells, there may be diagnostic confusion with MF. As noted in the definition above, this diagnosis may only be made if there is no history of or coexistence of patches and plaques typical of MF. In addition, histologically these lymphomas show dense, diffuse, or nodular infiltrates within the dermis with a tendency to infiltrate the subcutis. Epidermotropism is not prominent but may be present focally.

Primary cutaneous γδ T-cell lymphoma

As further described below, primary cutaneous γδ T-cell lymphoma (γδ CTCL) is an aggressive CTCL with a βF1–, CD3+, CD2+, CD4–, CD8–, CD5–, CD7+/–,

CD56+ immunophenotype with strong expression of cytotoxic granule-associated proteins. As the name implies, they show a clonal rearrangement of the TCR γ gene. TCR β may be rearranged or deleted but is not expressed. EBV is generally negative. So, these immunophenotypic differences should easily separate it from primary cutaneous CD4+ small/medium-sized pleomorphic T-cell lymphoma, which is defined as CD4+, negative for cytotoxic granule-associated proteins, and with a TCR clonal rearrangement.

Extranodal NK/T-cell lymphoma, nasal type

Likewise, primary cutaneous CD4+ small/medium-sized pleomorphic T-cell lymphoma should be distinguished from extranodal NK/T-cell lymphoma, nasal type, based on the differences in immunophenotypic features. Again, the latter group of lymphomas is most often sCD3–, CD2+, CD56+, and EBV+. The TCR is usually in germline configuration, it but may be rearranged in rare cases with a cytotoxic T-cell phenotype. Primary cutaneous CD4+ small/medium-sized pleomorphic T-cell lymphoma demonstrates a clonal TCR gene rearrangement.

Subcutaneous panniculitis-like T-cell lymphoma

SPTCLs show an α/β+, CD3+, CD4–, CD8+ T-cell phenotype, with expression of cytotoxic granule-associated proteins (ie, TIA-1, granzyme B, and perforin), in contrast to primary cutaneous CD4+ small/medium-sized pleomorphic T-cell lymphoma, which is CD4+ by definition and does not express cytotoxic granule-associated proteins.

Comparison of FCI to immunophenotyping by paraffin immunohistochemistry

Although FCI may be helpful in defining the T-cell phenotype in this provisional subtype of primary cutaneous lymphoma, paraffin IHC staining is also quite helpful in cases in which histopathologic correlation is particularly important or when there is a limited tissue biopsy. In addition, paraffin IHC staining is helpful in determining the presence or absence of cytotoxic granule-associated proteins (ie, TIA-1, granzyme B, and perforin) in the differential diagnosis of this entity.

Primary Cutaneous Aggressive Epidermotrophic CD8+ Cytotoxic TCL

Definition

Primary cutaneous aggressive epidermotropic CD8+ CTCL is characterized by a proliferation of epidermotropic CD8+ cytotoxic T-cells and aggressive clinical behavior [Berti 1999, Agnarsson 1990]. The neoplastic cells are small-medium or medium-large with pleomorphic or blastic nuclei. Differentiation from other types of CTCL expressing a CD8+ cytotoxic T-cell phenotype, as observed in >50% of patients with pagetoid reticulosis and in rare cases of MF, LyP, and C-ALCL, is based on the clinical presentation and clinical behavior [Berti 1999]. In these latter conditions, no difference in clinical presentation or prognosis between CD4+ and CD8+ cases is found. Epidermotropism is often pronounced, ranging from a linear distribution to a pagetoid pattern throughout the epidermis. Invasion and destruction of adnexal skin structures are commonly seen. Angiocentricity and angioinvasion may be present. Tumor cells are small-medium or medium-large with pleomorphic or blastic nuclei [Berti 1999]. There is no difference in survival between cases with a small- or large-cell morphology [Bekkenk 2003].

Typical Immunophenotype

The tumor cells have a βF1+, CD3+, CD8+, granzyme B+, perforin+, TIA-1+, CD45RA+, CD45RO–, CD2–, CD4–, CD5–, CD7–/+ phenotype [Santucci 2003, Massone 2004, Bekkenk 2003, Berti 1999, Agnarsson 1990]. EBV is generally negative. The neoplastic cells show clonal TCR gene rearrangements.

Differential Diagnosis

Hypopigmented MF

Clinically, these lymphomas are characterized by the presence of localized or disseminated eruptive papules, nodules, and tumors showing central ulceration and necrosis or by superficial, hyperkeratotic patches and plaques [Santucci 2003, Berti 1999]. Most cases of MF are CD4+, and as previously discussed, cytotoxic granule-associated proteins are not expressed in the early patch/plaque lesions of MF.

Primary cutaneous γδ T-cell lymphoma

The clinical features of primary cutaneous aggressive epidermotropic CD8+ CTCL are very similar to those observed in patients with a cutaneous γ/δ T-cell lymphoma (γ/δ CTCL). In addition, γ/δ CTCL may have 3 major histopathologic patterns of involvement: epidermotropic, dermal, and subcutaneous. However, γ/δ CTCL has a CD4–/CD8– immunophenotype, although CD8 may be expressed in rare cases of γ/δ CTCL [de Wolf-Peeters 2000, Toro 2003]. However, other immunophenotypic differences should help distinguish these entities (ie, CD2-negativity in primary cutaneous aggressive epidermotropic CD8+ CTCL and CD2-positivity in γ/δ CTCL).

Primary cutaneous small-medium CD4+ T-cell lymphoma

As discussed previously, this lymphoma is defined by its characteristic immunophenotype, CD3+, CD4+, CD8–, CD30–, which should easily distinguish it from the immunophenotype of primary cutaneous aggressive epidermotropic CD8+ CTCL.

Extranodal NK/T-cell lymphoma, nasal type

The aggressive clinical course and angiocentricity and angioinvasion that may be encountered in primary cutaneous aggressive epidermotropic CD8+ CTCL may cause diagnostic confusion with extranodal NK/T-cell lymphoma, nasal type. However, in NK/T-cell lymphoma, sCD3 is generally negative, CD8 is negative, EBV is almost always positive, and CD2 is usually positive with CD56-positivity.

Subcutaneous panniculitis-like T-cell lymphoma

Although these lymphomas have overlapping immunophenotypic features, CD3+ and CD8+ with expression of cytotoxic granule-associated proteins, these 2 entities are usually distinguished by their histologic features (epidermotrophic in the CD8+ aggressive lymphoma and subcutaneous in SPTCL) and clinical courses (aggressive in the CD8+ epidermotrophic lymphoma and indolent in SPTCL).

Comparison of FCI to Immunophenotyping by Paraffin Immunohistochemistry

Although FCI may be helpful in defining the T-cell phenotype in this provisional subtype of primary cutaneous lymphoma, paraffin IHC staining is also quite helpful in cases in which histopathologic correlation is particularly important or when there is a limited tissue biopsy. In addition, paraffin IHC staining is helpful in determining the presence of cytotoxic granule-associated proteins (ie, TIA-1, granzyme B, and perforin) and the absence of EBV by EBER-ISH in the differential diagnosis of this entity.

Primary Cutaneous γδ T-Cell Lymphoma (Aggressive)

Definition

Cutaneous γ/δ T-cell lymphoma (γ/δ CTCL) is a lymphoma composed of a clonal proliferation of mature, activated γ/δ T cells with a cytotoxic phenotype. The neoplastic cells are generally medium- to large-sized with coarsely clumped chromatin. Large blastic cells with vesicular nuclei and prominent nucleoli are distinctly infrequent. This group includes cases previously known as SPTCL with a γ/δ phenotype. A similar and possibly related condition may present primarily in mucosal sites [Arnulf 1998]. Whether cutaneous and mucosal γδ TCL are all part of a single disease (ie, muco-cutaneous γ/δ TCL) is not yet clear [de Wolf-Peeters 2000, Jaffe 2003]. Distinction between "primary" and "secondary" cutaneous cases is not useful in this group, since both groups have a very grim prognosis.

Typical Immunophenotype

The tumor cells characteristically have a βF1−, CD3+, CD2+, CD5−, CD7+/−, CD56+ immunophenotype with strong expression of cytotoxic granule-associated proteins. Most cases lack both CD4 and CD8, though CD8 is expressed in some cases. The cells show clonal rearrangement of the TCR γ gene. TCR β may be rearranged or deleted, but it is not expressed. EBV is generally negative. Expression of the γδ TCR is easily and better assessed by FCI than by paraffin IHC staining.

Differential Diagnosis

Other T-cell lymphomas primarily involving skin

As discussed previously, 3 major histologic patterns of involvement may be present in the skin: epidermotropic, dermal, and subcutaneous. Often more than 1 histologic pattern is present in the same patient in different biopsy specimens or within a single biopsy specimen [Toro 2003, Berti 1991]. The neoplastic cells are generally medium to large in size with coarsely clumped chromatin. Large blastic cells with vesicular nuclei and prominent nucleoli are infrequent. Apoptosis and necrosis are common, often with angioinvasion. The subcutaneous cases may show rimming of fat cells, similar to SPTCL of α/β origin. The distinctions between γ/δ CTCL, SPTCL, and primary cutaneous CD8+ epidermotrophic TCL have already been discussed in the appropriate sections above. Distinguishing γ/δ CTCL from extranodal NK/T-cell lymphoma, nasal type is

usually made by the lack of sCD3 in the NK/T-cell lymphoma, although there are rare cases with a cytotoxic T-cell immunophenotype. EBV-positivity is characteristic of NK/T-cell lymphoma, whereas γ/δ CTCL is generally EBV−. They both have an aggressive clinical course.

Contribution of Paraffin Immunohistochemistry

In frozen sections, the cells are strongly positive for TCR-δ. If only paraffin sections are available, the absence of βF1 may be used to infer a γ/δ origin under appropriate circumstances [Salhany 1998, Jones 2002]. In addition, paraffin IHC staining may be useful in demonstrating the presence of cytotoxic granule-associated proteins and the absence of EBV by EBER-ISH.

Extranodal NK/T-Cell Lymphoma, Nasal Type (Aggressive)

Definition

Extranodal NK/T-cell lymphoma, nasal type, is a nearly always an EBV+ lymphoma of small, medium, or large cells usually with an NK-cell or more rarely a cytotoxic T-cell phenotype. The skin is the second most common site of involvement after the nasal cavity/nasopharynx. Skin involvement may be a primary or secondary manifestation of the disease. Since both groups show an aggressive clinical behavior and require the same type of treatment, the distinction between "primary" and "secondary" cutaneous involvement seems unnecessary [Santucci 2003, Natkunam 1999, Herling 2004b, El Shabrawi-Caelen 2000, Miyamoto 1998]. Therefore, the WHO classification-derived term "extranodal NK/T-cell lymphoma, nasal type," rather than "(primary) cutaneous NK/T-cell lymphoma, nasal type," is maintained. This lymphoma will be discussed in more detail in the section below regarding other extranodal lymphomas.

Primary Cutaneous Peripheral T-Cell Lymphoma, Unspecified (Aggressive)

Definition

PTCL, unspecified, in the WHO classification represents a heterogeneous group including all T-cell neoplasms that do not fit into any of the better defined subtypes of T-cell lymphoma/leukemia. For the remaining diseases that do not fit into any of the above accepted or provisional entities, the designation PTCL, unspecified, is maintained. In all cases, a diagnosis of MF must be excluded by a complete clinical examination and an accurate clinical history.

Immunphenotype

Most cases show an aberrant CD4+ T-cell phenotype with variable loss of pan-T-cell antigens. CD30 staining is negative or restricted to a few scattered tumor cells. Rare cases may show co-expression of CD56. Expression of cytotoxic granule-associated proteins is not common [Bekkenk 2003].

Extranodal NK/T-Cell Lymphoma, Nasal Type

Definition

Extranodal NK/T-cell lymphoma (NK/TCL), nasal type is a predominantly extranodal lymphoma characterized by a broad morphologic spectrum. The infiltrate is often angiocentric with prominent necrosis and vascular destruction. It is designated NK/T (rather than NK) cell lymphoma, because while most cases appear to be NK-cell neoplasms (EBV+ CD56+), rare cases show an EBV+ CD56– cytotoxic T-cell phenotype. The qualifier "nasal-type" refers to the fact that the nasal cavity is the most common site of involvement. However, other extranodal sites may also be involved.

Typical Immunophenotype and Variations

Most nasal-type NK/TCLs are thought to be of true NK cell origin, as evidenced by the typical immunophenotype: CD2+, CD56+, surface CD3–, CD4–, CD5–, CD8–, and no evidence of clonal TCR gene rearrangements. However, unlike normal NK cells, these tumors are usually CD7– and CD16–. The tumor cells express

the ε chain of CD3 in their cytoplasm and, therefore, often stain positively for CD3 by IHC staining of paraffin sections [Mason 1989]. A representative case is demonstrated in [f14.10]. A subset of tumors has evidence of T-cell lineage [Natkunam 1999]. This T-cell subset may demonstrate CD8-positivity and be negative for CD56. These cases also typically exhibit clonal TCR gene rearrangements, supporting the true T-cell origin.

A common feature of all cases is the expression of cytotoxic granule-associated proteins (ie, TIA-1, granzyme B, or perforin) and EBV. The WHO classification recommends that although CD56 may be negative (as in the rare T-cell cytotoxic subtype), the diagnosis should not be made in the absence of cytotoxic granule-associated protein expression or in the absence of EBV-positivity.

Contribution of FCI

FCI may be particularly helpful in distinguishing surface CD3-negativity/positivity and cytoplasmic CD3-positivity, as well as in defining the remainder of the NK/T-cell immunophenotype.

Differential Diagnosis

Inflammatory/reactive conditions

Admixed nonneoplastic inflammatory cells are characteristic of this lymphoma, and if the neoplastic cells are small, these inflammatory cells can make the diagnosis of malignancy problematic, particularly in small biopsy samples. An important clue to the diagnosis of malignancy in small cell cases is infiltration of the underlying bone of the nasal septum and extensive ulceration; bone infiltration

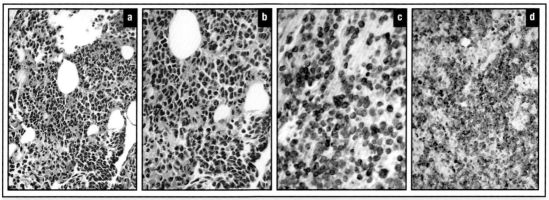

[f14.10] This case demonstrates a typical extranodal NK/T-cell lymphoma of "nasal" type. The clinical history reveals a 74-year-old male who presents with an abrupt onset of inability to walk and stand with a T3 lesion by MRI. A soft tissue (T3 epidural) biopsy is performed. H&E sections **a, b** demonstrate the characteristic morphology. Flow cytometric analysis was not performed (and thus not available for demonstration). Immunohistochemical stains reveal positivity of the malignant cells for cytoplasmic CD3 **c**, TIA-1 **d**, CD5, CD56, perforin, granzyme B, and EBV-in-situ-hybridization (all, not demonstrated). The diagnosis of extranodal NK/T-cell lymphoma, nasal type, is made.

is extremely uncommon in inflammatory conditions and should be considered highly suggestive of the presence of lymphoma. Demonstration of aberrant loss of T-cell antigens (ie, CD5 and CD7), CD56 expression, cytotoxic granule-associated protein expression, and EBV (EBER-ISH) positivity are helpful in establishing the diagnosis of lymphoma. These cases illustrate that NK/TCL should be considered in the differential diagnosis of atypical inflammatory infiltrates in the nasal cavity and sinuses.

DLBCL

NK/TCL should be distinguished from diffuse large B-cell lymphomas (DLBCLs) involving this site. FCI will typically reveal a monoclonal B-cell population in DLBCL. However, one should keep in mind that if a complete immunophenotypic profile is not available by FCI, occasional cases of NK/TCL may express CD20 in association with the additional B-cell marker, CD79a. By applying a complete immunophenotypic profile by FCI and/or IHC staining, demonstration of the remainder of the immunophenotype helps clarify this aberrant B-cell marker expression.

ALCL

One confusing feature may be the expression of CD30 in cases of NK/TCL, which is usually expressed in a subset of NK/TCL tumor cells, likely as a feature of histologic progression [Natkunam 2000]. However, occasional cases of NK/TCL with CD30 expression will also show uniform large cell morphologic features. Most large cell variants usually demonstrate a range of cytomorphologic features and variable rather than strong, uniform CD30 staining as seen in ALCL. Although ALCL may also express CD56 and exhibit angioinvasion [Sioutos 1992, Macgrogan 1996], tumor cells are uniformly and strongly positive for CD30 and rarely positive for EBV [Herling 2004b, Herbst 1997]. These features, combined with the otherwise typical immunophenotypes and genetic and clinical features, will aid in an accurate diagnosis.

Aggressive NK-cell leukemia with tissue involvement

One of the controversial issues at the present time is the relationship between disseminated nasal-type NK/TCL with a BM/leukemic phase [Soler 1994, Chang 2002], and aggressive NK-cell leukemia that can rarely secondarily involve the skin [Imamura 1990, Radonich 2002, Nava 2005].

Since these 2 tumors have a similar phenotype, and both diseases are often associated with a

hemophagocytic syndrome, some authors believe that aggressive NK-cell leukemia represents a leukemic form of nasal type NK/TCL, similar to the relationship between lymphoblastic lymphoma and leukemia [Chan 2001, Chan 1997, Chan 1998].

However, since nasal-type NK/TCL only rarely involves the BM and PB (aggressive NK-cell leukemia typically has PB involvement with patchy infiltration of the BM), and nasal-type NK/TCL has a much higher incidence of skin involvement (aggressive NK-cell leukemia has much less frequent involvement of the skin), it has been suggested that these 2 diseases are different [Oshimi 2005]. In addition, nasal-type NK/TCL only infrequently involves lymph nodes, whereas lymphadenopathy is common in aggressive NK-cell leukemia. Clinically, aggressive NK-cell leukemia typically occurs in young patients, and nasal-type NK/TCL is a disease of middle-aged to older adults.

CD4+/CD56+ hematodermic tumor (alias blastoid natural killer cell lymphoma)

As mentioned previously, the neoplastic cells of CD4+/CD56+ hematodermic tumor (HDT) are tumors of plasmacytoid dendritic cell lineage and express CD4 and CD56 in the absence of lineage-specific markers of T cells, B cells, or myelomonocytic markers. Expression of EBV antigens actually excludes a diagnosis of HDT [Suzuki 1997].

Contribution of FCI and Comparison to IHC Immunophenotyping

Extranodal NK/TCLs of nasal type may be defined by FCI, as described in the immunophenotypic features above. ISH staining may be particularly useful when there is a limited tissue biopsy. In addition, ISH staining is effective in demonstrating expression of cytotoxic granule-associated proteins and EBV (EBER-ISH).

Enteropathy-Associated T-Cell Lymphoma

Definition

Enteropathy-associated T-cell lymphoma (ETL) is a tumor of intraepithelial T lymphocytes showing varying degrees of transformation (morphologically) but usually composed of large lymphoid cells. It is a rare type of T-cell lymphoma, often associated with a history of celiac disease, usually arising in the jejunum, but can involve other gastrointestinal (GI) tract sites (ie, stomach and colon).

Typical Immunophenotype with Morphologic and Immunophenotypic Subgroups

Enteropathy-associated T-cell lymphoma is typically CD3+, CD5−, CD7+, CD8−/+, CD4−, CD103+, and demonstrates expression of cytotoxic granule-associated proteins. The intraepithelial lymphocytes in the adjacent enteropathic mucosa may show an abnormal immunophenotype, usually CD3+, CD5−, CD8−, CD4−, and are identical to the immunophenotype of the lymphoma. In almost all cases, a varying proportion of the neoplastic cells demonstrate expression of CD30. A representative case is demonstrated in [f14.11].

There are 2 histologic groups of ETL that correlate with clinical and immunophenotypic features. Pleomorphic-anaplastic ETL is usually associated with a history of celiac disease, histologic evidence of enteropathy, and is most often CD56−. Monomorphic ETL often occurs without a history of celiac disease, has variable histologic evidence of enteropathy, and is usually CD56+ and CD8+. There is no described association with EBV. ETL typically demonstrates clonally rearranged TCR β and γ genes. Comparative genomic hybridization has shown recurrent chromosomal gains and losses that are characteristic of ETL and uncommon in other T-cell lymphomas, providing useful ancillary data for the diagnosis of ETL. These are tabulated in [t14.2]. Gains of chromosome 9q33-q34 are the hallmark genetic alteration in ETL, occurring in up to 70% of cases [Zettl 2002, Deleeuw 2007].

Contribution of FCI

FCI is particularly useful in demonstrating the aberrant T-cell immunophenotype in ETL and demonstrating expression of CD103.

Differential Diagnosis

MALT and other primary B-cell lymphomas of the GI tract

The presence of intraepithelial lymphocytes in ETL may cause diagnostic confusion with primary B-cell lymphomas of the GI tract, including those of mucosa-associated lymphoid tissue origin. However, the B-cell immunophenotype of these latter lymphomas should clearly distinguish them from ETL.

Other T-cell lymphomas primarily involving the GI tract: γδ T-cell lymphoma and NK/T-cell lymphoma

γδ T-cell lymphoma and NK/TCL may be more problematic in the differential diagnosis of ETL, due to overlapping morphologic and immunophenotypic features. In a setting of celiac disease, the differential diagnosis is clearer. However, in other situations, the differential diagnosis between ETL and γδ T-cell lymphoma may rely on demonstration of a TCR β gene rearrangement (ie, demonstrated in ETL), a characteristic cytogenetic finding (ie, gains of chromosome 9q33-q34 in ETL), or the presence/absence of EBV (absent in ETL and detected in a significant proportion of mucosal γδ T-cell lymphomas) [Arnulf 1998]. Likewise, ETL may be differentiated from the subset of NK/TCL with a T-cell cytotoxic immunophenotype by the demonstration of EBV in NK/TCL.

Comparison of FCI to immunophenotyping by paraffin immunohistochemistry

IHC staining may be useful in the diagnosis of ETL in limited tissue biopsies and in the differential diagnosis with other TCLs, by demonstrating the presence of cytotoxic granule-associated proteins and the absence of EBV (EBER-ISH) in ETL.

Hepatosplenic T-cell Lymphoma (and Other Non-Cutaneous γδ T-Cell Lymphomas)

Definition

Hepatosplenic T-cell lymphoma (HSTCL) is an extranodal and systemic neoplasm derived from cytotoxic T cells usually of γδ T-cell receptor type, medium in size, and demonstrating marked sinusoidal infiltration of spleen, liver, and BM. Mucosal γδ T-cell lymphomas are regarded as a subset of activated and cytotoxic (ie, TIA-1+, granzyme B+, and perforin+) T-cell lymphomas with heterogeneous clinicopathologic features.

Typical Immunophenotype

The neoplastic cells of HSTCL are most frequently CD2+, CD3+, CD4−, CD5− (rarely +), CD7+/−, CD8− (rarely + with CD4-), CD56+ (rarely negative), CD16+/−, CD57− (rarely +), and usually CD25− and CD30−. The neoplastic cells of HSTCL also usually have an inactive (or immature) cytotoxic profile (ie, positive for TIA-1 and negative for granzyme B and perforin) [Gaulard 1990, Vega 2001, Cooke 1996, Boulland 1997]. A representative case is demonstrated in [f14.12]. Most cases of HSTCL demonstrate γδ TCR. Expression of the γδ TCR is easily and better assessed by FCI than by paraffin IHC staining. However, as mentioned previously, if only paraffin sections are available, the

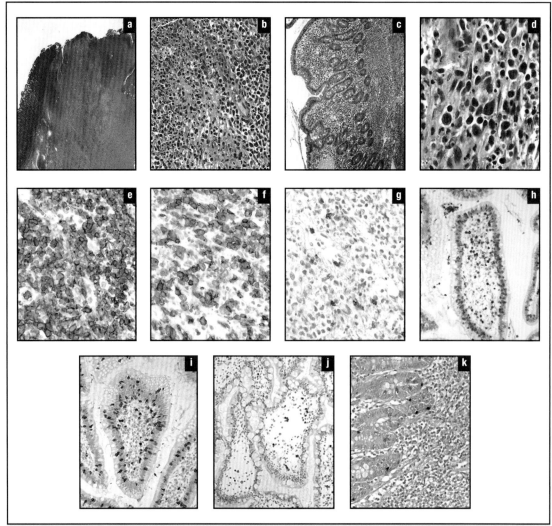

[f14.11] This case demonstrates a typical case of enteropathy-associated T-cell lymphoma. The clinical history reveals a 58-year-old male with history of celiac disease who presents with ileal perforation. Three years before, he had also had an episode of small intestinal perforation. A resection of a segment of small intestine is performed. The low power H&E section of the small intestine **a** shows ulceration and focal perforation. Higher power **b** demonstrates a patchy, multifocal infiltrate of medium-sized and large atypical lymphoid cells, with occasional large bizarre cells on a background of cellular debris and inflammatory cells. H&E section of the small intestine away from the lymphoma **c** demonstrates villous blunting. Flow cytometric analysis was not performed (and thus not available for demonstration). By immunohistochemical staining, the malignant cells **d** are positive for CD3, CD2 **e**, CD8, variable CD30 **f**, diffuse TIA-1, and diffuse granzyme B, and are negative for CD4, CD5 **g**, CD56, CD20, CD15, ALK, and EBER. The intraepithelial lymphocytes are CD3+, CD2+ **h**, CD8+ **i**, CD4–, CD5– **j**, and CD56– with a subset EBER+ **k**. The molecular results of PCR on paraffin-embedded tissue shows no clonal TCR rearrangement. Diagnosis is made of enteropathy-associated T-cell lymphoma, classical type arising in celiac disease.

absence of βF1 may be used to infer a $\gamma\delta$ origin under the appropriate circumstances [Salhany 1998, Jones 2002]. In addition, although most cases express the $\gamma\delta$ TCR, some cases express the $\alpha\beta$ TCR. $\alpha\beta$ HSTCL has clinicopathologic and cytogenetic features similar to those of $\gamma\delta$ HSTCL cases and, therefore, is currently considered a variant of the disease [Lai 2000, Macon 2001, Suarez 2000]. Isochromosome 7q is a consistent cytogenetic abnormality in HSTCL that expresses the $\gamma\delta$ TCR [Alonsozana 1997]. The same abnormality has also been found in HSTCL cases expressing the $\alpha\beta$ TCR [Lai 2000, Macon 2001, Suarez 2000].

As mentioned in the definition above, the neoplastic cells of mucosal $\gamma\delta$ TCL have a similar immunophenotype to HSTCL, but are TIA-1+, granzyme B+, and perforin+, in contrast with the non-activated cytotoxic immunophenotype of HSTCL. As mentioned previously, EBV is detected in a significant proportion of mucosal cases [Arnulf 1998].

Contribution of FCI

FCI is particularly useful in establishing the immunophenotype of the neoplastic cells in HSCTL and mucosal γδ TCL and in demonstrating the γδ TCR in these lymphomas.

Differential Diagnosis

Hepatosplenic type: CLL, hairy cell leukemia and variant, and other chronic B-cell lymphoproliferative disorders

Although splenic involvement by CLL, hairy cell leukemia (HCL), and its variant (HCL-V) may morphologically mimic hepatosplenic γδ TCL, the distinctive

B-cell immunophenoypes of these disorders should clearly distinguish these entities from HSTCL.

T-LGLL and mature T-cell leukemias

On the other hand, T-cell large granular lymphocytic leukemia (T-LGLL) or other mature T-cell leukemias, composed of medium-sized neoplastic cells, involving the spleen may be more problematic in the differential diagnosis of HSTCL. Hepatosplenic T-cell lymphoma is more frequent in younger patients and has a more aggressive clinical course than T-LGLL. Also, it differs from T-LGLL in immunophenotype (most cases are CD4–/CD8–) and by the presence of isochromosome 7q [Alonsozana 1997].

Mucosal sites: MALT and other primary B-cell lymphomas of the GI tract

Although mucosal involvement by MALT-lymphoma, CLL/SLL, mantle cell lymphoma, or other small B-cell lymphomas primarily involving the GI tract may morphologically mimic mucosal γδ TCL, the distinctive

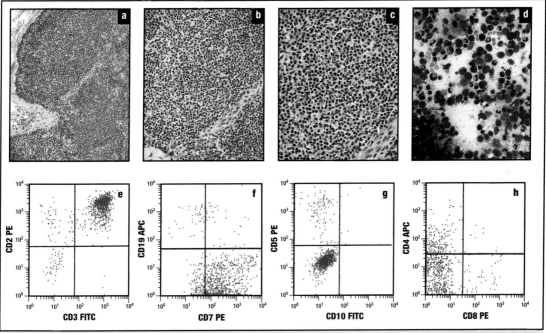

[f14.12] This case demonstrates a typical case of hepatosplenic T-cell lymphoma. The clinical history reveals a 21-year-old male who presents with hemolytic anemia associated with left cervical lymphadenopathy, ascites, and splenomegaly. He had initially presented to an outside hospital with fevers, stomach ache, vomitting, and a petechial rash. The patient also reported a significant weight loss. The H&E sections **a-c** of the lymph node demonstrate the morphology. The bone marrow aspirate **d** demonstrates the abnormal lymphoid cells. By flow cytometric analysis of the bone marrow aspirate, the lymphocyte region (17% of the marrow cells) is composed of 83% T cells with a subset showing an aberrant immunophenotype. The aberrant T cells express CD3 **e**, CD2 **e**, and heterogeneous CD7 **f** with loss of CD5 **g** and no significant expression of either CD4 **h** or CD8 **h**. The cytogenetic results show isochromosome 7q, and molecular analysis identified TCR γ gene rearrangement. Diagnosis of hepatosplenic T-cell lymphoma is made.

B-cell immunophenotypes of these B-cell disorders should clearly distinguish these entities from mucosal γδ TCL.

Other primary T-cell lymphomas of the GI tract: enteropathy-associated T-cell lymphoma and NK/T-cell lymphoma

Enteropathy-associated T-cell lymphoma and NK/TCL may be more problematic in the differential diagnosis of mucosal γδ TCL, due to overlapping morphologic and immunophenotypic features. In a setting of celiac disease, the differential diagnosis is clearer. However, in other situations, the differential diagnosis between mucosal γδ TCL and ETL may rely on demonstration of a TCR ß gene rearrangement (ie, demonstrated in ETL), a characteristic cytogenetic finding (ie, gains of chromosome 9q33-q34 in ETL), or the presence/absence of EBV (absent in ETL and detected in a significant proportion of mucosal γδ T-cell lymphomas) [Arnulf 1998]. The differential diagnosis between mucosal γδ T-cell lymphoma and a primary NK/TCL of the GI tract may be even more problematic, since the subset of NK/TCL with a cytotoxic T-cell immunophenotype may have overlapping immunophenotypic features, and they both are typically EBV+. In this situation, demonstration of a γδ TCR would support a mucosal γδ TCL.

Comparison of FCI to Immunophenotyping by Paraffin Immunohistochemistry

FCI is extremely useful in defining the immunophenotypes of the γδ TCLs and in distinguishing them from the entities in their differential diagnosis. Expression of the γδ TCR is easily and better assessed by FCI than by paraffin IHC staining. However, paraffin IHC staining may be quite useful in limited biopsy specimens and in evaluating for the presence/absence of cytotoxic-associated proteins and EBV (EBER-ISH). As already mentioned, if only paraffin sections are available, the absence of βF1 may be used to infer a γδ origin under the appropriate circumstances [Salhany 1998, Jones 2002].

Primary Extranodal Peripheral T-Cell Lymphoma, Unspecified

Definition

PTCL, unspecified, in the WHO classification, represents a heterogeneous group including all T-cell neoplasms that do not fit into any of the better-defined subtypes of T-cell lymphoma/leukemia. For the remaining diseases that do not fit into any of the above

accepted extranodal lymphomas, the designation PTCL, unspecified is maintained. Of course, secondary extranodal involvement by a malignant lymphoma primarily arising in a nodal or cutaneous site must be excluded from this designation.

Nodal Angioimmunoblastic T-Cell Lymphoma (AITL)

Definition

Angioimmunoblastic T-cell lymphoma (AITL) is a peripheral (mature) T-cell lymphoma characterized by systemic disease and a polymorphous infiltrate involving lymph nodes, with a prominent proliferation of high endothelial venules and follicular dendritic cells (FDCs). Patients with AITL often have profound immune dysfunction and immunodeficiency. The polymorphous infiltrate is composed of small- to medium-sized lymphocytes usually with clear to pale cytoplasm and distinct cell membranes, small "reactive" lymphocytes, eosinophils, plasma cells, histiocytes, and increased numbers of FDCs in the later stages of the disease. Partial nodal involvement with hyperplastic follicles may be observed in early AITL and at relapse. The natural disease progression of AITL reveals subsequently regressed follicles, or no identifiable follicles, associated with prominent FDC expansion encircling vessels. "High-grade" histologic "transformation" is not infrequent, occurring in up to 23% of cases, and most often EBV-associated and of B-cell origin [Attygalle 2007].

Typical Immunophenotype with the Contribution of FCI

The infiltrates are composed of an admixture of CD4+ and CD8+ cells. Although CD4+ cells usually outnumber CD8+ cells, and the neoplastic cells are usually (if not always) CD4+, there is usually a normal CD4:CD8 ratio [Namikawa 1987]. The neoplastic T cells of AITL have been shown to characteristically express CD10 in up to 80%-90% of cases [Namikawa 1987, Attygalle 2002, Chen 2006, Reichard 2006, Stacchini 2007]. Although phenotypic aberrances are not described in the WHO classification of AITL, flow cytometric studies have clearly demonstrated an immunophenotypic profile of CD2+, CD4+ with immunophenotypic aberrancies (CD10 co-expression or loss of pan T-cell antigens, CD3 and CD7, in the great majority of cases—96%) [Stacchini 2007, Lee 2003, Merchant 2006]. Of further interest, this characteristic immunophenotype is apparently maintained in extranodal sites, including BM, and even in morphologically less definitive biopsy specimens [Merchant 2006]. Subsequent to the identification of CD10 on the neoplastic cells of AITL, CXCL13 (a marker of follicular helper T cells) has also been shown to be characteristically expressed by these neoplastic T cells. This marker (by itself) is more sensitive (100%) and specific than CD10 alone [Dupuis 2006, Grogg 2006, Ortonne 2007]. The plasma cells are usually polyclonal; although some cases may show clonal plasma cell populations [Balague 2007]. It has been recommended that monoclonal plasma cell populations forming tumor masses should be regarded as plasma cell neoplasms or plasmacytomas [Warnke 2007]. The FDCs are CD21+, which is the most sensitive marker for extracellular FDCs in the setting of AITL [Troxell 2005]. A representative case of AITL is demonstrated in [f14.13].

In addition, there may be numerous interfollicular CD20+ large cells scattered and in small aggregates. These are typically EBV+ by EBER-ISH and demonstrate a B-cell clone by molecular studies. However, molecular findings should not be used to determine whether a large B-cell proliferation fulfills the criterion for lymphoma, since up to 30% of AITL will demonstrate a B-cell clone by molecular studies, even in the absence of a recognizable B-cell proliferation [Tan 2006]. DLBCL may be diagnosed in AITL when there are sheets of monoclonal large B cells [Warnke 2007]. In the limited literature on this topic, 70% of B-cell proliferations in AITL are EBV+ by EBER-ISH [Higgins 2000, Lome-Maldonado 2002, Ohshima 1994, Weiss 1992]. A T-cell clone may be identified in up to 80% of cases. The cytogenetic findings in AITL are tabulated in [t14.2]. The most common cytogenetic abnormalities are trisomy 3, trisomy 5, and an additional X chromosome [Kaneko 1988, Schlegelberger 1994].

Differential Diagnosis

Reactive lymphoid hyperplasia and T-zone lymphoma

Early AITL typically shows follicular hyperplasia and may be confused with reactive lymphoid hyperplasia. Recent reports have suggested the demonstration of a CD10+ T-cell population may aid in the diagnosis of this specific type of T-cell lymphoma [Attygalle 2002, Attygalle 2004, Yuan 2002]. However, as has been discussed previously, CD10+ T cells exist in lymphoblastic lymphoma/leukemia and thymoma, and it has more recently been shown there is a normal small subset of CD10+ peripheral T cells that may exist in

reactive lymphoid proliferations as well as B-cell lymphoma [Cook 2003]. Although CD10-positivity may be demonstrated in reactive lymphoid proliferations, the flow cytometric detection of a CD10+/CD3–/CD2+/CD4+/CD8–/CD7– population in correlation with morphology is highly specific for early AITL, rather than a reactive lymphoid hyperplasia.

Differentiation from a T-zone lymphoma (TZL) may be more problematic and even controversial. TZL is a rare subtype of nodal peripheral T-cell lymphoma according to the Kiel classification [Lennert 1978] and was first described by Lennert and Mohri in 1978 [Lennert 1978]. Histologically, involved lymph nodes show expanded T zones infiltrated by uniform, small- to medium-sized T cells with abundant pale to clear cytoplasm accompanied by a proliferation of other T-zone constituents (ie, interdigitating dendritic cells that are S100+ and factor XIIIa+) and high endothelial venules [Krajewski 1988, Siegert 1994, Lennert 1986, Nakamura 1991, Liang 1987, Takagi 1992, Hasui 1992]. Immunohistologically, the neoplastic cells express the pan-T-cell antigens: CD3, CD4, and CD45RO. TCR genes are clonally rearranged in most cases. The most frequently observed cytogenetic abnormality is trisomy 3 [Schlegelberger 1996, Schlegelberger 1994, Lakkala Paranko 1987, Godde Salz 1981]. Later phases of the disease are associated with the absence of the follicles [Pinkus 1992]. Kazakov et al reported that a case with an inconspicuous B-cell reaction in the early stage of the disease (papular lesions), while in the advanced stage of the disease (subcutaneous nodules), was characterized by clusters of CD20+ CD79a+ cells expressing Bcl-2 protein and scattered networks of dermal dendritic cells (CD21+) corresponding to remnants of the follicles [Kazakov 2002]. TZL has an aggressive clinical course with a tendency to early dissemination and is notably resistant to treatment [Helbron 1979]. Based on these descriptions, it seems TZL may actually represent early AITL, and the clinical significance of distinguishing these entities seems clinically irrelevant.

Peripheral T-cell lymphoma, unspecified (PTCL-U), and composite lymphoma of PTCL with DLBCL

A number of PTCL lymphomas may show some but not all features of AITL, and even when a feature is present, it may not be sufficiently well developed to provide convincing support for a diagnosis of AITL. In addition, there are cases that display all of the histologic and immunophenotypic features of AITL but occur in extranodal locations, or the patients lack the clinical

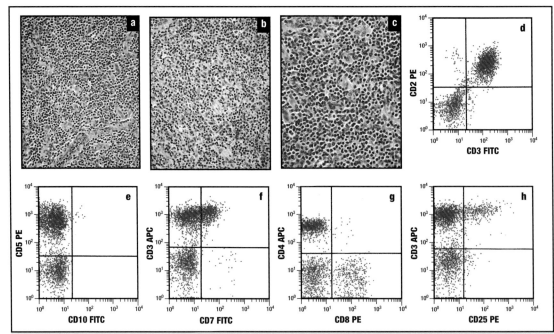

[f14.13] This case demonstrates a typical case of angioimmunoblastic T-cell lymphoma. The clinical history reveals a 67-year-old male who presents with a 1-month history of night sweats, cough, lymphadenopathy, and hepatosplenomegaly. A right axillary lymph node biopsy is performed. H&E sections of the lymph node **a-c** reveal the characteristic morphology. By flow cytometric analysis of the lymph node suspension, the lymphocyte region (93% of cells in the suspension) is composed of 68% T cells with an aberrant immunophenotype. The aberrant T cells express CD3 **d, f, h**, CD2 **d**, and CD5 **e** with partial loss of CD7 **f**. There is a normal CD4:CD8 ratio of 2:1 **g**. There is no significant expression of CD25 **h**. The cytogenetic results are normal. The diagnosis is made of angioimmunoblastic T-cell lymphoma.

syndrome of AITL. It is difficult to know whether such cases belong in the AITL category or in PTCL-U. Although a small number of cases of PTCL-U may show CD10+ of the neoplastic cells [Stacchini 2007], the specific flow cytometric detection of a CD10+/CD3–/CD2+/CD4+/CD8–/CD7– neoplastic population or expression of CXCL13 by IHC staining should help establish a diagnosis of AITL in these diagnostically challenging cases. Although CXCL13 has been demonstrated in a subset (30%) of PTCL-U, all of these cases showed borderline features with AITL [Dupuis 2006].

An AITL with a DLBCL, as defined earlier, would be differentiated from a composite lymphoma composed of a peripheral TCL and a DLBCL by the criteria required for a diagnosis of AITL in the peripheral TCL component, as previously discussed.

Primary cutaneous and extranodal T-cell lymphomas (skin and/or extranodal involvement by AITL)

Skin manifestations of AITL are frequent, sometimes as first manifestations of the disease. Thus, AITL with skin involvement at presentation may be diagnostically confused with primary cutaneous lymphomas. CXCL13

IHC staining has been shown to be particularly helpful in establishing a diagnosis of AITL in such cases. Neoplastic AITL CXCL13+ T cells localize in the skin, and an accurate diagnosis of AITL may be rendered in skin specimens using CXCL13 IHC staining on paraffin-embedded tissues [Ortonne 2007].

Likewise, extranodal involvement by AITL at presentation may cause diagnostic confusion with primary extranodal T-cell lymphomas. However, it has been demonstrated that in addition to the differences in the T-cell immunophenotypes of the neoplastic cells in these various lymphomas already discussed previously, the neoplastic cells of AITL retain their CD10-positivity in extranodal dissemination [Attygalle 2004]. The neoplastic cells in ETL and NK/TCL are characteristically CD10–.

Comparison of FCI to Immunophenotyping by Paraffin Immunohistochemistry

Although a loss of CD3 staining may be identified by visually comparing regions of slides stained for CD3, CD5, and CD20, this phenomenon is analyzed more objectively and sensitively by FCI. In addition, FCI allows for multi-color analysis, which is important in detecting a CD10+/CD3–/CD2+/CD4+/CD8–/CD7– neoplastic population. Also, in a subset of cases, demonstrably weaker surface CD3 expression resulting in dual CD3+ T-cell subpopulations may be noted by FCI.

However, the composition of routine lymphoma FCI panels may not be optimized for revealing this phenotypic anomaly directly, emphasizing the need to be vigilant for this possibility in suggestive cases. One caveat of particular importance concerns the risk of overlooking an aberrant population of CD3- T cells, if selective CD3 gating strategies are used for FCI. By extension, losses of other pan–T-cell antigens, most notably CD7, are not infrequent in AILT, and, although not specific for AILT, if present in a major subpopulation, this feature should prompt the use of a more comprehensive set of anti-T-cell antibodies in diagnostic FCI.

FCI not only allows for multi-color analysis in order to precisely define the immunophenotype of the neoplastic cells in AITL but is also technically advantageous for the identification of small subsets of phenotypically aberrant cells in a large background of inflammatory cells or hematopoietic precursors in the bone marrow. In particular, FCI has been shown to identify immunophenotypically aberrant T-cell subsets, including those with a loss of CD3 and/or co-expression of CD10, in a significant proportion (82%) of cases that did not show aggregates of neoplastic clear cells.

Comprehensive FCI with multiple surface marker antibody combinations and appropriate gating analysis techniques are more likely to successfully identify these subsets of aberrant clones and, therefore, guide key additional investigations (ie, molecular studies for T-cell receptor clonality) for an earlier and more accurate diagnosis of AILT.

On the other hand, CD21+ FDCs are best evaluated in AITL by IHC staining. In addition, CXCL13 expression is only evaluated by IHC staining at this time.

Peripheral T-Cell Lymphoma, Unspecified (PTCL-U)

Definition

Peripheral T-cell lymphoma, unspecified (PTCL-U) is basically a diagnosis of exclusion and represents a collective group of T-cell lymphomas that do not belong to any of the better-defined entities in the WHO classification.

Immunophenotypic Variations

T-cell-associated antigens are positive; and aberrant T-cell phenotypes are common. Most nodal cases are CD4+ and CD8–. CD30 may be variably expressed in large cell variants but not to the degree and uniformity as seen in CD30+ anaplastic large cell lymphoma (ALCL), which is discussed below. Expression of cytotoxic granule-associated proteins is rare in nodal cases. EBV is usually absent in the neoplastic cells but may be present in reactive bystander cells of predominantly B-cell or, more rarely, T-cell lineage. TCR genes are clonally rearranged in most cases. No single consistent chromosomal abnormality has been identified in this heterogeneous group of lymphoma.

Contribution of FCI

FCI is extremely useful in defining an aberrant T-cell immunophenotype by multi-color analysis or in determining clonality by TCR Vβ analysis in PTCL-U. The absence of an aberrant T-cell immunophenotype may greatly aid in evaluating T-cell lymphoma mimics, which are discussed below.

Differential Diagnosis

AITL

This differential diagnosis has been discussed in detail in the discussion above regarding AITL.

T-cell lymphoma mimics

Anticonvulsant-associated lymphoproliferative disorder

Arene oxide-producing anticonvulsant drugs (ie, phenytoin, carbamazepine, and phenobarbital) may induce a lymphadenopathy with varying degrees of architectural effacement and preferential involvement of the parafollicular areas similar to T-cell lymphoma. The cellular infiltrates include numerous large immunoblasts with occasional nuclear atypia and frequent mitoses. Eosinophils, plasma cells, and neutrophils are also present. Atypical large, transformed lymphocytes with Reed-Sternberg nuclei may be seen. Immunophenotyping reveals the immunoblasts to be predominantly of B-cell or, more rarely, of T-cell lineage. Monoclonality of B-cell and T-cell type has been reported [Katzin 1990, Warnke 2007]. The lymphadenopathy will regress upon withdrawal of the drug. One may avoid this pitfall by acquiring a reliable clinical history and being aware of these anticonvulsant-induced changes.

Kikuchi-Fujimoto disease

Kikuchi-Fujimoto disease is a subacute necrotizing lymphadenopathy, which may demonstrate a marked proliferation composed of histiocytes and immunoblasts associated with apoptosis, karyorrhetic debris, and necrosis, simulating a malignant lymphoma. The histiocytes will stain with CD68, and the lymphocytes in the involved zones are predominantly CD8+ T cells. A rather large study of 56 consecutive cases of Kikuchi-Fujimoto disease to determine the pattern of TCR rearrangement revealed that except for 1 unusual case with recurrent lymphadenopathy, none had a monoclonal β or γ rearrangement [Lin 2002]. Eight cases had a polyclonal pattern at both β and γ loci; 20 cases, a mixed polyclonal β and oligoclonal γ pattern; and 27 cases, an oligoclonal pattern at both loci. The high frequency of oligoclonality did not indicate an early-stage T-cell lymphoma in evolution, as confirmed by spontaneous resolution of the lymphadenopathy in all cases within 6 months. Rather, it is consistent with reports of oligoclonal T cells in a variety of immune reactions. This study concluded that, in the vast majority of cases, absence of a monoclonal TCR rearrangement excludes the possibility of T-cell lymphoma, and the presence of an oligoclonal pattern implies a benign immune reaction. Lack of a monoclonal T-cell population in Kikuchi lymphadenitis at the time of initial examination may be used as a diagnostic criterion to exclude the possibility of T-cell lymphoma.

Mastocytosis

Systemic mastocytosis may involve nodal sites in a paracortical pattern and thus mimic early involvement by a T-cell lymphoma. As described in Chapter 18, neoplastic mast cells do not express B-lineage or T-lineage associated antigens, but instead express CD2, CD117, and CD25 by FCI, greatly aiding in the distinction of these 2 entities.

Comparison of FCI to Immunophenotyping by Paraffin Immunohistochemistry

As mentioned previously, FCI may be particularly helpful in defining an aberrant immunophenotype. However, when FCI is not available or there is a limited biopsy specimen, IHC staining may also aid in evaluating for an aberrant T-cell immunophenotype. In addition, IHC staining may be particularly useful in

determining the cell of origin of immunoblasts in the T-cell lymphoma mimics and in recognizing the numerous histiocytes by CD68 IHC staining in Kikuchi-Fujimoto disease.

Anaplastic Large Cell Lymphoma

Definition and Morphologic Variants

Anaplastic large cell lymphoma (ALCL) is defined by the WHO classification as a T-cell lymphoma consisting of lymphoid cells that are commonly large with abundant cytoplasm and pleomorphic, often horseshoe-shaped nuclei. The cells are strongly and uniformly CD30+, and most cases express cytotoxic granule-associated proteins. The majority are positive for the ALCL kinase (ALK) protein. Primary systemic ALCL must be distinguished from primary cutaneous ALCL and other T-cell and B-cell non-Hodgkin lymphomas with anaplastic features and/or CD30 expression. The most frequent histologic variants include the common variant (70%), the lymphohistiocytic variant (10%, seen more frequently in adolescents), and the small cell variant (5%-10%, seen more frequently in pediatric patients). Other less frequent histologic variants have been described and include the following: sarcomatoid, myxoid, neutrophil-rich, eosinophil-rich, hypocellular, giant cell-rich, "signet-ring" like, and mucinous. Although, ALCL most commonly presents as a tissue mass, a leukemic form also exists.

Typical Immunophenotype and Variations

According to the WHO classification, the neoplastic cells of ALCL are strongly CD30+ on the cell membrane and in the paranuclear (Golgi) region (not simply diffuse, cytoplasmic). Only those of T-cell or null-cell immunophenotype are included in ALCL, according to the WHO classification. The great majority of ALCLs express one or more T-cell antigens. Those of T-cell lineage commonly show an aberrant T-cell immunophenotype. They are often CD3−, CD5−, and CD7−, and do not express TCRs, suggesting defective T-cell signaling [Bonzheim 2004]. CD2 and CD4 are more useful; CD4 is expressed more than CD8. A subset of cases is dual CD4−/CD8− [Stein 2000]. Some may show a "null-cell" immunophenotype (defined as negative for all T-cell, B-cell, histiocytic, and plasmacytic antigens) but generally reveal a TCR gene rearrangement. Most cases exhibit positivity for the cytotoxic granule-associated proteins. The neoplastic cells are variably positive for CD45 (LCA) (up to one-third may be negative, particularly by IHC staining) and CD45RO (UCHL-1). CD25 has also been shown to be strongly expressed by ALCL (frozen tissue, IHC staining).

ALK expression is detectable in 60%-85% of cases. ALK over-expression may appear as nuclear and cytoplasmic, cytoplasmic only, or rarely membranous staining. In the majority of cases that have the t(2;5)/NPM-ALK translocation, ALK staining is both nuclear and cytoplasmic. In cases with variant translocations, the ALK staining may be cytoplasmic only or membranous. No differences have been found between NPM-ALK+ ALCLs and ALCLs showing variant translocations involving ALK and fusion partners other than NPM [Falini 1999, Gascoyne 1999, Shiota 1995]. The overall 5-year survival rate in ALK+ALCL is close to 80%, in contrast to only 40% in ALK-ALCLs.

The majority of ALCLs are positive for EMA with a staining pattern similar to CD30, although in some cases, only a proportion of the malignant cells are positive.

CD15 expression is rarely observed, and when present, only a small proportion of the neoplastic cells stain. ALCL is generally negative for EBV (EBER-ISH and LMP1); rare cases have been described with EBV-positivity. A representative case is demonstrated in [f14.14].

Contribution of FCI

FCI of ALCL has been successful in detecting the neoplastic cells in ALCL in up to 96% of cases. The majority of cases show neoplastic cells with high side light scatter properties, similar to monocytes or granulocytes. Thus, light scatter gating on the typical lymphoid regions may yield false-negative results in a substantial number of cases. In addition, CD45 (LCA) is also expressed in the great majority (ie, 95%) of cases (a higher percentage than by IHC staining). The great majority of cases studied in the literature (ie, 96%) have shown CD30 expression with an aberrant T-cell population in 94% of cases. CD2 (72% of cases) and CD4 (63%-80% of cases) are the most commonly expressed T-cell antigens with less frequent expressions of CD3 (32%-40% of cases), CD7 (32% of cases), CD5 (26-32% of cases), and CD8 (21% of cases) [Juco 2003, Dunphy 2000, Kesler 2007]. In addition, and somewhat unexpectedly, 59% of ALCL cases have demonstrated CD13 expression; 1 CD13+ ALCL was also CD33+, and 2 others, also CD15+. One simply needs to be aware of this recognized aberrant expression that may occur in ALCL to avoid a possible misdiagnosis of granulocytic sarcoma. CD25 has been demonstrated in 88% of cases by FCI.

FCI is particularly suitable for immunophenotyping body fluids, fine needle aspirates, PB specimens, BM aspirates, and tissue biopsies when an ample tissue is available for ancillary studies. FCI also allows for multicolor analysis to define the co-expression of CD30 on an aberrant T-cell population.

Differential Diagnosis

Primary cutaneous CD30+ lymphoproliferative disorder and cutaneous ALCL

CD30+ ALCL may occur as a primary cutaneous form or as a systemic form. The primary cutaneous form of ALCL is characteristically ALK– and has a more favorable prognosis than systemic ALCL. However, systemic CD30+ ALCLs, which are associated with the t(2;5) (p23;q35) chromosomal translocation and express ALK, are associated with a better survival. Initially, clusterin was considered a useful marker in distinguishing primary cutaneous and systemic ALCL; however clusterin may be expressed in both forms but is clearly not expressed in HL. On the other hand, CD44v6 (a variant form of CD44, which is a multifunctional cell surface adhesion molecule), has been shown to be an independent marker of the systemic form of ALCL [Liang 2002].

Classical Hodgkin lymphoma

The cells of anaplastic lymphoma may morphologically resemble some forms of classical Hodgkin lymphoma (cHL) cells, and the eosinophil-rich and lymphohistiocytic variants of ALCL may cause even more diagnostic confusion with cHL. In addition, cHL cells generally show strong Golgi staining with CD30 and are CD45 (LCA)-negative, as are some cases of ALCL. However, FCI does not reveal an aberrant T-cell population in cHL. The neoplastic cells of cHL are negative for all T-cell markers. In addition, IHC staining may demonstrate CD20 expression in the cHL cells in up to 67% of cHL cases, and in 97% of cHL cases, the neoplastic cells express Pax-5, which encodes for a B-cell-specific transcription factor [Torlakovic 2002]. EMA is generally negative in cHL or if positive only focally and weakly. cHL are all ALK–. ALK expression is virtually specific for ALCL. It is absent from all postnatal normal human tissues (except rare cells in the brain) and from human neoplasms other than ALCL (except inflammatory myofibroblastic tumor and rare ALK+ DLBCLs with plasmablastic morphology, as discussed below). EBV is positive in the great majority of cHL cases, as

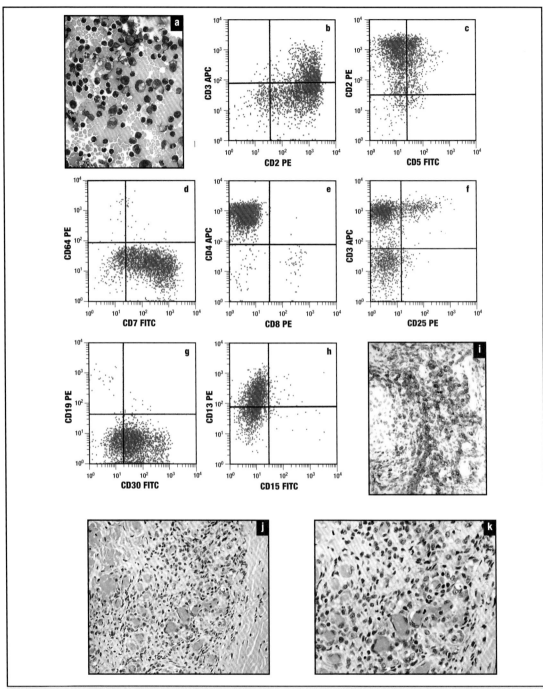

[f14.14] This case demonstrates a CD30+ anaplastic large cell lymphoma with myeloid antigen expression. The clinical history reveals a 19-year-old female who presents with a history of a right ischial bone-based lesion, upon which an FNA is performed. The patient also has co-existent skin lesions, one of which is also biopsied. The FNA cytomorphology of the right ischial bone lesion **a** is demonstrated. By flow cytometric analysis of the FNA specimen, the "expanded" lymphocyte region (ie, increased number of cells within a "lymphoid" region composed of a mixture of small to large lymphoid cells) is composed of 93% T cells with an aberrant immunophenotype. The aberrant T cells express CD2 **b, c**, dim/partial CD3 **b**, dim/partial CD5 **c**, CD7 **d**, and CD4 **e** without CD8 **e** or significant CD25 **f**. The aberrant T cells definitively express CD30 **g** and aberrant CD13 **h** without any additional myelomonocytic markers expressed (not demonstrated). The CD30 immunohistochemical stain **i** is demonstrated, as are the H&E sections of the subsequent skin biopsy **j, k**. The cytogenetic analysis reveals ALK rearrangement by FISH. The diagnosis of anaplastic large cell lymphoma with myeloid antigen expression is made.

is CD15 with optimal IHC staining. Lastly, expression of clusterin may be demonstrated in systemic ALCL [Wellmann 2000] and in a substantial subset of cutaneous ALCL [Lae 2002], but not in any cases of cHL.

T-cell and B-cell NHLs with CD30 expression

Non-Hodgkin lymphomas of non-ALCL type may reveal CD30 staining, but the staining is generally not as intense or diffuse. Barry et al reported the co-expression of CD30 and CD15 in at least a subset of the neoplastic cells in cases of PTCL [Barry 2003]. Two distinct groups were identified based on morphologic and immunophenotypic features. The first group had histologic features mimicking cHL with CD30+, CD15+ Reed-Sternberg-like cells in an inflammatory background of varied extent and composition. The background lymphoid cells showed minimal cytologic atypia. The RS-like cells were negative for CD20 and CD79a, and CD45 expression was absent in 80% of cases. The RS-like cells expressed CD25 and at least 1 T-cell-associated marker in all cases. The background T-cell population showed convincing subset predominance in 80% of cases, loss of T-cell-associated antigens in 60% of cases, and coexpression of CD30 and CD15 in 20% of cases. The second group had morphologic features more in keeping with PTCL than cHL. The proportion of neoplastic cells co-expressing CD30 and CD15 varied. Loss of T-cell antigens was noted in all cases, CD4 predominated in 80% of cases, and 50% of cases expressed CD45. PCR analysis revealed clonal TCR γ chain gene rearrangements in 82% of cases, but no immunoglobulin heavy (IgH) chain gene rearrangements. ISH studies for EBV were negative in all cases. In some PTCL cases, the overlap with cHL may be striking, and combined immunophenotypic and molecular studies are often necessary to confirm the diagnosis. These cases had a worse prognosis than cHL and ALCL.

B-cell NHLs may also demonstrate CD30-positivity, also not as uniform or strong as in ALCL. The majority is of large cell or immunoblastic morphology; a third of small noncleaved cell lymphomas express CD30. However, CD30 may be stronger and more uniform in primary mediastinal B-cell lymphoma (discussed below), sinusoidal CD30+ large B-cell lymphoma (discussed below), and DLBCL, anaplastic variant (discussed below).

Primary mediastinal large B-cell lymphoma

This differential diagnosis was discussed in detail in Chapter 12 in the section on primary mediastinal large B-cell lymphoma.

TCRLBCL

The differential diagnoses of T-cell rich large B-cell lymphoma and the lymphohistiocytic-rich variant of ALCL were discussed in detail in Chapter 12 in the section on DLBCL.

Anaplastic variant of DLBCL and ALK+ DLBCL

The differential diagnoses of the anaplastic variant of DLBCL, ALK+ DLBCL, and ALCL were discussed in detail in Chapter 12.

Primary effusion lymphoma

This differential diagnosis was discussed in detail in Chapter 12 in the section on primary effusion lymphoma.

Sinusoidal CD30+ large B-cell lymphoma

Some of the characteristic features of ALCL, such as CD30 antigen expression and the presence of large pleomorphic lymphoid cells infiltrating lymph node sinuses, may be found in a rare variant of DLBCL [Lai 2000]. Necrosis and admixed granulocytes are also frequently seen in such cases. The neoplastic cells in such cases are positive for CD30 and CD20 or CD79a and are ALK−. ISH for EBV may be positive in a small subset of these neoplasms. These neoplasms may be distinguished from ALCL due to their B-lineage and lack of ALK expression. Although 2 cases tested were EMA−, it is unclear how this variant differs from the anaplastic variant of DLBCL with a sinusoidal growth pattern [Li 2002].

Sarcoma and inflammatory myofibroblastic tumor

The sarcomatoid and myxoid variants of ALCL may mimic soft tissue sarcomas, most commonly pleomorphic rhabdomyosarcoma, malignant fibrous histiocytoma, pleomorphic liposarcoma, and inflammatory myofibroblastic tumor. Rare cases of rhabdomyosarcoma may be ALK+. Inflammatory myofibroblastic tumors frequently co-express ALK and alpha-smooth muscle actin. CD30 is negative in inflammatory myofibroblastic tumor and rhabdomyosarcoma. Malignant fibrous histiocytoma and pleomorphic liposarcoma are CD30− and ALK−.

Metastatic carcinoma, mesothelioma, and melanoma

CD30 expression may be encountered in embryonal carcinoma, focally in seminoma and seminomatous components of mixed germ cell tumors (occurring with and without co-localized expression of cytokeratin), pancreatic carcinomas, salivary gland tumors, and malignant mesothelioma [Hittmair 1996, Dunphy 2000]. In addition, EMA is positive in carcinoma as well as in mesothelioma and is frequently expressed in ALCL. Cytokeratin is positive in carcinoma, in mesothelioma (mesothelioma is also calretinin+), and in rare cases of aggressive, large B-cell lymphomas [Lasota 1996]. In addition, a rare case of B-cell anaplastic large cell lymphoma (ie, anaplastic variant of DLBCL), confirmed by immunohistochemistry and Southern blot immunoglobulin gene rearrangement analysis, has been reported to contain neoplastic cells immunoreactive for cytokeratin, using antibodies CAM 5.2, M20, MAK 6, and KS-B17.2. Bands corresponding to cytokeratin 18 and cytokeratins 18 and 8 were seen on Western blot immunoanalysis using antibodies KS-B17.2 and CAM 5.2 [Frierson 1994]. However, all of these cases are ALK–. There are no reported cases of ALCL (according to WHO criteria) with cytokeratin-positivity.

Morphologically malignant melanoma may mimic ALCL; however the immunophenotype of malignant melanoma is as follows: CD30–, ALK–, HMB.45+, MART1+, and S-100+.

Leukemia and granulocytic sarcoma

As mentioned previously, ALCL may express myelomonocytic markers (ie, CD13, CD15, and CD33), but the expression of CD30, variable expression of T-cell markers, and lack of immature markers should distinguish ALCL from granulocytic sarcoma.

Reactive conditions: Immunoblastic proliferations

CD30 staining may also be observed in benign immunoblastic proliferations [Segal 1994]. However, the CD30 staining is not as strong or uniform, and there is no evidence of an aberrant T-cell or monoclonal B-cell population. ALK is negative.

Comparison of FCI to IHC Immunophenotyping

The contributions of FCI in the diagnosis of ALCL have been discussed previously. An obvious drawback to IHC analysis is that it is not well suited to the analysis of fluid specimens, such as body fluids, peripheral blood or bone marrow aspirate specimens, or samples obtained by fine-needle aspiration. IHC analysis is also relatively insensitive compared with flow cytometry. Thus, dim antigen expression detected by FCI may often be negative by IHC analysis. For example, CD45 (LCA) is commonly positive in ALK+ ALCL when assessed by flow cytometry as previously discussed, but it can be negative in a subset of cases by IHC analysis. However, a potential drawback to a flow cytometric approach is that certain antigens are expressed intracellularly (ie, ALK and the cytotoxic granule-associated proteins) and require cell permeabilization for analysis. On the other hand, IHC staining is well suited to the analysis of ALK+ ALCL tissue specimens, and many pathologists consider this approach the method of choice. Most of the antibodies essential for diagnosis of ALK+ ALCL are reactive in routinely fixed, paraffin-embedded tissue sections, and some of these antibodies (ie, ALK and cytotoxic granule-associated proteins) are optimized for this approach to immunophenotypic diagnosis. In addition, a study comparing the detection of t(2;5) in CD30+ ALCL by IHC, FISH, and RT-PCR techniques in paraffin-embedded tissue demonstrated that IHC studies, using antibody ALK1, and FISH for ALK gene rearrangement are equally effective in identifying patients with ALCL who have a favorable outcome.

CD4+CD56+ Hematodermic Tumor, Alias "Blastic NK-Cell Lymphoma"

Definition

CD4+CD56+ hematodermic tumor (HDT) is composed of cells with a lymphoblast-like morphology and derives from plasmacytoid dendritic cells. Although this entity is not of NK-cell origin, it is included in this chapter since it previously would have been classified within the category of "blastic NK-cell lymphoma." Frequent sites of disease include skin (60%) and PB/BM (70%). The overall prognosis is poor in HDT, despite multiagent chemotherapy and/or radiation.

Typical Immunophenotype

The neoplastic cells in CD4+CD56+ HDT are typically positive for CD45, HLA-DR, CD43, CD4, and CD56 [Reichard 2005]. The pDC markers, CD123 (strong, >90% of cases), TCL-1 (90% of cases), CD45RA, blood dendritic cell antigen (BCDA)-2 (expressed in more mature cases), and myxovirus A (MxA) may be detected by FCI and/or IHC staining [Pilichowska 2007].

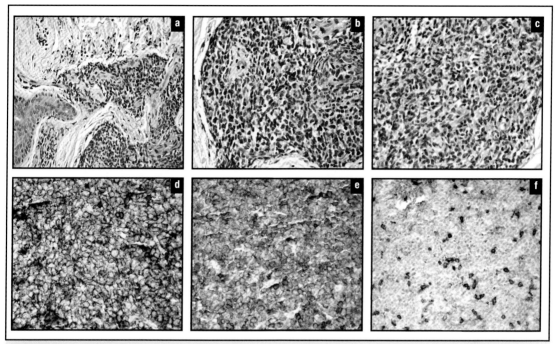

[f14.15] This case demonstrates a typical case of hematodermic tumor. The clinical history reveals a 68-year-old male with a supposed history of "NK/T-cell lymphoma" who presents with a new nodule on the right arm. A punch biopsy of the skin from the right forearm is performed. The H&E sections of the skin punch biopsy **a-c** demonstrate the characteristic morphology. Flow cytometric analysis was not performed (and thus not available for demonstration). Immunohistochemical stains reveal positivity of the malignant cells for CD4 (not demonstrated), CD43 **d**, CD45 **e**, and CD56 (not demonstrated), and negativity for CD3 **f**, CD5, CD7, CD8, CD30, CD34, CD57, myeloperoxidase, CD79a, CD20, and TdT (all, not demonstrated). Diagnosis is made of hematodermic tumor.

There may also be a subset of cases with CD2 positivity, weak CD7 positivity, weak CD33 positivity, TdT positivity (up to 50% of cases), as well as CD68 positivity. All cases are otherwise negative for EBV (EBER-ISH), B cell, T cell, myeloid, and NK-cell markers. TCRγ gene rearrangement is negative in these cases. Although clonal rearrangements of the TCR genes are lacking in HDTs, occasional cases with clonal or oligoclonal TCRγ or TCRδ chain gene rearrangements have been reported, perhaps related to blast state and the expression of TdT [Liu 2004, Aoyama 2001]. A representative case is demonstrated in **[f14.15]**.

Expression of EBV antigens, myeloperoxidase, lysozyme, PAX-5, CD20, CD22, and TCR protein should exclude a diagnosis of HDT [Herling 2007]. Although there is no single defining genetic abnormality described, complex structural chromosomal abnormalities have been demonstrated. By far, the most frequently observed is deletion 5q (up to 72% of cases), followed in decreasing frequency by alterations of 13q, 12p, and 6q, and losses of chromosomes 15 and 9 [Brody 1995, Kameoka 1998, Petrella 1999, DiGiuseppe 1997, Leroux 2002,

Hallermann 2004] (see **[t14.2]**). Trisomies of chromosomes 8 and 21 and monosomy 7 are rare in HDTs, in contrast to AML and MDS [Bernasconi 2002, Rigolin 1997].

Contribution of FCI

FCI allows for multicolor analysis, which is particularly important in defining the "lineage-negative" immunophenotype of the neoplastic cells of CD4+CD56+ HDT.

Differential Diagnosis

Primary cutaneous T-cell lymphoma and NK/T-cell lymphoma, nasal type

Once recognized, the distinction of HDT from NK-cell malignancies is relatively straightforward [Bekkenk 2004]. Although both tumor types express CD56, angioinvasion of tumor cells and expression of CD2, cytoplasmic CD3, EBV, and cytotoxic granule-associated proteins, such as granzyme B and perforin, support a diagnosis of an NK-cell tumor. In addition, the absence of CD123, TCL1 [Herling 2003], and CD45RA in NK-cell malignancies may be used to resolve discordant results for other markers. Although rare NK-like T-cell malignancies may express CD4 and CD56, the absence of a clonal TCR gene rearrangement in HDTs is most helpful in excluding a T-cell lymphoma.

Leukemia cutis

More challenging is the distinction of HDTs from myeloproliferative disorders with monocytic differentiation, given the propensity of these tumors to occur in the skin [Bekkenk 2004]. CD4 may be expressed in the monocytic lineage and in myelomonocytic tumors [Petrella 2002, Knapp 1989]. CD56 is expressed in 20% to 30% of AML and is associated with skin involvement and the French-American-British M5 monocytic subtype [Di Bona 2002, Delgado 2002, Kuwabara 1999]. CD56 may also be detected in chronic myeloid leukemias showing blastic transformation of a monocytic immunophenotype along with skin manifestation [Kaddu 1999]. Furthermore, CD4 and CD56 expression may be dim in HDT, and the myeloid-associated molecules CD33 [Garnache-Ottou 2005] and CD68 [Petrella 2005] are seen in significant proportions of prototypic HDT cases. As stated earlier, CD33 may be expressed in s subset of HDT cases. Overall, it is advisable to include additional myeloid lineage-specific markers, such as MPO, markers for pDC (DC2) differentiation, like CD123 or BDCA-2, and other discriminating markers, such as TCL1 and lysozyme, in the diagnostic panel.

At this point, it is worth considering how CD4+/CD56+/CD123+ HDT stands in relationship to CD7+/CD56+ myeloid/natural killer cell precursor acute leukemia, which is discussed in detail in Chapter 10. This distinct entity was described in 1997 by Suzuki et al and is characterized by the following immunophenotype: CD7+, CD33+, CD34+, CD56+, and frequently HLA-DR+ [Suzuki 1997]. A subset of these cases is cCD3+ by flow cytometry with additional cases cCD3+ by Northern blotting. The majority show germline configurations of the TCR β and γ chain genes and Ig heavy chain gene. They are characteristically negative for MPO by cytochemical staining and negative for other NK, T-cell, and B-cell markers by FCI. This distinct entity would have previously been classified within the category of "blastic NK-cell lymphoma" (now termed CD4+, CD56+ HDT) and its unique biology obscured.

Comparison of FCI to IHC Immunophenotyping

Although FCI offers the advantage of defining the "lineage-negative" immunophenotype in HDT, paraffin IHC may be useful in limited biopsy specimens, and for the evaluation of markers not available for or routinely analyzed by FCI (ie, BDCA-2, MxA protein, EBV-EBER-ISH, cytotoxic granule-associated proteins) and important in the differential diagnosis of HDT.

References

Abo T, Balch CM [1981] A differentiation antigen of human NK and K cells identified by a monoclonal antibody (HNK-1). *J Immunol* 127:1024-1029.

Agnarsson BA, Vonderheid EC, Kadin ME [1990] Cutaneous T-cell lymphoma with suppressor/cytotoxic (CD8) phenotype: Identification of rapidly progressive and chronic subtypes. *J Am Acad Dermatol* 22:569-577.

Ahmad E, Kingma DW, Jaffe ES, et al [2005] Flow cytometric immunophenotypic profiles of mature gamma delta T-cell malignancies involving peripheral blood and bone marrow. *Cytometry B Clin Cytom* 67:6-12.

Alonsozana EL, Stamberg J, Kumar D, et al [1997] Isochromosome 7q: The primary cytogenetic abnormality in hepatosplenic gammadelta T-cell lymphoma. *Leukemia* 11:1367-1372.

Aoyama Y, Yamane T, Hino M, et al [2001] Blastic NK-cell lymphoma/leukemia with T-cell receptor gamma rearrangement. *Ann Hematol* 80:752-754.

Arnulf B, Copie-Bergman C, Delfau-Larue MH, et al [1998] Nonhepatosplenic gammadelta T-cell lymphoma: A subset of cytotoxic lymphomas with mucosal or skin localization. *Blood* 91:1723-1731.

Attygalle A, Al-Jehani R, Diss TC, et al [2002] Neoplastic T cells in angioimmunoblastic T-cell lymphoma express CD10. *Blood* 99:527-633.

Attygalle A, Diss TC, Munson P, Isaacson PG, Du MQ, Dogan A [2004] CD10 expression in extranodal dissemination of angioimmunoblastic T-cell lymphoma [abstract]. *Am J Surg Pathol* 28:54-61.

Attygalle A, Kyriakou C, Dupuis J, et al [2007] Histologic evolution of angioimmunoblastic T-cell lymphoma in consecutive biopsies: Clinical correlation and insights into natural history and disease progression. *Am J Surg Pathol* 31:1077-1088.

Balague O, Martinez A, Colomo L, et al [2007] Epstein-Barr virus negative clonal plasma cell proliferations and lymphomas in peripheral T-cell lymphomas: A phenomenon with distinctive clinicopathological features. *Am J Surg Pathol* 31:1310-22.

Barry TS, Jaffe ES, Sorbara L, Raffeld M, Pittaluga S [2003] Peripheral T-cell lymphomas expressing CD30 and CD15. *Am J Surg Pathol* 27:1513-1522.

Basarab T, Fraser-Andrews EA, Orchard G, et al [1998] Lymphomatoid papulosis in association with mycosis fungoides: A study of 15 cases. *Br J Dermatol* 139:630-638.

Beck RC, Stahl S, O'Keefe CL, et al [2003] Detection of mature T-cell leukemias by flow cytometry using anti-T-cell receptor V beta antibodies. *Am J Clin Pathol* 120:785-794.

Bekkenk M, Geelen FAMJ, van Voorst Vader PC, et al [2000] Primary and secondary cutaneous CD30-positive lymphoproliferative disorders: long-term follow-up data of 219 patients and guidelines for diagnosis and treatment: a report from the Dutch Cutaneous Lymphoma Group. *Blood* 95:3653-3661.

Bekkenk MW, Vermeer MH, Jansen PM, et al [2003] Peripheral T-cell lymphomas unspecified presenting in the skin: Analysis of prognostic factors in a group of 82 patients. *Blood* 102:2213-2219.

Bekkenk MW, Jansen PM, Meijer CJ, et al [2004] CD56+ hematological neoplasms presenting in the skin: A retrospective analysis of 23 new cases and 130 cases from the literature. *Ann Oncol* 15:1097-1108.

Beljaards RC, Meijer CJLM, Scheffer E, et al [1989] Prognostic significance of CD30 (Ki-1/Ber-H2) expression in primary cutaneous large-cell lymphomas of T-cell origin: a clinicopathologic and immunohistochemical study in 20 patients. *Am J Pathol* 135:1169-1178.

Bernasconi P, Boni M, Cavigliano PM, et al [2002] Molecular genetics of acute myeloid leukemia. *Ann N Y Acad Sci* 963:297-305.

Berti E, Cerri A, Cavicchini S, et al [1991] Primary cutaneous gamma/delta lymphoma presenting as disseminated pagetoid reticulosis. *J Invest Dermatol* 96:718-723.

Berti E, Tomasini D, Vermeer MH, Meijer CJLM, Alessi E, Willemze R [1999] Primary cutaneous CD8-positive epidermotropic cytotoxic T-cell lymphoma: A distinct clinicopathologic entity with an aggressive clinical behaviour. *Am J Pathol* 155:483-492.

Bonzheim I, Geissinger E, Roth S, et al [2004] Anaplastic large cell lymphomas lack the expression of T-cell receptor molecules or molecules of proximal T-cell receptor signaling. *Blood* 104:3358-3360.

Boulland ML, Kanavaros P, Wechsler J, et al [1997] Cytotoxic protein expression in natural killer cell lymphomas and in alpha beta and gamma delta peripheral T-cell lymphomas. *J Pathol* 183:432-439.

Boulland ML, Wechsler J, Bagot M, et al [2000] Primary CD30-positive cutaneous T-cell lymphomas and lymphomatoid papulosis frequently express cytotoxic proteins. *Histopathology* 36:136-144.

Brito-Babapulle V, Matutes E, Catovsky D. Classification of T-cell disorders. *Atlas Genet Cytogenet Oncol Haematol*. February 2001. URL:http//www.infobiogen.fr/services/chromcancer/Anomalies/TcellClassifID2079.html

Brody JP, Allen S, Schulman P, et al [1995] Acute agranular CD4-positive natural killer cell leukemia: Comprehensive clinicopathologic studies including virologic and in vitro culture with inducing agents. *Cancer* 75:2474-2483.

Burg G, Dummer R, Wilhelm M, et al [1991] A subcutaneous delta-positive T-cell lymphoma that produces interferon gamma. *N Engl J Med* 325:1078-1081.

Catovsky D, Ralfkiaer E, Muller-Hermelink HK [2001] T-cell prolymphocytic leukaemia. In: Jaffe ES, Harris NL, Stein H, et al, eds. *Pathology and Genetics of Tumours of Haematopoietic and Lymphoid Tissues*. Lyon, France: IARC Press; 195-198. World Health Organization Classification of Tumours.

Chan JK, Sin VC, Wong KF, et al [1997] Nonnasal lymphoma expressing the natural killer cell marker CD56: A clinicopathologic study of 49 cases of an uncommon aggressive neoplasm. *Blood* 89:4501-4513.

Chan JK [1998] Natural killer cell neoplasms. *Anat Pathol* 3:77-145.

Chan JKC, Jaffe ES, Ralfkiaer E [2001] Extranodal NK/T-cell lymphoma, nasal type. In: Jaffe ES, Harris NL, Stein H, et al, eds [2001] *Pathology and Genetics of Tumours of Haematopoietic and Lymphoid Tissues*. Lyon, France: IARC Press; 204-207. World Health Organization Classification of Tumours.

Chang SE, Lee SY, Choi JH, et al [2002] Cutaneous dissemination of nasal NK/T-cell lymphoma with bone marrow, liver and lung involvement. *Clin Exp Dermatol* 27:120-122.

Chen W, Kesler MV, Karandikar NJ, McKenna RW, Kroft SH [2006] Flow cytometric features of angioimmunoblastic T-cell lymphoma. *Clinical Cytometry* 708:142-148.

Chott A, Vonderheid EC, Olbricht S, et al [1996] The dominant T cell clone is present in multiple regressing skin lesions and associated T-cell lymphomas of patients with lymphomatoid papulosis. *J Invest Dermatol* 106:696-700.

Ciccone E, Ferrini S, Bottino C, et al [1988] A monoclonal antibody specific for a common determinant of the human T cell receptor gamma/delta directly activates CD3+WT31- lymphocytes to express their functional program(s). *J Exp Med* 168:1-11.

Cook JR, Craig FE, Swerdlow SH [2003] Benign CD10-positive T cells in reactive lymphoid proliferations and B-cell lymphomas. *Mod Pathol* 16:879-885.

Cooke CB, Krenacs L, Stetler-Stevenson M, et al [1996] Hepatosplenic T-cell lymphoma: A distinct clinicopathologic entity of cytotoxic gamma delta T-cell origin. *Blood* 88:4265-4274.

de Bruin PC, Beljaards RC, van Heerde P, et al [1993] Differences in clinical behaviour and immunophenotype between primary cutaneous and primary nodal anaplastic large cell lymphoma of T- or null cell phenotype. *Histopathol* 23:127-135.

de Wolf-Peeters C, Achten R [2000] Gamma-delta T-cell lymphomas: A homogeneous entity? *Histopathology* 36:294-305.

DeCoteau JF, Butmarc JR, Kinney MC, et al [1996] The t(2;5) chromosomal translocation is not a common feature of primary cutaneous CD30+ lymphoproliferative disorders: Comparison with anaplastic large-cell lymphoma of nodal origin. *Blood* 87:3437-3441.

Deleeuw RJ, Zettl A, Klinker E, et al [2007] Whole genome analysis and HLA genotyping of enteropathy-associated T-cell lymphoma reveals two distinct lymphoma subtypes. *Gastroenterology* 132:1902-1911.

Delgado J, Morado M, Jimenez MC, et al [2002] CD56 expression in myeloperoxidase-negative FAB M5 acute myeloid leukemia. *Am J Hematol* 69:28-30.

Di Bona E, Sartori R, Zambello R, et al [2002] Prognostic significance of CD56 antigen expression in acute myeloid leukemia. *Haematologica* 87:250-256.

DiGiuseppe JA, Louie DC, Williams JE, et al [1997] Blastic natural killer cell leukemia/lymphoma: A clinicopathologic study. *Am J Surg Pathol* 21:1223-1230.

Dunphy CH, Popovic WJ [1995] True T-cell chronic lymphocytic leukemia: Case report and review of the literature. *Cell Vision* 2:491-494.

Dunphy CH, Gardner LJ, Bee CS [2000a] Malignant mesothelioma with CD30-positivity. A case report and review of the literature. *Arch Pathol Lab Med* 124:1077-1079.

Dunphy CH, Gardner LJ, Manes JL, Bee CS, Taysi K [2000b] CD30+ anaplastic large-cell lymphoma with aberrant expression of CD13: Case report and review of the literature. *J Clin Lab Anal* 14:299-304.

Dupuis J, Boye K, Martin N, et al [2006] Expression of CXCL13 by neoplastic cells in angioimmunoblastic T-cell lymphoma (AITL): A new diagnostic marker providing evidence that AITL derives from follicular helper T cells. *Am J Surg Pathol* 30:490-494.

El Shabrawi-Caelen L, Cerroni L, Kerl H [2000] The clinicopathologic spectrum of cytotoxic lymphomas of the skin. *Semin Cutan Med Surg* 19:118-123.

El Shabrawi-Caelen L, Kerl H, Cerroni L [2004] Lymphomatoid papulosis: Reappraisal of clinicopathologic presentation and classification into subtypes A, B, and C. *Arch Dermatol* 140:441-447.

Epling-Burnette PK, Painter JS, Chaurasia P, et al [2004] Dysregulated NK receptor expression in patients with lymphoproliferative disease of granular lymphocytes. *Blood* 103:3431-3439.

Esin S, Shigematsu M, Nagai S, et al [1996] Different percentages of peripheral blood gamma delta + T cells in healthy individuals from different areas of the world. *Scand J Immunol* 43:593-596.

Falini B, Pileri S, Zinzani PL, et al [1999] ALK+ lymphoma: Clinico-pathological findings and outcome. *Blood* 93:2697-2706.

Farag SS, Caligiuri MA [2006] Human natural killer cell development and biology. *Blood Rev* 20:123-137.

Felgar RE, Salhany KE, Macon WR, et al [1999] The expression of TIA-1+ cytolytic-type granules and other cytolytic lymphocyte-associated markers in CD30+ anaplastic large cell lymphomas (ALCL): Correlation with morphology, immunophenotype, ultrastructure, and clinical features. *Hum Pathol* 30:228-236.

Fink-Puches R, Chott A, Ardigo M, et al [2004] The spectrum of cutaneous lymphomas in patients less than 20 years of age. *Pediatr Dermatol* 21:525-533.

Fitzgerald JE, Ricalton NS, Meyer AC, et al [1995] Analysis of clonal CD8+ T cell expansions in normal individuals and patients with rheumatoid arthritis. *J Immunol* 154:3538-3547.

Friedmann D, Wechsler J, Delfau MH, et al [1995] Primary cutaneous pleomorphic small T-cell lymphoma. *Arch Dermatol* 131:1009-1015.

Frierson, Jr. HF, Bellafiore FJ, Gaffey MJ, McCary WS, Innes, Jr. DJ, Williams ME [1994] Cytokeratin in anaplastic large cell lymphoma. *Modern Pathol* 7:317-321.

Garnache-Ottou F, Chaperot L, Biichle S, et al [2005] Expression of the myeloid-associated marker CD33 is not an exclusive factor for leukemic plasmacytoid dendritic cells. *Blood* 105:1256-1264.

Gascoyne RD, Aoun P, Wu D, et al [1999] Prognostic significance of anaplastic lymphoma kinase (ALK) protein expression in adults with anaplastic large cell lymphoma. *Blood* 93:3913-3921.

Gaulard P, Bourquelot P, Kanavaros P, et al [1990] Expression of the alpha/beta and gamma/delta T-cell receptors in 57 cases of peripheral T-cell lymphomas; Identification of a subset of gamma/delta T-cell lymphomas. *Am J Pathol* 137:617-628.

Gellrich S, Wernicke M, Wilks A, et al [2004] The cell infiltrate in lymphomatoid papulosis comprises a mixture of polyclonal large atypical cells (CD30-positive) and smaller monoclonal T cells (CD30-negative). *J Invest Dermatol* 122:859-861.

Gentile TC, Hadlock KG, Uner AH, et al [1998] Large granular lymphocyte leukaemia occurring after renal transplantation. *Br J Haematol* 101:507-512.

Godde Salz E, Schwarze EW, Stein H, et al [1981] Cytogenetic findings in T-zone lymphoma. *J Cancer Res Clin Oncol* 101:81-89.

Gorczyca W, Weisberger J, Liu Z, et al [2002] An approach to diagnosis of T-cell lymphoproliferative disorders by flow cytometry. *Clinical Cytometry* 50:177-190.

Grogg KL, Attygalle AD, Macon WR, Remstein ED, Kurtin PJ, Dogan A [2006] Expression of CXCL13, a chemokine highly upregulated in germinal center T-helper cells, distinguishes angioimmunoblastic T-cell lymphoma from peripheral T-cell lymphoma, unspecified. *Mod Pathol* 18:1101-1107.

Hallermann C, Middel P, Griesinger F, et al [2004] CD4+ CD56+ blastic tumor of the skin: Cytogenetic observations and further evidence of an origin from plasmocytoid dendritic cells. *Eur J Dermatol* 14:317-322.

Hasui K, Sato E, Sakae K, et al [1992] Immunohistological quantitative analysis of S100 protein-positive cells in T-cell malignant lymphomas, especially in adult T-cell leukemia/lymphomas. *Pathol Res Pract* 188:484-489.

Helbron D, Brittinger G, Lennert K [1979] T-zone lymphoma—clinical symptoms, therapy, and prognosis (author's transl). *Blut* 39:117-131.

Herbst H, Sander C, Tronnier M, et al [1997] Absence of anaplastic lymphoma kinase (ALK) and Epstein-Barr virus gene products in primary cutaneous anaplastic large cell lymphoma and lymphomatoid papulosis. *Br J Dermatol* 137:680-686.

Herling M, Teitell MA, Shen RR, et al [2003] TCL1 expression in plasmacytoid dendritic cells (DC2s) and the related CD4+ CD56+ blastic tumors of skin. *Blood* 101:5007-5009.

Herling M, Khoury JD, Washington LT, et al [2004a] A systematic approach to diagnosis of mature T-cell leukemias reveals heterogeneity among WHO categories. *Blood* 104:328-335.

Herling M, Rassidakis GZ, Jones D, et al [2004b] Absence of Epstein-Barr virus in anaplastic large cell lymphoma: A study of 64 cases classified according to World Health Organization criteria. *Hum Pathol* 35:455-459.

Herling M, Patel KA, Khalili J, et al [2006] TCL1 shows a regulated expression pattern in chronic lymphocytic leukemia that correlates with molecular subtypes and proliferative state. *Leukemia* 20:280-285.

Herling M, Jones D [2007] CD4+/CD56+ hematodermic tumor: The features of an evolving entity and its relationship to dendritic cells. *Am J Clin Pathol* 127:687-700.

Higgins JP, van de Rijn M, Jones CD, et al [2000] Peripheral T-cell lymphoma complicated by a proliferation of large B cells. *Am J Clin Pathol* 114:236-247.

Hittmair A, Rogatsch H, Hobisch A, Mikuz G, Feichtinger H [1996] CD30 expression in seminoma. *Hum Pathol* 27:1166-1171.

Hoffmann T, De Libero G, Colonna M, et al [2000] Natural killer-type receptors for HLA class I antigens are clonally expressed in lymphoproliferative disorders of natural killer and T-cell type. *Br J Haematol* 110:525-536.

Hoque SR, Child FJ, Whittaker SJ, et al [2003] Subcutaneous panniculitis-like T-cell lymphoma: A clinicopathological, immunophenotypic and molecular analysis of six patients. *Br J Dermatol* 148:516-525.

Imamura N, Kusunoki Y, Kawa-Ha K, et al [1990] Aggressive natural killer cell leukaemia/lymphoma: Report of four cases and review of the literature: Possible existence of a new clinical entity originating from the third lineage of lymphoid cells. *Br J Haematol* 75:49-59.

Jaffe ES, Krenacs L, Raffeld M [2003] Classification of cytotoxic T-cell and natural killer cell lymphomas. *Semin Hematol* 40:175-184.

Jones D, Dang NH, Duvic M, Washington LT, Huh YO [2001] Absence of CD26 expression is a useful marker for diagnosis of T-cell lymphoma in peripheral blood. *Am J Clin Pathol* 115:885-892.

Jones D, Vega F, Sarris A, Medeiros LJ [2002] CD4-CD8-"Double-negative" cutaneous T-cell lymphomas share common histologic features and an aggressive clinical course. *Am J Surg Pathol* 26:225-231.

Juco J, Holden JT, Mann KP, Kelley LG, Li S [2003] Immunophenotypic analysis of anaplastic large cell lymphoma by flow cytometry. *Am J Clin Pathol* 119:205-212.

Kaddu S, Beham-Schmid C, Zenahlik P, et al [1999] CD56+ blastic transformation of chronic myeloid leukemia involving the skin. *J Cutan Pathol* 26:497-503.

Kadin M, Nasu K, Sako D, Said J, Vonderheid E [1985] Lymphomatoid papulosis: A cutaneous proliferation of activated helper T cells expressing Hodgkin's disease associated antigens. *Am J Pathol* 119:315-325.

Kadin ME, Vonderheid EC, Sako D, et al [1987] Clonal composition of T cells in lymphomatoid papulosis. *Am J Pathol* 126:13-17.

Kameoka J, Ichinohasama R, Tanaka M, et al [1998] A cutaneous agranular CD2- CD4+ CD56+ "lymphoma": Report of two cases and review of the literature. *Am J Clin Pathol* 110:478-488.

Kaneko Y, Masaki N, Sakurai M, et al [1988] Characteristic karyotypic pattern in T-cell lymphoproliferative disorders with reactive "angioimmunoblastic lymphadenopathy with dysproteinemia-type" features. *Blood* 72:413-421.

Katzin WE, Julius CJ, Tubbs RR, et al [1990] Lymphoproliferative disorders associated with carbamazepine. *Arch Pathol Lab Med* 114:1244-1248.

Kaudewitz P, Stein H, Dallenbach F, et al [1989] Primary and secondary cutaneous Ki-1+ (CD30+) anaplastic large cell lymphomas: Morphologic, immunohistologic, and clinical characteristics. *Am J Pathol* 135:359-367.

Kazakov DV, Kempf W, Michalis S, et al [2002] T-zone lymphoma with cutaneous involvement: A case report and review of the literature. *Br J Dermatol* 146:1096-1100.

Kazatchkine MD [1995] Nomenclature for T-cell receptor (TCR) gene segments of the immune system: WHO-IUIS Nomenclature Sub-Committee on TCR Designation. *Immunogenetics* 42:451-453.

Kelemen K, Guitart J, Kuzel TM, Goolsby CL, Peterson LC [2008] The usefulness of CD26 in flow cytometric analysis of peripheral blood in Sézary syndrome. *Am J Clin Pathol* 129:146-156.

Kesler MV, Paranjape GS, Asplund EL, McKenna RW, Jamal S, Kroft. SH [2007] Anaplastic large cell lymphoma: A flow cytometric analysis of 29 cases. *Am J Clin Pathol* 128:314-322.

Kinney MC, Jones D [2007] Cutaneous T-cell and NK-cell lymphomas: The WHO-EORTC classification and the increasing recognition of specialized tumor types. *Am J Clin Pathol* 127:670-86.

Knapp W, Stockinger H, Majdic O [1989] Antibody-defined cell surface molecules of the immune system. *Curr Opin Immunol* 2:884-891.

Kondo H, Watanabe J, Iwasaki H [2001] T-large granular lymphocyte leukemia accompanied by an increase of natural killer cells (CD3-) and associated with ulcerative colitis and autoimmune hepatitis. *Leuk Lymphoma* 41:207-212.

Krajewski AS, Myskow MW, Cachia PG, et al [1988] T-cell lymphoma: Morphology, immunophenotype and clinical features. *Histopathology* 13:19-41.

Kumar S, Pittaluga S, Raffeld M, et al [2005] Primary cutaneous CD30-positive anaplastic large cell lymphoma in childhood: Report of 4 cases and review of the literature. *Pediatr Dev Pathol* 8:52-60.

Kummer JA, Vermeer MH, Dukers DF, Meijer CJLM, Willemze R [1997] Most primary cutaneous CD30-positive lymphoproliferative disorders have a CD4-positive cytotoxic T-cell phenotype. *J Invest Dermatol* 109:636-640.

Kuwabara H, Nagai M, Yamaoka G, et al [1999] Specific skin manifestations in CD56 positive acute myeloid leukemia. *J Cutan Pathol* 26:1-5.

Lae ME, Ahmed I, Macon WR [2002] Clusterin is widely expressed in systemic anaplastic large cell lymphoma but fails to differentiate primary from secondary cutaneous anaplastic large cell lymphoma. *Am J Clin Pathol* 118:773-779.

Lai R, Larratt LM, Etches W, et al [2000a] Hepatosplenic T-cell lymphoma of alphabeta lineage in a 16-year-old boy presenting with hemolytic anemia and thrombocytopenia. *Am J Surg Pathol* 24:459-463.

Lai R, Medeiros LJ, Dabbagh L, Formenti KS, Coupland RW [2000b] Sinusoidal CD30-positive large B-cell lymphoma: A morphologic mimic of anaplastic large cell lymphoma. *Mod Pathol* 13:223-228.

Lakkala Paranko T, Franssila K, et al [1987] Chromosome abnormalities in peripheral T-cell lymphoma. *Br J Haematol* 66:51-60.

Lamberson C, Hutchison RE, Shrimpton AE [2001] A PCR assay for detecting clonal rearrangement of the TCR-gamma gene. *Mol Diagn* 6:117-124.

Lanier LL, Phillips JH, Hackett J Jr, et al [1986] Natural killer cells: Definition of a cell type rather than a function. *J Immunol* 137:2735-2739.

Lanier LL [1998] NK cell receptors. *Annu Rev Immunol* 16:359-393.

Lasota J, Hyjek H, Koo CH, Blonski J, Miettinen, M [1996] Cytokeratin-positive large-cell lymphomas of B-cell lineage. A study of five phenotypically unusual cases verified by polymerase chain reaction. *Am J Surg Pathol* 20:346-354.

Lee P-S, Lin C-N, Chuang S-S [2003] Immunophenotyping of angioimmunoblastic T-cell lymphomas by multiparameter flow cytometry. *Pathol Res Pract* 199:539-545.

Leibson PJ [1998] Cytotoxic lymphocyte recognition of HLA-E: Utilizing a nonclassical window to peer into classical MHC. *Immunity* 9:289-294.

Lennert K [1978] Classification of non-Hodgkin's lymphomas. In: Lennert K, ed. *Malignant Lymphomas Other Than Hodgkin's Disease*. 1st ed. Berlin: Springer-Verlag; 83-109.

Lennert K, Mohri N [1978] Malignant lymphoma, lymphocytic, T-zone type (T-zone lymphoma). In: Lennert K, ed. *Malignant Lymphomas Other Than Hodgkin's Disease*. 1st ed. Berlin: Springer-Verlag; 196-209.

Lennert K, Feller AC, Godde Salz E [1986] Morphologie, Immunhistochemie und Genetik peripherer T-Zellen-Lymphome. *Onkologie* 9:97-107.

Leroux D, Mugneret F, Callanan M, et al [2002] CD4(+), CD56(+) DC2 acute leukemia is characterized by recurrent clonal chromosomal changes affecting 6 major targets: A study of 21 cases by the Groupe Français de Cytogenetique Hematologique. *Blood* 99:4154-4159.

Li X, Lu H, Yang J, et al [2002] A clinicopathologic study of CD30-positive sinusoidal large B-cell lymphoma. *Zhongua Bing Li Xue Za Zhi* 31:305-308.

Li Y, Braylan RC, Al-Quran SZ [2007] Flow-cytometric assessment of T-cell clonality in clinical specimens. *Lab Medicine* 38:477-482.

Liang R, Todd D, Chan TK, et al [1987] Peripheral T-cell lymphoma. *J Clin Oncol* 5:750-755.

Liang X, Golitz LE, Smoller BR, et al [2002] Association of expression of CD44v6 with systemic anaplastic large cell lymphoma: Comparison with primary cutaneous anaplastic large cell lymphoma. *Am J Clin Pathol* 117:276-282.

Lima M, Almeida J, Santos AH, et al [2001] Immunophenotypic analysis of the TCRVbeta repertoire in 98 persistent expansions of CD3(+)/TCR-alphabeta(+) large granular lymphocytes: Utility in assessing clonality and insights into the pathogenesis of the disease. *Am J Pathol* 159:1861-1868.

Lima M, Almeida J, Dos Anjos Teixeira M, et al [2003] TCRalphabeta+/CD4+ large granular lymphocytosis: A new clonal T-cell lymphoproliferative disorder. *Am J Pathol* 163:763-771.

Lin CW, Chang CL, Li CC, Chen YH, Lewe WH, Hsu SM [2002] Spontaneous regression of Kikuchi lymphadenopathy with oligoclonal T-cell populations favors a benign immune reaction over a T-cell lymphoma. *Am J Clin Pathol* 117:627-635.

Liu XY, Atkins RC, Feusner JH, et al [2004] Blastic NK-cell-like lymphoma with T-cell receptor gene rearrangement. *Am J Hematol* 75:251-253.

Lome-Maldonado C, Canioni D, Hermine O, et al [2002] Angioimmunoblastic T-cell lymphoma (AILD-TL) rich in large B cells and associated with Epstein-Barr virus infection: A different subtype of AILD-TL? *Leukemia* 16:2134-2141.

Lotzova E, Ades EW [1989] Natural killer cells: Definition, heterogeneity, lytic mechanism, functions and clinical application: Highlights of the Fifth International Workshop on natural killer cells, Hilton Head Island, NC, March 1988. *Nat Immun Cell Growth Regul* 8:1-9.

Loughran TP, Kadin ME, Starkebaum G, et al [1985] Leukemias of large granular lymphocytes: Association with clonal chromosomal abnormalities and autoimmune neutropenia, thrombocytopenia, and hemolytic anemia. *Annals of Internal Medicine* 102:169-175.

Loughran TP [1993] Clonal diseases of large granular lymphocytes. *Blood* 82:1-14.

Lundell R, Hartung L, Hill S, et al [2005] T-cell large granular lymphocyte leukemias have multiple phenotypic abnormalities involving pan-T-cell antigens and receptors for MHC molecules. *Am J Clin Pathol* 124:937-946.

Macgrogan G, Vergier B, Dubus P, et al [1996] CD30-positive cutaneous large cell lymphomas: A comparative study of clinicopathologic and molecular features of 16 cases. *Am J Clin Pathol* 105:440-450.

Macon WR, Levy NB, Kurtin PJ, et al [2001] Hepatosplenic alphabeta T-cell lymphomas: A report of 14 cases and comparison with hepatosplenic gammadelta T-cell lymphomas. *Am J Surg Pathol* 25:285-296.

Makishima H, Ishida F, Saito H, et al [2003] Lymphoproliferative disease of granular lymphocytes with T-cell receptor gamma delta-positive phenotype: Restricted usage of T-cell receptor gamma and delta subunit genes. *Eur J Haematol* 70:212-218.

Mason DY, Cordell J, Brown M, et al [1989] Detection of T cells in paraffin wax embedded tissue using antibodies against a peptide sequence from the CD3 antigen. *J Clin Pathol* 42:1194-1200.

Massone C, Chott A, Metze D, et al [2004] Subcutaneous, blastic natural killer (NK), NK/T-cell and other cytotoxic lymphomas of the skin: A morphologic, immunophenotypic and molecular study of 50 patients. *Am J Surg Pathol* 28:719-735.

Masuko-Hongo K, Kato T, Suzuki S, et al [1998] Frequent clonal expansion of peripheral T cells in patients with autoimmune diseases: A novel detecting system possibly applicable to laboratory examination. *J Clin Lab Anal* 12:162-167.

McCoy JP Jr, Overton WR, Schroeder K, et al [1996] Immunophenotypic analysis of the T cell receptor V beta repertoire in CD4+ and CD8+ lymphocytes from normal peripheral blood. *Cytometry* 26:148-153.

Merchant SH, Amin MB, Viswanatha DS [2006] Morphologic and immunophenotypic analysis of angioimmunoblastic T-cell lymphomas: Emphasis on phenotypic aberrancies for early diagnosis. *Am J Clin Pathol* 128:29-38.

Miyamoto T, Yoshino T, Takehisa T, Hagari Y, Mihara M [1998] Cutaneous presentation of nasal/nasal type T/NK cell lymphoma: Clinicopathological findings of four cases. *Br J Dermatol* 139:481-487.

Morice WG, Kurtin PJ, Leibson PJ, et al [2003] Demonstration of aberrant T-cell and natural killer-cell antigen expression in all cases of granular lymphocytic leukaemia. *Br J Haematol* 120:1026-1036

Morice WG, Kimlinger T, Katzmann JA, et al [2004] Flow cytometric assessment of TCR- Vβ expression in the evaluation of peripheral blood involvement by T-cell lymphoproliferative disorders: A comparison with conventional T-cell immunophenotyping and molecular genetic techniques. *Am J Clin Pathol* 121:373-383.

Morice WG, Katzmann JA, Pittelkow MR, et al [2006] A comparison of morphologic features, flow cytometry, TCR-Vβ analysis, and TCR-PCR in qualitative and quantitative assessment of peripheral blood involvement by Sézary syndrome. *Am J Clin Pathol* 125:364-374.

Naeim, F [2001] Chronic lymphoid leukemias. In: *Atlas of Bone Marrow and Blood Morphology*. Philadelphia, PA: WB Saunders. (pp. 98-116),

Nakamura S, Suchi T [1991] A clinicopathologic study of node-based, low-grade, peripheral T-cell lymphoma: Angioimmunoblastic lymphoma, T-zone lymphoma, and lymphoepithelioid lymphoma. *Cancer* 67:2566-2578.

Namikawa R, Suchi T, Ueda R, et al [1987] Phenotyping of proliferating lymphocytes in angioimmunoblastic lymphadenopathy and related lesions by the double immunoenzymatic staining technique. *Am J Pathol* 127:279-287.

Nascimento AF, Pinkus JL, Pinkus GS [2004] Clusterin, a marker for anaplastic large cell lymphoma: Immunohistochemical profile in hematopoietic and nonhematopoietic malignant neoplasms. *Am J Clin Pathol* 121:709-717.

Natkunam Y, Smoller BR, Zehnder JL, Dorfman RF, Warnke RA [1999] Aggressive cutaneous NK and NK-like T-cell lymphomas: Clinicopathologic, immunohistochemical, and molecular analyses of 12 cases. *Am J Surg Pathol* 23:571-581.

Natkunam Y, Warnke RA, Haghighi B, et al [2000] Coexpression of CD56 and CD30 in lymphomas with primary presentation in the skin: Clinicopathologic, immunohistochemical and molecular analyses of seven cases. *J Cut Pathol* 27:392-399.

Nava VE, Jaffe ES [2005] The pathology of NK-cell lymphomas and leukemias. *Adv Anat Pathol* 12:27-34.

Nijsten T, Curiel-Lewandrowski C, Kadin ME [2004] Lymphomatoid papulosis in children: A retrospective cohort study of 35 cases. *Arch Dermatol* 140:306-312.

O'Malley DP [2007] T-cell large granular leukemia and related proliferations. *Am J Clin Pathol* 127:850-859.

Ohshima K, Takeo H, Kikuchi M, et al [1994] Heterogeneity of Epstein-Barr virus infection in angioimmunoblastic lymphadenopathy type T-cell lymphoma. *Histopathology* 25:569-579.

Ortonne N, Buyukbabani N, Delfau-Larue M-H, Bagot M, Wechster J [2003] Value of the CD8-CD3 ratio for the diagnosis of mycosis fungoides. *Mod Pathol* 16:857-862.

Ortonne N, Dupuis J, Plonquet A, et al [2007] Characterization of CXCL13+ neoplastic T cells in cutaneous lesions of angioimmunoblastic T-cell lymphoma (AITL). *Am J Surg Pathol* 31:1068-1076.

Oshimi K, Kawa K, Nakamura S, et al [2005] NK-cell neoplasms in Japan. *Hematology* 10:237-245.

Pancake BA, Zucker-Franklin D, Coutavas EE [1995] The cutaneous T-cell lymphoma, mycosis fungoides, is a human T-cell lymphotropic virus-associated disease. *J Clin Invest* 95:547-554.

Pancake BA, Wassef EH, Zucker-Franklin D [1996] Demonstration of antibodies to human T-cell lymphotropic virus-1 tax in patients with the cutaneous T-cell lymphoma, mycosis fungoides, who are seronegative for antibodies to the structural proteins of the virus. *Blood* 88:3004-3009.

Pascal V, Schleinitz N, Brunet C, et al [2004] Comparative analysis of NK cell subset distribution in normal and lymphoproliferative disease of granular lymphocyte conditions. *Eur J Immunol* 34:2930-2940.

Petrella T, Dalac S, Maynadie M, et al, for the Groupe Français d'Etude des Lymphomes Cutanes (GFELC) [1999] CD4+ CD56+ cutaneous neoplasms: A distinct hematological entity? *Am J Surg Pathol* 23:137-146.

Petrella T, Comeau MR, Maynadie M, et al [2002] "Agranular CD4+ CD56+ hematodermic neoplasm" (blastic NK-cell lymphoma) originates from a population of CD56+ precursor cells related to plasmacytoid monocytes. *Am J Surg Pathol* 26:852-862.

Petrella T, Bagot M, Willemze R, et al [2005] Blastic NK-cell lymphomas (agranular CD4+CD56+ hematodermic neoplasms): A review. *Am J Clin Pathol* 123:662-675.

Pilichowska ME, Fleming MD, Pinkus JL, Pinkus GS [2007] CD4+/CD56+ hematodermic neoplasm ("blastic natural killer cell lymphoma"): Neoplastic cells express the immature dendritic cell marker BDCA-2 and produce interferon. *Am J Clin Pathol* 128:445-453.

Pinkus GS, Said JW [1992] Peripheral T-cell lymphomas. In: Knowles DM, ed. *Neoplastic Hematopathology*. 1st ed. Baltimore: Williams & Wilkins: 837-868.

Posnett DN, Sinha R, Kabak S, et al [1994] Clonal populations of T cells in normal elderly humans: The T cell equivalent to "benign monoclonal gammopathy." *J Exp Med* 179:609-618. Erratum in: *J Exp Med.* 1994;179:1077. 1994; 179:609-618.

Radonich MA, Lazova R, Bolognia J [2002] Cutaneous natural killer/T-cell lymphoma. *J Am Acad Dermatol* 46:451-456.

Ralfkiaer E [1991] Immunohistological markers for the diagnosis of cutaneous lymphomas. *Semin Diagn Pathol* 8:62-72.

Ralfkiaer E [1994] Controversies and discussion on early diagnosis of cutaneous T-cell lymphoma: Phenotyping. *Dermatol Clin* 12:329-334.

Reichard KK, Burks EJ, Foucar K, et al [2005] CD4(+) CD56(+) lineage-negative malignancies are rare tumors of plasmacytoid dendritic cells. *Am J Surg Pathol* 29:1274-1283.

Reichard KK, Schwartz EJ, Higgins JP, Narasimhan B, Warnke RA, Natkunam Y [2006] CD10 expression in peripheral T-cell lymphomas complicated by a proliferation of large B-cells. *Mod Pathol* 19:337-343.

Rigolin GM, Cuneo A, Roberti MG, et al [1997] Myelodysplastic syndromes with monocytic component: Hematologic and cytogenetic characterization. *Haematologica* 82:25-30.

Rosenberg WM, Moss PA, Bell JI [1992] Variation in human T cell receptor V beta and J beta repertoire: Analysis using anchor polymerase chain reaction. Eur *J Immunol* 22:541-549.

Saffer H, Wahed A, Rassidakis GZ, et al [2002] Clusterin expression in malignant lymphomas: A survey of 266 cases. *Mod Pathol* 15:1221-1226.

Saito T, Matsuno Y, Tanosaki R, et al [2002] Gamma delta T-cell neoplasms: A clinicopathological study of 11 cases. *Ann Oncol* 13:1792-1798.

Salhany KE, Macon WR, Choi JK, et al [1998] Subcutaneous panniculitis-like T-cell lymphoma: Clinicopathologic, immunophenotypic, and genotypic analysis of alpha/beta and gamma/delta subtypes. *Am J Surg Pathol* 22:881-893.

Santucci M, Pimpinelli N, Massi D, et al [2003] Cytotoxic/natural killer cell cutaneous lymphomas: Report of EORTC Cutaneous Lymphoma Task Force Workshop. *Cancer* 97:610-627.

Sasaki K, Sugaya M, Fujita H, et al [2004] A case of primary cutaneous anaplastic large cell lymphoma with variant anaplastic lymphoma kinase translocation. *Br J Dermatol* 150:1202-1207.

Schlegelberger B, Himmler A, Godde E et al [1994] Cytogenetic findings in peripheral T-cell lymphomas as a basis for distinguishing low-grade and high-grade lymphomas. *Blood* 83:505-511.

Schlegelberger B, Zhang Y, Weber-Matthieson K, Grote W [1994] Detection of aberrant clones in nearly all cases of angioimmunoblastic lymphadenopathy with dysproteinemia-type T-cell lymphoma by combined interphase and metaphase cytogenetics. *Blood* 84:2640-2648.

Schlegelberger B, Feller AC [1996] Classification of peripheral T-cell lymphomas: Cytogenetic findings support the updated Kiel classification. *Leuk Lymphomq* 20:411-416.

Segal GH, Kjeldsberg CR, Smith GP, Perkins SL [1994] CD30 antigen expression in florid immunoblastic proliferations: A clinicopathologic study of 14 cases. *Am J Clin Pathol* 102:292-298.

Scmenzato G, Zambello R, Starkebaum G, et al [1997] The lymphoproliferative disease of granular lymphocytes: Updated criteria for diagnosis. *Blood* 89:256-260.

Shichishima T, Kawaguchi M, Ono N, et al [2004] Gammadelta T-cell large granular lymphocyte (LGL) leukemia with spontaneous remission. *Am J Hematol* 75:168-172.

Shiota M, Nakamura S, Ichinohasama R, et al [1995] Anaplastic large cell lymphoma expressing the novel chimeric protein p80NPM/ALK: A distinct clinicopathologic entity. *Blood* 86:1954-1960.

Siegert W, Nerl C, Engelhard M, et al [1994] Peripheral T-cell non-Hodgkin's lymphomas of low malignancy: Prospective study of 25 patients with pleomorphic small cell lymphoma, lymphoepitheloid cell (Lennert's) lymphoma and T-zone lymphoma. *Br J Haematol* 87: 529-534.

Sioutos N, Kadin ME [1992] Perivascular Ki-1 + lesions. *Int J Hematol* 55:275-279.

Sokolowska-Wojdylo M, Wenzel J, Gaffal E, et al [2005] Absence of CD26 expression on skin-homing CLA+CD4+ T lymphocytes in peripheral blood is a highly sensitive marker for early diagnosis and therapeutic monitoring of patients with Sézary syndrome. *Experimental Dermatology* 30:702-706.

Soler J, Bordes R, Ortuno F, et al [1994] Aggressive natural killer cell leukaemia/lymphoma in two patients with lethal midline granuloma. *Br J Haematol* 86:659-662.

Stacchini A, Demurtas A, Aliberti S, et al [2007] The usefulness of flow cytometric CD10 detection in the differential diagnosis of peripheral T-cell lymphomas. *Am J Clin Pathol* 128:854-864.

Stein H, Foss HD, Durkop H, et al [2000] CD30+ anaplastic large cell lymphoma: A review of its histopathologic, genetic, and clinical features. *Blood* 96:3681-3695.

Steinhoff M, Hummel M, Anagnostopoulos I, et al [2002] Single-cell analysis of CD30+ cells in lymphomatoid papulosis demonstrates a common clonal T-cell origin. *Blood* 100:578-584.

Suarez F, Wlodarska I, Rigal-Huguet F, et al [2000] Hepatosplenic alphabeta T-cell lymphoma: An unusual case with clinical, histologic, and cytogenetic features of gammadelta hepatosplenic T-cell lymphoma. *Am J Surg Pathol* 24:1027-1032.

Suzuki R, Yamamoto K, Seto M, et al [1997] CD7+ and CD56+ myeloid/natural killer cell precursor acute leukemia: A distinct hematolymphoid disease entity. *Blood* 90:2417-2428.

Takagi N, Nakamura S, Ueda R, et al [1992] A phenotypic and genotypic study of three node-based, low-grade peripheral T-cell lymphomas: Angioimmunoblastic lymphoma, T-zone lymphoma, and lymphoepithelioid lymphoma. *Cancer* 69:2571-2582.

Tan B, Warnke R, Arber D [2006] The frequency of B- and T-cell clones and EBV in T-cell lymphomas: A comparison between AILT and PTCL-NOS. *J Mol Diagn* 8:466-475.

Tarazona R, DelaRosa O, Alonso C, et al [2000] Increased expression of NK cell markers on T lymphocytes in aging and chronic activation of the immune system reflects the accumulation of effector/senescent T cells. *Mech Aging Dev* 121:77-88.

Teitell MA, Lones MA, Perkins SL, et al [2005] TCL1 expression and Epstein-Barr virus status in pediatric Burkitt lymphoma. *Am J Clin Pathol* 124:569-575.

ten Berge RL, Oudejans JJ, Ossenkoppele GJ, et al [2000] ALK expression in extranodal anaplastic large cell lymphoma favours systemic disease with (primary) nodal involvement and a good prognosis and occurs before dissemination. *J Clin Pathol* 53:445-450.

Torlakovic E, Torlakovic G, Nguyen PL, Brunning RD, Delabie J [2002] The value of anti-Pax-5 immunostaining in routinely fixed and paraffin-embedded sections. A novel pan pre-B and B-cell marker. *Am J Surg Pathol* 26:1343-1350.

Toro JR, Liewehr DJ, Pabby N, et al [2003] Gammadelta-T-cell phenotype is associated with significantly decreased survival in cutaneous T-cell lymphoma. *Blood* 101:340/-3412.

Trinchieri G [1989] Biology of natural killer cells. *Adv Immunol* 47:187-376.

Troxell ML, Schwartz EJ, van de Rijn M, et al [2005] Follicular dendritic cell immunohistochemical markers in angioimmunoblastic T-cell lymphoma. *Appl Immunohistochem Mol Morphol* 13:297-303.

Valbuena JR, Herling M, Admirand JH, et al [2005] T-cell prolymphocytic leukemia involving extramedullary sites. *Am J Clin Pathol* 123:456-464.

van den Beemd R, Boor PP, van Lochem EG, et al [2000] Flow cytometric analysis of the Vbeta repertoire in healthy controls. *Cytometry* 40:336-345.

Vega F, Medeiros LJ, Bueso-Ramos C, et al [2001] Hepatosplenic gamma/delta T-cell lymphoma in bone marrow; a sinusoidal neoplasm with blastic cytologic features. *Am J Clin Pathol* 116:410-419.

Vergier B, Beylot-Barry M, Pulford K, et al [1998] Statistical evaluation of diagnostic and prognostic features of CD30+ cutaneous lymphoproliferative disorders: A clinicopathologic study of 65 cases. *Am J Surg Pathol* 22:1192-1202.

von den Driesch P, Coors EA [2002] Localized cutaneous small to medium-sized pleomorphic T-cell lymphoma: A report of 3 cases stable for years. *J Am Acad Dermatol* 46:531-535.

Vonderheid EC, Sobel EL, Nowell PC, et al [1985] Diagnostic and prognostic significance of Sézary cells in peripheral blood smears from patients with cutaneous T-cell lymphoma. *Blood* 66:358-366.

Vonderheid EC, Bernengo MG, Burg G, et al [2002] Update on erythrodermic cutaneous T-cell lymphoma: Report of the International Society for Cutaneous Lymphomas. *J Am Acad Dermatol* 46:95-106.

Warnke RA, Jones D, His ED [2007] Morphologic and immunophenotypic variants of nodal T-cell lymphomas and T-cell lymphoma mimics. *Am J Clin Pathol* 127:511-527.

Warren HS, Christiansen FT, Witt CS [2003] Functional inhibitory human leucocyte antigen class I receptors on natural killer (NK) cells in patients with chronic NK lymphocytosis. *Br J Haematol* 121:793-804.

Weiss LM, Jaffe ES, Liu XF, et al [1992] Detection and localization of Epstein-Barr viral genomes in angioimmunoblastic lymphadenopathy and angioimmunoblastic lymphadenopathy-like lymphoma. *Blood* 79:1789-1795.

Wellmann A, Thieblemont C, Pittaluga S, et al [2000] Detection of differentially expressed genes in lymphomas using cDNA arrays: Identification of clusterin as a new diagnostic marker for anaplastic large-cell lymphomas. *Blood* 96:398-404.

Whittam LR, Calonje E, Orchard G, Fraser-Andrews EA, Woolford A, Russell-Jones R [2000] CD8-positive juvenile onset mycosis fungoides: An immunohistochemical and genotypic analysis of six cases. *Br J Dermatol* 143:1199-1204.

Willemze R, Beljaards RC [1993] Spectrum of primary cutaneous CD30+ lymphoproliferative disorders: A proposal for classification and guidelines for management and treatment. *J Am Acad Dermatol* 28:973-980.

Willemze R, Kerl H, Sterry W, et al [1997] EORTC classification for primary cutaneous lymphomas: A proposal from the Cutaneous Lymphoma Study Group of the European Organization for Research and Treatment of Cancer (EORTC). *Blood* 90:354-371.

Witzig TE, Phyliky RL, Li CY, et al [1986] T-cell chronic lymphocytic leukemia with a helper/inducer membrane phenotype: A distinct clinicopathologic subtype with a poor prognosis. *Am J Hematol* 21:139-155.

Wong N, Wong KF, Chan JKC, et al [2000] Chromosomal translocations are common in natural killer-cell lymphoma/leukemia as shown by spectral karyotyping. *Human Pathology* 31:771-774.

Yokote T, Akioka T, Oka S, et al [2005] Flow cytometric immunophenotyping of adult T-cell leukemia/lymphoma using CD3 gating. *Am J Clin Pathol* 124:199-204.

Yuan C, Vergilio J, Harris N, Bagg A [2002] Angioimmunoblastic T-cell lymphoma. A neoplasm of intrafollicular CD10+, BCL-6+, CD4+ memory T cells [abstract] *Mod Pathol* 15:1125.

Zambello R, Trentin L, Ciccone E, et al [1993] Phenotypic diversity of natural killer (NK) populations in patients with NK-type lymphoproliferative disease of granular lymphocytes. *Blood* 81:2381-2385.

Zettl A, Ott G, Makulik A, et al [2002] Chromosomal gains at 9q characterize enteropathy-associated T-cell lymphoma. *Am J Pathol* 161:1635-1645.

14

15 Hodgkin Lymphoma

Chapter Contents

Classification

- Classical Hodgkin lymphoma
- Nodular sclerosis classical Hodgkin lymphoma
- Mixed cellularity classical Hodgkin lymphoma
- Lymphocyte-rich classical Hodgkin lymphoma
- Lymphocyte-depleted classical Hodgkin lymphoma
- Nodular lymphocyte predominant Hodgkin lymphoma

Introduction

Although flow cytometric immunophenotyping (FCI) has been widely used in immunophenotyping non-Hodgkin lymphomas (NHLs), it has not been embraced as widely in Hodgkin lymphoma (HL). This difference in practice is most likely due to the fact that the neoplastic cells in HL are generally relatively scarce, more difficult to detect by FCI, and are often bound by normal T cells, and that immunohistochemical (IHC) staining is the standard, preferred method of immunophenotyping in HL. However, in fine needle aspirate (FNA) or limited biopsy specimens, material may not be available for IHC staining and an alternative method of immunophenotyping is desired in such cases.

Due to the scarcity of neoplastic cells, HL may be underdiagnosed by FCI. The detection by FCI of expressions of CD15 and CD30 by the neoplastic cells of classical HL (cHL) has been recognized for some time [Dunphy 2000]. However, one should also keep in mind that there have been reported cases of granulomatous adenitis, in which a few cells with a cHL immunophenotype were erroneously detected and diagnosed as HL by FCI [Ravoet 2004]. Nevertheless, the potential of FCI to properly recognize the neoplastic cells of cHL is continuing to improve and will be discussed in detail. In addition, FCI of the T-regulatory cells and inflammatory infiltrates in HL may also have diagnostic usefulness in HL.

Classical Hodgkin Lymphoma

Definition

Classical Hodgkin lymphoma is a monoclonal lymphoid neoplasm composed of mononuclear Hodgkin cells and multinucleated Reed-Sternberg (RS) cells residing in an infiltrate containing a variable mixture of non-neoplastic small lymphocytes, eosinophils, neutrophils, histiocytes, plasma cells, fibroblasts, and collagen fibers.

Typical Immunophenotype

The immunophenotypic and genetic features of the neoplastic cells in cHL are similar in the histologic subtypes, outlined above in the classification. They are CD30+, CD45 (LCA)–, CD15+ (may be expressed by only a minority of the neoplastic cells), CD20+ (up to 40% of cases, variable intensity and on a minority of the neoplastic cells), Pax-5+ (97% of cases) [Torlakovic 2002], and generally negative for all T-cell antigens, epithelial membrane antigen (EMA; <5% of cases and weak), Oct2, BOB.1, and ALK. EBV (LMP1 and EBNA-1) may be detected, most frequently in mixed cellularity cHL (approximately 75% of cases) and least often in nodular sclerosis cHL (10%-40% of cases). Most cases demonstrate immunoglobulin (Ig) gene rearrangement. Conventional cytogenetic and FISH studies show aneuploidy and hypertetraploidy; there are no recurrent or specific chromosomal abnormalities in cHL. A representative case is demonstrated in **[f15.1]**.

Contributions of FCI

Identification and purification of cHL cells from lymph nodes by flow cytometry and FC sorting

The neoplastic cells of cHL generally fall within a region of high forward light scatter (due to their large size), increased side light scatter (due to their intermediate degree of cytoplasmic complexity and granularity), and CD45-negativity. CD15 and CD30 expressions by the neoplastic cells of cHL may be detected by FCI

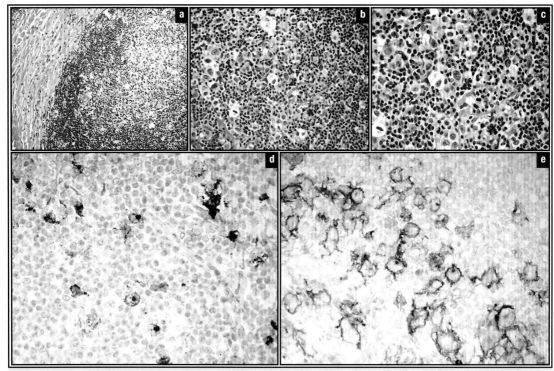

[f15.1] This case demonstrates a classical Hodgkin lymphoma, nodular sclerosis subtype. The clinical history reveals a 21-year-old female presents with a left supraclavicular mass, which is biopsied. H&E sections of the lymph node **a-c** reveal the characteristic cytomorphology and histological features. Flow cytometric analysis of the lymph node fails to reveal an aberrant T-cell or monoclonal B-cell population. By immunohistochemical staining, the malignant cells reveal the characteristic Golgi staining with CD15 **d** and intense positivity for CD30 **e**. The diagnosis of classical Hodgkin lymphoma, nodular sclerosis subtype, is made.

[Dunphy 2000]. However, not only are the neoplastic cells of cHL often scarce in FC suspensions prepared from tissue specimens, but they are often bound by normal T cells. Nevertheless, Fromm et al have recently described the disruption of the interaction between RS cells and the normal T cells by adding "blocking" antibodies, allowing for purification and identification of the RS cells from the tissue suspensions. By this approach, flow cytometry enabled the identification RS cells in 89% of cHL cases [Fromm 2006]. This technique may be particularly suited to FNA or limited biopsy specimens, in which IHC staining is not able to be performed. Although Fromm et al did not demonstrate any RS-cell population in non-cHL neoplasms or in reactive lymph nodes, correlation with histology and/or cytomorphology continues to be the mainstay for a reliable diagnosis, and FCI findings should never be interpreted in a vacuum.

Analysis of T-regulatory cells and inflammatory infiltrates in the diagnosis of cHL

In addition to the identification of RS-cell populations by FCI in the diagnosis of cHL, FC analysis of the T-regulatory cells and inflammatory infiltrates in tissue specimens may also be useful in establishing a diagnosis of cHL. A recent FC study of the inflammatory infiltrates in cHL vs and reactive lymph nodes has demonstrated, in general, a significant difference in the number (increased percentage) of CD4+, bright CD25+ regulatory T cells in cHL as compared to reactive lymph nodes (9% in cHL vs 2% in reactive lymph nodes) [Hudnall 2008]. A subsequent FC study of the T-regulatory cells in cHL, B-cell NHLs, and benign cases further demonstrated that the mean CD152 expression in the CD4+, CD25+ T-regulatory cells was also higher in cHL than in B-NHLs and benign cases. In this study, mean CD152 in CD4+, CD25+ T-regulatory cells were distinguished cHL from benign cases with 79% sensitivity and 100% specificity, and from B-cell NHLs with 71% sensitivity and 90% specificity [Bosler 2008]. See **[f15.2]**.

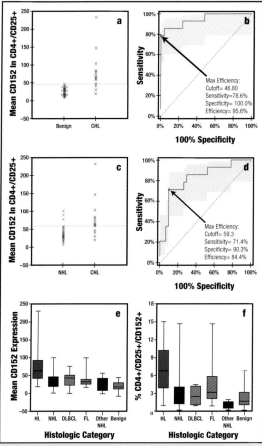

[f15.2] Dot plots **a, c** and ROC curves **b, d** of mean CD152 expression in CD4+CD25+ lymphocytes comparing HL vs benign **a, b** and NHL **c, d**. Box and whisker plots of mean CD152 expression **e** and percentage of lymphocytes co-expressing CD4, CD25, and CD152 **f** in HL, all NHLs combined, diffuse large B-cell lymphoma, follicular lymphoma, and benign cases. The middle line corresponds to the median value, while box edges denote the 25th and 75th percentiles, and bars are the maximum and minimum. *Reprinted with permission of* [Bosler 2008].

Differentiation from NHL and detection of composite lymphoma (ie, cHL and NHL)

FCI should be routinely performed on specimens suspected of cHL, not only to consider the above contributions of FCI to the diagnosis of cHL, but also to exclude a B-cell NHL (which will most often reveal a monoclonal B-cell population) or T-cell NHL (which may reveal an aberrant T-cell immunophenotype), and to exclude the co-existence of cHL with a B-cell NHL or T-cell NHL. Such a case is demonstrated in [f15.3]. In addition, FCI is recommended even when considering relapse of cHL, since a NHL may occur after therapy for cHL [Borchmann 2006].

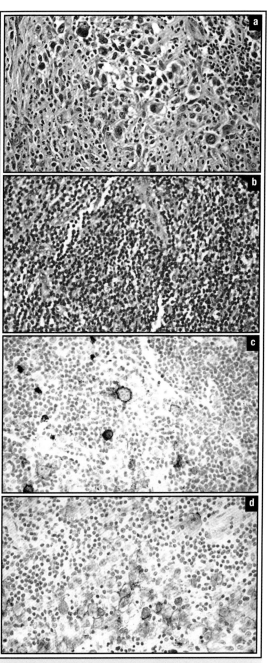

[f15.3] This case demonstrates a composite lymphoma, composed of classical Hodgkin lymphoma (cHL), nodular sclerosis subtype and follicular lymphoma (FL), grade 1. The clinical history reveals a 63-year-old female presents with a right neck mass, which is biopsied. H&E sections reveal the characteristic histological features of cHL **a** and adjacent to the cHL is an area with the characteristic morphology of FL **b**. Flow cytometric analysis was not performed (and thus not able to be demonstrated). Immunohistochemical staining reveals positivity of the malignant cells within the cHL with CD15 **c** and CD30 **d**. They are negative for CD45, CD3, and CD20 (not demonstrated). Bcl-2 stains the neoplastic follicles depicted in **b** (not demonstrated). The diagnosis of composite lymphoma, classical Hodgkin lymphoma and follicular lymphoma (Grade1), is made.

Differential Diagnosis

Diffuse large B-cell lymphoma (DLBCL) or large T-cell lymphoma, including anaplastic large cell lymphoma (ALCL)

The presence of a monoclonal B-cell population by FCI virtually excludes a stand-alone diagnosis of cHL. Likewise, a significant aberrant T-cell population with significant loss of pan T-cell antigens would exclude a stand-alone diagnosis of cHL. CD30 expression may also be demonstrated by FCI in the neoplastic cells of ALCL, but these are generally associated with a significant aberrant T-cell population and CD45-positivity by FCI.

In addition, when a monoclonal or aberrant B-cell population or an aberrant T-cell population, characterized by a loss of a T-cell antigen, is identified, cHL may be excluded only after correlation with the histology, in order to exclude the possibility of a composite lymphoma. In cases in which FCI data are diagnostic, microscopic observations may provide additional information, not only due to sampling, but also due to patterns of involvement and the cytological features of the malignant cells. Correlation with histologic and cytomorphologic features is always required.

Nodular lymphocyte-predominant HL (NLPHL)

The neoplastic cells of NLPHL are also often quite scarce and not routinely detected by FCI. Although classical RS cells are not encountered in NLPHL, there may be diagnostic confusion. As will be discussed below, a double-positive CD4+CD8+ T-cell population is commonly found in approximately 60% of NLPHL cases [Rahemtullah 2006]. However, a double-positive CD4+CD8+ T-cell population may also be identified in a minor subset (6%) of cHL cases.

Contribution of paraffin IHC staining

CHL may be distinguished from diffuse large B-cell lymphoma (DLBCL) [particularly the T-cell-rich (TCR) and lymphohistiocytic-rich (LHR) variants] and ALCL (particularly the LHR variant) primarily by IHC staining. The neoplastic cells of cHL are CD45–, intensely CD30+, and typically CD15+ with CD20-positivity in up to 40% of cases. EMA is generally negative. The CD20-positivity in cHL is also less intense and not as uniform as seen in the TCR– and LHR-rich variants of DLBCL. The neoplastic cells of the lymphohistiocytic-rich variant of ALCL are uniformly and intensely positive for CD30, may variably express T-cell antigens, are EMA+ in 80% of cases, and are uniformly negative for all B-cell markers. See [t15.1].

t15.1 Comparison of Immunophenotypic Profiles of cHL, NLPHL, and ALCL						
Subtype	T-Cell Markers	CD20	CD79a	PAX5	Oct2	BOB.1
cHL	–	+ (40%)	+ (20%)	+ (97%)	–	–
NLPHL	–	+	+	+	+	+
ALCL-O	– (CD43V+)	–	–	–	–	–
ALCL-T	V+	–	–	–	–	–

(continued on next page)

CHL may also be distinguished from NLPHL primarily by IHC staining. This differential diagnosis is discussed below in the section regarding NLPHL (subsection regarding the contribution of paraffin IHC staining). Also see **[t15.1]**.

Nodular Lymphocyte-Predominant HL

Definition

NLPHL is a monoclonal B-cell neoplasm characterized by a nodular and diffuse polymorphous proliferation of scattered large neoplastic cells known as popcorn or L&H (lymphocytic and/or histiocytic RS cell variants). These neoplastic cells reside in large spherical meshworks of follicular dendritic cell (FDC) processes filled with non-neoplastic lymphocytes.

Typical Immunophenotype

L&H cells are positive for CD45, CD20, CD79a, BCL6, Oct2, and BOB.1 in virtually all cases, for J chain and CD75 in most cases [Poppema 1980, Stein 1986], and for EMA in approximately half of cases [Anagnostopoulos 2000]. They lack CD15 and CD30 in nearly all cases [Dunphy 1997]. In tissue sections, the L&H cells are typically "ringed" by CD3+ T cells and to a lesser extent by CD57+ cells. Ig gene rearrangements are detected in

DNA of isolated single L&H cells. EBV is negative. A representative case is demonstrated in **[f15.4]**.

Limitations and Contribution of FCI

As mentioned previously, the neoplastic cells of NLPHL are often quite scarce and not routinely detected by FCI. Purification and identification of L&H cells by FC techniques has not been reported, as in the neoplastic cells of cHL. Nevertheless, FCI has identified a double-positive CD4+CD8+ T-cell population in approximately 60% of NLPHL cases [Rahemtullah 2006]. See **[f15.5]**. However, this double positive population may also be encountered in approximately 40% of cases of progressive transformation of germinal centers (PTGCs) (which may be morphologically difficult to distinguish form NLPHL) in approximately 6% of cHL cases, and in approximately 4% of cases of nonspecific-reactive hyperplasia (RH). Although this finding is not entirely specific, it is important to recognize that this double-positive CD4+CD8+ population is commonly encountered in NLPHL, in order to avoid a misdiagnosis of a T-cell lymphoma. In addition, this population may be a clue to the diagnosis of NLPHL, particularly in cases with limited tissue.

t15.1 Comparison of Immunophenotypic Profiles of cHL, NLPHL, and ALCL (Continued)						
Subtype	CD15	CD30	CD45	EMA	LMP and EBNA-1	ALK
cHL	+ (80%, may be on minority of cells)	+ (100%) strong	– (<5%+)	– (<5%+)	+ (75%-MCHL; 10%-40%-NSHL)	–
NLPHL	– (rare+)	+ (19%) focal	+	+ (50%)	–	–
ALCL-0	– (0%-20%+)	+	V+	+ (80%)	–	+ (60%-85%)
ALCL-T	– (0%-20%+)	+	V+	+ (80%)	–	+ (60%-85%)

0, null cell immunophenotype; ALCL, anaplastic large cell lymphoma; cHL, classical Hodgkin lymphoma; MCHL, mixed cellularity cHL; NLPHL, nodular lymphocyte predominant Hodgkin lymphoma; NSHL, nodular sclerosis cHL; T, T-cell immunophenotype; V, variably.

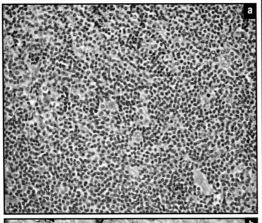

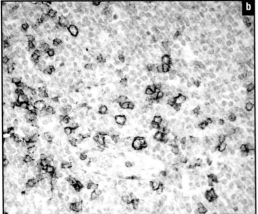

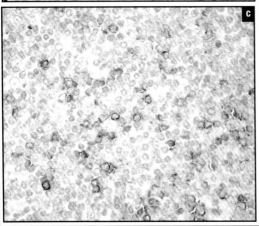

[f15.4] This case demonstrates a typical case of nodular lymphocyte-predominant Hodgkin lymphoma. The clinical history reveals a 58-year-old female who presents with splenomegaly, anemia, and left inguinal lymphadenopathy, which is biopsied. H&E section of the lymph node **a** reveals the characteristic morphology. Flow cytometric analysis of the lymph node fails to reveal an aberrant T-cell or monoclonal B-cell population. Immunohistochemical staining reveals positivity of the malignant cells with CD45 (not demonstrated) and CD20 **b**. The malignant cells are "ringed" by CD57+ cells **c**. The diagnosis of lymphocyte-predominant Hodgkin lymphoma is made.

Differentiation from NHL

FCI should be routinely performed on tissues suspected of NLPHL, not only to detect the abnormal population as described above, but also to exclude a B-cell or T-cell NHL. A prominent population of monoclonal B cells should make one consider a B-cell NHL, and a significantly aberrant T-cell population (other than double positive CD4+CD8+) should make one consider a T-cell NHL.

Differential Diagnosis

PTGC

Morphologically, PTGC and NLPHL may be diagnostically challenging. Unfortunately, FCI will not reveal a monoclonal B-cell population in either case, and a double-positive CD4+CD8+ T-cell population is encountered in approximately 40% of PTGC cases and 60% of NLPHL cases—a significant overlap. This differential diagnosis primarily relies on histology combined with IHC staining, which should reveal the characteristic immunophenotype in NLPHL, as described above.

Lymphocyte-rich cHL

The lymphocyte-rich cHL (LRHL) may have a nodular pattern and be diagnostically confused with NLPHL. However, the neoplastic cells of LRHL maintain the immunophenotype of cHL. See [t15.1].

TCRBCL

It is not currently clear whether a purely diffuse form of LPHL exists. Many lesions likely represent TCRBCL. This differential diagnosis is primarily discussed in the following subsection regarding the contribution of paraffin IHC staining.

Contribution of Paraffin IHC Staining

Paraffin IHC immunophenotyping may be widely applied in recognizing NLPHL and differentiating it from PTGC, lymphocyte-rich cHL, and TCRBCL.

TCRBCL may be better defined by paraffin IHC staining, since these lymphomas typically do not reveal a monoclonal B-cell population by FCI due to the low number of malignant cells relative to the background cells. These DLBCLs are characterized by a background rich (>80% background cells) in lymphocytes, with or without a histiocytic component. This group of DLBCLs represents a heterogeneous group and by paraffin IHC staining, the scattered large malignant B-cells have the following immunophenotype: CD20+,

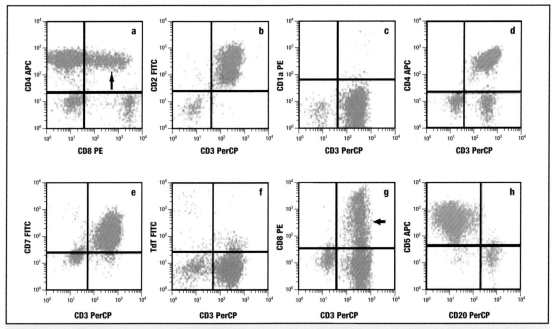

[f15.5] Analysis of T-cell antigen expression in nodular lymphocyte-predominant Hodgkin lymphoma (NLPHL) with double-positive T cells. A case of NLPHL **a** shows the characteristic double-positive population with bright CD4 **a** and variable dim CD8 **g** expression (arrows) constituting 20% of T cells. Further analysis demonstrates that all T cells express CD2 **b** and CD7 **e**, and no CD20–CD5– population is observed, indicating that all T cells express CD5 **h**. Finally, no subgroup of T cells shows positive staining for CD1a **c** or terminal deoxynucleotidyl transferase (TdT) **f**, markers of immature thymocytes. (APC, allophycocyanin; FITC, fluorescein isothiocyanate; PE, phycoerythrin; PerCP, peridinin chlorophyll protein.). *Reprinted with permission from [Rahemtullah 2006].*

CD10–/+ (25%-50%), CD5 (10%), bcl-2+ (30%-50%), and bcl-6+ (majority of cases). A representative case was demonstrated in [f12.37]. As alluded to previously, the distinction of TCRBCL from a pure, diffuse type of LPHL may not be possible and has been a matter of controversy [McBride 1996, Rudiger 1998, Schmidt 1990]. As discussed above, the L&H cells are typically ringed by CD3+ and/or CD57+ lymphocytes by paraffin IHC staining. However, areas within NLPHL may have a diffuse pattern, characterized by scattered L&H cells set in a diffuse background of reactive T cells with a loss of CD57+ T cells, as well as a loss of the follicular dendritic cell meshwork. So unless the characteristic ringing of L&H cells by CD3 or CD57 is clearly demonstrated, the distinction of LPHL with a diffuse pattern from TCR-DLBCL primarily relies on the presence of a nodular component of LPHL existing in association with the diffuse areas in the same biopsy. In the absence of a nodular component of LPHL, a purely diffuse pattern would be regarded as TCRBCL. In the report of NLPHL by Fan et al, the diffuse pattern of LPHL (TCRBCL-like) was significantly more common in cases that recurred than in those without recurrence, and the predominance of a diffuse pattern was even

a stronger prediction of recurrence [Fan 2003]. Thus, although the distinction between TCRBCL and pure, diffuse LPHL has been controversial, a predominant diffuse pattern in LPHL seems important to recognize.

References

Anagnostopoulos I, Hansmann ML, Franssila K, et al [2000] European Task Force on Lymphoma project on lymphocyte predominance Hodgkin disease: Histologic and immunohistologic analysis of submitted cases reveals 2 types of Hodgkin disease with a nodular growth pattern and abundant lymphocytes. *Blood* 96:1889-1899.

Borchmann P, Behringer K, Josting A, et al [2006] Secondary malignancies after successful primary treatment of malignant Hodgkin's lymphoma. *Pathologe* 27:47-52.

Bosler DS, Douglas-Nikitin VK, Harris VN, Smith MD [2008] Detection of T-regulatory cells has a potential role in the diagnosis of classical Hodgkin lymphoma. *Cytometry B Clin Cytom* 74:227-235.

Dunphy CH, Wolaniuk JW, and Glauber JG [1997] Nodular lymphocyte-predominant Hodgkin's disease with CD15, CD20, and LCA coexpression. *Cell Vis J Anal Morphol* 4:347-350.

Dunphy CH [2000] Contribution of flow cytometric immunophenotyping to the evaluation of tissues with suspected lymphoma? *Cytometry* 42:296-306.

Fan Z, Natkunam Y, Bair E, Tibshirani R, Warnke RA [2003] Characterization of variant patterns of nodular lymphocyte predominant Hodgkin lymphoma with immunohistologic and clinical correlation. *Am J Surg Pathol* 27:1346-1356.

Fromm JR, Kussick SJ, Wood BL [2006] Identification and purification of classical Hodgkin cells from lymph nodes by flow cytometry and flow cytometric cell sorting. *Am J Clin Pathol* 126:764-780.

Hudnall SD, Betancourt E, Barnhart E, Patel J [2008] Comparative flow immunophenotypic features of the inflammatory infiltrates of Hodgkin lymphoma and lymphoid hyperplasia. *Clinical Cytometry* 74B:1-8.

McBride JA, Rodriguez J, Luthra R, et al [1996] T-cell-rich B-cell lymphoma simulating lymphocyte-rich Hodgkin disease. *Am J Surg Pathol* 20:193-201.

Poppema S [1980] The diversity of the immunological staining pattern of Sternberg-Reed cells. *J Histochem Cytochem* 28:788-791.

Rahemtullah A, Reichard KK, Preffer FI, Harris NL, Hasserjian RP [2006] A double positive CD4+CD8+ T-cell population is commonly found in nodular lymphocyte predominant Hodgkin lymphoma. *Am J Clin Pathol* 126:805-814.

Ravoet C, Demartin S, Gerard R, et al [2004] Contribution of flow cytometry to the diagnosis of malignant and non-malignant conditions in lymph node biopsies. *Leuk Lymphoma* 45:1587-1593.

Rudiger T, Jaffe ES, Delsol G, et al [1998] Workshop report on Hodgkin disease and related disease ('gray zone' lymphoma). *Ann Oncol* 9(suppl 5):S31-S38.

Schmidt U, Metz KA, Leder LD, et al [1990] T-cell-rich B-cell lymphoma and lymphocyte predominant Hodgkin disease: Two closely related entities? *Br J Haematol* 2:398-403.

Stein H, Hansmann ML, Lennert K, Brandtzaeg P, Gatter KC, Mason DY [1986] Reed-Sternberg and Hodgkin cells in lymphocyte-predominant Hodgkin's disease of nodular subtype contain J chain. *Am J Clin Pathol* 86:292-297.

Torlakovic E, Torlakovic G, Nguyen PL, Brunning RD, Delabie J [2002] The value of anti-Pax-5 immunostaining in routinely fixed and paraffin-embedded sections. A novel pan pre-B and B-cell marker. *Am J Surg Pathol* 26:1343-1350.

16 Immunodeficiency-Associated Lymphoproliferative Disorders

Chapter Contents

Classification

- Lymphoproliferative diseases associated with primary immune disorders
- Lymphomas associated with infection by the human immunodeficiency virus (HIV)
- Post-transplant lymphoproliferative disorders (PTLDs)
- Methotrexate (MTX)-associated lymphoproliferative disorders (Other iatrogenic immunodeficiency-associated lymphoproliferative disorders, 2008)

Introduction

The WHO classification recognizes these 4 broad clinical settings of immunodeficiency (as outlined above) associated with an increased incidence of lymphoma and other lymphoproliferative disorders (LPDs). The primary immune disorders are discussed individually. The primary immune disorders with their flow cytometric findings and the significance of the findings are outlined in **[t16.1]**. The lymphomas occurring more specifically in HIV+ patients are discussed in detail, as are the PTLDs. **[t16.2]** outlines the lymphomas and lymphoproliferative disorders associated with the 4 broad clinical settings of immunodeficiency.

Lymphoproliferative Diseases Associated with Primary Immune Disorders

Autoimmune Lymphoproliferative Syndrome (ALPS; Canale-Smith Syndrome)

Definition

Autoimmune lymphoproliferative syndrome (ALPS; Canale-Smith syndrome) is a disorder of lymphocyte homeostasis, usually associated with germline Fas mutations (including mutations in CD95, CD95L, and caspases 8 and 10) [Straus 2001]. Fas (CD95/APO-1) is a cell surface receptor initiating programmed cell death, or apoptosis, of activated lymphocytes. There is an associated 15-fold and 50-fold increase in risk for developing non-Hodgkin lymphomas (NHLs) and Hodgkin lymphomas (HLs), respectively. Investigation of patients with Fas mutations (and their families) has demonstrated that all have defective lymphocyte apoptosis. Thus, there appears to be a significant role of Fas-mediated apoptosis in preventing B-cell and T-cell lymphomas.

Lymphocyte phenotypes

The cells in ALPS are T cells with the following immunophenotype: CD3+/dual negative CD4 and CD8 (DNTCs)/CD45RO–/CD45RA+/CD43+/CD57+/CD16–/CD56–/TIA-1(±)/perforin(±) [Lim 1998, Warnke 2007]. CD25 is negative. They usually bear $\alpha\beta$ T-cell receptors (TCRs), but rare cases may show positivity for $\gamma\delta$ TCRs [van den Berg 2003]. Another characteristic finding in up to 70% of patients is a coexistent polyclonal B-cell lymphocytosis (20%-40% of total lymphocytes) with expansion of CD5+ B cells. EBV is typically negative [Lim 1998]. A representative case of ALPS is demonstrated in **[f16.1]**.

Characteristics of associated lymphoproliferative diseases

A significant feature of lymphoma in ALPS is its diversity. Patients are at increased risk of developing NHL (15-fold; B- and T-cell types) and HL (50-fold; particularly nodular lymphocyte predominant HL). The preponderance of B-cell malignancies is notable given the fact that apoptosis in both T and B cells is abnormal in ALPS and the major non-malignant cell types that expand in ALPS are DNTCs, which are believed to be mature T cells that have lost expressions of their CD4 and CD8 co-receptors [Fisher 1995, Sneller 1997, Lenardo 1999]. Therefore, Fas defects do not appear to shift the distribution between T and B lymphoid malignancies.

t16.1 The Contribution of FCI in Primary Immune Disorders

Disorder	FCI findings	Clinical Significance
ALPS	CD3+/CD4–/CD8–/CD45RO–/ CD45RA+/ CD43+/CD57+/ CD16–/CD56–/ TIA-1±/perforin± Co-existent polyclonal B lymphocytosis	Diagnosis Immunophenotype lymphomas
CVID	Normal # of PB sIg+, CD20+B cells; 50% of cases: deficiency of CD4/normal # CD8 cells or normal # of CD4/ increased # CD8 cells	Patients with increased CD8 cells may benefit from cimetidine therapy Immunophenotype lymphomas
AT	Increase in cells with the $\gamma\delta$ TCR	Detect increase in $\gamma\delta$ TCR+ cells Immunophenotype T-cell neoplasms
X-LPS1	Increase in PB CD8+ cells	Detect increase in CD8+ cells Immunophenotype B-NHLs
WAS	Gradual decline in CD3+ cells	Detect total CD3+ cell count to predict infectious complications Immunophenotype lymphomas
SCID	Lymphopenia with marked ↓ T cells; PB B cells IP as cord blood B cells (CD1c+, CD38+, and CD23+)	Detect decreased # of PB T cells Define "cord blood" IP of PB B cells Immunophenotype LPDs
Chronic active EBV infection	Massive expansion ↑ CD8+/ TCRαβ+ T cells, >90% with an activated T-cell IP 33: up-regulation of CD2, CD11a, CD11b, CD11c, CD38, CD45RO, and HLA-DR, and down-regulation of CD3, CD7, CD28, and CD45RA CD16–, CD56–, and CD57–	Detect increased activated T cells Immunophenotype clonal T-cell expansions

ALPS, autoimmune lymphoproliferative syndrome; AT, ataxia telangiectasis; CVID, common variable immunodeficiency; EBV, Epstein-Barr virus; FCI, flow cytometric immunophenotyping; IP, immunophenotype; LPDs, lymphoproliferative disorders; PB, peripheral blood; SCID, severe combined immunodeficiency syndrome; sIg, surface immunoglobulin; TCR, T-cell receptor; WAS, Wiskott-Aldrich syndrome; X-LPS1, X-linked lymphoproliferative syndrome

Contribution of FCI

Flow cytometric immunophenotyping (FCI) is most useful for defining the DNTCs by multi-color analysis and in immunophenotyping the malignant lymphomas that may develop in ALPS.

Common Variable Immunodeficiency

Definition

Common variable immunodeficiency (CVID), also known as common variable or late-onset hypogamma-globulinemia, is a clinically heterogeneous group of disorders characterized by markedly reduced serum levels

t16.2 Immunodeficient Disorders & Associated Lymphomas/LPDs

Disorder	Associated Lymphomas/LPDs
ALPS	NHL (15-fold; B- & T-cell types) & HL (50-fold; particularly NLPHL)
CVID	Mainly DLBCLs related to GCB cells, but T-cell NHLs & HLs may also develop
AT	T-cell neoplasms
X-LPS1	B-cell NHLs, particularly extranodal
WAS	Most often EBV-associated diffuse, aggressive B-cell NHLs; also cases not associated with EBV and EBV-associated HLs
SCID	Clonal T-cell proliferations in SCID patients treated with retroviral therapy
Chronic active EBV infection	Clonal T-cell proliferations, often with a cytotoxic T-cell IP (ie, CD3+, CD8+, CD4–, and cytotoxic granule-associated proteins+).
HIV infection	Vast majority of B-cell origin 3 main groups: 1. polymorphic LPs (5%) 2. systemic NHL & HL of various subtypes (including BL, DLBCL, PCNSL, & MALT lymphoma and cHL-MCHL & LDHL most commonly, but also NSHL), that also occur in immunocompetent pts (>85%) 3. lymphomas occurring more specifically in HIV+ pts (PBL of the oral cavity (3%) and PEL (4%).
Post transplant	PTLDs (see text for classification)
MTX therapy	Most commonly DLBCL (35%), cHL (25%) or HL-like lesions; also FL, LPL, BL, MCL, PTCL, & polymorphic PTLD-like lesion; commonly extranodal (not CNS); approximately 50% are EBV-associated, the frequency of which depends on the particular subtype—rates highest in HL (approximately 75% of cases).

ALPS, autoimmune lymphoproliferative syndrome; AT, ataxia telangictasia; BL, Burkitt lymphoma; CNS, central nervous system; CVID, common variable immunodeficiency; DLBCL, diffuse large B-cell lymphoma; EBV, Epstein-Barr virus; FL, follicular lymphoma; GCB, germinal center B; HIV, human immunodeficiency virus; IP, immunophenotype; LP, lymphoid proliferations; LPDs, lymphoproliferative disorders; LPHL, lymphocyte-depleted HL; LPL, lymphoplasmacytic lymphoma; MALT, mucosa-associated lymphoid tissue; MCHL, mixed cellularity HL; MCL, mantle cell lymphoma; MTX, methotrexate; NHL, non-Hodgkin lymphoma; NLPHL, nodular lymphocyte-predominant HL; NSHL, nodular sclerosis HL; PBL, plasmablastic lymphoma; PCNSL, primary central nervous system lymphoma; PEL, primary effusion lymphoma; PTCL, peripheral T-cell lymphoma; PTLDs, post-transplant LPDs; pts, patients; SCID, severe combined immunodeficiency syndrome; WAS, Wiskott-Aldrich syndrome; X-LPS1, X-linked lymphoproliferative syndrome.

of immunoglobulin (Ig)G, variably reduced serum levels of other Igs, and an increased incidence of infections [Hermans 1976, Rosen 1984, Weiss 1991, Yocum 1991].

The common defect in CVID is a block in the normal differentiation of B lymphocytes into antibody-producing plasma cells [Hermans 1976, Rosen 1984, Waldmann 1988, Waldman 1974]. Patients with CVID may develop benign lymphoid lesions (ie, atypical lymphoid hyperplasia, reactive lymphoid hyperplasia, and chronic granulomatous inflammation) [Sander 1992], as well as malignant lymphomas (mainly diffuse large B-cell lymphomas—DLBCLs—but also T-cell NHLs and

HLs). The actual increased risk is probably not as high as originally quoted, since earlier studies did not include immunophenotypic and molecular genetic analyses, and more recently, mucosa-associated lymphoid tissue (MALT) lymphomas have been also been recognized in this setting and may have been included as "atypical lymphoid hyperplasias" in older studies [Cunningham-Rundles 2002, Desar 2006]. More recent studies quote an increased risk of 12-fold to 15-fold [Mellemkjaer 2002].

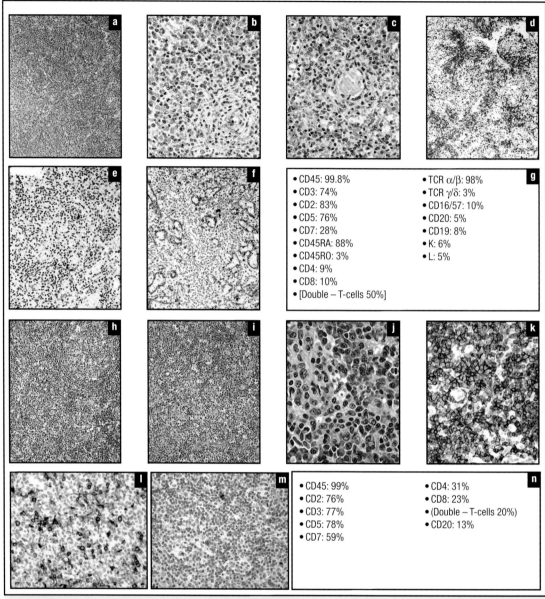

- CD45: 99.8%
- CD3: 74%
- CD2: 83%
- CD5: 76%
- CD7: 28%
- CD45RA: 88%
- CD45RO: 3%
- CD4: 9%
- CD8: 10%
- [Double – T-cells 50%]

- TCR α/β: 98%
- TCR γ/δ: 3%
- CD16/57: 10%
- CD20: 5%
- CD19: 8%
- K: 6%
- L: 5%

- CD45: 99%
- CD2: 76%
- CD3: 77%
- CD5: 78%
- CD7: 59%

- CD4: 31%
- CD8: 23%
- (Double – T-cells 20%)
- CD20: 13%

[f16.1] This case demonstrates the pathologic features in a patient with autoimmune lymphoproliferative syndrome (ALPS). The clinical history reveals a 6-year-old male with autoimmune hemolytic anemia, idiopathic thrombocytopenia purpura, generalized lymphadenopathy, and marked splenomegaly since the first year of life. Viral serology is negative. There is no evidence of opportunistic infections. Patient has a history of poor response to steroids. To ameliorate thrombocytopenia, splenectomy was performed at age 2.5. Three years later, a cervical lymph node biopsy is performed to rule out lymphoma. H&E sections of the diffusely enlarged, congested spleen (1040 g) reveal an atypical proliferation of lymphocytes in various stages of immunoblastic transformation and plasma cells; no apoptotic bodies are identified **a–c**. T cells are identified with CD3 immunohistochemical staining **d**; however, they are negative for CD4 **e** and CD8 **f**. The reported flow cytometric data of the splenic tissue **g** are provided. H&E sections of the subsequent lymph node biopsy **h–j** reveal expansion of the paracortex by an atypical proliferation of lymphocytes seen in various stages of transformation (from small to medium and large transformed immunoblastic cells) and many plasma cells. Follicles with germinal centers, not particularly enlarged or activated, are present. Macrophages with apoptotic bodies are seen within the germinal centers but not in the paracortex. T cells are again identified with CD3 immunohistochemical staining **k**; however, most are negative for CD4 **l** and CD8 **m**. The reported flow cytometric data of the lymph node **n** are provided. The molecular results show EBER by ISH (EBV-RNA): negative; PCR TCR-gamma and IgH genes: polyclonal; genomic sequencing point mutation in APT1 gene encoding apoptosis receptor Fas/APO-1/CD95 by SSCP PCR analysis. Cytogenetic results demonstrate normal male karyotype with decreased apoptosis in FHA stimulated PB T-cells (<1% cell death) after FAS ligand. Diagnosis of autoimmune lymphoproliferative syndrome (ALPS; Canale-Smith syndrome) due to mutation in APT-1 gene (ALPS Ia) is made.

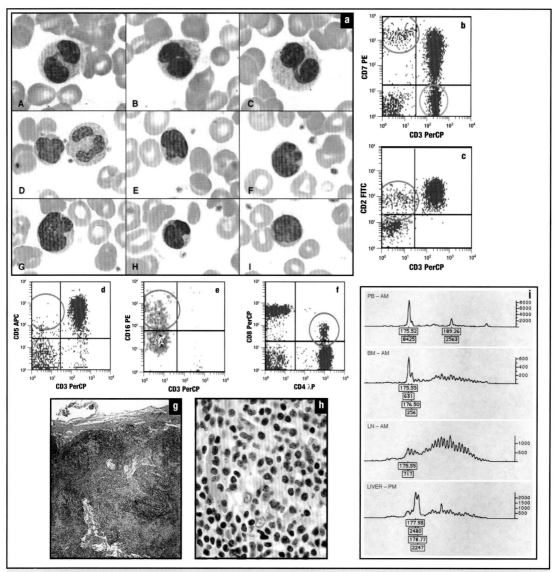

[f16.2] This case demonstrates the pathologic features in a patient with common variable immunodeficiency. The clinical history reveals a 43-year-old Caucasian male with common variable immunodeficiency (CVID), complicated at various times by autoimmune hemolytic anemia, thrombocytopenia, and neutropenia, who is noted to have a peripheral blood lymphocytosis with a WBC of 8,300 × 10^3/mm^3 (8,300 × 10^9/L) (72% lymphocytes); hemoglobin and platelet counts are normal. Wright-Giemsa stain [×1000] of the peripheral blood smear **a** reveals atypical bilobated mononuclear cells [inserted **A-C**] as well as atypical lymphocytes with irregular nuclei, some with azurophilic granules [inserted **D-I**]. Flow cytometric analysis of the peripheral blood **b-f** shows a predominance (90%) of T cells, most of which are immunophenotypically normal, TCR α-β positive, and with a CD4:CD8 ratio of 1:1. Seen are subpopulations of CD2+, CD7+, CD16+, CD3–, CD5–, and NK cells **b-e** (blue circles). CD56 is also positive on these cells (not demonstrated); CD4+, CD8(dim)+ cells **f** (purple circle); and CD3+, CD7+ cells **b** (green circle). There is no expression of CD1a, CD10, or TdT; and CD3–, CD16/56+ NK-cells. A subsequent bone marrow showed an interstitial and nodular immunophenotypically normal T-cell lymphocytosis (30%), without overt histologic features of lymphoma. A subsequent lymph node biopsy reveals abnormal architecture with loss of follicles and focally prominent sclerosis **g**. Cytologically, most of the nodal parenchyma consists of small mature appearing lymphocytes and intermediate-sized immunoblasts, but no overt evidence of lymphoma **h**. Flow cytometric analysis of the lymph node biopsy (not demonstrated) reveals a predominant population of T lymphocytes with a CD4:CD8 ratio of 2.3:1. The majority of the CD4+ cells are CD45RO+, CD45–, and CD62L–. Neither the population of dual positive CD4+CD8+ T cells, nor the CD7– T-cells, evident peripherally, are detected. TCRG PCR using capillary electrophoresis **i** shows apparently identical monoclonal peaks in peripheral blood, bone marrow, and liver, but not overtly in the lymph node. The cytogenetic results are normal, 46, XY. Diagnosis of systemic atypical T-cell proliferation with common T-cell clone, arising in a patient with CVID is made. *AM, antemortem; PM, postmortem.*

Lymphocyte Phenotypes

Although CVID often involves a defect intrinsic to B lymphocytes [Spickett 1990], patients with CVID usually have a normal number of circulating B lymphocytes and express recognizable anti-surface Ig and CD20, and approximately half of CVID patients demonstrate abnormal expressions of T-cell markers (including a deficiency of CD4/normal numbers of CD8 cells, or normal numbers of CD4/increased numbers of CD8 cells) [Ichikawa 1982, Reinherz 1979, Reinherz 1981, Gupta 1982]. Of note, in patients with increased CD8 cells, cimetidine therapy may result in a decrease in CD8 cells with a concomitant increase in serum Igs [White 1985, Segal 1989].

Characteristics of associated lymphoproliferative diseases

As mentioned previously, malignant lymphomas developing in CVID are mainly DLBCLs, but T-cell NHLs and HLs may also develop in this setting. Such a case is demonstrated in [f16.2]. Many of the DLBCLs appear to be histogenetically related to germinal center B cells [Ariatti 2000].

Contribution of FCI

Based on the findings described above, FCI may be useful in pinpointing a specific diagnosis, in determining possible therapeutic options, and in immunophenotyping the malignant lymphomas that may develop in CVID.

Ataxia Telangiectasia

Definition

Ataxia telangiectasia (AT) is a rare condition associated with a marked decrease in serum IgA, IgG2, and IgE, and poor cell-mediated immune responsiveness [Ammann 1982]. These patients may develop T-cell neoplasms (ie, precursor T-cell lymphoblastic leukemia/lymphoma and T-prolymphocytic leukemia).

Lymphocyte phenotypes

Patients with AT demonstrate an increase in cells with the γδ TCR.

Characteristics of associated lymphoproliferative diseases

These patients may develop T-cell neoplasms, as mentioned previously.

Contribution of FCI

FCI may be useful in detecting the increase in cells with the γδ TCR and in immunophenotyping the T-cell neoplasms that may develop in AT.

X-Linked Lymphoproliferative Syndrome-1 (Duncan Syndrome)

Definition

This syndrome is characterized by a marked depression of the immune response to EBV [Purtilo 1990]. Despite the nomenclature, not all cases are due to X-linked inheritance. Most patients with X-linked lymphoproliferative syndrome die of an EBV-induced B-cell lymphoproliferation after exposure to infectious mononucleosis (IM) [Schuster 1990]. Those who survive IM are usually left with hypogammaglobulinemia or may develop B-cell NHLs.

Lymphocyte phenotypes

There is an increase in CD8+ T cells in the peripheral blood (PB).

Characteristics of associated lymphoproliferative diseases

Patients with X-linked lymphoproliferative syndrome are prone to develop B-cell NHLs, particularly in extranodal sites (eg, the terminal ileum).

Contribution of FCI

FCI is useful in confirming an increase in PB CD8+ T cells and in immunophenotyping the B-cell NHLs that may develop in Duncan syndrome.

Wiskott-Aldrich Syndrome

Definition

Wiskott-Aldrich syndrome (WAS) is a condition characterized by the following triad: eczematoid dermatitis, thrombocytopenia, and recurrent infections with opportunistic infections [Blease 1968]. Immunologic studies reveal normal IgG, decreased IgM, elevated IgA and IgE levels, and decreased T-cell function. Patients with WAS often have an increased susceptibility (7%) to the development of NHLs.

Lymphocyte phenotypes

After developing relatively normal proportions of T lymphocytes during infancy, children with WAS show a gradual decline in T cell numbers, both in the

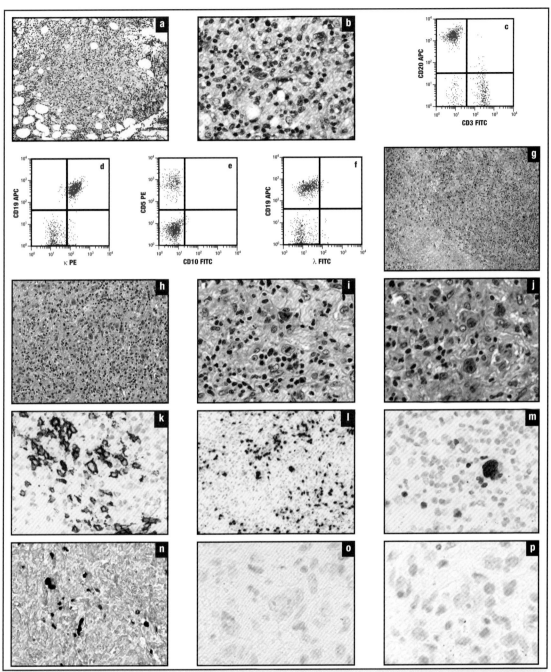

[f16.3] This case demonstrates an age-related EBV-associated B-cell lymphoproliferative disorder. The clinical history reveals a 79-year-old female with fatigue, fever, weight loss, treated for multiple UTIs without improvement. There is no known autoimmune or immunodeficiency disorder, and her HIV status is negative. CT and PET scans reveal multistation lymph node enlargement and splenic infiltration, "compatible with lymphoma." EBV viral load is elevated (7798 copies/mL). Bone marrow biopsy is performed. H&E sections of the bone marrow biopsy **a, b** reveal the large abnormal lymphoid cells. The flow cytometric data of the bone marrow aspirate is provided **c-f**, revealing a monoclonal κ B-cell population (CD5–, CD10–, CD23–). H&E sections of the subsequent lymph node biopsy **g-j** reveal obliteration of the normal architecture with areas of necrosis and large abnormal lymphoid cells, some with "Hodgkin-like" cytomorphological features. By immunohistochemical staining, the abnormal lymphoid cells are positive for CD20 **k**, PAX-5 **l**, bcl-6, MUM1 **m**, and EBV-in-situ hybridization **n**, and are negative for CD15 **o** and CD30 **p**. Molecular results reveal a clonal immunoglobulin heavy chain rearrangement, negative for T cell gene rearrangement. The diagnosis of age-related EBV-associated B-cell lymphoproliferative disorder is made.

peripheral blood and in lymphoid organs [Gotoff 1967]. Although the CD4:CD8 ratio remains normal, CD43 expression (normally expressed by T cells) is markedly decreased in these patients [Park 1991].

Characteristics of associated lymphoproliferative diseases

Lymphomas developing in WAS are most often diffuse aggressive B-cell neoplasms, resembling those seen in human immunodeficiency virus (HIV) infections and the post-transplantation setting and often associated with EBV. However, there are cases not associated with EBV and also EBV-associated HLs that may develop in these patients [Kroft 1998, Sasahara 2001].

Contribution of FCI

FCI may be particularly useful in following the total number of CD3+ cells (to aid in predicting infectious complications) and in immunophenotyping the malignant lymphomas that may develop in WAS.

Severe Combined Immunodeficiency Syndrome

Definition

Severe combined immunodeficiency (SCID) is the most severe immunodeficiency syndrome, characterized by lymphopenia, a primary defect in T-cell lineage (markedly decreased T cells), and the absence of serum immunoglobulin (Ig)G, IgA, and IgM. Retroviral gene therapy in X-linked SCID patients has been associated with the development of lymphoproliferative disorders.

Lymphocyte imuunophenotypes

The peripheral blood lymphocytes express CD1c, CD38, and CD23. They are usually present on cord blood B cells but only on a small subset of adult B lymphocytes [Small 1989].

Characteristics of associated lymphoproliferative diseases

There have been reports of uncontrolled exponential clonal proliferation of mature T cells (with $\gamma\delta$ + or $\alpha\beta$ + TCRs) in SCID patients treated with retroviral therapy. The clones showed retrovirus vector integration in proximity to the LMO2 proto-oncogene promoter, leading to aberrant transcription and expression of LMO2. Thus, retrovirus vector insertion can trigger deregulated clonal T-cell proliferations with unexpected frequency,

most likely driven by retrovirus enhancer activity on the LMO2 gene promoter [Hacein-Bey-Abina 2003].

Contribution of FCI

FCI is particularly useful in detecting the decreased numbers of T cells in the peripheral blood, in defining the "cord blood" immunophenotype of the peripheral blood B cells, and in immunophenotyping the lymphoproliferative disorders that may develop in SCID.

Chronic Active EBV

Definition

Chronic active EBV infection is also included in this section, since it may be considered a pathogen-specific type of immune dysfunction in patients who seem to have a specific inability to clear an EBV infection (that most other individuals would be able to handle without adverse effects). Recent studies have suggested mutations in the perforin gene as a specific mechanism for susceptibility to chronic active EBV infection and hemophagocytosis [Warnke 2007]. Such infections have been most commonly associated with clonal T-cell proliferations [Gaillard 1992, Jones 1988, Kanegane 1998, Kanegane 1999, Nakagawa 2002].

Lymphocyte phenotypes

A relatively recent and comprehensive study of the immunophenotype and TCR-V repertoire of peripheral blood T-cells from 28 patients with acute infectious mononucleosis was performed by flow cytometry using 3- and 4-color combinations of monoclonal antibodies directed against a large panel of T- and NK-cell associated markers, activation- and adhesion-related molecules and TCR-Vβ, –Vγ and –Vδ families [Lima 2003]. Nearly all patients (27/28) showed a massive expansion of CD8+/TCR$\alpha\beta$+ T cells, the majority (>90%) of which displayed an immunophenotype compatible with T-cell activation, including up-regulation of CD2, CD11a, CD11b, and CD11c adhesion molecules, CD38, CD45RO and HLA-DR together with down-regulation of CD3, CD7, CD28, and CD45RA. The natural killer cell antigens (ie, CD16, CD56, and CD57) were all negative. Of note, small expansions of 1 or more TCR-Vβ families accounting for $12 \pm 7\%$ of either the CD8+/TCR$\alpha\beta$+ or the CD4+/TCR$\alpha\beta$+ T-cell compartment were found in 12 of 14 patients studied. The results of this study provide evidence for extensive T-cell activation during acute EBV infection.

Characteristics of associated lymphoproliferative diseases

As mentioned earlier, chronic active EBV infections are most often complicated by clonal T-cell proliferations, which often have a cytotoxic T-cell immunophenotype (ie, CD3+, CD8+, CD4−, and cytotoxic granule-associated proteins+). They are typically negative for CD30 and CD56 and may demonstrate (or be negative for) a TCR β gene rearrangement [Nakagawa 2002].

Contribution of FCI

FCI is particularly useful in determining the presence of activated T cells as described above by multi-color analysis, as well as in immunophenotyping the clonal T-cell proliferations that may develop in the setting of chronic active EBV infections.

Age-Related EBV-Associated B-Cell Lymphoproliferative Disorders

Definition

There is a newly recognized clinicopathologic disease entity occurring in elderly patients with EBV-associated B-cell lymphoproliferative disorders (B-LPDs) showing similarities in many respects to immunodeficiency-associated LPDs but without evidence of an underlying immunodeficiency [Oyama 2003, Shimoyama 2006]. Therefore, the nosological category of senile or age-related EBV+ B-LPD has been proposed for these patients. It has been asserted that this disease may be related to immunological deterioration as a result of the aging process (ie, senescence in immunity) [Shimoyama 2008]. This new disease entity is characterized pathologically by centroblasts, immunoblasts, and Reed-Sternberg-like giant cells with varying degrees of reactive components, often posing diagnostic problems histologically.

Typical immunophenotype

The EBV+ B cells are usually CD20+ or CD79a+ and show light chain restriction. Those with immunoblastic or plasmacytoid features lack CD20 expression and demonstrate cytoplasmic Ig. LMP1 and EBNA2 have been positive in the large atypical cells in 94% and 28% of the tested cases, respectively [Oyama 2003, Shimoyama 2006, Oyama 2007]. The large atypical cells are also positive for CD30 in 75% of cases but not CD15. Clonality of the Ig genes and EBV is usually detected by genotypic techniques and are helpful in distinguishing polymorphous age-related B-LPD from IM and EBV+ reactive B-LPD in the middle-aged or elderly patients,

the atypical clinical findings of the latter having been reported recently by Kojima et al [Kojima 2007]. A representative case is demonstrated in **[f16.3]**.

Contribution of FCI

FCI may be particularly helpful in detecting a monoclonal B-cell immunophenotype.

Lymphomas Associated with Infection by HIV

Approximately 1%-6% of HIV+ patients develop lymphoma each year.

Classifications

The vast majority of lymphomas developing in HIV+ patients are of B-cell origin.

The classification of HIV-associated lymphomas may be broadly divided into 3 main groups:

1. polymorphic lymphoid proliferations (resembling polymorphic post-transplant lymphoproliferative disorder-PTLD, to be discussed in section C) (5% of all HIV-associated lymphomas)

2. systemic NHL and HL of various histological subtypes (including Burkitt lymphoma-BL, DLBCL, primary central nervous system lymphoma-PCNSL, and MALT lymphoma as well as classical HL-mixed cellularity and lymphocyte-depleted most commonly, but also nodular sclerosis subtype), also occurring in immunocompetent patients (>85%)

3. lymphomas occurring more specifically in HIV+ patients, including plasmablastic lymphoma of the oral cavity (PBL) (3%) and primary effusion lymphoma (PEL) (4%) [Tran 2008]

Oncogenic viral infections are undoubtedly implicated in lymphomagenesis. For example, EBV is found in 60% of HIV-associated lymphomas with the highest incidence in PCNSL (100%) followed by HL (close to 100%), PEL (90%), the immunoblastic variant of DLBCL (80%), PBL (50%), and BL (30%). The following discussion will be limited to those lymphomas occurring specifically in HIV+ patients.

Primary Effusion Lymphoma

Definition

Primary effusion lymphoma is a neoplasm of large B cells usually presenting as serous effusions without detectable tumor masses. The neoplastic cells may exhibit a range of appearances, from large immunoblastic or plasmablastic cells to more anaplastic morphology. Some neoplastic cells may even resemble Reed-Sternberg cells. The WHO classification states that PEL is universally associated with human herpes virus 8 (HHV-8)/Kaposi sarcoma herpes virus (KSHV), most often occurring in the setting of immunodeficiency (eg, HIV infection, post-transplantation).

By definition, there is no discrete contiguous lymphomatous mass associated with the effusion. However, it should be recognized there is an extra-cavitary variant of PEL represented by KSHV+ solid lymphomatous presentations, indistinguishable morphologically, immunophenotypically, and genotypically [Chadburn 2004]. There are no associated effusions in these patients.

Typical immunophenotype

The neoplastic cells of PEL typically express CD45 but are negative for pan-B-cell markers (eg, CD19, CD20, and CD79a) as well as sIg and cIg and most T-cell markers. Activation and plasma cell-related markers (eg, CD30, CD38, and CD138) are usually expressed. EBV genome is also detected in the majority of cases [Sepp 1990].

A representative case of PEL was demonstrated in [f12.43]. A representative case of a "solid," or extra-cavitary variant, of PEL within bone marrow is demonstrated in [f16.4].

Variant immunophenotype

Aberrant expression of cCD3, as well as CD7 and CD56, have been reported in PEL [Polski 2000, Beaty 1999]. Of note, the extra-cavitary variant of PEL appears to express B-cell associated antigens (25%) and Ig (25%) slightly more often than the PELs (<5% and 15%, respectively).

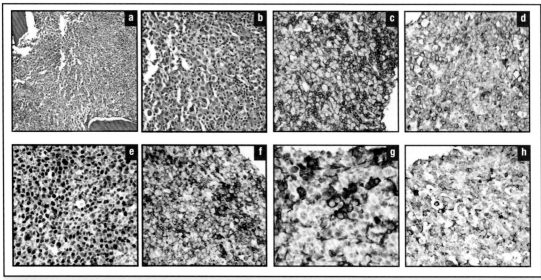

[f16.4] This case demonstrates a rare primary effusion lymphoma, solid variant. The clinical history reveals a 27-year-old HIV+ male who presents with a history of CNS toxoplasmosis and CMV retinitis, complicated by hypotension, thrombocytopenia, anemia, coagulopathy, fevers, and hypoxic respiratory failure. A BM biopsy is performed. CBC data include WBC 3.4 × 10³/mm³ (3.4 × 10⁹/L), Hgb 10.1 g/dL, Plt 30 × 10³/mm³ (30 × 10⁹/L). H&E sections of the bone marrow biopsy **a, b** reveal sheets of large abnormal lymphoid-appearing cells. The bone marrow did not aspirate for a specimen to analyze by flow cytometric analysis. By immunohistochemical staining, the large abnormal cells are positive for CD45 **c**, CD30 **d**, MUM1 **e**, CD2 **f**, equivocal CD4 **g**, and subset epithelial membrane antigen **h**. The cytogenic results show numerous structural and numerical abnormalities, including rearrangements involving chromosomes 1 and 9, and deletions of chromosome 6. Molecular results identify a clonal Ig heavy chain gene rearrangement. The diagnosis of primary effusion lymphoma, solid variant is made.

Contribution of FCI

FCI is particularly useful in determining the typical lack of T-cell and B-cell markers by multi-color analysis.

Differential diagnosis

Diffuse large B-cell lymphoma with high grade features and Burkitt lymphoma

The distinction between PEL and involvement of a body fluid by a DLBCL with high grade features or a BL relies primarily on the absence of a contiguous or other primary site of lymphomatous involvement. In addition, DLBCL with high-grade features and BL both have a mature B-cell immunophenotype with expression of surface B-cell antigens and are typically negative for CD30, CD138, and T-cell antigens.

Anaplastic large B-cell lymphoma (ALCL) (see [t12.3])

Due to the anaplastic features of (and expression of CD30 by) the neoplastic cells of PEL, ALCL should be considered in the differential diagnosis. However, the neoplastic cells of PEL typically express CD138 (not encountered in anaplastic CD30+ LCL) and are uniformly ALK–. Although some cases of PEL may demonstrate an aberrant rearrangement of TCR genes, cases of PEL typically demonstrate rearranged and mutated Ig genes. ALCLs typically demonstrate a rearrangement of TCR but do not demonstrate an Ig gene rearrangement or mutation.

Plasmablastic lymphoma and plasmablastic plasmacytoma (see [t12.3])

Since the neoplastic cells of PEL may appear plasmablastic and express CD138, differential diagnoses should also include PBL and plasmablastic plasmacytoma. This distinction again is primarily based on sole body cavity involvement with no contiguous mass or other site of disease. In addition, although the neoplastic cells of PEL may appear plasmablastic and express CD138, they typically do not demonstrate cytoplasmic expression of Ig or light chains, as seen in PBL and plasmablastic plasmacytoma.

Contribution of paraffin immunohistochemical (IHC) immunophenotyping

Although PEL is a primary lymphoma arising within a body cavity as an effusion, cell blocks may be prepared for IHC staining. The nuclei of the neoplastic cells are positive for the HHV8/KSHV-associated latent protein by IHC staining [Dupin 1999]. In addition, EBER positivity by in-situ hybridization (ISH) may also be demonstrated in PEL. Other lymphomas that may be included in the differential diagnosis of PEL are negative for HHV8.

Plasmablastic Lymphoma of the Oral Cavity

Definition

PBL is an uncommon, recently described B-cell-derived lymphoma that displays distinctive affinity for extranodal presentation in the oral cavity or jaw. The tumors display a diffuse growth pattern composed of large cells with eccentric nuclei containing single, central, and prominent nucleoli associated with deeply basophilic cytoplasm containing a paranuclear hof. PBL is strongly associated with HIV infection but has been reported in HIV-negative individuals [Folk 2006]. Most cases of AIDS-related PBL have an immunophenotype and tumor suppressor gene expression profile virtually identical to plasmablastic plasmacytoma or plasmablastic plasma cell myeloma (PCM), and unlike DLBCL [Vega 2005]. These results question the WHO classification of PBL as a variant of DLBCL.

Typical immunophenotype with variations

Cases of PBL and plasmablastic PCM have been shown to have nearly identical immunophenotypes, being positive for CD138 and CD38 and negative for CD20, corresponding to a plasma cell immunophenotype. The only significant difference demonstrated between PBL and PCM is the presence of EBV-encoded RNA, being positive in all PBL cases tested and negative in all PCM cases. There is no association with KSHV/HHV8. A representative case of PBL was demonstrated in [f12.31],.

Contribution of FCI

FCI is particularly useful in determining the typical lack of T-cell and B-cell markers by multi-color analysis. CD138 may also be detected by FCI.

Differential diagnosis

DLBCL, including ALK+ DLBCL (or DLBCL of plasmacytic type) and the anaplastic variant of DLBCL

ALK+ DLBCL (also referred to as DLBCL of plasmablastic type) may be diagnostically confused with PBL, based on overlapping morphological and immunophenotypic features. ALK+ DLBCL is characterized by the following immunophenotype by IHC staining: ALK+, CD30–, CD20–, EMA+, and CD138+, and monoclonal cytoplasmic Ig or light chain, best demonstrated by ISH staining. Although cases of ALK+ DLBCL (or DLBCL of plasmacytic type) have not been reportedly HIV+, PBL may also occur in HIV-negative patients. The main immunophenotypic difference between these 2 entities is the ALK-positivity in the DLBCL of plasmacytic type and ALK-negativity in PBL.

The anaplastic variant of DLBCL is a CD30+ diffuse anaplastic lymphoma of B-cell origin [Maes 2001] and may have morphological features overlapping with PBL. The distinction is based primarily on the B-cell immunophenotype in the anaplastic variant of DLBCL and the plasma cell immunophenotype (ie, CD138-positivity and monoclonal cytoplasmic Ig or light chain) in PBL.

Anaplastic large cell lymphoma

PBL may have overlapping morphological features with anaplastic large cell lymphoma (ALCL). The distinction is based on the plasma cell immunophenotype in PBL and the T-cell or "null" cell immunophenotype characteristic of ALCL in the WHO classification.

Plasmablastic plasmacytoma

Plasmablastic plasmacytoma has an identical immunophenotype to PBL. A representative case of plasmablastic plasmacytoma was demonstrated in [f12.32]. Plasmablastic plasmacytoma is most often distinguished from PBL by the presence of EBV-encoded RNA, being positive in all PBL cases tested and negative in all plasmacytoma cases.

Primary effusion lymphoma

This differential was discussed in the section above regarding PEL.

Burkitt lymphoma

BL with plasmacytoid differentiation should also be considered in the differential diagnosis of PBL. However, in this variant of BL, typically only a subset of neoplastic cells shows plasmacytoid differentiation.

The immunophenotypic features of ALCL, the anaplastic variant of DLBCL, DLBCL of plasmablastic type (ALK+ DLBCL), PBL, and plasmablastic plasmacytoma, as well as PEL are compared in [t12.3].

Contribution of FCI and comparison with IHC immunophenotyping

Paraffin IHC staining for CD138 and IHC staining for κ and λ light chains or ISH for κ and λ light chain mRNA may be particularly useful in the diagnosis of PBL. EBV-encoded RNA may also be readily evaluated by ISH in the differential diagnosis of a plasmablastic plasmacytoma vs a PBL. ALK staining may also be useful in excluding an ALK+ DLBCL or ALK+ ALCL.

Post-Transplant Lymphoproliferative Disorders

Classification

1. Early lesions
   Reactive plasmacytic hyperplasia
   IM-like

2. Polymorphic PTLD

3. Monomorphic PTLD
   B-cell neoplasms
     DLBCL
     BL
     Plasma cell myeloma
     Plasmacytoma-like lesions
   T-cell neoplasms
     Peripheral T-cell lymphoma,
       not otherwise specified
     Other types

4. HL and HL-like PTLD

PTLD is a heterogeneous syndrome ranging from a benign, self-limited form of lymphoproliferation with many features of a florid viral infection at 1 end of the spectrum to an aggressive, widely disseminated lymphoma, most often of B-cell immunophenotype.

Plasmacytic hyperplasia characteristically involves the oropharynx or nodal sites. Immunophenotypic studies show an admixture of polyclonal B cells, plasma cells, and T cells. It is nearly always polyclonal, usually contains multiple EBV infection events, and lacks oncogene and tumor suppressor gene alterations.

Polymorphic PTLDs may arise nodally or extranodally, are composed of a mixture of B and T cells, are most often monoclonal, usually contain a single form of EBV, and lack oncogene and tumor suppressor gene alterations.

Monomorphic B-cell PTLDs show B-cell associated antigen expression with monotypic Ig expression in 50% of cases. DLBCL of immunoblastic type and plasma cell myeloma represent widely disseminated disease of monoclonal origin containing a single form of EBV and alterations of 1 or more oncogene or tumor suppressor genes (ie, *N-ras*, p53, *c-myc*).

Monomorphic T-cell PTLDs show expression of T-cell markers and may show variable expressions of CD4 or CD8, CD56, or CD30 and either $\alpha\beta$ or $\gamma\delta$ TCRs.

HL and HL-like PTLDs show expression of CD15 and CD30, as classical HL. However, HL-like PTLDs often demonstrate an atypical immunophenotype with B-cell antigen expression [Harris 1997].

Representative cases of the various subtypes of PTLD are demonstrated in **[f16.5]**, **[f16.6]**, and **[f16.7]**.

Patients with lymphomatous-PTLD appear to have a more aggressive clinical course and poorer outcomes than lymphomas in immunocompetent hosts [Meije 2002]. Approximately 90% are of B-cell origin, and

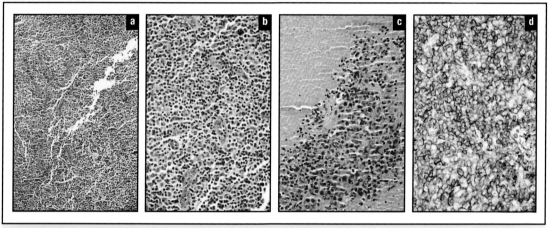

[f16.5] This case demonstrates a post-transplantation lymphoproliferative disorder exhibiting co-existing polymorphic and monomorphic subtypes. The clinical history reveals a 20-year-old female with a history of AML, status post unrelated donor peripheral blood stem cell transplant presents with bilateral cervical lymphadenopathy and an increased EBV viral load. H&E sections of the lymph node reveal polymorphic morphology **a, b** and monomorphic morphology **c** in other areas. Flow cytometric analysis of the lymph node fails to reveal a monoclonal B-cell or significantly aberrant T-cell population. By immunohistochemical staining, the monomorphic cells are positive with CD20 **d**. The molecular results show no clonal IGH gene rearrangement; there was no amplifiable DNA for TCR gamma gene rearrangement analysis. Cytogenetic results are normal. Diagnosis of post-transplant lymphoproliferative disorder, polymorphic and monomorphic subtypes, is made.

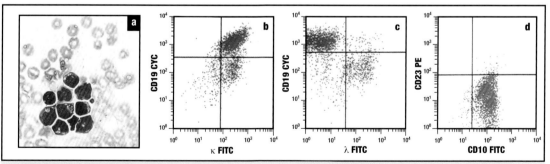

[f16.6] This case demonstrates a rare post-transplantation Burkitt lymphoma. The clinical history reveals a 32-year-old white male who has cystic fibrosis and is 4.5 years status post double lung transplant and subsequent immunosuppression. His post-transplant course was complicated by nonrecurrent EBV viremia. He presents with a 6-week history of early satiety, nausea, watery diarrhea (brief course), generalized malaise, and myalgias associated with a 20-pound weight loss. Examination reveals no lymphadenopathy, normoactive bowel sounds with mild tenderness to deep palpation in the right upper quadrant. CT scan reveals a large soft tissue mass in the region of the porta hepatis, which displaces the liver and celiac axis vessels, and hypodense lesions of the liver, spleen and left kidney. A fine needle aspiration (FNA) under CT-guidance is obtained. The FNA cytomorphology **a** demonstrates the classical morphology of Burkitt lymphoma. Flow cytometric analysis of the FNA specimen reveals a monoclonal B-cell population expressing CD19 **b, c** and restricted κ **b** and CD10 **d**. The cytogenetic results reveal karyotype 46, XY, t(8;14)(q24;q32). Every cell analyzed contains the 8;14 translocation commonly associated with Burkitt lymphoma. Diagnosis is made of post-transplant Burkitt lymphoma.

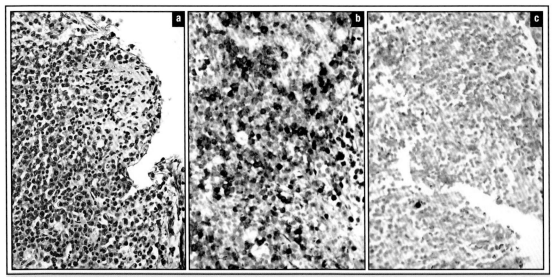

[f16.7] This case demonstrates a post-transplantation disorder of monomorphic, monoclonal plasmacytic origin. The clinical history reveals a 19-year-old male with a history of a liver transplant (10 years previously for biliary atresia) who presents with ascites, a pleural effusion, and lymphadenopathy, which is biopsied. The H&E section **a** reveals a monotonous population of plasma cells. Flow cytometric analysis was not performed (and thus not available for demonstration). By in-situ hybridization, monoclonal κ staining is demonstrated **b**; λ staining is absent **c**. The diagnosis of post-transplant lymphoproliferative disorder, monomorphic subtype, plasmacytic origin, is made.

the majority of these are EBV-associated. T-cell PTLD is generally EBV–, and, in common with non-EBV-associated B-cell PTLD, tend to occur late (>1 year) after solid-organ transplantation. HL and HL-like PTLDs are virtually all EBV+.

Contribution of FCI in Comparison to Molecular and IHC Techniques

In this diagnostic scheme, determination of clonality is obviously important in PTLDs to categorize the process and to manage the treatment of the patient. Analysis of clonality may be determined by genotypic techniques; however, analysis of clonality in PTLDs by immuno-phenotyping has primarily consisted of IHC studies, which have usually yielded indeterminate results. Recent studies determining clonality in PTLDs by FCI have demonstrated the value of routinely performing FCI in suspected cases [Dunphy 2002]. In fact, FCI has been shown to be useful for identifying a clonal process in PTLDs with negative results by genotypic studies. It is recommended that FCI and genotypic studies be routinely performed in PTLDs to detect a clonal process.

Methotrexate (MTX)-Associated Lymphoproliferative Disorders

Definition

This group of lymphoproliferative disorders is defined as a lymphoid proliferation or lymphoma in a patient immunocompromised with MTX, typically for treatment of an autoimmune disease (eg, rheumatoid arthritis, psoriasis, dermatomyositis), which may resemble DLBCL, HL, or polymorphic PTLD. These lymphoproliferative disorders are EBV-related and may regress with cessation of MTX therapy. In addition, there is no definitive epidemiological evidence as to the extent to which MTX increases the risk of lymphoma in such patients, if at all. No excessive risk of lymphoma was observed in 1 retrospective study or in several longitudinal studies of patients receiving MTX, even after long-term follow-up [Moder 1995, Kremer 1997, Weinblatt 1998]. The issue of causality is confounded by the estimated 2-fold increased risk of lymphoma (particularly NHL) in patients with rheumatoid arthritis [Hakulinen 1985, Franklin 2006]. The strongest evidence for causality is the fact that at least partial regression of lymphoma occurs upon withdrawal of MTX, in approximately 60% of reported cases [Salloum 1996, Kamel 1993]. The majority of these have been EBV+ [Salloum 1996].

Characteristics of Associated Lymphoproliferative Diseases

The lymphoproliferative disorders observed are variable and most commonly include DLBCL (35%), HL (25%), or HL-like lesions. Also encountered are follicular lymphoma, lymphoplasmacytic lymphoma, Burkitt lymphoma, mantle cell lymphoma, peripheral T-cell lymphoma, and a picture analogous to polymorphic PTLD [Tran 2008]. Extranodal presentation appears common, but in contrast to HIV+ patients, high frequencies of neurological involvement are not seen [Georgescu 1999]. Approximately 50% of these lymphoproliferative disorders are EBV-associated [Salloum 1996]. The frequency of EBV infection within the malignant cell varies between the various subtypes, with rates highest in HL (approximately 75% of cases).

Immunophenotypes

The immunophenotypes mirror those of similar histological types not associated with MTX therapy, including the HL-like lesion with CD20-positivity, CD30-positivity, and CD15-negativity of the large cells.

Contribution of FCI and IHC Immunophenotyping

FCI is useful, and IHC staining has its role, as in similar histological types not associated with MTX therapy.

References

Ammann J, Wara DW, Pillarisetty RJ, et al [1982] The prevalence of autoantibodies in T-cell, B-cell, and phagocytic immunodeficiency disorders. *Clin Immnol Immunopathol* 23:145-151.

Ariatti C, Vivenza D, Capello D, et al [2000] Common-variable immunodeficiency-related lymphomas associate with mutations and rearrangements of BCL-6: Pathogenetic and histogenetic implications. *Hum Pathol* 31:871-873.

Beaty MW, Kumar S, Sorbara L, Miller K, Raffeld M, Jaffe ES [1999] A biophenotypic human herpes virus 8-associated primary bowel lymphoma. *Am J Surg Pathol* 23:992-994.

Blease RM, Strober W, Brown W, et al [1968] The Wiskott-Aldrich syndrome. A disorder with a possible defect in antigen processing or recognition. *Lancet* 1:1056-1061.

Chadburn A, Hyjek E, Mathew S, Cesarman E, Said J, Knowles DM [2004] KSHV-positive solid lymphomas represent an extra-cavitary variant of primary effusion lymphoma. *Am J Surg Pathol* 28:1401-1416.

Cunningham-Rundles C, Cooper DL, Duffy TP, et al [2002] Lymphomas of mucosal-associated lymphoid tissue in common variable immunodeficiency. *Am J Hematol* 69:171-178.

Desar IM, Keuters M, Raemaekers JM, et al [2006] Extranodal marginal zone (MALT) lymphoma in common variable immunodeficiency: A report of two cases and a brief review of the literature. *Neth J Med* 64:136-140.

Dunphy CH, Gardner LJ, Grosse LE, Evans HL [2002] Flow cytometric immunophenotyping in posttransplant lymphoproliferative disorders. *Am J Clin Pathol* 117:24-29.

Dupin N, Fisher C, Kellam P, et al [1999] Distribution of human herpes virus-B latently infected cells in Kaposi's sarcoma, multicentric Castleman's disease, and primary effusion lymphoma. *Proc Natl Acad Sci USA* 96:4546-4551.

Fisher GH, Rosenberg FJ, Straus SE, et al [1995] Dominant interfering Fas gene mutations impair apoptosis in a human autoimmune lymphoproliferative syndrome. *Cell* 81:935-946.

Folk GS, Abbondanzo SL, Childers EL, Foss RD [2006] Plasmablastic lymphoma: A clinicopathologic correlation. *Ann Diagn Pathol* 10:8-12.

Franklin J, Lunt M, Bunn D, Symmons D, Silman A [2006] Incidence of lymphoma in a large primary care derived cohort of cases of inflammatory polyarthritis. *Ann Rheum Dis* 65:617-622.

Gaillard F, Mechinaud-Lacroix F, Papin S, et al [1992] Primary Epstein-Barr virus infection with clonal T-cell lymphoproliferation. *Am J Clin Pathol* 98:324-333.

Georgescu L, Paget SA [1999] Lymphoma in patients with rheumatoid arthritis: what is the evidence of a link with methotrexate? *Drug Saf* 20:475-487.

Gotoff SP, Amirmikri E, Liebner EJ [1967] Ataxia telangiectasia: neoplasia, untoward response to X-irradiation and tuberous sclerosis. *Am J Dis Child* 114:617-625.

Gupta S [1982] T-cell subpopulations defined with monoclonal antibodies in patients with primary immunodeficiency. *Immuno Letters* 4:129-133.

Hacein-Bey-Abina S, Von Kalle C, Schmidt M, et al [2003] LM02-associated clonal T cell proliferation in two patients after gene therapy for SCID-X1. *Science* 302:415-419.

Hakulinen T, Isomaki H, Knekt P [1985] Rheumatoid arthritis and cancer studies based on linking nationwide registries in Finland. *Am J Med* 78:29-32.

Harris NL, Ferry JA, Serdlow SH [1997] Posttransplant lymphoproliferative disorders: summary of Society of Hematopathology Workshop. *Semin Diagn Pathol* 14:8-14.

Hermans PE, Diaz-Buxo JA, Stobo JD [1976] Idiopathic late-onset immunoglobulin deficiency: Clinical observations in 50 patients. *Am J Clin Med* 61:221-237.

Ichikawa Y, Gonzaleez EB, Daniels JC [1982] Suppressor cells of mitogen-induced lymphocyte proliferation in the peripheral blood of patients with common variable hypogammaglobulinemia. *Clin Immunol Immunopathol* 25:252-263.

Jones JF, Shurin S, Abramowsky C, et al [1988] T-cell lymphomas containing Epstein-Barr viral DNA in patients with chronic Epstein-Barr virus infections. *N Engl J Med* 318:733-741.

Kamel OW, van de Rijn M, Weiss LM, et al [1993] Brief report: Reversible lymphomas associated with Epstein-Barr virus occurring during methotrexate therapy for rheumatoid arthritis and dermatomyositis. *N Engl J Med* 328:1317-1321.

Kanegane H, Bhatia K, Gutierrez M, et al [1998] A syndrome of peripheral blood T-cell infection with Epstein-Barr virus (EBV) followed by EBV-positive T-cell lymphoma. *Blood* 91:2085-2091.

Kanegane H, Miyawaki T, Yachie A, et al [1999] Development of EBV-positive T-cell lymphoma following infection of peripheral blood T-cells with EBV. *Leuk Lymphoma* 34:603-607.

Katano H, Ali MA, Patera AC, et al [2004] Chronic active Epstein-Barr virus infection associated with mutations in perforin that impair its maturation. *Blood* 103:1244-1252.

Kojima M, Kashimura M, Itoh H et al [2007] Epstein-Barr virus-related reactive lymphoproliferative disorders in middle-aged or elderly patients presenting with atypical features. A clinicopathological study of six cases. *Pathol Res Pract* 203: 587-591.

Kremer JM [1997] Safety, efficacy, and mortality in a long-term cohort of patients with rheumatoid arthritis taking methotrexate: follow-up after a mean of 13.3 years. *Arthritis Rheum* 40:984-985.

Kroft SH, Finn WG, Singleton TP, Ross CW, Sheldon S, Schnitzer B [1998] Follicular large cell lymphoma with immunoblastic features in a child with Wiskott-Aldrich syndrome: An unusual immunodeficiency-related neoplasm not associated with Epstein-Barr virus. *Am J Clin Pathol* 110:95-99.

Lenardo M, Chan KM, Hornung F, et al [1999] Mature T lymphocyte apoptosis - immune regulation in a dynamic and unpredictable antigenic environment. *Annu Rev Immunol* 17:221-253.

Lim MS, Straus SE, Dale JK, et al [1998] Pathological findings in human autoimmune lymphoproliferative syndrome. *Am J Pathol* 153:1541-1547.

Lima M, Teixeira Mdos A, Queirós ML, et al [2003] Immunophenotype and TCR-Vbeta repertoire of peripheral blood T-cells in acute infectious mononucleosis. *Blood Cells* Mol Dis 30:1-12.

Maes B, Anastasopoulou A, Kluin-Nelemans JC, et al [2001] Among diffuse large B-cell lymphomas, T-cell-rich/histiocyte-rich BCL and CD30+ anaplastic B-cell subtypes exhibit distinct clinical features. *Ann of Oncol* 12:853-858.

Meije E, Dekke AW, Weersink AJ, Rozenberg-Arska M, Verdonck LF [2002] Prevention and treatment of Epstein-Barr virus-associated lymphoproliferative disorders in recipients of bone marrow and solid organ transplants. *Br J Haematol* 119:596-607.

Mellemkjaer L, Hammarstrom L, Andersen V, et al [2002] Cancer risk among patients with IgA deficiency or common variable immunodeficiency and their relatives: A combined Danish and Swedish study. *Clin Exp Immunol* 130:495-500.

Moder KG, Tefferi A, Cohen MD, Menke DM Luthra HS [1995] Hematologic malignancies and the use of methotrexate in rheumatoid arthritis: A retrospective study. *Am J Med* 99:276-281.

Nakagawa A, Masafumi I, Saga S [2002] Fatal cytotoxic T-cell proliferation in chronic active Epstein-Barr virus infection in childhood. *Am J Clin Pathol* 117:283-290.

Oyama T, Ichimura K, Suzuki R, et al [2003] Senile EBV+ B-cell lymphoproliferative disorders: A clinicopathologic study of 22 patients. *Am J Surg Pathol* 27:16-26.

Oyama T, Yamamoto K, Asano N, et al [2007] Age-related EBV-associated B-cell lymphoproliferative disorders constitute a distinct clinicopathologic group: A study of 96 patients. *Clin Cancer Res* 13:5124-5132.

Park JH, Rosenstein YJ, Remold-O'Donnell E, et al [1991] Enhancement of T-cell activation by the CD43 molecule whose expression is defective in Wiskott-Aldrich syndrome. *Nature* 350:706-709.

Polski JM, Evans HL, Grosso LE, Popovic WJ, Taylor L, Dunphy CH [2000] CD7 and CD56-positive primary effusion lymphoma in a human immunodeficiency virus-negative host. *Leukemia and Lymphoma* 39:633-639.

Purtilo DT, Okano M, Grierson HL [1990] Immune deficiency as a risk factor in Epstein-Barr virus-induced malignant diseases. *Environ Health Perspect* 88:225-230.

Reinherz EL, Rubinstein AJ, Geba RS, et al [1979] Abnormalities of immunoregulatory cells in disorders of immune function. *N Engl J Med* 301:1018-1022.

Reinherz EL, Geha R, Wohl EM, et al [1981] Immunodeficiency associated with loss of T4+ inducer T-cell function. *N Engl J Med* 304:811-816.

Rosen FS, Cooper MD, Wedgwood RJP [1984] The primary immunodeficiencies (second of two parts). *N Engl J Med* 311:300-310.

Salloum E, Cooper DL, Howe G, et al [1996] Spontaneous regression of lymphoproliferative disorders in patients treated with methotrexate for rheumatoid arthritis and other rheumatic diseases. *J Clin Oncol* 14:1943-1949.

Sander CA, Medeiros LJ, Weiss LM, Yano T, Sneller MC, Jaffe ES [1992] Lymphoproliferative lesions in patients with common variable immunodeficiency syndrome. *Am J Surg Pathol* 16:1170-1182.

Sasahara Y, Fujie H, Kumaki S, Ohashi Y, Minegishi M, Tsuchiya S [2001] Epstein-Barr virus-associated Hodgkin's disease in a patient with Wiskott-Aldrich syndrome. *Acta Paediatr* 90:1348-1351.

Schuster V, Kreth HW, Muller-Hermelink HK, et al [1990] Epstein-Barr virus infection rapidly progressing to monoclonal lymphoproliferative disease in a child with selective immunodeficiency. *Eur J Pediatr* 150:48-53.

Segal R, Dayan M, Epstein N, et al [1989] Common variable immunodeficiency. A family study and therapeutic trial with cimetidine. *J Allergy Clin Immunol* 84:753-761.

Sepp N, Schuler G, Romani N, et al [1990] "Intravascular lymphomatosis" (angioendotheliomatosis): Evidence for a T-cell origin in two cases. *Hum Pathol* 21:1051-1058.

Shimoyama Y, Oyama T, Asano N et al [2006] Senile Epstein-Barr virus associated B-cell lymphoproliferative disorders: A mini review. *J Clin Exp Hematop* 46:1-4.

Shimoyama Y, Yamamoto K, Asano N, Oyama T, Kinoshita T, Nakamura S [2008] Age-related Epstein-Barr virus-associated B-cell lymphoproliferative disorders: Special references to lymphomas surrounding this newly recognized clinicopathologic disease. *Cancer Sci* 99:1085-1091.

Small TN, Keever C, Collins N, et al [1989] Characterization of B cells in severe combined immunodeficiency disease. *Hum Immunol* 25:181-193.

Sneller MC, Wang J, Dale JK, et al [1997] Clinical, immunologic, and genetic features of an autoimmune lymphoproliferative syndrome associated with abnormal lymphocyte apoptosis. *Blood* 89:1341-1348.

Spickett GP, Webster AD, Farrant J [1990] *Cell*ular abnormalities in common variable immunodeficiency. *Immunodefic Rev* 2:199-219.

Straus SE, Jaffe ES, Puck JM, et al [2001] The development of lymphomas in families with autoimmune lymphoproliferative syndrome with germline Fas mutations and defective lymphocyte apoptosis. *Blood* 98:194-200.

Tran H, Cheung C, Gill D, et al [2008] Methotrexate-associated mantle-cell lymphoma in an elderly man with myasthenia gravis. *Nat Clin Pract Oncol* 5:234-238.

Tran H, Nourse J, Hall S, Green M, Griffiths L, Gandhi MK [2008] *Blood Review*s May 2 [Epub ahead of print].

van den Berg A, Tamminga R, de Jong D, Maggio E, Kamps W, Poppema S [2003] Fas gene mutation in a case of autoimmune lymphoproliferative syndrome type 1A with accumulation of $\gamma\delta$+ T cells. *Am J Surg Pathol* 27:546-553.

Vega F, Chang CC, Medeiros LJ, et al [2005] Plasmablastic lymphomas and plasmablastic plasma cell myelomas had nearly identical immunophenotypic profiles. *Mod Pathol* 18:806-815.

Waldman TA, Durm M, Broder S, et al [1974] Role of suppressor T cells in pathogenesis of common variable hypogammaglobulinemia. *Lancet* 2:609-613.

Waldmann TA [1988] Immunodeficiency diseases: Primary and acquired. In: Samter M, Talmage Dw, Frank MM, Austen KF, Claman HN, eds. *Immunological Diseases.* Vol 1, 4th ed Boston: Little, Brown and Company :411-465.

Warnke RA, Jones D, and His ED [2007] Morphologic and immunophenotypic variants of nodal T-cell lymphomas and T-cell lymphoma mimics. *Am J Clin Pathol* 127:511-527.

Weinblatt ME, Maier AL, Fraser PA, Coblyn JS [1998] Longterm prospective study of methotrexate in rheumatoid arthritis: Conclusion after 132 months of therapy. *J Rheumatol* 25:238-242.

Weiss LM, Chen YY [1991] Effects of different fixatives on detection of nucleic acids from paraffin-embedded tissues by the in situ hybridization using oligonucleotide proteins. *J Histochem Cytochem* 39:1237-1242.

White WB, Ballow M [1985] Modulation of suppressor cell activity by cimetidine in patients with common variable hypogammaglobulinemia. *N Engl J Med* 312:198-202.

Yocum MW, Kelso JM [1991] Common variable immunodeficiency: The disorder and treatment. *Mayo Clin Proc* 66:83-96.

17 Histiocytic and Dendritic Cell Neoplasms

Chapter Contents

Classification

- Histiocytic sarcoma
- Langerhans cell histiocytosis and sarcoma
- Interdigitating dendritic cell sarcoma/tumor (No tumor, 2008)
- Follicular dendritic cell sarcoma/tumor (No tumor, 2008)
- Dendritic cell sarcoma, not otherwise specified (Not categorized as such, 2008; see below)
  - (Fibroblastic reticular cell tumor, 2008)
  - (Indeterminate dendritic cell tumor, 2008)
  - (Disseminated juvenile xanthogranuloma, 2008)

Histiocytic Sarcoma

Definition

Histiocytic sarcoma is a malignant proliferation of cells showing morphologic and immunophenotypic features similar to those of mature histiocytes. There is expression of at least 1 histiocytic marker (without accessory/dendritic cell markers). Neoplastic proliferations associated with acute monocytic leukemia (ie, monocytic sarcoma) are excluded.

Immunophenotype

By definition, there is expression of at least 1 "histiocytic marker," including CD68 (KP-1 or more specifically, PG-M1), lysozyme, CD11c, and CD14. Since these markers (except CD14, a monocyte-specific marker) may also be expressed by myeloid cells, there must be absence of myeloperoxidase (MPO), CD33, and CD34. CD45, CD45RO, and HLA-DR are also usually expressed, as is CD4. There may be weak or focal expression of S-100 protein, but the neoplastic cells are negative for accessory/dendritic cell markers (ie, CD1a, CD21, CD23, CD35), CD30, HMB-45, epithelial membrane antigen-EMA, or keratin). Histiocytic sarcoma lacks immunoglobulin (Ig) and T-cell receptor (TCR) gene rearrangements. A representative case is demonstrated in [f17.1], with listmode output available on the accompanying disk.

Contribution of FCI

Flow cytometric immunophenotyping (FCI) may be useful in detecting CD11c, CD14, CD4, CD45 (LCA), and HLA-DR on the neoplastic cells, and excluding expressions of CD1a, MPO, CD33, CD34, as well as B-cell and other T-cell antigens.

Differential Diagnosis

Langerhans and dendritic cell sarcomas

Histiocytic sarcoma may be distinguished from Langerhans and dendritic cell sarcomas by the lack of expression of accessory/dendritic cell markers, including CD1a, CD21, CD23, and CD35. The differential expression of markers in histiocytic and dendritic cell neoplasms is outlined in [t17.1].

Large cell lymphomas including ALCL

Histiocytic sarcoma may be differentiated from large cell lymphomas of B-cell origin by the lack of B-cell antigens and expression of at least 1 histiocytic marker. It may be differentiated from large cell lymphomas of T-cell origin by the lack of T-cell markers (except CD4) and from anaplastic large cell lymphoma, by the lack of CD30 expression and the lack of a TCR gene rearrangement.

Leukemia cutis (monocytic sarcoma)

Histiocytic sarcoma may be differentiated from monocytic sarcoma primarily by the lack of expression of CD33 in histiocytic sarcoma. Although histiocytic sarcoma does not express CD34, CD34 expression is also often not expressed in monocytic sarcoma.

Non-hematopoietic malignancies

Histiocytic sarcoma may be differentiated from carcinoma by the lack of EMA and cytokeratin expressions and from malignant melanoma, by the lack of HMB-45 expression.

t17.1 Expression of Markers in Histiocytic and Dendritic Cell Neoplasms

Neoplasm	CD68	Lyso-zyme	CD11c	CD14	CD45	HLA-DR	CD4	S-100	CD1a	Langerin	FDC	EMA
Histiocytic sarcoma	(±)*	(±)*	(±)*	(±)*	usual+	usual+	usual+	wk/focal+	–	20%+	–	–
LCH	var/wk+	var/wk+	–	–	var/wk+	usual+	usual+	+	+	+	–	–
LCS	(±)	(±)	–	–	(±)	usual+	usual+	+	+	focal+	–	–
IDC sarcoma	wk+	wk+	+	–	wk+	usual+	–	+	–	–	–	–
FDC sarcoma	var+	–	–	–	var+	usual+	–	var+	–	–	(±)†	often +

FDC, follicular dendritic cell; IDC, interdigitating cell; LCS, Langerhans cell sarcoma; LCH, Langerhans cell histiocytosis.
*Histiocytic sarcoma is defined by expression of at least 1 histiocytic marker (ie, CD68, lysozyme, CD11c, or CD14).
†FDC sarcoma is defined by expression of at least 1 FDC marker (ie, CD21, CD23, or CD35).
FDC sarcoma may show variable expressions of CD19 and CD20. All of these neoplasms are negative for myeloperoxidase, CD33, CD34, CD30, cytokeratins, and HMB-45. None show Ig or TCR gene rearrangements.
FDC markers include CD21, CD23, and CD35.

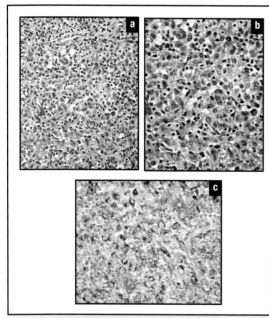

[f17.1] This case demonstrates a histiocytic sarcoma. The clinical history reveals a 9-year-old male who presents with left finger and arm masses associated with left axillary lymphadenopathy, which is biopsied. H&E sections of the lymph node **a, b** reveal the characteristic morphology. Flow cytometric analysis was not performed (and thus is not available for demonstration). By immunohistochemical staining, the malignant cells are intensely positive for CD68 **c**. They are negative for CD1a and show weak, focal positivity for S-100 (both, not demonstrated). The cytogenetic results show a balanced t(Y;7). The diagnosis of histiocytic sarcoma is made.

Comparison of FCI with Paraffin IHC Immunophenotyping

FCI is especially useful in defining the immunophenotype in histiocytic sarcoma by multi-color analysis (ie, detecting co-expressions of CD11c, CD14, CD45, HLA-DR, and CD4 and excluding expressions of CD1a, MPO, CD33, and CD34 as well as B-cell and other T-cell antigens by the neoplastic cells). However, paraffin IHC staining may also be useful in detecting histiocytic markers that are not generally (or not able to be) analyzed by FCI, including CD68, lysozyme, and CD45RO, and in excluding expressions of CD21, CD23, CD35, and CD30.

Langerhans Cell Histiocytosis and Langerhans Cell Sarcoma

Definitions

Langerhans cell histiocytosis (LCH) is a neoplastic proliferation of Langerhans cells, with expression of CD1a, S-100 protein, and the presence of Birbeck granules by ultrastructural examination. Langerhans cell sarcoma (LCS) is a neoplastic proliferation of Langerhans cells with overtly malignant cytologic features. LCS may be considered a higher grade variant of LCH and may present as such de novo or progress from antecedent LCH.

Immunophenotypes

As described in the definition, the neoplastic cells of LCH express CD1a and S-100 protein. Birbeck granules may now be detected by IHC expression of langerin [Lau 2008]. The neoplastic cells of LCH are also usually positive for vimentin, HLA-DR, and CD4 and may be variably and weakly positive for CD45, CD68, and lysozyme. They are negative for B-cell and T-cell (except CD4) antigens, CD30, MPO, CD34, and EMA, as well as CD21, CD23, and CD35. The immunophenotype of LCS is almost identical to LCH with more focal positivity of CD1a and more frequent expressions of CD68, lysozyme, and CD45. A representative case of LCH is demonstrated in [f17.2], with the listmode output available on the accompanying disk.

Contribution of FCI

FCI may be particularly useful in defining the immunophenotype of the neoplastic cells of LCH and/or LCS by multi-color analysis (ie, detecting co-expression of CD1a, HLA-DR, CD4, and possibly CD45, and excluding expression of myelomonocytic markers CD11c, CD14, CD33, and MPO, as well as CD34 and B-cell and other T-cell antigens by the neoplastic cells).

Differential Diagnosis

Systemic mastocytosis

The neoplastic cells of LCH may be quite difficult to morphologically distinguish from those of mastocytosis in histologic sections. Neoplastic mast cells do not express CD1a, langerin, S-100 protein, or CD4, but instead, express CD2, CD117, and CD25 by FCI, greatly aiding in the distinction of these 2 entities.

T-cell large granular lymphocytic leukemia

Infiltration by the neoplastic cells of LCH may histologically resemble those of T-cell large granular lymphocytic leukemia (T-LGLL). The immunophenotype of T-cell LGLL is as follows: CD2+, CD3+, CD4−, CD8+, CD16+/−, CD56−/+, CD57+). Thus, by FCI, T-LGLLs should be clearly distinguished immunophenotypically from LCH (ie, CD1a+, CD4+, and negative for all other T-cell antigens and all natural killer cell antigens).

Hairy cell leukemia

The neoplastic cells of LCH may also histologically resemble those of hairy cell leukemia (HCL). Hairy cell leukemia is a mature B-cell leukemia, which is typically

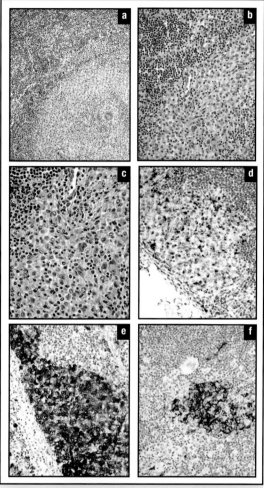

[f17.2] This case demonstrates a Langerhans cell histiocytosis. The clinical history reveals a 55-year-old female who presents with a 3-4 month history of an enlarged right cervical lymph node, which is biopsied. H&E sections of the lymph node **a-c** reveal the characteristic morphology. Flow cytometric analysis was not performed (and thus is not available for demonstration). By immunohistochemical staining, the characteristic cells are variable/weakly positive for CD68 **d** and strongly positive for S-100 **e** and CD1a **f**. The diagnosis of Langerhans cell histiocytosis is made.

strongly positive for CD11c, CD103, and CD25. Thus, by FCI, HCL should be easily distinguished from LCH, which is negative for all B-cell markers, as well as CD11c.

Histiocytic sarcoma, large cell lymphoma, and precursor T-cell lymphoblastic lymphoma/leukemia

Langerhans cell sarcoma may histologically resemble histiocytic sarcoma or a large cell lymphoma of B-cell or T-cell origin. However, in contrast to histiocytic sarcoma, LCS is negative for histiocytic markers, CD11c and CD14, and expresses CD1a. Langerin may be expressed in up to 20% of histiocytic sarcomas [Lau 2008]. In contrast to large cell lymphoma of B-cell origin, LCS is negative for all B-cell markers. In contrast to large cell lymphoma of T-cell origin (including anaplastic large cell lymphoma), LCS is negative for all T-cell markers (except CD4) and CD30, and does not reveal a TCR gene rearrangement. Although CD1a is expressed by LCS and may be expressed by precursor T-cell lymphoblastic lymphoma/leukemia, these 2 entities may be distinguished by the lack of pan T-cell antigens (ie, CD2, CD5, and CD7) as well as TdT (and CD34) in LCS.

Comparison of FCI with IHC Immunophenotyping

Although FCI may be useful in defining the immunophenotype of the neoplastic cells in LCH and LCS, paraffin IHC staining may also be useful in detecting CD1a and langerin (a highly specific and sensitive marker of the Langerhans cell) as well as S-100 protein, and in excluding expressions of CD14, CD21, CD23, CD35, and CD30. In addition, mast cell tryptase may be evaluated by IHC staining in differentiating LCH from systemic mastocytosis (positive in systemic mastocytosis); DBA.44 and TRAP IHC staining may be evaluated in differentiating LCH from HCL (both positive in HCL).

Interdigitating Dendritic Cell Sarcoma (DCS), Follicular DCS, and DCS, NOS

Definitions

Interdigitating dendritic cell (IDC) sarcoma is a neoplastic proliferation of spindle to ovoid cells with phenotypic features similar to those of IDCs. Follicular dendritic cell (FDC) sarcoma is a neoplastic proliferation of spindle to ovoid cells showing morphologic and phenotypic features of FDCs. The designation of sarcoma/tumor in these neoplasms is used because of the variable cytologic grade clinical behavior encountered in these neoplasms. In the previous WHO classification, dendritic cell sarcoma (DCS), not otherwise categorized, applied to those dendritic cell neoplasms that did not fall into the other well-defined categories and was a diagnosis of exclusion. However, the 2008 WHO classification, no longer includes this category and has separated out 2 new entities: Fibroblastic reticular cell tumor (originating from stromal-derived dendritic cells and indeterminate dendritic cell tumor (originating from myeloid-derived dendritic cells).

Immunophenotypes

The neoplastic cells of IDC sarcoma consistently express S-100 protein, vimentin, and strong CD11c and are variably, weakly positive for CD45, CD68, and lysozyme. They are negative for CD1a, langerin, markers of FDCs (ie, CD21, CD23, and CD35), MPO, CD33, CD34, all B-cell and T-cell antigens, CD30, EMA, and cytokeratins.

The neoplastic cells of FDC sarcoma are positive for at least 1 of the FDC markers (ie, CD21, CD35, and CD23), are usually positive for vimentin and HLA-DR, and are often positive for EMA. They are variably positive for S-100 protein, CD68, and CD45, as well as CD19 and CD20 [Fonseca 1998]. They are consistently negative for CD1a, langerin, lysozyme, MPO, CD33, CD34, T-cell antigens, other B-cell antigens, CD30, HMB.45, and cytokeratins. IDC and FDC sarcomas lack Ig and TCR gene rearrangements. Representative cases of IDC and FDC sarcomas/tumors are demonstrated in [f17.3] and [f17.4], respectively, with listmode output available on the accompanying disk.

Contribution of FCI

FCI is helpful in determining the presence of strong CD11c expression and lack of expressions of CD1a, CD33, MPO, and CD34, as well as B-cell and T-cell antigens by the neoplastic cells of IDC sarcoma.

FCI is useful in determining the lack of expressions of CD1a, CD33, MPO, and CD34, as well as other B-cell and T-cell antigens by the neoplastic cells of FDC sarcoma.

Differential Diagnosis

Sarcomas of other origin

Sarcomas of other origin may be distinguished from IDC and FDC sarcomas by their expression of lineage specific markers (eg, smooth muscle actin-SMA in leiomyosarcoma) and their lack of FDC markers (to differentiate from FDC sarcoma) and S-100 protein and CD11c expression (to differentiate from IDC sarcoma).

FDC sarcoma: inflammatory pseudotumor

The cells of inflammatory pseudotumor, or myofibroblastic tumor, are most often (ie, 90%) positive for SMA, muscle-specific actin, calponin and fibronectin [Qiu 2008], and are only weakly or focally positive for FDC markers.

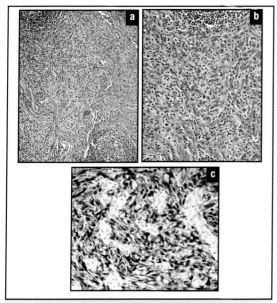

[f17.3] This case demonstrates an interdigitating cell sarcoma. The clinical history reveals a 15-year-old male who presents with a right neck (unresponsive to antibiotic therapy), which is biopsied. H&E sections of the lymph node **a, b** reveal the characteristic morphology. Flow cytometric analysis was not performed (and thus is not available for demonstration). By immunohistochemical staining, the characteristic cells are intensely positive for S-100 **c**, and negative for smooth muscle actin, desmin, CD21, CD35, and CD1a (none is demonstrated). Diagnosis of interdigitating cell sarcoma is made.

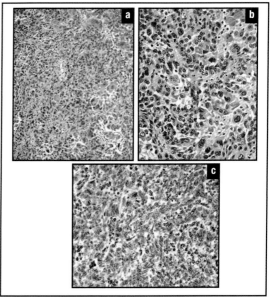

[f17.4] This case demonstrates a follicular dendritic cell sarcoma. The clinical history reveals a 28-year-old female presents with an abdominal mass (located between the lesser curvature of the stomach and the left lobe of the liver), which is biopsied. H&E sections of the lymph node **a, b** reveal the characteristic morphology. Flow cytometric analysis was not performed (and thus is not available for demonstration). By immunohistochemical staining, the characteristic cells are strongly positive for vimentin **c** and CD21 (not demonstrated) and negative for desmin, smooth muscle actin, S-100, CD1a, and all other markers analyzed (none is demonstrated). The diagnosis of follicular dendritic cell sarcoma is made.

Hodgkin lymphoma

Lymphocyte-depleted classical Hodgkin lymphoma (cHL) may be differentiated from FDC and IDC sarcomas by the expressions of CD15 and CD30, and lack of expressions of S-100 protein, CD11c, CD68, and lysozyme by the neoplastic cells of cHL.

Large cell lymphomas

Since some lymphomas may have a spindle pattern (ie, ALCL), and CD19 and CD20 may be expressed by FDC sarcomas, ALCL and large cell lymphomas of B-cell origin should be considered in the differential diagnosis of FDC sarcomas. In addition, since IDC sarcomas have a paracortical pattern in lymph nodes, large cell lymphomas of T-cell origin and sinusoidal large B-cell lymphomas should be considered in the differential diagnosis of IDC sarcoma. However, large cell lymphomas of B-cell origin do not express CD21 or CD35, EMA, S-100 protein, or CD68 and generally show an Ig gene rearrangement. Large cell lymphomas of T-cell origin show variable expression of T-cell antigens and

generally show a TCR gene rearrangement; ALCL also shows strong, uniform expression of CD30 in addition to a TCR gene rearrangement.

Non-hematopoietic neoplasms

FDC and IDC sarcomas may be differentiated from metastatic carcinoma and malignant melanoma by their negativity for cytokeratins and HMB.45, respectively.

Comparison of FCI to IHC Immunophenotyping

IHC staining is helpful in demonstrating expressions of CD21 and CD35 as well as frequent expression of EMA in the neoplastic cells of FDC sarcoma, and in demonstrating the consistent expression of S-100 protein in IDC sarcoma. IHC staining is also useful in distinguishing the differential diagnoses as discussed above (ie, SMA, muscle-specific actin, calponin, and fibronectin in sarcomas and myofibroblastic tumor, CD15 and CD30 in cHL, cytokeratins in metastatic carcinoma, and HMB-45 in malignant melanoma).

Disseminated Juvenile Xanthogranuloma

Definition

Disseminated juvenile xanthogranuloma (JXG) is a histiocytic proliferation, with clonality demonstrated in occasional cases.

Immunophenotype

The proliferating cells of JXG express vimentin, surface CD14, CD68 (coarse, granular pattern), and surface and cytoplasmic CD163. S100 is variably expressed (< 20% of cases), and CD1a and Langerin are negative.

Additional Applications of FC to Dendritic Cells

Dendritic Cell Vaccines in Cancer

In recent trials, dendritic cells have demonstrated the ability to promote an effective anti-tumor immune response and sensitize glioma cells to chemotherapy [Luptrawan 2008]. In addition, there is strong evidence that vaccination with tumor-lysate pulsed DCs results in the induction of a specific immune response in patients suffering from medullary thyroid carcinoma [Stift 2004]. FCI offers the ability to isolate dendritic cells by their absence of expression of CD14, CD19, CD3, and CD16, and their typical expressions of CD13 and CD33 [Thomas 1993]. A flow cytometric method to purify and sort dendritic cells is provided by Freudenthal et al [1990] and may be considered in preparing dendritic cell vaccines.

References

Fonseca R, Yamakawa M, Nakamura S, et al [1998] Follicular dendritic cell sarcoma and interdigitating reticulum cell sarcoma: A review. *Am J Hematol* 59:161-167.

Freudenthal PS, Steinman RM [1990] The distinct surface of human blood dendritic cells, as observed after an improved isolation method. *Proc Natl Acad Sci* 87:7698-7702.

Lau SK, Chu PG, Weiss LM [2008] Immunohistochemical expression of Langerin in Langerhans cell histiocytosis and non-Langerhans cell histiocytic disorders. *Am J Surg Pathol* 32:615-619.

Luptrawan A, Liu G, Yu JS [2008] Dendritic cell immunotherapy for malignant gliomas. *Rev Recent Clin Trials* 3:10-21.

Qiu X, Montgomery E, Sun B [2008] Inflammatory myofibroblastic tumor and low-grade myofibroblastic sarcoma: A comparative study of clinicopathologic features and further observations on the immunohistochemical profile of myofibroblasts. *Hum Pathol* 39:846-856.

Stift A, Sachet M, Yagubian R, et al [2004] Dendritic cell vaccination in medullary thyroid carcinoma. *Clin Cancer Res* 10:2944-2953.

Thomas R, Davis S, Lipsky PE [1993] Isolation and characterization of human peripheral blood dendritic cells. *J Immunol* 150:821-834.

18 Mastocytosis

Chapter Contents

Classification

- Cutaneous mastocytosis
- Indolent mastocytosis
- Systemic mastocytosis with associated clonal, hematological non-mast-cell lineage disease
- Aggressive systemic mastocytosis
- Mast cell leukemia
- Mast cell sarcoma
- Extracutaneous mastocytoma

Introduction

Mastocytosis is currently included in the myeloproliferative neoplasms in the 2008 WHO classification, and is defined as a proliferation of mast cells (MCs) and their subsequent accumulation in 1 or more organ systems. The manifestations of mastocytosis are heterogeneous, ranging from cutaneous lesions that may spontaneously regress to highly aggressive neoplasms associated with multisystem involvement and short survival times. In cutaneous mastocytosis (CM), the mastocytosis is limited to the skin. In systemic mastocytosis (SM), at least 1 extracutaneous organ is involved with or without cutaneous involvement. SM is commonly diagnosed in adults and includes the following 4 major categories:

1. indolent SM (ISM), the most common form, representing approximately two-thirds of all cases and involving mainly skin and bone marrow-BM)

2. a unique subcategory termed SM with an associated non-mast cell clonal hematological disease (SM-AHNMD), representing approximately 25%-33% of SM cases), most commonly (80%-90%) associated with myeloid disorders including all defined disease entities: myelodysplastic syndromes, myelodysplastic/myeloproliferative (MDS/MPN) diseases, myeloproliferative neoplasms, and acute myeloid leukemias (AMLs). Most common among these

are the MDS/MPN diseases, specifically chronic myelomonocytic leukemia (CMML). Associated lymphoid malignancies comprise only about 10%-20% of all AHNMDs, with plasma cell myelomas being most frequent within this group. Rare cases of acute and chronic "lymphoid" leukemia, as well as hairy cell leukemia (HCL) have also been reported. The clinical course of SM-AHNMD patients is mainly determined by the "AHNMD." Rarely, infiltrates of SM have been detected only after successful chemotherapy of an AML.

3. aggressive SM (ASM, representing approximately 5% of all SM cases), usually presenting without skin lesions

4. mast cell leukemia (MCL), probably representing the rarest variant of human leukemia

The extremely rare localized extracutaneous mast cell neoplasms may either present as a benign tumor (termed extracutaneous mastocytoma) or as a malignancy (termed mast cell sarcoma).

Diagnosis

The diagnosis of mastocytosis requires the demonstration of multi-focal clusters or aggregates of MCs in an adequate biopsy specimen. If the MCs are loosely scattered without forming aggregates, a definitive diagnosis may require demonstration of an aberrant immunophenotype (as will be described in the section below), detection of point mutations of kit (recurring genetic abnormalities encountered in mastocytosis), or perhaps additional biopsies. The neoplastic cells in mastocytosis may morphologically resemble normal MCs but more frequently show abnormal cytologic features (ie, more spindle-shaped with reniform or indented nuclei). In addition, neoplastic MCs may have more abundant "clear" cytoplasm, resembling histiocytes or the neoplastic cells of hairy cell leukemia in tissue sections. In smear preparations, neoplastic MCs may contain so few granules in their cytoplasm that they may not even be recognized as MCs, especially in immature MCs, as encountered in MCL. MCL is defined as showing at least 20% atypical, immature MCs in the BM. The atypical, immature MCs are characterized by bilobed nuclei (sometimes with prominent nucleoli) with relatively poorly granulated cytoplasm, as described above. As mentioned previously, the extremely rare localized extracutaneous MC neoplasms may either present as a benign tumor (termed extracutaneous mastocytoma) or as a malignancy (termed mast cell sarcoma). The benign tumor is composed of mature MCs, and the malignant version is composed of highly atypical, immature MCs. The immunophenotype of the neoplastic MCs is similar in various sites (ie, BM vs extramedullary sites) [Hahn 2007] and in all of the above neoplasms, and is described in the section below.

Immunophenotype of Neoplastic Mast Cells

Normal MCs lack myeloperoxidase (MPO) but demonstrate napthol ASD chloroacetate esterase (CAE). They express CD45, CD33, CD68, and CD117 (basophils do not express CD117) [Chin-Yang 2001], and lack CD14, CD15, and CD16, as well as T-cell and B-cell antigens (except CD22) [Escribano 2002].

Neoplastic MCs show a similar immunophenotype to normal MCs, but they also aberrantly express CD2 and CD25. Aberrant expressions of CD25 and/or CD2 serve as a minor criterion for making the diagnosis of SM per WHO guidelines [Jordan 2001, Sotlar 2004, Valent 2001a]. A representative case is demonstrated in **[f18.1]**, with listmode output available on the accompanying disk. In addition, CD25 expression by cutaneous MCs from adults presenting with urticaria pigmentosa (UP) correlates with underlying or subsequent SM, or may help define limited involvement by CM [Hollmann 2008]. CD25 is typically expressed by cutaneous MCs in all patients with associated systemic mastocytosis, compared to 25% of patients with limited CM. Additional immunophenotypic differences between normal/reactive MCs and neoplastic MCs are further discussed in detail in the section below regarding the contribution of flow cytometric immunophenotyping (FCI).

Neoplastic MCs may lack expression of CAE if they are poorly granulated, as described previously. However, they will demonstrate MC tryptase, even in cases with extremely immature, agranular neoplastic MCs, that

are CAE- and toluidine blue-negative [Horny 1998]. As alluded to earlier, mastocytosis is characterized by activating (usually somatic) point mutations of the *c-kit* proto-oncogene commonly involving exon 17 (most frequently the imatinib-resistant D816V) [Horny 2007].

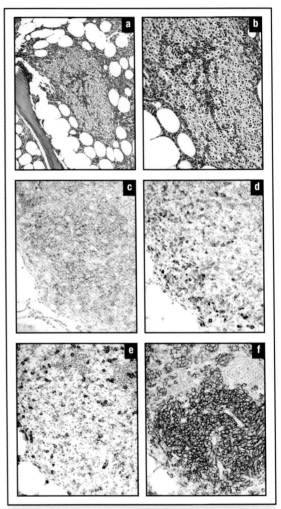

[f18.1] This case demonstrates a systemic mastocytosis. The clinical history reveals a 72-year-old female presents with multiple lytic bone lesions and a negative serum protein electrophoresis. A BM biopsy is performed. CBC data include WBC 5.4 × 10³/mm³ (5.4 × 10⁹/L), Hgb 10.7 g/dL, Plt 267 ×10³/mm³ (267 × 10⁹/L). H&E sections of the bone marrow biopsy **a, b** reveal the nodules of mast cells. Flow cytometric analysis fails to reveal a neoplastic population. By immunohistochemical staining, the mast cells are positive for CD117 **c** and mast cell tryptase **d**, show weak/equivocal staining for CD2 **e**, but show strong staining for CD25 **f**. The cytogenic results are normal. Molecular results are positive for the *c-Kit* Asp816Va1 mutation. The diagnosis of systemic mastocytosis is made.

Contribution of FCI and Comparison to Paraffin IHC Staining

Immunophenotyping of MCs may be accomplished by FCI or paraffin IHC staining. FCI techniques allow for the identification, enumeration, and exact immunophenotypical characterization by multi-color analysis of BMMCs. MCs are usually present in only low numbers in BM specimens. However, FCI is well-suited for the analysis of single-cell suspensions, even when such cells are present at very low frequencies due to the multi-parametric analytical capabilities of this technology. BMMCs may be specifically identified and accurately enumerated using FCI [Orfao 1996, Escribano 2000]. BMMCs may be clearly identified by FCI on the basis of their light-scatter properties (ie, increased side light scatter due to increased granularity as mature granulocytes) and strong CD117 expression. These CD117high cells are negative for the CD34 antigen; in addition, they are CD33+ and express significant amounts of the high affinity IgE receptor (FcεRI). It should also be kept in mind that neoplastic MCs express abnormally lower levels of CD117 (ie, moderate expression rather than strong expression as observed in normal and reactive MCs). Nevertheless, the single immunologic marker best suited for the identification of normal and neoplastic MCs is CD117. Despite the fact that CD117 may also be found in CD34+ hematopoietic stem and progenitor cells, myeloid precursors, CD56bright natural killer cells, and neoplastic cells of other hematologic malignancies as well as cells in non-hematopoietic tissues, MCs express uniquely higher amounts of CD117 as compared with other CD45+ hematopoietic cells [Escribano 1998]. To distinguish MCs from other CD117+ non-hematopoietic cells, counterstaining with CD45 is highly recommended. These specific antigen expression patterns, when associated with light scatter parameters, allow for the specific and sensitive identification of MCs, even when present in small numbers, provided an appropriate combination of fluorochrome-conjugated monoclonal antibodies is used in a direct immunofluorescence assay [Escribano 2000]. As mentioned previously, MCs display strong CD33 expressions, are FcεRI+, and CD34−; these markers may improve the identification of CD117high, CD45low MCs [Orfao 1996, Escribano 2000]. However, since CD117 will mark normal/reactive and neoplastic MCs, simultaneous staining for additional markers is usually required to clearly distinguish between normal/reactive and neoplastic MCs.

By FCI, it has been demonstrated that normal/reactive BMMCs and neoplastic BMMCs differ most significantly in expression of the following markers: CD2 and CD25. Thus, the most characteristic aberrant immunophenotypic feature of neoplastic BMMCs is the aberrant expression of CD2 and CD25 antigens [Escribano 1995, Escribano 1997]. In addition, normal BMMCs do not express CD16, CD35, CD41a, and CD41b, whereas neoplastic MCs may express CD16 (subset, 20%), uniformly may moderately express CD35 (also weakly expressed by "reactive" BMMCs), and may also express CD41a and CD41b (subset, 45%) [Escribano 2001]. In comparison to normal/reactive MCs, neoplastic MCs also show abnormally high levels of the CD11c complement receptor [Nuñez 2002], the CD59 complement regulatory molecule [Nuñez 2002], the CD63 lysosomal membrane antigen [US-Canadian consensus recommendations 1997], the CD69 early-activation antigen [Diaz-Agustin 1999], and CD88, a complement-related marker [Escribano 2004].

Among the antigens showing aberrant expression by neoplastic MCs, CD25 appears to be the most sensitive, specific, and user-friendly. However, it is recommended that aberrant or differential stronger expression of at least 1 additional marker from those mentioned above (ie, CD2, CD11c, CD35, CD59, CD63, and/or CD69) should also be demonstrated.

Despite the fact that different techniques may be used for the analysis of the expression of the antigens referred to above by neoplastic MCs, FCI is the preferred method because it allows sensitive detection and quantitative evaluation of antigen expression in large numbers of MCs, even when they are present in a sample at very low frequencies. Moreover, FCI has also been successfully applied for the immunophenotypical analysis of MCs from other tissue samples such as lymph nodes, spleen, and ascitic fluid [Escribano 2000].

From a technical point of view, a number of critical parameters have to be taken into consideration [Escribano 2000]; among these are the sample quality, dispersion of tissue particles, choice of monoclonal antibodies and fluorochromes, and/or the high light scatter and nonspecific auto-fluorescence of neoplastic MCs [Escribano 1997]. The CD117 and CD45 monoclonal antibody clones and fluorochrome conjugates must be selected carefully. For the detection of CD45, HLE-1 (Becton-Dickinson Biosciences [BDB], San Jose, CA) and J33 (Beckmann Coulter [BC], Miami, FL) conjugated with the peridin-chlorophyl protein/cyanine 5.5 or the phycoerythrin (PE)/cyanine 5 fluorochrome tandems may be considered reference reagents for users of bench-top BDB and BC FC instruments

[Gratama 2000]. For the sensitive detection of CD117, the 104D2 (BDB; DakoCytomation, Glostrup, Denmark) monoclonal antibody clone could be considered the reference reagent. In general, CD117-PE conjugates are brighter and provide a clear stain for MCs. However, the use of other new CD117 conjugates (eg, CD117-APC) instead of CD117-PE is recommended once assessment of the reactivity for a marker that may be dimly expressed on neoplastic MCs (ie, CD2) is performed. PE should be used preferentially for the weakest antigen (ie, CD2), since it has been clearly demonstrated that the percentage of CD2+ cases varies significantly depending on the fluorochrome conjugate used: 66.6% vs 86.5% for the CD2-FITC and CD2-PE reagents, respectively. Despite the higher sensitivity of the CD2-PE reagent in neoplastic MCs, as compared to CD2-FITC, it has been consistently negative in normal/reactive MCs. In [t18.1], a list of monoclonal antibody clones and fluorochrome conjugates that have been used successfully in combination with

CD45 and CD117 for the FC immunophenotypic characterization of normal/reactive vs neoplastic MCs is provided. As for the specific identification of rare cells (such as mast cells), the use of a Boolean gating strategy, such as those shown in [f18.2] and [f18.3], is recommended for the identification of MCs, and it avoids the need to use isotypic controls. Evaluation of baseline autofluorescence levels specifically for mast cells, especially when characterization of expression of 1 or more markers is evaluated, may be easily achieved by staining cells in a separate tube with the same CD45, CD117 fluorochrome-conjugated monoclonal antibody combination. The minimum FCI panel recommended for the diagnosis of mastocytosis includes CD2, CD25, CD45, and CD117 monoclonal antibodies, and a tube as described above to evaluate baseline auto-fluorescence levels specifically for the MC population under study. The differential expression of markers evaluated by FCI in normal, reactive, and neoplastic MCs is outlined in [t18.2].

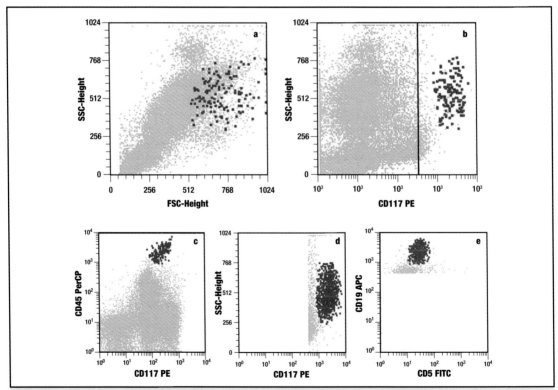

[f18.2] Representative bivariate dot plots of data acquisition for the identification of BM MC in a case of indolent systemic mastocytosis. **a-c** In the first step, 50,000 events/tube were acquired, corresponding to the total nucleated BM cells. In the second step, acquisition through a live gate drawn on CD117+/++ cells was performed **d**, and only the events included in this region (R1) were stored **e**. Data were acquired and analyzed with CellQuest software (Becton-Dickinson Biosciences); events corresponding to mast cells are shown as blue dots in all bivariate dot plots. *Reprinted with permission of Wiley-Liss, Inc, a subsidiary of John Wiley & Sons, Inc.*

t18.1 List of Antigens Whose Expression Has Been Extensively Analyzed on Mast Cells from Mastocytosis and Specific Information about the Exact Clones, Fluorochrome Conjugates, and Sources*

	Clone	Fluorochrome	Ig subclass	Sources[†]
CD2	S5.2	FITC, PE	IgG_{2a}	BDB
CD11b	D12	PE	IgG_{2a}	BDB
CD11c	S-HCL-3	PE	IgG_{2b}	BDB
CD11c	3.9	FITC, PE	IgG_1	Caltag
CD13	TÜK 1	FITC	IgG_1	Caltag
CD25	2A3	FITC, PE	IgG_1	BDB
CD33	P67.6	FITC, PE	IgG_1	BDB
CD34	8G12	FITC, PE, APC	IgG_1	BDB
CD35	E 11	FITC	IgG_1	Cymbus Biotechnology
CD38	HIT 2	FITC	IgG_1	Caltag
CD38	HB7	FITC	IgG_1	BDB
CD45	2D1	PerCP	IgG_1	BDB
CD45	J33	PECy5	IgG_1	Beckmann Coulter
CD59	MEM 43	FITC	IgG_{2a}	Cymbus
CD59	P282 (H19)	PE	IgG_{2a}	BDB
CD63	CLBGran/12	FITC	IgG_1	Beckmann Coulter
CD69	L78	FITC, APC	IgG_1	BDB
CD71	LO1.1	FITC	IgG_{2a}	BDB
CD88	W17/1	FITC	IgG_1	Serotec
CD117	104D2	PE, APC	IgG_1	DakoCytomation, BDB
CD117	YB5.B8	APC	IgG_1	BDB Pharmingen
CD138	BB4	FITC	IgG_1	
Bcl-2	124	FITC	IgG_1	DakoCytomation
Anti-IgE	Polyclonal	FITC		Biosource

FITC, fluorescein isothiocyanate; Ig, immunoglobulin; PE, phycoerythrin; PECy5, PE/cyanine 5.

*The reagents listed have been tested in 3- or 4-color combinations of monoclonal antibodies in which CD45 and CD117 stainings were used consistently for the specific identification of mast cells.

[†]Beckmann Coulter, Miami, FL; Becton-Dickinson Biosciences (BDB), San Jose, CA; Biosource, Camarillo, CA; Caltag, San Francisco, CA Cymbus Biotechnology, Southamption, UK; DakoCytomation, Glostrup, Denmark Serotec, Oxford, UK). *Reprinted with permission of Wiley-Liss, Inc., a subsidiary of John Wiley & Sons, Inc.*

t18.2 Differential Antigen Expression of Surface Antigens on BM Mast Cells

Surface Antigen	Normal MCs	Reactive MCs	Neoplastic MCs
CD2	–	–	Wk to mod+ (100%)
CD11c	Wk+ (71%)	ND	Wk to mod+ (100%)
CD13	Wk+ (33%)	ND	Wk+ (75%)
CD14	–	–	–
CD15	–	–	–
CD16	–	–	Wk+ (20%)
CD19	–	–	–
CD20	–	–	–
CD22	Wk+ (60%)	Wk+ (50%)	Wk+ (60%)
CD25	–	–	Mod+ (100%)
CD33	Mod to strong+ (100%)	Mod to strong+ (100%)	Strong pos (100%)
CD34	–	–	–
CD35	–	Wk+	Mod+ (100%)
CD41a	–	ND	Wk+ (45%)
CD42b	–	ND	Wk+ (45%)
CD45	Mod+ (100%)	Mod+ (100%)	Mod+ (100%)
CD59*	+	+	Very high levels
CD63	Mod+ (100%)	Mod+ (100*)	Strong+ (100%)
CD69	Wk+ (100%)	Wk+ (100%)	Mod to strong+ (100%)
CD88*	+	Pos	Very high levels
CD117	Strong+(100%)	Strong+ (100%)	Mod+ (100%)
FcεRI	Mod to strong+ (100%)	Mod to strong+ (100%)	Mod+ (100%)

BM, bone marrow; MCs, mast cells;mod, moderate; –, negative; +, positive; wk, weak.
*CD59 and CD88 are expressed at higher levels on neoplastic MCs than on normal and reactive MCs.

FCI of MCs should be applied in the following situations:

1. evaluation of BMMCs from all adult patients with suspected mastocytosis at diagnosis

2. all mastocytosis cases with suspected involvement of peripheral blood (PB) and/or other tissues

3. follow-up mastocytosis cases with suspected disease progression, due to significant changes in total blood cell counts and/or the leukocyte differential, the appearance of PB dysplasia, the presence of circulating MCs, and/or increases in serum tryptase levels and organomegalies

4. pediatric mastocytosis cases with persistent disease (ie, without significant regression after puberty) or progressive (adult form) disease before puberty develops (ie, increase in serum tryptase levels and/or organomegalies)

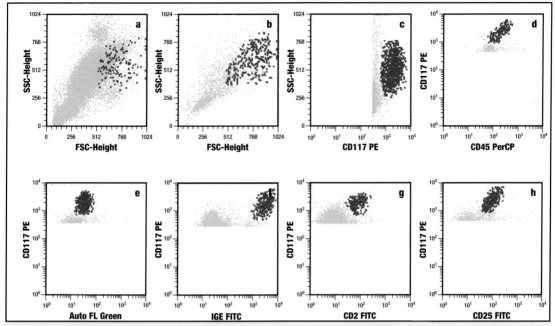

[f18.3] Representative bivariate dot plots of data analysis of BM MC from the same case of indolent systemic mastocytosis shown in **[f18.1]** using the PAINT-A-Gate Pro software program (Becton-Dickinson Biosciences). **a** Events corresponding to the whole BM cellularity (first step of data acquisition) are shown. **b-h** These correspond to gated CD117+ cells. MC (blue dots) display high side scatter and autofluorescence levels **c-e** and express the high-affinity IgE receptor **e**. In addition, CD2 and CD25 antigens are aberrantly expressed on MC **g, h**. *Reprinted with permission of Wiley-Liss, Inc, a subsidiary of John Wiley & Sons, Inc.*

5. follow-up of minimal residual disease in patients undergoing cytoreductive therapy, recommended as interval monitoring of CD25 expression on BMMCs, generally for aggressive SM disease subtypes [Pardanani 2004, Escribano 1997, Elliott 2004]

6. incidental mastocytosis with an associated clonal hematological non-MC lineage disease [Escribano 2004]

7. immunophenotyping an associated clonal hematological non-MC lineage disease

Since mastocytosis may be associated with BM fibrosis and limited tissue specimens may be available for evaluation of suspected mastocytosis, IHC staining may be necessary for the evaluation of the presence of neoplastic MCs. In all such cases of suspected mastocytosis, a limited IHC panel of at least 3 of the following markers is recommended:

1. anti-tryptase is highly specific and sensitive (with the exception of both neoplastic tryptase+

myeloblasts and basophils), and therefore allows screening for both the number of loosely scattered MCs and immediate detection of even small compact MC infiltrates. One should keep in mind there may be background staining with tryptase in extramedullary tissues.

2. antibodies against KIT (CD117) to confirm the presence of MC in such cases. Although anti-KIT antibodies are highly non-specific (ie, KIT is also expressed by hematopoietic stem cells, melanocytes, germ cells, and CAJAL cells), they have been found to be of superior sensitivity, allowing verification of tryptase+ cells as MCs without significant background-staining. CD117 typically reveals a granular, cytoplasmic staining pattern, suggesting that stem cell growth factor is localized within MC granules [Akin 2002]. This localization would also explain the somewhat decreased expression of CD117 by FCI in some neoplastic MCs (ie, those with decreased granularity).

3. antibodies against CD25, a very non-specific antigen, being expressed by activated T cells and by certain B-cell malignancies (like HCL), should also be applied in all cases of suspected SM, since as previously discussed, neoplastic MCs co-express CD25. CD25 IHC staining is of particular diagnostic value in the BM, since CD25+ lymphatic cells are either rare or absent, and the CD25-reactivity of megakaryocytes may be easily used as an internal positive control.

Because of a lower sensitivity for the detection of neoplastic MCs and the presence of CD2+ T cells in almost all tissue infiltrates of mastocytosis, the diagnostic value of anti-CD2 antibodies by IHC staining is even more limited when compared to FCI. It has been reported that screening for CD2 expression by IHC staining may have a relatively low diagnostic value because a significant proportion of neoplastic MCs stain negatively, since CD2 expression by neoplastic BMMCs is generally weak [Jordan 2001, Sotlar 2004, Horny 2002].

Differential Diagnosis

Cutaneous Mastocytosis

Urticaria pigmentosa

Urticaria pigmentosa (UP) is a clinicopathologic term used to describe reddish-brown cutaneous macules and papules, characterized histologically by MC infiltration of the papillary and upper reticular dermis and reactive basal hyperpigmentation of the overlying epidermis. Although typically a benign, self-limited disorder of childhood, a significant proportion (up to 30%) of adolescent and adult-onset UP represents cutaneous involvement by underlying SM. It has been demonstrated that aberrant CD25 expression by cutaneous MCs highly correlates with an underlying or subsequent development of SM and may also define limited CM (in approximately 20% of cases). Thus, the detection of aberrant expression of CD25 by cutaneous MCs may be useful for stratifying adult patients presenting with UP for additional clinical evaluation.

Systemic Mastocytosis

Reactive mastocytosis

Mast cells may be increased as a reactive mastocytosis (RM) in various hematologic disorders and malignant neoplasms. RM cannot be distinguished from SM based solely on the quantity of mast cells, since it has been determined that there are no statistical differences in mast cell numbers in RM and SM. However, SM usually reveals dyspoietic mast cells (ie, decreased cytoplasmic granules and uneven granule distribution) and other dyspoietic bone marrow elements (ie, erythroid, myeloid, and megakaryocytic cells), which aid in the distinction between reactive mastocytosis and SMCD [Stevens 2001]. However, note also that in very rare instances, there may be a focal and/or diffuse collagen fibrosis of the BM, containing an abundance of loosely scattered, spindle-shaped MCs lacking both expression of CD25 and an activating point mutation of *c-kit*. This condition must be regarded as reactive, representing an important mimicker of mastocytosis and perhaps termed "fibromastocytic lesion" [Horny 2007].

SM associated with eosinophilia (SM-eos) vs SM-CEL vs chronic eosinophilic leukemia (CEL) with RM

Eosinophilia (BM and/or peripheral blood) commonly accompanies SM (in 20%-40% of cases, termed SMeos) [Mutter 1963, Lawrence 1991, Travis 1988, Pardanani 2002]. In addition, the associated eosinophilia may be clonal in a subset of these cases [Pardanani 2003]. In fact, up to 50% of SM-eos patients carry the *FIP1L1-PDGFRA* fusion oncogene, which results from an 800-kb interstitial deletion of chromosome 4q12, thereby generating a constitutively active PDGFRA tyrosine kinase [Cools 2003]. The demonstrable presence of the *FIP1L1-PDGFRA* gene within cells of multiple hematopoietic lineages including MCs should discriminate between SM with a reactive eosinophilia and SM-CEL [Robyn 2006]. In addition, such cases lack the point mutation D816V (KIT), a finding clearly in contrast to all other subtypes of SM-AHNMD carrying D816V in almost all cases. These patients exhibit clinical and histologic features of myeloproliferation and generally have an elevated serum tryptase level, but may lack pathognomonic clusters of atypical MCs in the BM on routine staining [Pardanani 2004, Klion 2003, Klion 2004, Pardanani 2003]. This category of neoplastic MCs and coexistent clonal eosinophils not only includes classical cases of SM-CEL characterized by multifocal compact diagnostic MC infiltrates and criteria for both SM and CEL, but also cases of CEL containing loosely scattered CD25+ abnormal MCs but not fulfilling the diagnostic criteria of SM. In fact, in the current literature, *FIP1L1-PDGFRA*+ cases have been variably classified as a unique subtype of SM [Pardanani 2004, Pardanani 2003], as a "myeloproliferative variant" of hypereosinophilic syndrome [Pardanani 2004, Klion 2003], as CEL [Bain 2004], or as a myelomastocytic-overlap syndrome [Valent 2001b]. Given the sensitivity of this disorder to imatinib therapy, it is currently recommended that all suspected SM-eos cases (ie, cases with clonal/abnormal MCs and clonal/abnormal eosinophils) be screened for the *FIP1L1-PDGFRA* fusion by either fluorescence in situ hybridization or reverse transcriptase polymerase chain reaction [Tefferi 2004a, Tefferi 2004b].

On the other hand, CEL with RM is characterized by CEL with associated normal mast cells by morphology as well as immunophenotypic and molecular genetic features.

Hairy Cell Leukemia

The neoplastic cells of HCL typically are Sg+ (M±D, G, or A) and demonstrate expression of B-cell lineage associated antigens (ie, CD19, CD20, CD22, and CD79a but not CD79b) with associated strong expressions of CD11c, CD103, and CD25. They are typically negative for CD5, CD10, and CD23. In addition, as mentioned previously, SM may be associated with HCL. To identify CD25-expressing atypical mast cells in HCL may be challenging since the neoplastic B cells usually strongly express CD25. However, HCL does not express CD117 or CD2. Multi-parametric FCI may be particularly useful in this situation.

Langerhans Cell Histiocytosis

In BM and tissue sections, the neoplastic cells of Langerhans cell histiocytosis (LCH) may strikingly resemble those of mastocytosis. However, as described in Chapter 17, the neoplastic cells of LCH likewise do not express CD117, mast cell tryptase, CD25, or CD2, but instead express dim CD45 and CD1a. Again, the differences in immunophenotypes by FCI greatly aid in the distinction of these 2 entities.

Large Granular Lymphocyte Leukemia (LGLL)

In BM and tissue sections, the neoplastic cells of LGLL may strikingly resemble those of mastocytosis. However, by FCI, these entities should be clearly distinguishable by their characteristic immunophenotypes: NK-LGL leukemia (CD2+, CD3–, CD4–, CD8+, CD16+, CD56+, CD57v) and T-LGL leukemia (CD2+, CD3+, CD4–, CD8+, CD16+/–, CD56–/+, CD57+). They do not express CD117 or mast cell tryptase.

Mast Cell Sarcoma

Mast Cell Leukemia

The aleukemic form of mast cell leukemia (MCL) is virtually indistinguishable from mast cell sarcoma.

Granulocytic Sarcoma

Other forms of acute leukemia may involve extramedullary sites. Mast cell sarcoma is MPO–, CD33+, weak CD13+ (subset), CD11c+, and negative for all additional myelomonocytic markers, but it is positive for MC tryptase.

Sarcomas

One should be able to distinguish mast cell sarcoma from other forms of sarcoma by its unique co-expression of CD117, CD2, and CD25 by FCI and expression of MC tryptase by IHC staining.

Large Cell Lymphomas

Large cell lymphomas of T-cell and B-cell origin should be easily distinguished from mast cell sarcoma, since MCS lacks expression of T-cell markers (except CD2), lacks expression of B-cell markers (except CD22), and uniquely co-expresses CD117, CD25, and CD2 as well as MC tryptase.

Mast Cell Leukemia

Mast Cell Sarcoma, Leukemic Phase

Mast cell sarcoma may progress to a leukemic phase and be indistinguishable from mast cell leukemia.

Other Forms of Acute Leukemia

Myelomastocytic leukemia (MML)

MML represents a rare advanced myeloid neoplasm (usually a myelodysplastic syndrome of RAEB type or even AML by WHO criteria) exhibiting more than 10% metachromatic immature cells (often metachromatic blasts) in the BM or PB but not fulfilling criteria for a diagnosis of SM. Many times, most cases of MML are cytomorphologically misdiagnosed as acute basophilic leukemia without adequate histopathologic and immunophenotypic analysis of a BM core biopsy. Histologically, there is an abundance of tryptase (or rarely, chymase) expressing cells, but there are no compact MC infiltrates; there is no aberrant immunophenotype of the MCs (ie, no co-expression of CD25); and there is no activating point mutation of *c-kit*. In most cases of MML, a significant increase in CD34+ progenitor/blast cells is detected. Tentatively, MML is best categorized as a subgroup within the MDS/MPN overlap diseases.

Tryptase+ AML

Tryptase+ AML is also a rare entity, characterized by strong expression of tryptase and less frequently KIT (CD117) by myeloblasts in an otherwise morphologically unremarkable AML (often subtypes FAB M1, M2, or M4-eo). Tryptase+ AML lacks the diagnostic criteria for SM. The separation of tryptase+ AML from MML is possible by counting metachromatic cells in PB and/or BM smears; the presence of more than 10% metachromatic cells with signs of MC differentiation argues for the diagnosis of MML [Valent 2002].

Basophilic leukemia (BAL)

BAL is an extremely rare variant of myeloid leukemia and until now could not be diagnosed histologically in BM core biopsy specimens. The neoplastic cells of BAL are negative for CD117 but do express detectable amounts of tryptase by IHC staining. However, a definitive diagnosis of BAL is only possible when basophil-related antibodies like 2D7 and/or BB1 are used for IHC analysis of a BM core biopsy specimen. In contrast to MC granules, metachromatic granules of basophils are water-soluble and therefore cannot be detected in routinely processed formalin-fixed tissues. In most published cases of BAL, the underlying disease has been classified as Ph+ CML. Recently, a unique case of secondary basophilic leukemia in a patient with Ph+ CML with associated SM was diagnosed retrospectively in an analysis of almost 200 cases of CML, using antibodies against 2D7 and BB1, respectively [Horny 2007].

References

Akin C, Jaffe ES, Raffeld M, et al [2002] An immunohistochemical study of the bone marrow lesions of systemic mastocytosis: Expression of stem cell factor by lesional mast cells. *Am J Clin Pathol* 118:242-247.

Bain BJ [2004] Relationship between idiopathic hypereosinophilic syndrome, eosinophilic leukemia, and systemic mastocytosis. *Am J Hematol* 77:82-85.

Chin-Yang L [2001] Diagnosis of mastocytosis: Value of cytochemistry and immunohistochemistry. *Leuk Res* 25:537-541.

Cools J, DeAngelo DJ, Gotlib J, et al [2003] A tyrosine kinase created by fusion of the PDGFRA and FIP1L1 genes as a therapeutic target of imatinib in idiopathic hypereosinophilic syndrome. *N Engl J Med* 348:1201-1214.

Diaz-Agustin B, Escribano L, Bravo P, Herrero S, Nunez R, Navalon R, Navarro L, Torrelo A, Cantalapiedra A, Del Castillo L, Villarrubia J, Navarro JL, San Miguel JF, Orfao A [1999] The CD69 early activation molecule is overexpressed in human bone marrow mast cells from adults with indolent systemic mast cell disease. *Br J Haematol* 106:400-405.

Elliott MA, Pardanani A, Li CY, Tefferi A [2004] Immunophenotypic normalization of aberrant mast cells accompanies histological remission in imatinib-treated patients with eosinophilia-associated mastocytosis. *Leukemia* 18:1027-1029.

Escribano L, Orfao A, Villarrubia J, et al [1995] Expression of lymphoid-associated antigens in mast cells: Report of a case of systemic mast cell disease. *Br J Haematol* 91:941-943.

Escribano L, Orfao A, Villarrubia J, et al [1997] Sequential immunophenotypic analysis of mast cells in a case of systemic mast cell disease evolving to a mast cell leukemia. *Cytometry* 30:98-102.

Escribano L, Orfao A, Díaz Agustín B, et al [1998] Indolent systemic mast cell disease in adults: Immunophenotypic characterization of bone marrow mast cells and its diagnostic implications. *Blood* 91:2731-2736.

Escribano L, Navalón R, Núñez R, Díaz Agustín B, Bravo P [2000] *Flow cytometry immunophenotypic analysis of human mast cells.* In: Robinson JP, Darzynkiewicz Z, Dean P, Orfao A, Rabinovitch P, Wheeless L, eds. *Current Protocols in Cytometry.* New York: John Wiley & Sons 6.6.1-6.6.18.

Escribano L, Diaz-Agustin B, Bellas C, et al [2001] Utility of flow cytometric analysis of mast cells in the diagnosis and classification of adult mastocytosis. *Leuk Res* 25:563-570.

Escribano L, Diaz-Agustin B, Nunez R, Prados A, Rodriguez R, Orfao A [2002] Abnormal expression of CD antigens in mastocytosis. *Int Arch Allergy Immunol* 127:127-132.

Escribano L, Diaz-Agustin B, Lopez A, et al [2004] Immunophenotypic analysis of mast cells in mastocytosis: When and how to do it. Proposals of the Spanish Network on Mastocytosis (REMA). *Cytometry B Clin Cytom* 58:1-8.

Gratama JW, Keeney M, Sutherland DR [2000] *Enumeration of CD34+ hematopoietic stem cells and progenitors cells.* In: Robinson JP, Darzynkiewicz Z, Dean P, Orfao A, Rabinovitch P, Wheeless L, eds. *Current Protocols in Cytometry.* New York: John Wiley & Sons 6.4.1-6.4.22.

Hahn HP, Hornicj JL [2007] Immunoreactivity for CD25 in gastrointestinal mucosal mast cells is specific for systemic mastocytosis. *Am J Surg Pathol* 31:1669-1676.

Hollmann TJ, Brenn T, Hornick JL [2008] CD25 expression on cutaneous mast cells from adult patients presenting with urticaria pigmentosa is predictive of systemic mastocytosis. *Am J Surg Pathol* 32:139-145.

Horny HP, Sillaber C, Menke D, Kaiserling E, Wehrmann M, Stehberger B, Chott A, Lechner K, Lennert K, Valent P [1998] Diagnostic value of immunostaining for tryptase in patients with mastocytosis. *Am J Surg Pathol* 22:1132-1140.

Horny HP, Valent P [2002] Histopathological and immunohistochemical aspects of mastocytosis. *Int Arch Allergy Immunol* 127:115-117.

Horny HP, Sotlar K, Valent P [2007] Mastocytosis: State of the art. *Pathobiology* 74:121-132.

Jordan JH, Walchshofer S, Jurecka W, et al [2001] Immunohistochemical properties of bone marrow mast cells in systemic mastocytosis: Evidence for expression of CD2, CD117/Kit, and bcl-x(L). *Hum Pathol* 32:545-552.

Klion AD, Noel P, Akin C, et al [2003] Elevated serum tryptase levels identify a subset of patients with a myeloproliferative variant of idiopathic hypereosinophilic syndrome associated with tissue fibrosis, poor prognosis, and imatinib responsiveness. *Blood* 101:4660-4666.

Klion AD, Robyn J, Akin C, et al [2004] Molecular remission and reversal of myelofibrosis in response to imatinib mesylate treatment in patients with the myeloproliferative variant of hypereosinophilic syndrome. *Blood* 103:473-478.

Lawrence JB, Friedman BS, Travis WD, Chinchilli VM, Metcalfe DD, Gralnick HR [1991] Hematologic manifestations of systemic mast cell disease: A prospective study of laboratory and morphologic features and their relation to prognosis. *Am J Med* 91:612-624.

Mutter RD, Tannenbaum M, Ultmann JE [1963] Systemic mast cell disease. *Ann Intern Med* 59:887-906.

Nuñez R, Escribano L, Schernthaner G, Prados A, Rodriguez-Gonzalez R, Diaz-Agustin B, Lopez A, Hauswirth A, Valent P, Almeida J, Bravo P, Orfao A [2002] Overexpression of complement receptors and related antigens on the surface of bone marrow mast cells in patients with systemic mastocytosis. *Br J Haematol* 120:257-265.

Orfao A, Escribano L, Villarrubia J, Velasco JL, Cerveró C, Ciudad J, Navarro JL, San Miguel JF [1996] Flow cytometric analysis of mast cells from normal and pathological human bone marrow samples. Identification and enumeration. *Am J Pathol* 149:1493-1499.

Pardanani A, Baek JY, Li CY, Butterfield JH, Tefferi A [2002] Systemic mast cell disease without associated hematologic disorder: A combined retrospective and prospective study. *Mayo Clin Proc* 77:1169-1175.

Pardanani A, Ketterling RP, Brockman SR, et al [2003] CHIC2 deletion, a surrogate for FIP1L1-PDGFRA fusion, occurs in systemic mastocytosis associated with eosinophilia and predicts response to imatinib therapy. *Blood* 102:3093-3096.

Pardanani A, Reeder T, Li CY, Tefferi A [2003] Eosinophils are derived from the neoplastic clone in patients with systemic mastocytosis and eosinophilia. *Leuk Res* 27:883-885.

Pardanani A, Brockman SR, Paternoster SF, et al [2004] FIP1L1-PDGFRA fusion: Prevalence and clinicopathologic correlates in 89 consecutive patients with moderate to severe eosinophilia. *Blood* 104:3038-3045.

Pardanani A, Kimlinger T, Reeder T, Li CY, Tefferi A [2004] Bone marrow mast cell immunophenotyping in adults with mast cell disease: A prospective study of 33 patients. *Leuk Res* 28:777-783.

Robyn J, Lemery S, McCoy JP, et al [2006] Multilineage involvement of the fusion gene in patients with FIP1L1/PDGFRA-positive hypereosinophilic syndrome. *Br J Haematol* 132:286-292.

Sotlar K, Horny HP, Simonitsch I, et al [2004] CD25 indicates the neoplastic phenotype of mast cells: A novel immunohistochemical marker for the diagnosis of systemic mastocytosis (SM) in routinely processed bone marrow biopsy specimens. *Am J Surg Pathol* 28:1319-1325.

Stevens EC, Rosenthal NS [2001] Bone marrow mast cell morphologic features and hematopoietic dyspoiesis in systemic mast cell disease. *Am J Clin Pathol* 116:177-182.

Tefferi A, Pardanani A [2004a] Systemic mastocytosis: Current concepts and treatment advances. *Curr Hematol Rep* 3:197-202.

Tefferi A, Pardanani A [2004b] Clinical, genetic, and therapeutic insights into systemic mast cell disease. *Curr Opin Hematol* 11:58-64.

Travis WD, Li CY, Bergstralh EJ, Yam LT, Swee RG [1988] Systemic mast cell disease: Analysis of 58 cases and literature review. *Medicine* (Baltimore) 67:345-368.P 80

US-Canadian consensus recommendations on the immunophenotypic analysis of hematologic neoplasia by flow cytometry; Bethesda, Maryland; 16-17 November 1995. *Cytometry*. 1997; 30: 213-274.

Valent P, Horny HP, Escribano L, et al [2001a] Diagnostic criteria and classification of mastocytosis: A consensus proposal. *Leuk Res* 25:603-625.

Valent P, Sperr WR, Samorapoompichit P, et al [2001b] Myelomastocytic overlap syndromes: Biology, criteria, and relationship to mastocytosis. *Leuk Res* 25:595-602.

Valent P, Samorapoompichit P, Sperr WR, Horny HP, Lechner K [2002] Myelomastocytic leukemia: Myeloid neoplasm characterized by partial differentiation of mast cell-lineage cells. *Hematol J* 3:90-94.

19 FCI for Fine Needle Aspirate Specimens

Chapter Contents

The cytomorphological features evaluated in specimens acquired by fine needle aspiration (FNA) combined with flow cytometric immunophenotyping (FCI) has been reported to be successful in evaluating sites for lymphomatous involvement in 75%-90% of cases. The detection of a monoclonal B-cell population or significant lack of light chain expression, or detection of an aberrant T-cell immunophenotype apply, as discussed in detail in Chapters 12 and 14, respectively. The specificity of combining FNA cytomorphology and FCI in diagnosing non-Hodgkin lymphomas (NHLs) has been repeatedly reported as 100%; however, the sensitivity is at best approximately 93% [Dong 2001, Dey 2006, Zeppa 2004]. False "negatives" in the diagnosis of NHL may result from the following scenarios: tumoral necrosis or sclerosis, partial tissue involvement, T-cell NHL without an aberrant immunophenotype, or a T-cell-rich or lymphohistiocytic-rich diffuse large B-cell lymphoma (TCR-DLBCL or LHR-DLBCL) without detectable monoclonal B cells.

The ability and limitations of this combined approach in classifying (or subtyping) and grading of NHLs will be discussed in detail in the appropriate section below. In addition, this combined approach in evaluating recurrent NHL, classical HL (cHL), other hematolymphoid neoplasms, and non-hematolymphoid malignancies will be discussed, as will the applications of ancillary studies. First, however, the unique specimen handling requirements of FNA specimens are discussed.

Recommended Triage Procedures for FNAs

Non-Lymph Node Specimens with Malignant Neoplasms Suspicious for Lymphoma and for FNAs of Lymph Node Specimens

The first pass of the FNA containing diagnostic material is retained for cytomorphological evaluation. The material from this first pass is expressed onto glass slides and smears are prepared, stained (1 slide for Diff-Quick stain, 1 slide for Papanicalou stain), and reviewed. If by cytomorphological examination, there is obvious carcinoma, at least 1 additional pass is obtained for preparation of a cell block. If by cytomorphological examination, there is a suspicion of lymphoma, a second pass is obtained and placed into Roswell Park Memorial Institute (RPMI) 1640 media (Cellgro media) for FCI. Additional passes may be obtained for additional material for FCI or other ancillary studies and for a FNA core biopsy (FNAB). A cytospin preparation of the flow cytometry specimen is Wright-stained and reviewed to assess for the quality of the specimen for FCI. It is recommended that the FNA flow cytometry specimen be analyzed as soon as possible after collection; however, if necessary, it may be refrigerated overnight for processing the next morning.

FNAs of Lymph Node Specimens

The same guidelines above apply to the triage of FNA specimens of lymph nodes in the following situations: if a previous history of lymphoma (NHL or classical HL), if suspicious for lymphoma by cytomorphological examination, if there is a clinical suspicion of lymphoma, or if the patient is >30 years of age. As mentioned previously in Chapter 15, FCI should be routinely performed on specimens suspected of cHL, not only to consider the contributions of FCI to the diagnosis of cHL as outlined in that chapter, but also to exclude a B-cell NHL (which will most often reveal a monoclonal or aberrant B-cell population) or T-cell NHL (which may reveal an aberrant T-cell immunophenotype), and to exclude the co-existence of cHL with a B-cell NHL or T-cell NHL. Such a case of composite lymphoma was demonstrated in [f15.3]. In addition, FCI is recommended even when considering relapse of cHL, since a NHL may occur after therapy for cHL.

Initial Diagnosis of NHL

Subclassification (Subtyping) and Grading of NHLs

Accurate subclassification of NHLs by FNA and FCI has been reported to be attainable in 71%-79% of positive cases [Dey 2006]. This subclassification is based on the abnormal, characteristic cytomorphology and immunophenotype, and thus is more likely attainable in certain subtypes of NHL. Subclassification is most easily, reliably attained in the following subtypes: small lymphocytic lymphoma/chronic lymphocytic leukemia (SLL/CLL and the large cell transformations), mantle cell lymphoma (MCL and the blastoid variants), Burkitt lymphoma (BL), plasma cell neoplasms, anaplastic large cell lymphoma (ALCL), and precursor T-cell and B-cell lymphoblastic neoplasms. Such cases (eg, CLL/SLL, MCL-classical and blastoid variants, BL-atypical and post-transplant cases, and ALCL) are

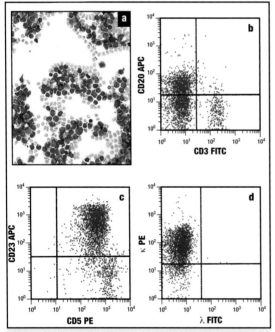

[f19.1] This case demonstrates an FNA specimen with SLL/CLL. The clinical history reveals a 65-year-old female who presents with a history of left breast carcinoma and CLL, and an enlarged left axillary lymph node, which is fine needle aspirated; the FNA is submitted for flow cytometric analysis. The FNA cytospin **a** reveals a mixture of lymphocytes with <30% large forms. Flow cytometric analysis of the FNA specimen reveals a monoclonal B-cell population with expression of CD19 (not demonstrated), CD20 **b**, CD23 **c**, CD5 **c**, and κ **d**. They do not express CD10 (not demonstrated) or λ **d**. The diagnosis of SLL is made.

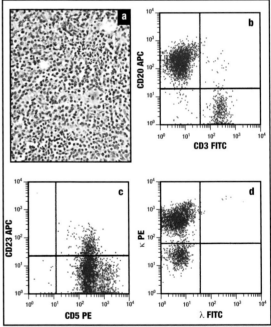

[f19.2] This case demonstrates a needle core biopsy specimen with mantle cell lymphoma. The clinical history reveals a 72-year-old male who presents with a large (9.5 × 7 × 5.7 cm) left abdominal mass, upon which a CT-guided core biopsy is performed. H&E section of the core needle biopsy **a** reveals a predominant population of small, slightly irregular lymphocytes. Flow cytometric analysis of a suspension prepared from the needle biopsy specimen reveals a monoclonal B-cell population with expression of CD19 (not demonstrated), CD20 **b**, CD5 **c** without significant CD23 **c**, and κ **d**. They do not express CD10 (not demonstrated) or λ **d**. The diagnosis is made of mantle cell lymphoma.

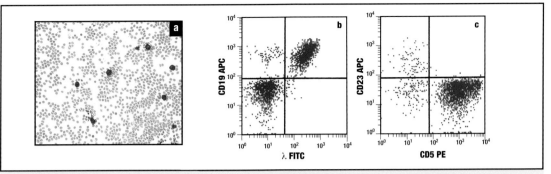

[f19.3] This case demonstrates an FNA specimen with mantle cell lymphoma. The clinical history reveals a 60-year-old male with a history of "mantle cell lymphoma" status post BM transplant who presents with an enlarging right neck mass, which undergoes fine needle aspiration. The FNA is submitted for flow cytometric analysis. The FNA cytospin **a** reveals a predominant population of large abnormal lymphocytes. Flow cytometric analysis of the FNA specimen reveals a monoclonal B-cell population with expression of CD19 **b** and λ **b**, CD20 (not demonstrated), and CD5 **c** without CD23 **c**. They do not express CD10 or κ (both, not demonstrated). The diagnosis of mantle cell lymphoma, blastoid variant, is made.

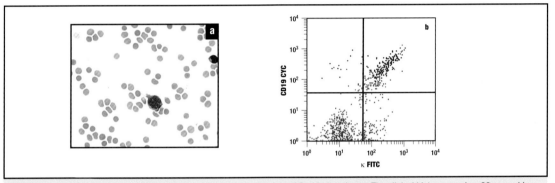

[f19.4] This case demonstrates an FNA specimen with an atypical variant of Burkitt lymphoma. The clinical history reveals a 38-year-old female with a history of ovarian Burkitt lymphoma (atypical variant) who presents with an abdominal mass, upon which fine needle aspiration is performed. The FNA is submitted for flow cytometric analysis. The FNA cytospin **a** reveals a population of large abnormal lymphocytes. Flow cytometric analysis of the FNA specimen reveals a monoclonal B-cell population with expression of CD19 **b** and κ **b**. FISH detects an abnormal signal pattern, consistent with an extra or rearranged copy of *myc*. The diagnosis of recurrent Burkitt lymphoma, atypical variant is made.

demonstrated in **[f19.1]**, **[f19.2]**, **[f19.3]**, **[f19.4]**, **[f16.5]**, and **[f14.14]**, respectively, with listmode output available on the accompanying disk. The accurate, reliable subclassification in these subtypes is due to the characteristic, uniform cytomorphology of the neoplastic cells and unique, characteristic immunophenotypes. Ancillary studies to support these specific subtypes [eg, t(11;14) in MCL, *c-myc* translocation in BL, t(2;5) in ALCL] may also be performed on FNA specimens, as will be discussed in the appropriate section below.

Accurate, reliable subclassification of other NHL subtypes [eg, marginal zone B-cell lymphoma, follicular lymphoma (FL)] is not as easily attained by this approach. For example, the relative lack of architecture that is able to be evaluated in FNA specimens is a major limitation in subtyping FLs. Not

only is FNA cytomorphology limited in its ability to diagnose FL, it is also limited in its ability to grade FLs. Merely counting the number of large cells may either overestimate or underestimate the number of large cells in the neoplastic population due to the presence of small and large reactive lymphocytes, the crushing of fragile large neoplastic cells, and the morphologic variability of transformed lymphoid cells. More recently, evaluation of grading FLs using TP slides has shown a significant upward trend in the number of centroblasts as the grades of FL increased. On the other hand, analysis of cell size by flow cytometry is not as reliable as using ThinPrep (TP) slides to distinguish grades of FL, especially Grade 2 vs Grade 3 [Brandao 2006]. In fact, although flow cytometry has the ability to analyze a large number of cells than by cytomorphological counting of large cells, flow cytometry has the propensity to underestimate the number of large cells due to their lower viability.

Even with TP slides, the grading of FLs by FNA combined with FCI, continues to be limited, due to the simple, undeniable fact that grading of FL by the WHO classification is based on the average number of centroblasts or large "transformed" cells in 10 neoplastic follicles at 40× high-power field (hpf) examination (ie, Grade 1: 0-5 centroblasts/hpf; Grade 2: 6-15 centroblasts/hpf; and Grade 3: >15 centroblasts/hpf) [Jaffe 2001]. It is important to accurately, reliably grade FLs, since grading of FL, in combination with clinical factors, is what ultimately effects prognosis and therapeutic decisions in these patients.

Although grading of FL is not entirely reliable by combining FNA and FCI, the evaluation of cell size by combining FCI and FNA cytomorphology does have diagnostic and clinical applications. The combined approach has been demonstrated to be useful in reliably diagnosing large cell lymphoma/transformation, if >40% large cells are present [Gong 2002].

Diagnostic Impact of Core Needle Biopsy

Since there are limitations, as discussed previously, regarding the subclassification and grading of NHLs, the question arises as to the contribution (or diagnostic impact) of obtaining and evaluating a core needle biopsy. A rather large retrospective study of 74 FNA specimens by Gong et al demonstrated no clear advantage in the diagnosis and classification of small B-cell NHLs by adding a core needle biopsy to FNA and FCI [Gong 2004]. However, a core needle biopsy was shown to be more useful in diagnosing DLBCL: 37% of cases were able to be diagnosed when a core needle biopsy was also available vs only 25% by FNA and FCI. Thus, a combined approach reduces the number of insufficient cases and is recommended in routine FNA practice.

Value of Fluorescent In-Situ Hybridization (FISH) and Polymerase Chain Reaction (PCR) Analysis in the Diagnosis of NHL by FNA

Although FNA specimens may not provide analyzable metaphases for conventional cytogenetic studies, they are well-suited to directed FISH analyses [eg, t(14;18) (or BCL2) for a definitive diagnosis of FL; t(11;14) (or BCL1) for MCL; a *c-myc* rearrangement for BL; t(2;5) for ALCL]. In addition, with proper handling and management of specimens, FNA can routinely provide samples adequate for molecular genetic studies. In a study by Safley et al [2004], of 30 FNAs with suspected hematolymphoid malignancies (20 diagnosed as B-cell NHL), the additional application of FISH and PCR analyses definitely subclassified 12 of the B-cell NHLs [ie, 4 FLs by BCL2 FISH or PCR, 2 MCLs by BCL1 FISH, and 50% of SLL (2/4) and DLBCL (4/8), [Safley 2004].

Evaluation of Recurrent NHL

The combined approach of FNA and FCI is also useful in evaluating tissues for recurrent involvement by an NHL. In a large, retrospective study of this approach in the evaluation of recurrent NHL, Chernoff et al demonstrated that 90% of recurrent cases were amenable to FNA [Chernoff 1992]. In addition, cytomorphology identified large cell transformation, as defined previously. A later study further indicated the findings of necrosis and numerous polymorphonuclear cells in this setting demand a tissue biopsy, since all of these cases represented recurrent NHL upon follow-up biopsy [Dunphy 1997].

Limitations of FNA Combined with FCI in the Evaluation of Primary and Recurrent Lymphomatous Involvement

As discussed previously, false negatives may result from the following situations [t19.1]: tumoral necrosis or sclerosis, partial tissue involvement, a T-cell NHL without an aberrant immunophenotype, or a T-cell-rich or lymphohistiocytic-rich diffuse large B-cell lymphoma (TCR-DLBCL or LHR-DLBCL) without detectable monoclonal B cells. In addition, there are limitations in definitive subclassification and grading of NHLs. Architecture (ie, follicular vs diffuse) cannot be determined by FNA cytomorphology. One should also exercise extreme caution in determining such architecture based only on a thin core needle biopsy. Core needle biopsies of lymph node specimens may be over-interpreted as large cell lymphoma (eg, if the needle happens to pass through a large, reactive germinal center, through an EBV-infected lymph node with marked reactive changes). As also previously mentioned, recurrent NHL is often associated with no definitive cytomorphological evidence of lymphomatous involvement but rather a background of necrosis and numerous polymorphonuclear cells, which demands a tissue biopsy. An initial diagnosis of classical HL also requires a tissue biopsy, even if it can be diagnosed by immunophenotyping of the FNA or core needle biopsy, in order to determine the subtype, which is based on architectural patterns.

Classical Hodgkin Lymphoma (cHL)

The combined approach using FNA and FCI is useful in evaluating tissues for involvement by cHL, either as an initial diagnosis or as a recurrence, primarily in excluding the presence of an NHL, either alone or as a composite lymphoma. The applications of FCI in diagnosing cHL have been discussed in detail in Chapter 15.

Composite Lymphoma

FNA and FCI may be useful not only in identifying a composite lymphoma of cHL and NHL but also in detecting a composite lymphoma of a B-cell NHL and a T-cell NHL.

Situations Requiring Biopsy, Based on FNA and FCI Results

The following situations require biopsies, based on FNA and FCI results, when evaluating for lymphomatous involvement [t19.1]: NHL of follicle center cell origin with a mixed cellular composition, indeterminate results, the presence of necrosis in the evaluation of an initial diagnosis of lymphoma, the presence of necrosis and polymorphonuclear cells in the evaluation of recurrent NHL, <10% neoplastic cells detected by FCI, a predominance of small cells detected by cytomorphology or by FCI with clinical signs of transformation, and evaluating for an initial diagnosis of or recurrence of cHL, due to the possibility of a composite lymphoma or a subsequent NHL after therapy for cHL.

Detecting Hematopoietic Malignancy Granulocytic Sarcoma Chloroma, Monocytic Sarcoma, Erythroid Sarcoma

As discussed in Chapters 12 and 14, involvement of tissue specimens by granulocytic, monocytic, or erythroid sarcomas should be considered in the differential diagnosis of NHLs of B-cell and T-cell origin, respectively, due to the similarities of the blasts to large cell lymphoma, the presence of lymphoglandular bodies, and the rarity of Auer rods and eosinophilic myelocytes. The combined approach of FNA and FCI may be quite useful in these differential diagnoses. The neoplastic cells of granulocytic sarcomas are typically distinguished by their variable expression of myelomonocytic markers, as AMLs (described in Chapter 10). They most commonly express CD13 and CD33 with variable expression of CD34 [Suh 2000] and are negative for CD10, CD20, and surface light chains. They may aberrantly express CD19 or T-cell antigens, as in AMLs (discussed in Chapter 10). Note that AMLs associated with

t(8;21) are also associated with PAX-5 nuclear positivity by immunohistochemical staining. The neoplastic cells of monocytic sarcomas, like AMLs with monocytic differentiation, typically show variable expression of CD13, CD11b, CD14, CD15, and CD33, with generally strong expressions of CD64 and HLA-DR. They are typically CD34−. The neoplastic cells of erythroid sarcoma may be distinguished from NHLs by their lack of B-cell and T-cell antigens and expression of glycophorin A; such a case was demonstrated in [f10.14]. Also, as mentioned previously, ALCL may express myelomonocytic markers, but the expression of CD30, variable expression of T-cell markers, and lack of immature markers should distinguish ALCL from granulocytic sarcoma.

t19.1 Evaluation of Lymphomatous Involvement by FNA and FCI: Limitations and Situations Requiring Large Incisional or Excisional Biopsy

Situations with "False-Negative" Results	Situations Requiring Large Incisional/ Excisional Bx
Tumoral necrosis	Grading of FL
Tumoral sclerosis	"Indeterminant" or suspicious results
T-NHL without an aberrant IP	Necrosis: "initial" evaluation for NHL
B-NHL with T-cell- or LH-rich background	Necrosis & numerous PMNs: evaluation for recurrent NHL
Classical HL	<10% neoplastic cells detected by FCI Predominance of small cells by cytomorphology or by FCI with signs of clinical transformation Evaluating for an initial dx or recurrence of cHL

bx, biopsy; cHL, classical Hodgkin lymphoma; dx, diagnosis; FCI, flow cytometric immunophenotyping FL, follicular lymphoma FNA, fine needle aspiration; IP, immunophenotype; LH, lymphohistiocytic; NHL, non-Hodgkin lymphoma; PMNs, polymorphonuclear cells

Determining Presence of Metastatic Non-Hematolymphoid Malignancy

A combined FCA and FCI approach may also be useful in determining the presence of a non-hematolymphoid malignancy by detecting cohesive malignant cells by cytomorphology and the presence of large, CD45– cells by FCI. However, one should keep in mind that some cases of large cell lymphoma may also be CD45–, particularly ALCL, so correlation with the cytomorphology and additional markers are necessary to exclude a diagnosis of lymphoma in such cases.

References

Borchmann P, Behringer K, Josting A, et al [2006] Secondary malignancies after successful primary treatment of malignant Hodgkin's lymphoma. *Pathologe* 27:47-52.

Brandao GDA, Rose R, Mckenzie S, Maslak P, Lin O [2006] Grading follicular lymphomas in fine-needle aspiration biopsies: The role of ThinPrep slides and flow cytometry. *Cancer Cytopathol* 108:319-323.

Chernoff WG, Lampe HB, Cramer H, Banerjee D [1992] The potential clinical impact of the fine needle aspiration/flow cytometric diagnosis of malignant lymphoma. *J Otolaryngology Suppl* 1:1-15.

Dey P, Amir T, Jassar AA, et al [2006] Combined applications of fine needle aspiration cytology and flow cytometric immunophenotyping for diagnosis and classification of non Hodgkin lymphoma. *Cytojournal* 3:24.

Dong HY, Harris NL, Preffer FI, Pitman MB [2001] Fine-needle aspiration biopsy in the diagnosis and classification of primary and recurrent lymphoma: A retrospective analysis of the utility of cytomorphology and flow cytometry. *Mod Pathol* 14:472-481.

Dunphy CH, Ramos R [1997] Combining fine-needle aspiration and flow cytometric immunophenotyping in evaluation of nodal and extranodal sites for possible lymphoma: A retrospective review. *Diagn Cytopathol* 16:200-206.

Gong JZ, Williams DC Jr, Liu K, Jones C [2002] Fine-needle aspiration in non-Hodgkin lymphoma: Evaluation of cell size by cytomorphology and flow cytometry. *Am J Clin Pathol* 117:880-888.

Gong JZ, Snyder MJ, Lagoo AS, et al [2004] Diagnostic impact of core-needle biopsy on fine-needle aspiration of non-Hodgkin lymphoma. *Diagn Cytopathol* 31:23-30.

Jaffe ES, Harris NL, Stein H, Vardiman JW [2001] *World Health Organization Classification of Tumours. Pathology and Genetics of Tumours of Haematopoietic and Lymphoid Tissues.* Lyon, France: IARC Press; 2001.

Safley AM, Buckley PJ, Creager AJ, et al [2004] The value of fluorescence in situ hybridization and polymerase chain reaction in the diagnosis of B-cell non-Hodgkin lymphoma by fine-needle aspiration. *Arch Pathol Lab Med* 128:1395-1403.

Suh YK, Shin HJC [2000] Fine-needle aspiration biopsy of granulocytic sarcoma: A clinicopathologic study of 27 cases. *Cancer Cytopathol* 90:364-372.

Zeppa P, Marion G, Troncone G, et al [2004] Fine-needle cytology and flow cytometry immunophenotyping and subclassification of non-Hodgkin lymphoma: A critical review of 307 cases with technical suggestions. *Cancer Cytopathol* 102:55-65.

20 FCI for Body Fluids

Chapter Contents

Introduction

The combined approach of cytomorphology with FCI is useful for evaluating serous effusions for lymphomatous or leukemic involvement, just as it is for evaluating fine needle aspiration specimens (see Chapter 19).. The detection of a monoclonal B-cell population or significant lack of light chain expression, or detection of an aberrant T-cell immunophenotype apply, as discussed in detail in Chapters 12 and 14, respectively. The detection of neoplastic myeloblasts, precursor B-cell lymphoblasts, and precursor T-cell lymphoblasts apply, as discussed in Chapters 10, 11, and 13, respectively.

The advantages of FCI (in comparison to cytomorphology alone or to combined cytomorphology and immunocytochemistry) are in the detection of a small population of monoclonal (or aberrant) cells (ie, neoplastic B cells, T cells, or myeloblasts) in a background of reactive cells (particularly useful in effusion samples in which the predominant cell population is often reactive T lymphocytes), increased diagnostic precision through evaluation of objective parameters, and the evaluation of multiple markers by multi-color analysis [Simsir 1999]. The combined approach with FCI has been demonstrated to establish recurrence in 50% of non-Hodgkin lymphoma (NHL) cases and to establish an initial diagnosis of NHL in a significant number of cases analyzed by this combined approach (ie, 69% of effusions diagnosed with lymphomatous involvement by this approach represented newly diagnosed NHL). In 36% of these newly diagnosed lymphomas, a tissue biopsy was obviated due to the ability to subclassify the NHL based on combining the cytomorphology and characteristic FCI features [Dunphy 1996]. The applications of this technique in detecting secondary or recurrent involvement of a serous effusion or cerebrospinal fluid (CSF) by an NHL, or establishing a new diagnosis of an NHL, which may obviate tissue biopsy, has significant therapeutic implications. In addition, this combined approach is also useful in evaluating involvement of serous effusions (including CSF) by acute leukemias and directing therapy [Hegde 2005, Bromberg 2007].

Suitable Specimens

All types of body fluids may be analyzed by FCI. It is recommended that the specimens be analyzed as soon as possible after collection; however, if necessary, the specimens may be refrigerated overnight for processing the next morning. If feasible, it is recommended a cell pellet be prepared from the body fluid specimen and placed into RPMI for processing the next day.

Non-Hodgkin Lymphoma

Primary Diagnosis and Subclassification

NHLs may present as a serous effusion but more often involve serous cavities secondarily. Similar to the combined FNA and FCI approach, combining body fluid cytomorphology and FCI may result in a reliable subclassification of a subset of NHLs. This subclassification is again based on the abnormal, characteristic cytomorphology and immunophenotype, and thus is more likely attainable in certain subtypes of NHL [ie, small lymphocytic lymphoma/chronic lymphocytic leukemia (SLL/CLL and the large cell transformations), mantle cell lymphoma (MCL and the blastoid variants), Burkitt lymphoma (BL), plasma cell neoplasms, anaplastic large cell lymphoma (ALCL), and precursor T-cell and B-cell lymphoblastic neoplasms]. The accurate, reliable subclassification in these subtypes is due to the characteristic, uniform cytomorphology of the neoplastic cells and unique, characteristic immunophenotypes. Representative cases are demonstrated in **[f20.1]**, **[f20.2]**, **[f20.3]**, **[f20.4]**, and **[f20.5]**.

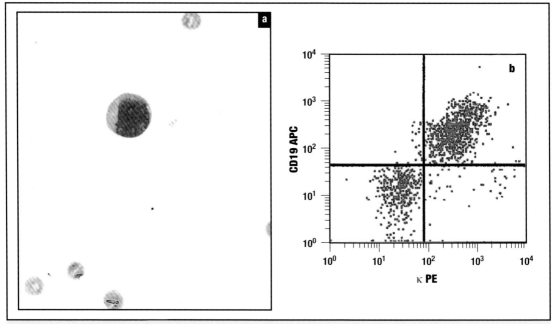

[f20.1] This case demonstrates a vitreous fluid with large B-cell lymphoma. The clinical history reveals an 80-year-old female who presents with a history of decreased vision and vitreitis in the left eye. Vitreous fluid is submitted for flow cytometric analysis. A fluid cytospin **a** reveals a population of large abnormal lymphoid cells. Flow cytometric analysis of the fluid reveals a monoclonal B-cell population with expression of CD19 **b** and κ **b**. The diagnosis of large cell lymphoma of B-cell origin is made.

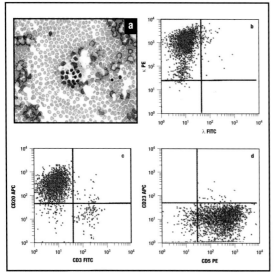

[f20.2] This case demonstrates a pleural fluid with mantle cell lymphoma. The clinical history reveals a 63-year-old female with a history of mantle cell lymphoma who presents with a pleural effusion. The pleural fluid is submitted for flow cytometric analysis. A fluid cytospin **a** reveals predominantly small lymphocytes. Flow cytometric analysis of the fluid reveals a monoclonal B-cell population with expression of CD19 (not demonstrated), CD20 **c**, CD5 **d** without CD23 **d**, and κ **b**. They do not express CD10 (not demonstrated) or λ **b**. The diagnosis of mantle cell lymphoma is made.

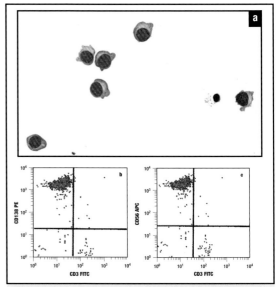

[f20.3] This case demonstrates a CSF with plasma cell dyscrasia. The clinical history reveals a 55-year-old female with a history of monoclonal λ myeloma, status post autologous and allogeneic stem cell transplants who presents with mental status changes. A CSF is submitted for flow cytometric analysis. A fluid cytospin **a** reveals sheets of plasma cells. Flow cytometric analysis of the fluid reveals that these cells express CD138 **b** and CD56 **c** with no bell markers of light chain expression (not demonstrated). The diagnosis of plasma cell myeloma is made.

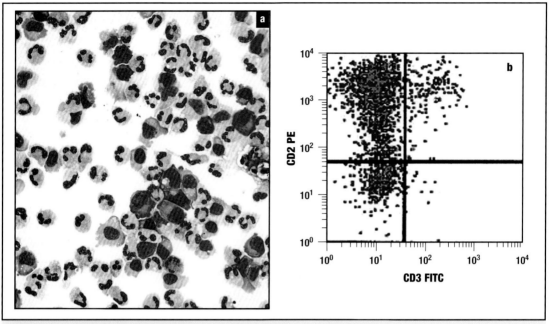

[f20.4] This case demonstrates a CSF with anaplastic large cell lymphoma. The clinical history reveals a 17-year-old male with a history of recurrent anaplastic large cell lymphoma who presents with fever, headache, and vomiting. A CSF specimen is submitted for flow cytometric analysis. A fluid cytospin **a** reveals sheets of anaplastic cells with polymorphonuclear cells in the background. Flow cytometric analysis of the fluid reveals that these anaplastic cells express CD2 **b** and CD45 (not demonstrated) without CD3 **b**. The diagnosis of recurrent anaplastic large cell lymphoma is made.

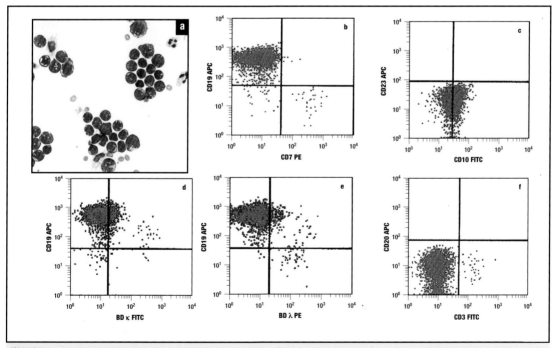

[f20.5] This case demonstrates a pleural fluid with Burkitt lymphoma. The clinical history reveals a 42-year-old male with an outside history of Burkitt lymphoma who presents with a pleural effusion. The pleural fluid is submitted for flow cytometric analysis. A fluid cytospin **a** reveals sheets of classical Burkitt lymphoma cells. Flow cytometric analysis of the fluid reveals a monoclonal B-cell population with expression of CD19 **b**, dim CD10 **c**, and dim κ **d**. They do not express CD20 **f**, CD23 **c**, or λ **e**. The diagnosis of Burkitt lymphoma is made.

NHL Restricted to Serous Effusions

Primary effusion lymphoma

Primary effusion lymphoma (PEL) is a neoplasm of large B cells usually presenting as serous effusions without detectable tumor masses. By definition, there is no discrete contiguous lymphomatous mass associated with the effusion. The WHO classification states that PEL is universally associated with human herpes virus 8 (HHV-8)/Kaposi sarcoma herpes virus (KSHV), most often occurring in the setting of immunodeficiency (eg, HIV infection, post-transplantation). This lymphoma

was discussed in detail in Chapter 12. A representative case of PEL was demonstrated in **[f12.43]**, with listmode output on the accompanying disk.

Detecting Hematopoietic Malignancy

This combined approach is also useful in evaluating involvement of various body cavities by acute leukemia, including those of precursor B-cell and precursor T-cell origin, as well as acute myeloid leukemias (AMLs). The same criteria apply as discussed in Chapters 13, 11, and 10, respectively. Representative cases are demonstrated in **[f20.6]**, **[f20.7]**, and **[f20.8]**.

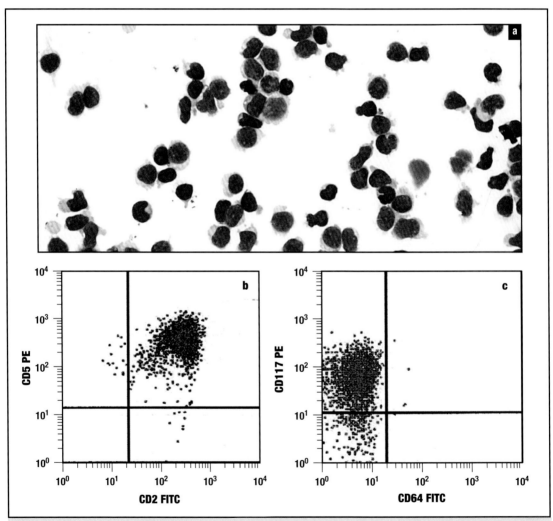

[f20.6] This case demonstrates a CSF with precursor T-cell lymphoblastic leukemia. The clinical history reveals a 67-year-old female with a history of precursor T-cell lymphoblastic leukemia, status post chemotherapy, who presents with an elevated WBC count in the CSF. A CSF specimen is submitted for flow cytometric analysis. A fluid cytospin **a** reveals sheets of blasts. By flow cytometric analysis of the fluid, the blasts express CD2, **b**, CD3 (not demonstrated), CD5 **b**, CD7 (not demonstrated), and CD117 **c**. They do not express HLA-DR, CD4, CD8, or other myelomonocytic antigens (except for CD64, all not demonstrated). The diagnosis of precursor T-cell lymphoblastic leukemia is made.

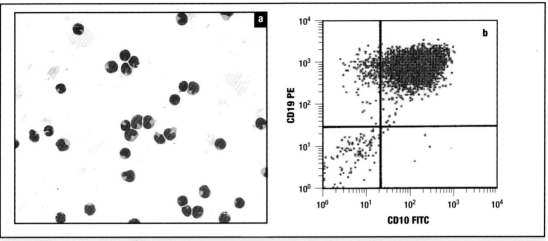

[f20.7] This case demonstrates a CSF with precursor B-cell lymphoblastic leukemia. The clinical history reveals a 34-month-old female with a history of precursor B-cell lymphoblastic leukemia presents with an increasing WBC count in the CSF. A CSF specimen is submitted for flow cytometric analysis. A fluid cytospin **a** reveals sheets of blasts. By flow cytometric analysis of the fluid, the blasts express CD19 and CD10 **b**. No additional markers could be analyzed. The diagnosis of precursor B-cell lymphoblastic leukemia is made

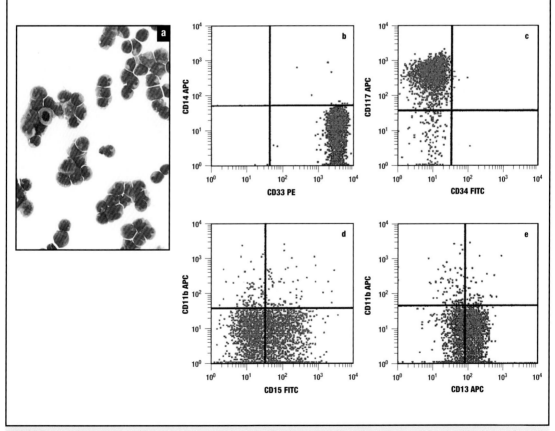

[f20.8] This case demonstrates a CSF with acute myeloid leukemia. The clinical history reveals a 65-year-old female with a history of AML, status post induction and consolidation, who presents with a 5-week history of progressive lower extremity pain. A CSF specimen is submitted for flow cytometric analysis. A fluid cytospin **a** reveals sheets of blasts. By flow cytometric analysis of the fluid, the blasts express CD33 **b**, CD117 **c**, CD15 **d**, CD13 **e**, and HLA-DR (not demonstrated). They do not express CD14 **b**, CD34 **c**, CD11b **d, e**, or CD64 (not demonstrated). The diagnosis of acute myeloid leukemia is made.

FISH and PCR to Diagnose NHL with Serous Effusions

Although body fluid specimens may not provide analyzable metaphases for conventional cytogenetic studies, they are well-suited to directed FISH analyses for diagnosing NHLs [eg, t(14;18) (or BCL2) for a definitive diagnosis of FL; t(11;14) (or BCL1) for MCL; a *c-myc* rearrangement for BL; t(2;5) for ALCL) and for acute myeloid leukemias [eg, translocations (8;21), (15;17), and abnormalities of inv (16) and 11q23 in AML; t(12;21), t(4;11), t(9;22) etc in precursor B-cell lymphoblastic leukemia]. In addition, with proper handling and management of specimens, body fluid specimens can routinely provide samples adequate for molecular genetic studies.

Determining Presence of Metastatic Non-Hematolymphoid Malignancy

This combined approach may also be useful in determining the presence of a non-hematolymphoid malignancy in a serous effusion, by detecting cohesive malignant cells by cytomorphology and the presence of large, CD45– cells by FCI. However, one should keep in mind that some cases of large cell lymphoma may also be CD45–, particularly ALCL, so correlation with the cytomorphology and additional markers are necessary to exclude a diagnosis of lymphoma in such cases.

Limitations

The primary unique limitations of using this combined approach in evaluating serous effusions for lymphomatous or leukemic involvement is the degree of lymphomatous (or leukemic) involvement and the cellularity of the specimen (particularly CSF specimens). This limitation should hopefully be addressed with the introduction of 9 (or more)-color FCI, in that lower volume and less cellular specimens may be more sensitively evaluated.

References

Bromberg JEC, Breems DA, Kraan J, et al [2007] CSF flow cytometry greatly improves diagnostic accuracy in CNS hematologic malignancies. *Neurology* 68:1674-1679.

Dunphy CH [1996] Combined cytomorphologic and immunophenotypic approach to evaluation of effusions for lymphomatous involvement. *Diagn Cytopathol* 15:427-430.

Hegde U, Filie A, Little RF, et al [2005] High incidence of occult leptomeningeal disease detected by flow cytometry in newly diagnosed aggressive B-cell lymphomas at risk for central nervous system involvement: The role of flow cytometry vs cytology. *Blood* 105:496-502.

Simsir A, Fetsch P, Stetler-Stevenson M [1999] Immunophenotypic analysis of non-Hodgkin's lymphomas in cytologic specimens: A correlative study of immunocytochemical and flow cytometric techniques. *Diagn Cytopathol* 20:278-284

Index

Numbers in *italics* refer to pages on which tables appear.
Numbers in **boldface** refer to pages on which figures appear.

A

α-naphthyl acetate esterase (ANAE),70, 116

Acidified serum lysis (Ham) test, 37

Acquired immunodeficiency syndrome (AIDS), 62, 173

Activated tissue histiocytes, 32

Acute basophilic leukemia, 76, 101

Acute erythroid leukemia, 76, 101

    erythroleukemia (erythroid/myeloid), 101

    pure erythroid leukemia, 101

Acute leukemias of ambiguous origin, **112**

Acute lymphoblastic leukemia (ALL), 56, **56**, 59, 60, 62, **62**, 65

Acute monoblastic and monocytic leukemia, 76, 101

Acute monocytic leukemia (AML)

    in de-novo AML, 101-102, **102-104, 106,** 106, **108,** 109, **109, 111, 114,** 115, 118, **119**

    in immunophenotyping, 309, **310**

    in normal vs abnormal findings, 56, 58-60, **62,** 69, 70

    in phenotypic markers, 21, 25-37, *39*

    in precursor B-cell neoplasm, 129

    in precursor neoplasms, 206

    transient myeloproliferative disorder, 36

Acute megakaryoblastic leukemia, 76, 101

Acute monocytic leukemias(AMoLs), 29, 70, 95, 96, 10-110

Acute myelogenous/myeloid leukemias (AML), 2, 12, 21, 23, **57,** 91, 92, 116-117, 289

    AML with maturation, 76, 101

    AML without maturation, 76, 101

Acute myelomonocytic leukemia (AMML), 29, 70, 76, 101, 109-110, 116, 118

Acute panmyelosis with myelofibrosis, 76, 101

Acute promyelocytic leukemia (APL), 23, 25, 27-28, 30, 56, **57,** 69, 76, 91, 101, 109, 118

Acute undifferentiated leukemia, 2008, 76

Adult T-cell leukemia/lymphoma (ATLL), 31, 37, 77, 216, 221-223, **222**

Aggressive NK-cell leukemia, 77, 220, **221**, 232

Alemtuzumab, 38

Alpha naphthyl butyrate esterase-ANBE, 99, 116

Anaplastic large cell lymphoma (ALCL)

    in FNA specimens, 302, 307

    in histiocytic and dendritic cell neoplasms, 283

    in Hodgkin Lymphoma, 259

    in immunophenotyping, 309, **309**

    in LPD, 276,

    in mature B-cell neoplasms, 172

    in mature T-cell and NK-cell neoplasms, **226,** 231, 240, **242,** 243

    in phenotypic markers, 27, 28, 33, 35, *39*

ANBE and α-naphthyl acetate esterase-ANAE, 99

Angioimmunoblastic T-cell lymphoma (AITL), 77, 236-239, **238,** 239

Anti-immunoglobulin antibody, 8

Antigens

    associated deficient, 37

    B-cell, 283, 286

    B-cell lineage-associated, 21

    B-cell lineage-restricted, 23

    CD61, 36

    CD7, 13

    erythrocyte-associated, 36

    hemoglobinuria (PNH)-associated deficient, 37

    intracellular, 8

    large granular lymphocyte-associated, 26

    leukocyte common (LCA), 19, 181

    lineage-associated, 24

    monocyte- and myeloid-associated, 27

    natural killer cell-associated, 26

    NK-cell, 69

    non-lineage, 31, *32,* 101

    non-myeloid, 83, 89

    pan-B cell, 23

    panhematopoietic cell, 19

    paroxysmal nocturnal hemoglobinuria (PNH)

    platelet-associated, 36

    progenitor cell-associated, 30

    sheep erythrocyte, 24

    T-cell, 24, 25, 203, 283, 286

    T-cell lineage-associated, 24, 26, 33, 130

Aplastic anemia (AA), 90